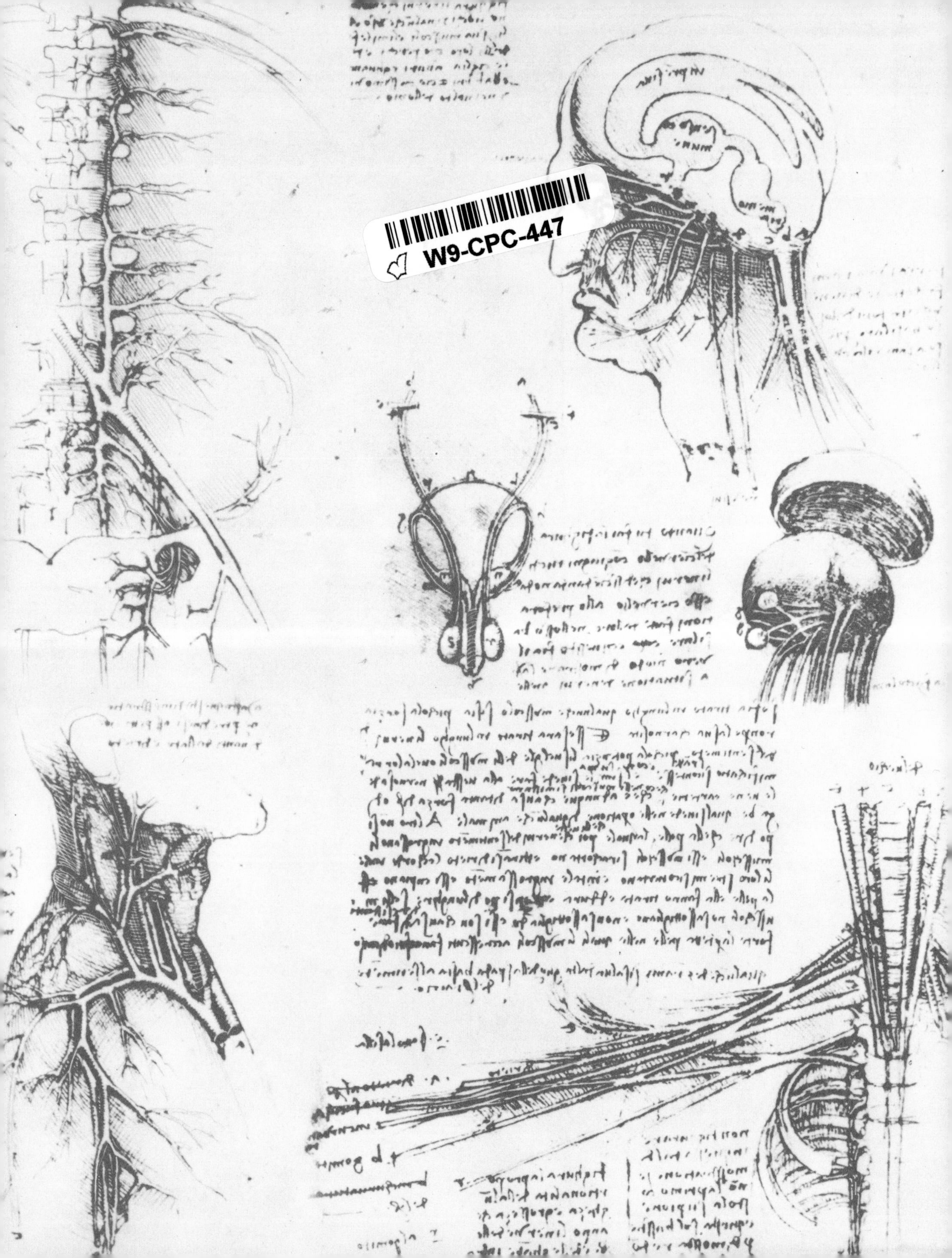

Sobotta / Figge · Atlas of Human Anatomy
Vol. 3

Sobotta/Figge

Atlas of Human Anatomy

Original Author Dr. med. Johannes Sobotta †, Professor and Director of the Anatomical Institute, University of Bonn, Germany

9th English Edition by Frank H. J. Figge †, Ph.D., Sc.D. (hon.), Professor Emeritus of Anatomy, School of Medicine, University of Maryland

Walther J. Hild, M.D., Professor and Chairman, Department of Anatomy
The University of Texas Medical Branch, Galveston, Texas

Based upon the 17th German Edition, edited by

Prof. Dr. med. Helmut Ferner, Director of the Anatomical Institute, University of Vienna, Austria
Prof. Dr. med. Jochen Staubesand, Director of the Anatomical Institute, University of Freiburg, Germany

Vol. 1: Regions, Bones, Ligaments, Joints and Muscles

Vol. 2: Visceral Anatomy

Vol. 3: Central Nervous System, Autonomic Nervous System
Sense Organs and Skin, Peripheral Nerves and Vessels

Urban & Schwarzenberg · Baltimore-Munich

Sobotta/Figge

Atlas of Human Anatomy

9th English Edition by Walther J. Hild, M.D., Professor and Chairman, Department of Anatomy
The University of Texas Medical Branch, Galveston, Texas

Based upon the 17th German Edition, edited by

Prof. Dr. med. Helmut Ferner, Director of the Anatomical Institute, University of Vienna, Austria
Prof. Dr. med. Jochen Staubesand, Director of the Anatomical Institute, University of Freiburg, Germany

Vol. 3

Central Nervous System, Autonomic Nervous System
Sense Organs and Skin, Peripheral Nerves and Vessels

443 Illustrations, mostly in color

Urban & Schwarzenberg · Baltimore-Munich 1977

The Original Author, Professor Dr. med. Johannes Sobotta, was born on January 31, 1869 in Berlin. He died on April 20, 1945 in Bonn, where he was Professor and Director of the Anatomical Institute, University of Bonn, Germany.

Address of the English editor:

Walther J. Hild, M.D., Professor and Chairman, Department of Anatomy,
The University of Texas Medical Branch, Galveston, Texas 77550

Addresses of the German editors:

Professor Dr. med. Helmut Ferner, Vorstand der I. Anatomischen Lehrkanzel der Universität,
Währingerstraße 13, A-1090 Wien, Austria

Professor Dr. med. Jochen Staubesand, Direktor des Anatomischen Instituts der Universität,
Albertstraße 17, 7800 Freiburg, Germany

The pictures on the end leaves are reprints of some of the anatomical illustrations of Leonardo da Vinci (1452–1519). They represent some of the anatomical subject matter depicted in this volume and illustrate how far the great artist and scholar of the Renaissance Period had progressed as a result of his own firsthand investigations of the anatomy of the human body.

German editions:

1. edition: J. F. Lehmanns Verlag, München 1907
2.–9. edition: J. F. Lehmanns Verlag, München 1914–1938
since 10. edition: Urban & Schwarzenberg, 1947
11. edition: 1949
12. edition: 1952
13. edition: 1956
14. edition: 1957
15. edition: 1960
16. edition: 1962 (ISBN 3-541-02836-X)
17. edition: 1973 (ISBN 3-541-02837-8)
3. reprint: 1975

Foreign editions:

English Version (with nomenclature in English)
SOBOTTA/FIGGE, Atlas of Human Anatomy
Urban & Schwarzenberg, München–Berlin–Wien, 9. edition 1974. (ISBN 3-541-06889-2)
1. reprint: Baltimore–Munich 1977

English Version (with nomenclature in Latin–PNA)
SOBOTTA/BECHER, Atlas of Human Anatomy
Urban & Schwarzenberg, München–Berlin–Wien, 9. edition 1975

Italian Version
Atlante di anatomia
USES, Firenze 1974

Japanese Version
Igaku-Shoin Ltd., Tokyo 1974

Portuguese Version
Atlas de Anatomia Humana
Editora Guanabara Koogan, Rio de Janeiro 1976

Spanish Version
Atlas de Anatomia
Ediciones Toray, Barcelona 1974

Turkish Version
Insan Anatomisi Atlasi
Urban & Schwarzenberg, München–Berlin–Wien 1973

In preparation:

French Version
Urban & Schwarzenberg, München–Wien–Baltimore 1977

Greek Version
Gregory Parisianos, Athen 1977

Persian Version
University of Tehran Press, Tehran/Iran

Arab. Version
Al Ahram, Cairo/Egypt

CIP-Kurztitelaufnahme der Deutschen Bibliothek

Sobotta, Johannes
Atlas of human anatomy / Sobotta-Figge. Orig. author Johannes Sobotta. – Baltimore, Munich [München] : Urban und Schwarzenberg.
Dt. Ausg. u. d. T.: Sobotta, Johannes: Atlas der Anatomie des Menschen.
[Nomenclature in English].
NE: Figge, Frank H. J. [Bearb.]; Sobotta-Figge, . . .
Vol. 3. Central nervous system, autonomic nervous system, sense organs and skin, peripheral nerves and vessels. – 9. Engl. ed. / by Walther J. Hild, based upon the 17. German ed. / by Helmut Ferner; Jochen Staubesand, 1. repr. – 1977.
ISBN 0-8067-1739-4 (Baltimore)
ISBN 3-541-71739-4 (München)

Printed in Germany by Kastner & Callwey, Buch- und Offsetdruckerei, München.

American Editor's Preface to the 9th Edition in English

During the revision of the Atlas for the 9th English Edition and after he had completed the work for the first and second volumes, Professor Frank H. J. Figge died suddenly. It was his wish, conveyed to me by Mrs. Rosalie Yerkes Figge and Mr. Michael Urban, that I should continue his work and arrange the translation of Volume III. I followed this request without hesitation because I felt that I owed this duty to my dear friend Frank who, together with his wife, had shown me so many personal and professional favors when I came to this country as an immigrant.

I welcome the decision by the publishers and Frank Figge to depart radically from previous English editions and to replace the Latin with anglicized nomenclature because education in classical languages of the prospective medical student today is minimal. However, the etymology appropriate for each volume is conveniently included to further the understanding of anatomical terms.

Due to the close cooperation of Mr. Michael Urban and Mr. Klaus Gullath of Urban & Schwarzenberg, the guaranteed publication at the scheduled time was possible, even in the face of delays caused by Professor Figge's untimely death. However, this schedule could not have been observed without the unflagging efforts of Mrs. Rosalie Yerkes Figge who, with her daughters, Rosalie Ann Figge Beasley and Barbara Figge Fox, continued to be responsible for the myriad technical details of preparing the manuscripts for Volumes I and II for publication, including the meticulous proofreading and indexing. I also wish to thank my secretary, Mrs. Jeannine Russell, for her willing and painstaking efforts in preparing the manuscript for volume 3, and to my colleagues in the Department of Anatomy for many valuable suggestions.

It is my hope and expectation that all this concerted and time-consuming work by many people will make Sobotta's unsurpassed illustrations even more useful to future students of anatomy.

Galveston, Texas, July 1974 — Walther J. Hild

Abstract of Preface to First German Edition

Experience with the work in the student anatomical laboratory, extending over a period of many years, has convinced the author of the advisability of presenting illustrations of the peripheral nervous system and of the blood vessels as they are seen by the student in his dissections, that is, nerves and vessels of any region in the same figure. For this reason in the majority of the figures, arteries and nerves, or arteries, veins and nerves, or arteries and veins were illustrated side by side in the same figure. Only occasionally a departure from this plan was necessary, when for the sake of clearness supplementary figures had to be added showing only the arteries or the nerves (as for instance in the case of the cranial nerves).

This method of illustrating anatomical dissections has the advantage that the student finds in a single illustration all the structures which he actually encounters in any particular stratum of the region which he dissects; otherwise the student must waste too much precious time in searching for each type of structure on different pages of the volume or even in different volumes. Moreover, as the structures are pictured in their natural relationship, this set of illustrations represents at the same time an atlas of topographical anatomy.

The simultaneous illustration of blood vessels and nerves made the use of colored illustrations an indispensable necessity. The arteries are shown in red, the veins in blue, and the nerves in yellow. The three-color plates employed in depicting the arteries, veins, and nerves, were used at the same time to reproduce in color, by means of the three-color process, the parts of the body in their natural colors; the object was to obtain illustrations in which individual types of structures could be readily distinguished from other types by their color.

In this volume of the atlas, as in Volumes I and II, text pages alternate with full-page plates. The text pages contain the explanation of these plates, some helpful diagrams, and brief descriptions of the essential structures; the descriptions, however, are sufficiently complete to serve the student as a convenient guide and means of quick orientation while he is working in the laboratory.

Würzburg, May 1906 J. Sobotta

Preface to the 17th German Edition

Unfortunately, the shortening of the time available to the student for dissection necessarily goes hand in hand with a significant decrease in anatomical education. More and more, first-hand dissection exercises are substituted by the study of illustrations, texts and schematic representations. However, it is self-evident that even the most accurate, excellent and didactically best illustration cannot substitute for the three-dimensional experience of the dissector's hand. That anatomical knowledge is retained most tenaciously that the student relates to its own dissection experiences. "This he can never learn from predissected preparations nor engravings and, therefore, there is for him only One anatomical museum of masterworks, only One anatomical atlas of highest accuracy, and only One textbook of admirable clarity – the human body".

More than a century has passed since Hyrtl wrote these words. They are as true today as ever!

The new edition of the third volume of Sobotta/Becher's atlas has been changed more than vols. one and two. The editors have omitted, for the most part, coherent text passages in order to make a clear distinction from textbooks of systemic anatomy and, at the same time, to gain space for the addition of new illustrations where this appeared desirable. The sections dealing with Central Nervous System, Skin, Peripheral Nerves and Vessels, especially those of head and neck have been considerably augmented.

Mrs. H. V. Eickstedt and Mr. K.-H. Hensel have been especially helpful with the arrangements.

Etymological explanations of anatomical terms have been considerably increased in volume 3. The index has been expanded by the inclusion of common-language and clinically used terms.

Dr. Alfred Bolliger (Zürich) deserves recognition for important angiological references to the illustrations of superficial veins of the lower extremity; Mr. Heinz Brehme (Institut für Humangenetik und Anthropologie der Universität Freiburg i. Br.) for making available and arranging illustrations of cutaneous ridge patterns; Dr. Herbert Schmidt (Pforzheim) for valuable arteriograms of the common carotid artery, abdominal aorta and common iliac artery.

Medical student G. Adelmann has been very helpful with proofreading, and Mrs. M. Engler has given considerable help with the preparation of the index for which we express our thanks again.

The publishing house of Urban and Schwarzenberg, especially Mr. M. Urban, Jr., Dr. R. Degkwitz and Mr. K. Gullath deserve recognition for their excellent cooperation and their thoughtful attitude toward various requests and wishes of the editors.

Vienna and Freiburg i. Br. — H. Ferner

June 1973 — J. Staubesand

Table of Contents

Abbreviations

ant.	=	anterior
a. or aa.	=	artery or arteries
caud.	=	caudal
cran.	=	cranial
dist.	=	distal
dors.	=	dorsal
ext.	=	external
gangl.	=	ganglion
inf.	=	inferior
int.	=	interior
lat.	=	lateral
lig. or ligg.	=	ligament or ligaments
longit.	=	longitudinal
m. or mm.	=	muscle or muscles
n. or nn.	=	nerve or nerves
obl.	=	oblique
post.	=	posterior
prox.	=	proximal
r. or rr.	=	ramus or rami
sup.	=	superior
superf.	=	superficial
transv.	=	transverse
v. or vv.	=	vein or veins

Etymology and Meaning of Anatomical Terms of Vol. III

accessory .... L. *accedere; nervus accessorius* so called because it is accessory to the vagus nerve
acetabulum .... L. *acetabulum* = small vessel to hold vinegar; cup-shaped socket of hipjoint
amygdaloid .... Gr. *amygdalē* = almond
aqueduct .... L. water conduit
arachnoid .... Gr. *arachnoidēs* from *ho arachnos* = the spider; spider web membrane covering brain and spinal cord
artery .... Latinized Gr., etymology uncertain. Probably from *aggeia ta aera terenta* = air-containing vessels. The ancients thought that the arteries contained air.
auricle .... L. diminutive of *auris* = ear; outer ear and also the ear of the heart

bulbus .... L. from the Gr. *ho bolbos* = onion

calcar avis .... L. = the spur of the rooster
calcarine .... Part of spur (from calcar)
callosum .... L. *callum* = horny skin
capillary .... L. *capillus*, hair of the scalp
cauda equina ...... horse's tail (L. *cauda* = tail; *equina*, adj. from *equus* = horse); name applied to the roots of the lumbar and sacral spinal nerves which are arranged around the caudal end of the spinal cord like the hair of a horse's tail
cava .... L. *cavus* = hollow *(venae cavae)*
cephalic .... Gr. *kephalikos* from *kephale* = head
cerebellum .... L. diminutive of *cerebrum*, the small brain
cerebrum .... L. brain; cerebral hemispheres
chiasma .... Gr. crossing or intersecting in the manner of an X
chorda tympani ... Cord of the middle ear cavity. Only nerve which is not called "*nervus*"; it received its name at a time when its nervous nature was not known.
chorioid .... Gr. *chorion* = a skin, membrane
ciliary .... L. *cilium* = eyelash
cingulum .... L. belt (from *cingere* = to gird or surround)
claustrum .... L. *claudere* = to close, bar
cluneal .... L. *clunis*, buttock
cochlea .... shell of a snail (Lat., but perhaps originally Gr.)
celiac .... Gr. *koilos* = hollow, referring to abdominal cavity
commissure .... L. *committere* = to connect
concha .... Gr. *conchē*, shell of a mussel
conjunctiva .... L. *conjungere* = to connect
cor .... L. *cor,* genitive, *cordis* = heart
corium .... L., but originally Gr. = skin
cornea .... L. *cornu* = horn
coronary .... L. *corona* = wreath, crown
corpus .... L. a body, mass or structure
crus .... L. leg (adj. *cruralis*)
culmen .... L. summit
cuneus .... L. a wedge (adj. *cuneatus*)
cutaneous .... L. *cutis* = skin

decussation .... L. *decussare* = to cross each other in the form of an X
dentate .... L. *dens* = tooth
diencephalon ..... Gr. *dia* = between + encephalon
ductus deferens ... L. from *de* = away a. *ferre* = to carry
dura mater .... L. *durus* = hard; *mater* = mother, protection

emboliform .... L. from the Gr. *ho embolos* = plug
encephalon .... Gr. from *he kēphalē* = the head, and *en* = in
epidermis .... Gr. *epi* = on top, and *derma* = skin
epigastric .... Gr. *epi* = above; *gaster* = stomach or belly

fasciculus .... L. diminutive of *fascis* = a bundle or bunch
fasciolar .... L. *fasciola* = a small band, diminutive of *fascia* = band
fastigial .... L. *fastigium*, gable
flaccid .... L. *flaccus*, flabby
flocculus .... L. diminutive of *floccus* = a flock or tuft (of wool)
fornix .... L. arch of a vault
fossa .... L. a ditch; in anatomy, a depressed area
fovea .... L. a pit; in anatomy, a depression of small diameter

ganglion .... Gr. swelling, node
gastroepiploic ..... Gr. *gaster* = stomach; Gr. *epiploon* = greater omentum
geniculate .... L. *geniculum* = a small knee
glomus .... L. a ball of thread
gluteus .... Gr. *gloutos* = buttocks
griseus .... L. gray
gyrus .... Gr. *gyros* = a convolution

habenula .... L. diminutive of *habena* = bridle, strap
helicotrema .... Gr. *helix* = snail, and *trema* = hole
hippocampus ...... Gr. from *hippos* = horse; and *kamptein* = to bend. Refers to the shape of the foot *(pes hippocampi)* of a legendary animal and is one of the fantastic names of the old nomenclature. At an earlier period the same structure was compared with Ammon's horns (amonites) and called cornu Ammonis.
hirci .... L. *hircus* = buck or he-goat. Hair of the axilla
hyaloid .... Gr. *hyaloeidēs* = like glass
hypoglossus ...... Gr. *hypo* = beneath, and *glossa* = tongue
hypothalamus ..... Gr. *hypo* = beneath. The part of the brain located beneath the thalamus

incus .... L. *cudere* = to beat; anvil, one of the ossicles of the ear
infundibulum ..... L. funnel
integument .... L. *integere* = to cover; clothe
iris .... Gr. *iris*. Gen. *iridis* = rainbow

lacuna .... L. *lacus* = lake
lanugo .... L. *lana* = wool; the fine primary hair
lenticular .... L. from *lens*, Gen. *lentis* = lentil
leptomeninx ...... Gr. *leptos* = soft, delicate
luteus .... L. yellow
lymph .... L. *lympha* = a clear liquid

mamilla .... L. diminutive from *mamma* = female, breast, nipple
medulla .... L. marrow
meninges .... Gr. (sing. *meninx*) = membrane
myenteric .... Gr. *mys* = muscle, *enteron* = gut. Nerve plexus in muscle layer of gut

nerve .... Latinized Gr. from *to neyron* = (at first) tendon; later, nerve
nucleus .... L. *nux* = nut, literally a kernel, designates an aggregation of nerve cells

obturator .... L. *obturare* = to stop up
operculum .... L. *operire* = to cover; lid or cover

pachymeninx ..... Gr. *pachys* = thick, firm; *meninx* = membrane
pallidus .... L. pale
palpebral .... L. *palpebra* = eyelid
pampiniform ...... L. *pampinus* = shoot of a vine, as in connection with plexus pampiniformis in spermatic cord
peduncle .... L. diminutive of *pes* = foot
pellucidus .... L. *pellucere* = to shine through
petrosal .... Gr. *petra* = rock; as applied to pars petrosa (hardest portion) of temporal bone
phrenic .... Gr. *phrenes* = diaphragm
pia mater .... L. *pius* = soft; *mater* = mother, in the sense of protection
pineal .... L. *pinus* = pine tree
plexus .... L. *plectere* = to interweave
pons .... L. bridge
pterygoid .... Gr. *pteryx* = wing
eidos = resemblance
pupil .... L. a little girl, a small doll; this name for the pupil is very ancient and refers to the diminutive mirror image which the observer sees of himself in the cornea of a (female) person confronting him. The pupil of the eye.

quadrigeminal .... L. *quadri* = combining form of *quattuor*, four, and *geminus* = twin or alike

ramus .... L. branch
raphe .... Gr. *rhaphe* = a seamlike junction or suture
rete .... L. network
rostral .... L. *rostrum* = beak; located towards the front end of the body
ruga ....L. wrinkle

sacculus .... L. a small sack, diminutive from *saccus* = a sack or bag
saphenous .... Hebrew or Aramaic, hidden; *vena saphena*, the hidden vein of lower extremity, so called because it does not show through the skin
scala .... L. staircase
scapha .... Gr. *scaphē* = boat; a boat-shaped depression
sclera .... Gr. *skleros* = hard
serratus .... L. *serra* = saw
sinus .... L. a cavity, a hollow, roundish recess
spinalis .... L. *spina* = thorn; used in the sense of belonging to the spinal column
splenius .... Gr. *splenion* = a bandage
stapes .... A late L. word from *stare* = to stand, and *pes* = foot; stirrup, one of the ossicles of the ear
striatus .... L. *stria* = stripe
suralis .... L. *sura* = calf; of the leg
sympathetic .... A division of the autonomic nervous system. Gr. *syn* = with and *pathos* = suffering, compassion

tapetum .... L. carpet, curtain
tarsus .... Gr. *tarsos* = a wickerwork frame. In the anatomy of the eye, it designates the cartilage of the eyelid; in the skeleton, the anklebones of the foot
tegmen .... L. cover or roof
telencephalon ..... Gr. *telos* = end + encephalon, endbrain or cerebral hemispheres
tenia .... L. band, stripe
tentorium .... L. tent, sheet stretched across, from *tendere* = to stretch
thalamus .... Gr. chamber; does not designate a cavity as the word would suggest, but two massive bodies forming the walls of the third ventricle.
tractus .... L. *trahere* = to drag or conduct; in neuroanatomy a large bundle of nerve fibers (larger than a fasciculus)
tragus .... Gr. *tragos* = a buck or he-goat; so named from the longer and thicker hair growing on that part of the outer ear and carrying the same name
tympanum .... Gr. *tympanon* = drum; the cavity of the middle ear

vagus .... L. wandering, roving; *nervus vagus*, so called because its branches extend as far as the abdomen although the nerve takes origin from the brain
vallecula .... L. diminutive of *valles* = valley
vas .... L. a vessel (pl. = *vasa*; gen. pl. = *vasorum*)
ventricle .... L. ventriculus = the belly; used to designate the cavities of the brain, and also the two great chambers of the heart
vesicalis .... L. *vesica* = bladder
vibrissa .... L. *vibrare* = to tremble or vibrate; hair of the nostril
vitreus .... L. *vitrum* = glass; translucent like glass
vorticose ....L. *vortex* = whirl

Central Nervous System

Brain

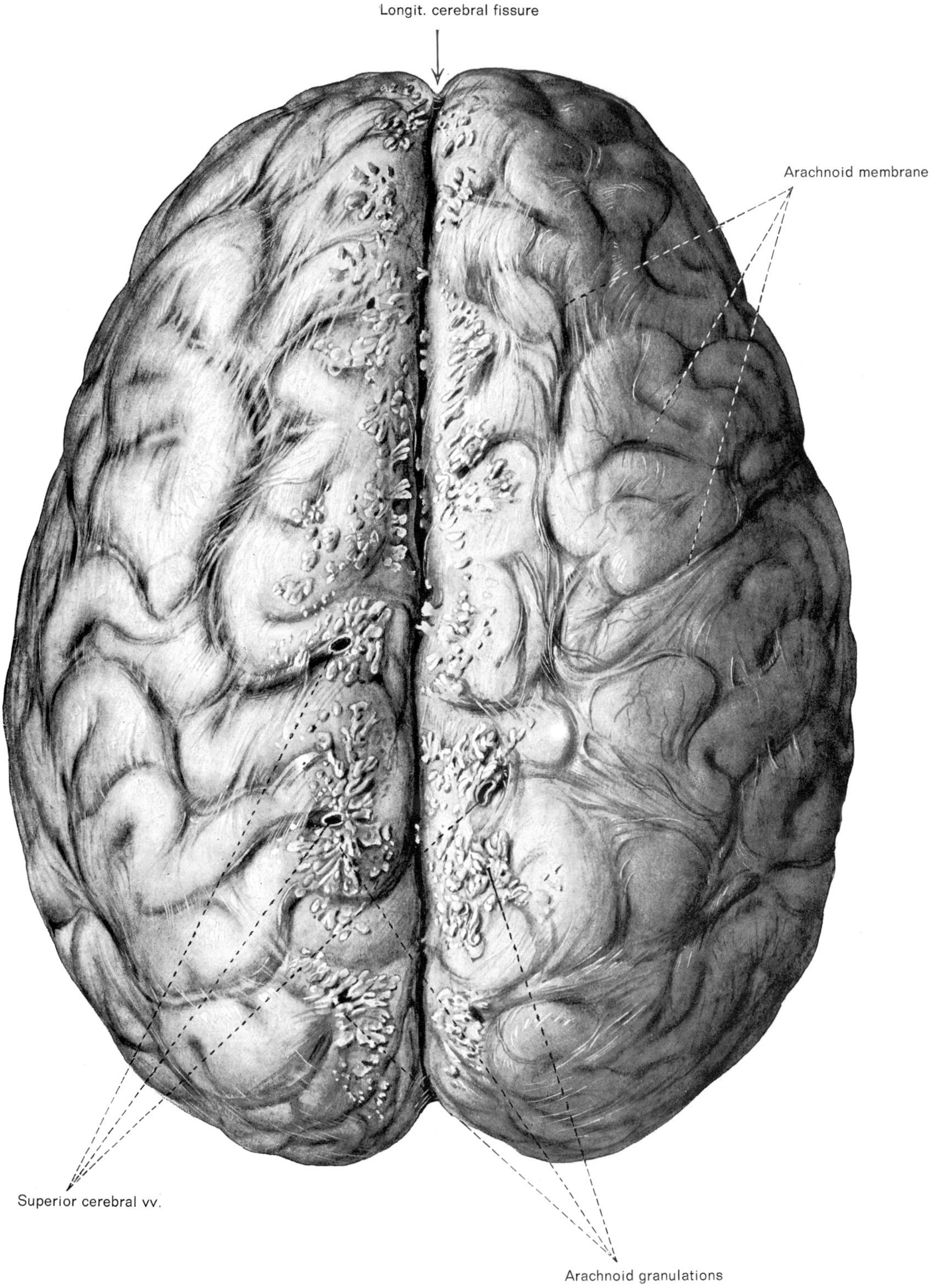
Longit. cerebral fissure
Arachnoid membrane
Superior cerebral vv.
Arachnoid granulations

Fig. 1. Telencephalon with leptomeninges seen from above.

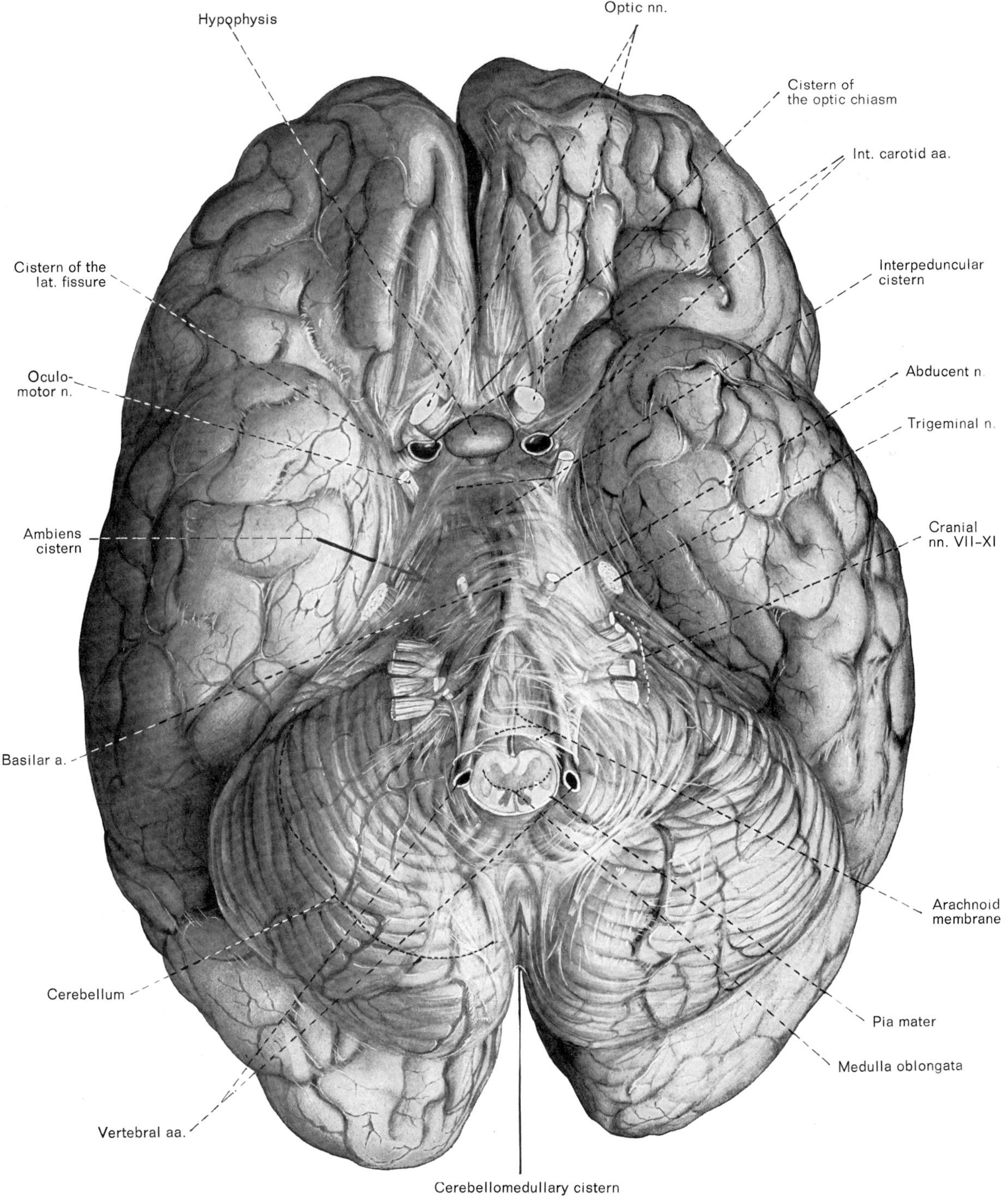
Hypophysis
Optic nn.
Cistern of
the optic chiasm
Int. carotid aa.
Cistern of the
lat. fissure
Interpeduncular
cistern
Oculo-
motor n.
Abducent n.
Trigeminal n.
Ambiens
cistern
Cranial
nn. VII–XI
Basilar a.
Arachnoid
membrane
Cerebellum
Pia mater
Medulla oblongata
Vertebral aa.
Cerebellomedullary cistern

Fig. 2. Brain with leptomeninges seen from below.

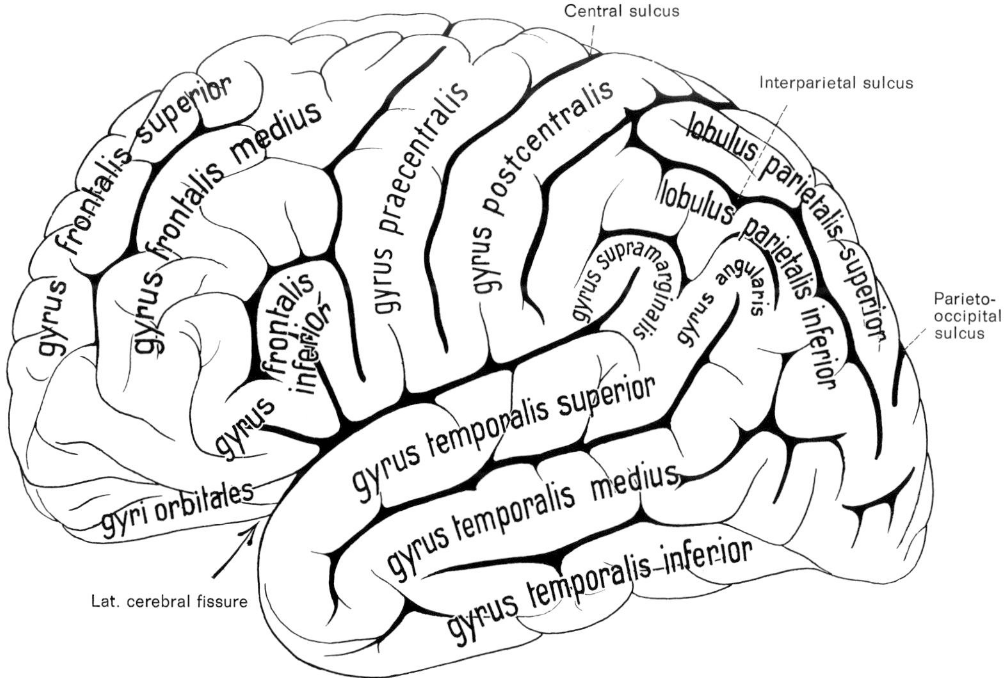
Central sulcus
Interparietal sulcus
Parieto-occipital sulcus
gyrus frontalis superior
gyrus frontalis medius
gyrus frontalis inferior
gyrus praecentralis
gyrus postcentralis
lobulus parietalis superior
lobulus parietalis inferior
gyrus supramarginalis
gyrus angularis
gyrus temporalis superior
gyrus temporalis medius
gyrus temporalis inferior
gyri orbitales
Lat. cerebral fissure

Fig. 3. Sulci and gyri of the pallium. Lateral view.

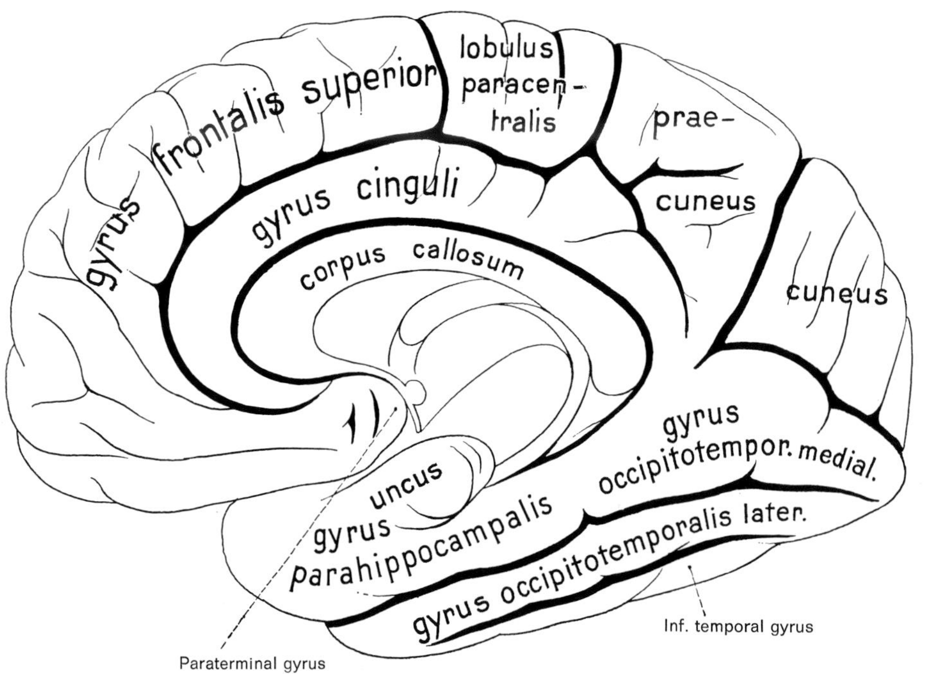
gyrus frontalis superior
lobulus paracentralis
praecuneus
cuneus
gyrus cinguli
corpus callosum
uncus
gyrus parahippocampalis
gyrus occipitotempor. medial.
gyrus occipitotemporalis later.
Inf. temporal gyrus
Paraterminal gyrus

Fig. 4. Sulci and gyri of the pallium. Medial view. The brain is halved in the median plane. The brain stem together with the cerebellum has been removed by an oblique section through the thalamus.

Fig. 5. Sulci and gyri of the pallium. Basal view. Brain stem and cerebellum have been removed. Hypophysis, olfactory tracts and optic nerves have been sectioned.

Fig. 6. The lobes of the telencephalon. The region of the frontal, frontoparietal and temporal opercula is shown by stippling.

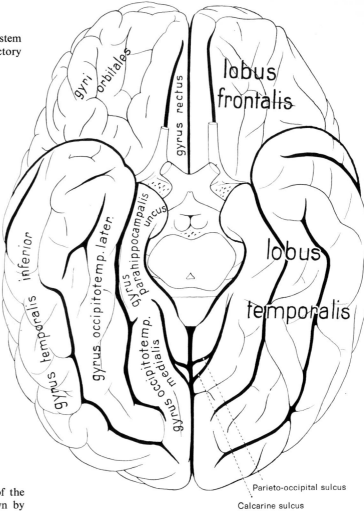

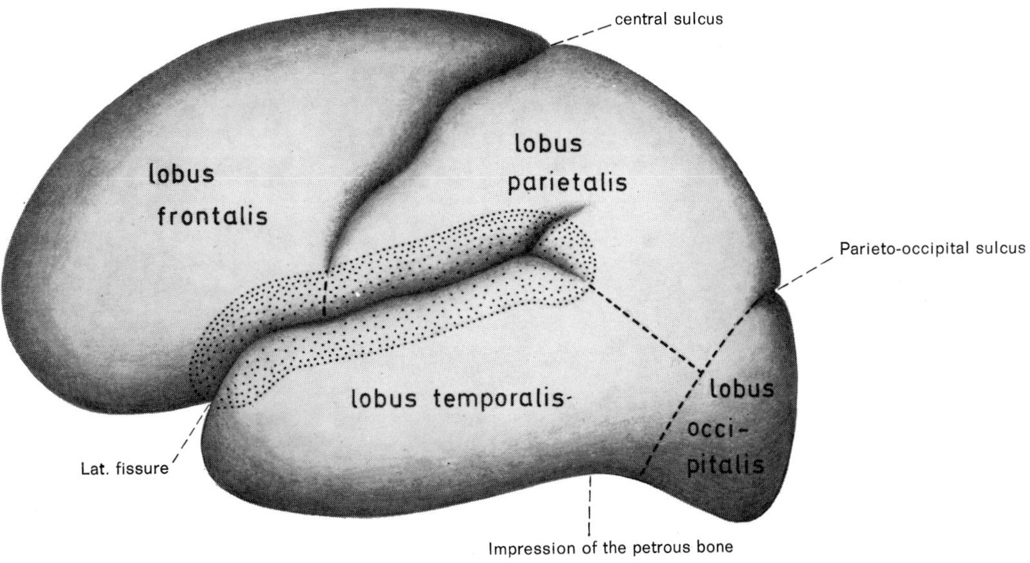
central sulcus
lobus frontalis
lobus parietalis
Parieto-occipital sulcus
lobus temporalis
lobus occi-pitalis
Lat. fissure
Impression of the petrous bone

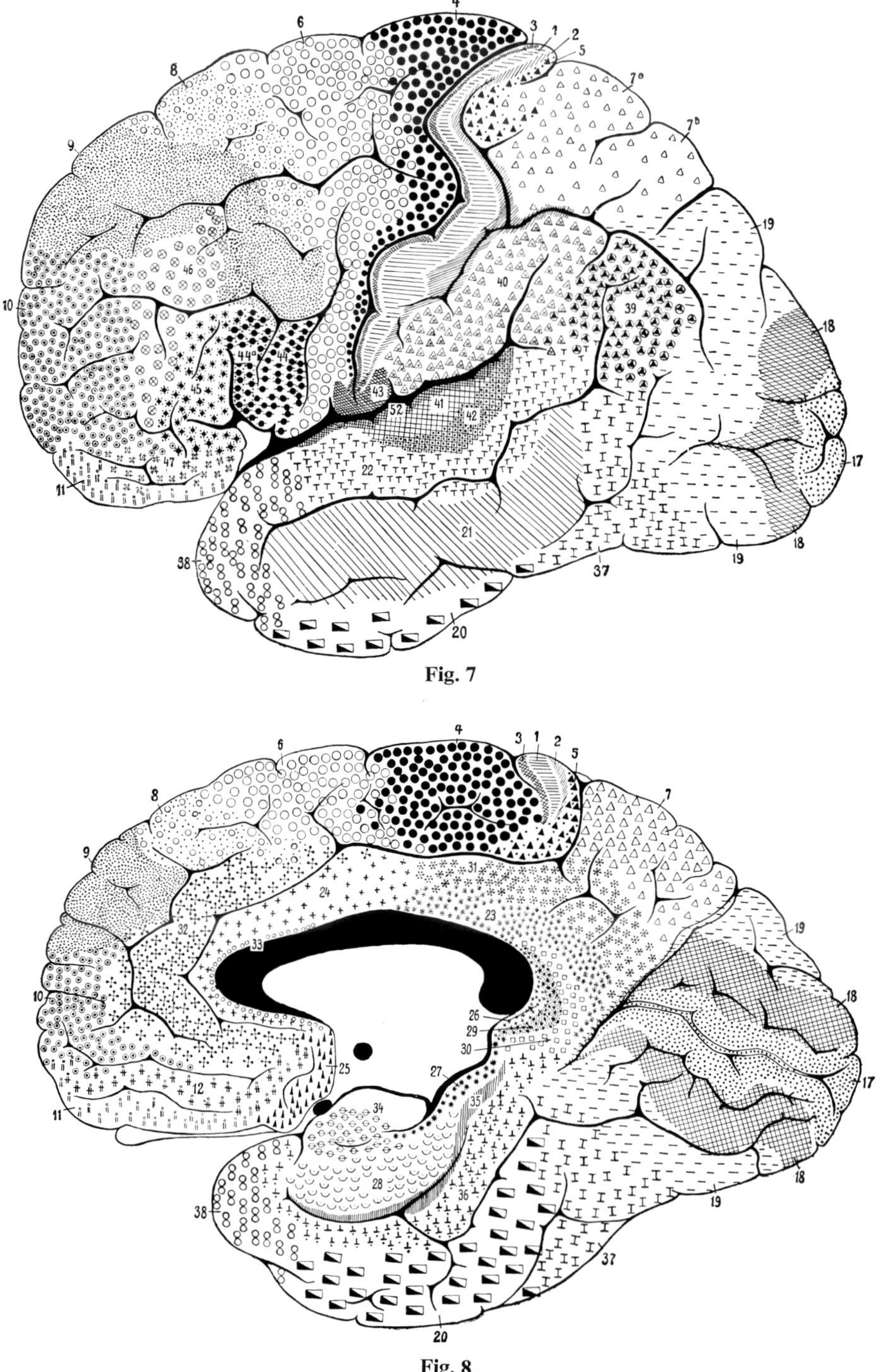

4
6
3
1
2
5
8
7a
7b
9
19
46
40
10
39
18
44
45
43
52
41
42
17
47
22
11
21
38
37
19
18
20

Fig. 7

4
6
3
1
2
5
8
7
9
31
24
23
19
32
33
10
18
26
29
30
25
27
17
11
12
34
35
28
36
18
19
38
37
20

Fig. 8

Figg. 7 and 8. Cytoarchitectonic cortical areas of the lateral (top) and medial (bottom) surface of the cerebral hemisphere, so-called brain charts (from *K. Brodmann:* Vergleichende Lokalisationslehre der Großhirnrinde. Barth, Leipzig 1909). The areas are numbered in the original manner and are marked by different symbols. These cytoarchitectonic cortical fields coincide only roughly with functional cortical areas.

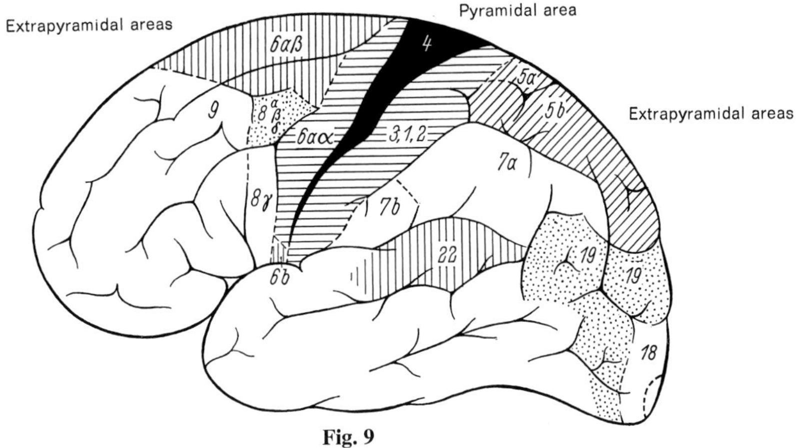
Extrapyramidal areas
Pyramidal area
Extrapyramidal areas
6aβ
4
5a
5b
9
6aα
3,1,2
7a
8γ
7b
22
19
19
6b
18

Fig. 9

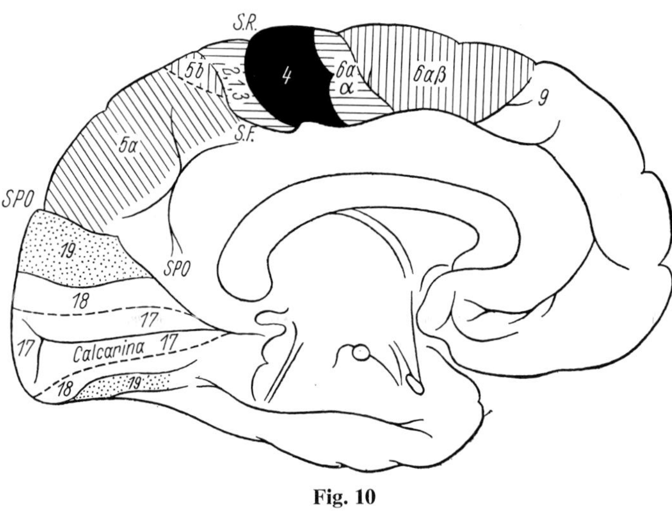
S.R.
5b
2,1,3
4
6a α
6aβ
9
S.F.
5a
SPO
19
SPO
18
17
Calcarina 17
17
18
19

Fig. 10

Figg. 9 and 10. Cortical motor areas of the human cerebral hemisphere. Lateral view (top), medial view (bottom). The pyramidal area is rendered in black, extrapyramidal areas 6aα, 6aβ, 3, 1, 2, 5a, 5b and 22 are hatched, motor areas for eye movements 8$\alpha\beta\delta$ and 19 are stippled; SR central sulcus; SPO parieto-occipital sulcus; SF cingulate sulcus (from *Bumke-Foerster* [ed.]: Handbuch der Neurologie, Vol. VI. Springer, Berlin 1936).

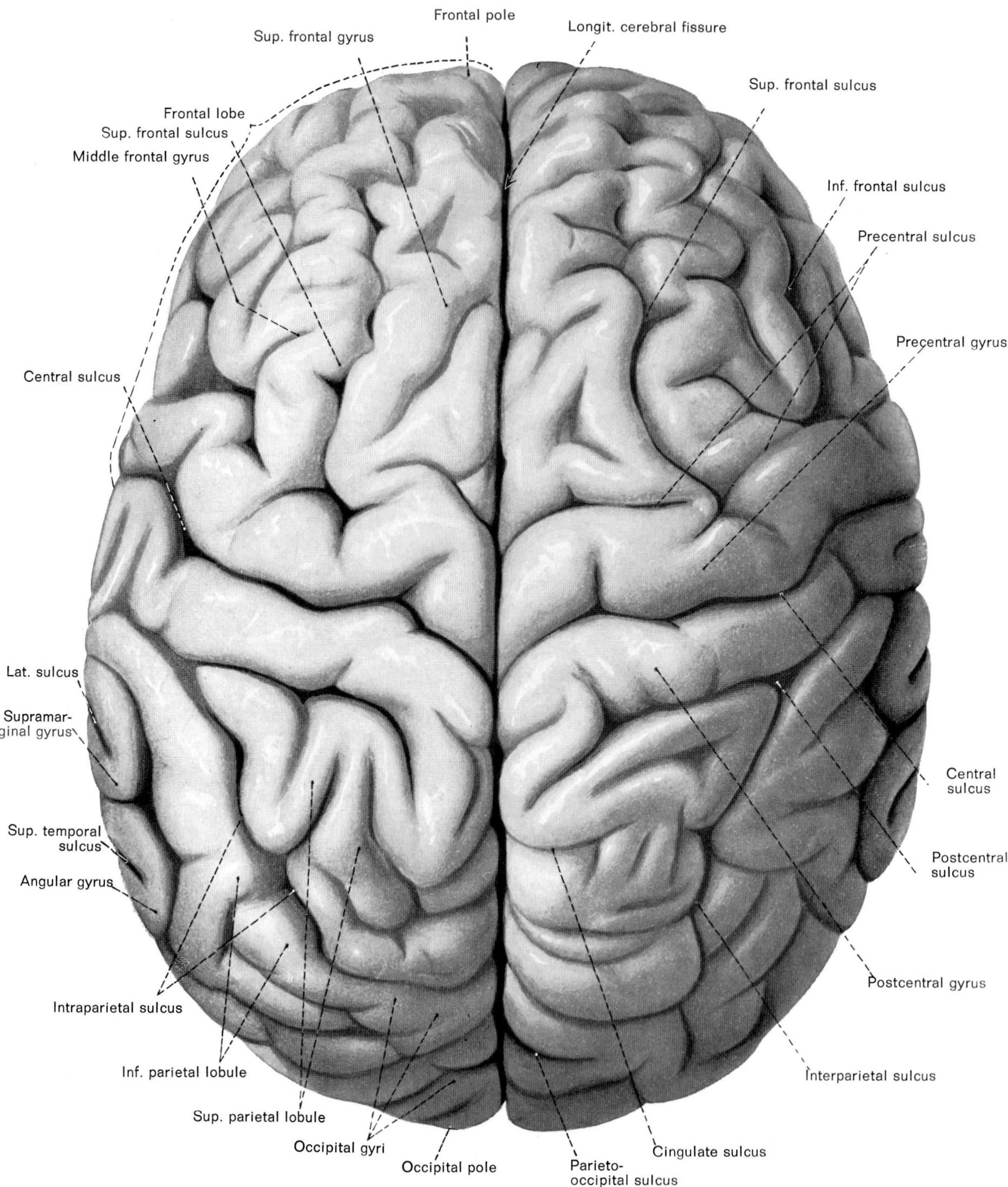
Frontal pole
Sup. frontal gyrus
Longit. cerebral fissure
Sup. frontal sulcus
Frontal lobe
Sup. frontal sulcus
Middle frontal gyrus
Inf. frontal sulcus
Precentral sulcus
Precentral gyrus
Central sulcus
Lat. sulcus
Supramar-
ginal gyrus
Central
sulcus
Sup. temporal
sulcus
Postcentral
sulcus
Angular gyrus
Postcentral gyrus
Intraparietal sulcus
Inf. parietal lobule
Interparietal sulcus
Sup. parietal lobule
Occipital gyri
Occipital pole
Cingulate sulcus
Parieto-
occipital sulcus

Fig. 11. Cerebral hemispheres after removal of the leptomeninges. View from above.

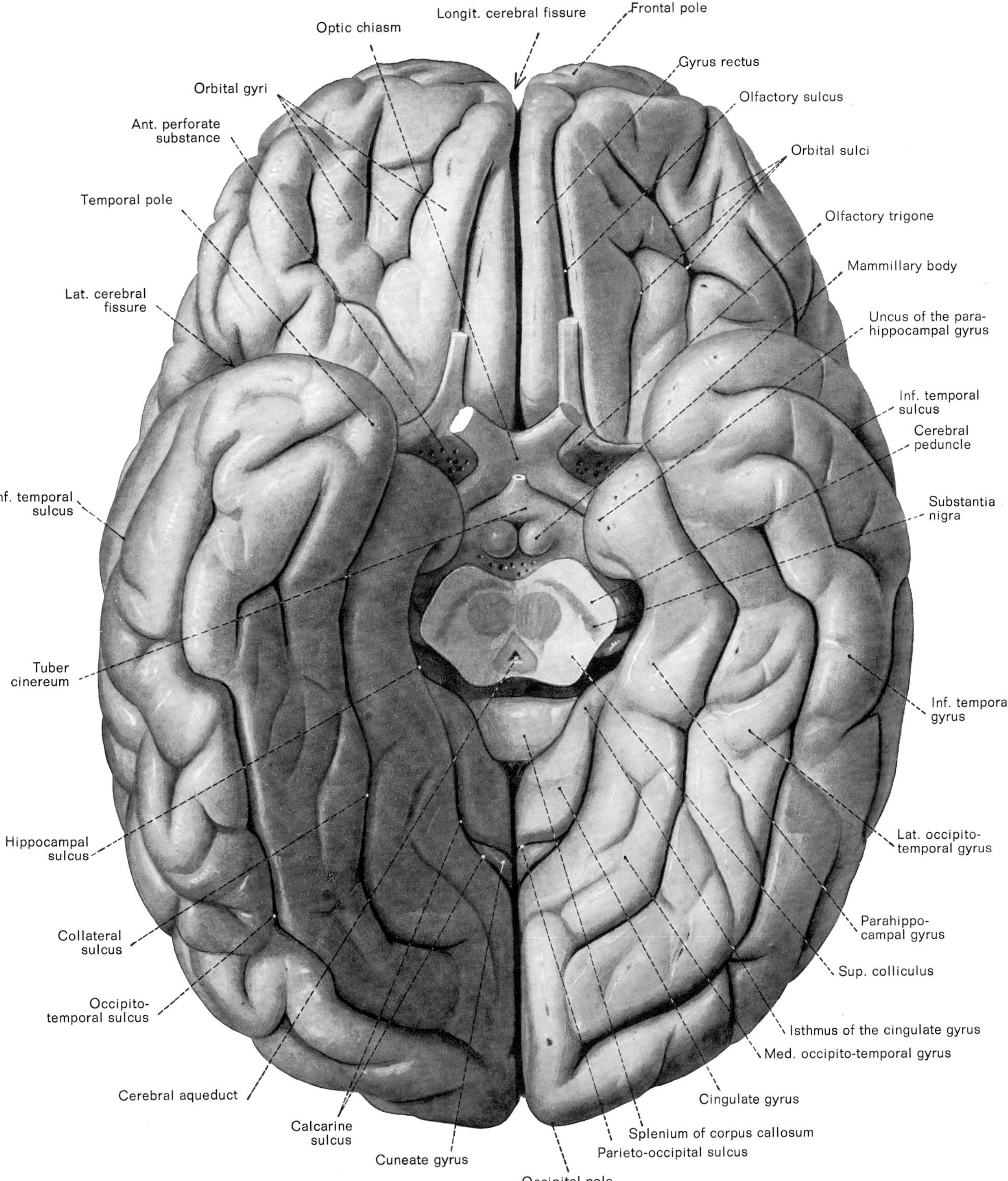
Optic chiasm
Longit. cerebral fissure
Frontal pole
Gyrus rectus
Orbital gyri
Olfactory sulcus
Ant. perforate substance
Orbital sulci
Temporal pole
Olfactory trigone
Mammillary body
Lat. cerebral fissure
Uncus of the para-hippocampal gyrus
Inf. temporal sulcus
Cerebral peduncle
Inf. temporal sulcus
Substantia nigra
Tuber cinereum
Inf. temporal gyrus
Hippocampal sulcus
Lat. occipito-temporal gyrus
Parahippo-campal gyrus
Collateral sulcus
Sup. colliculus
Occipito-temporal sulcus
Isthmus of the cingulate gyrus
Med. occipito-temporal gyrus
Cerebral aqueduct
Cingulate gyrus
Calcarine sulcus
Splenium of corpus callosum
Parieto-occipital sulcus
Cuneate gyrus
Occipital pole

Fig. 12. Cerebral hemispheres after removal of the leptomeninges. View from below. Brain stem and cerebellum have been removed by a cross section through the midbrain. The section through the midbrain reveals the red nucleus on both sides under the substantia nigra.

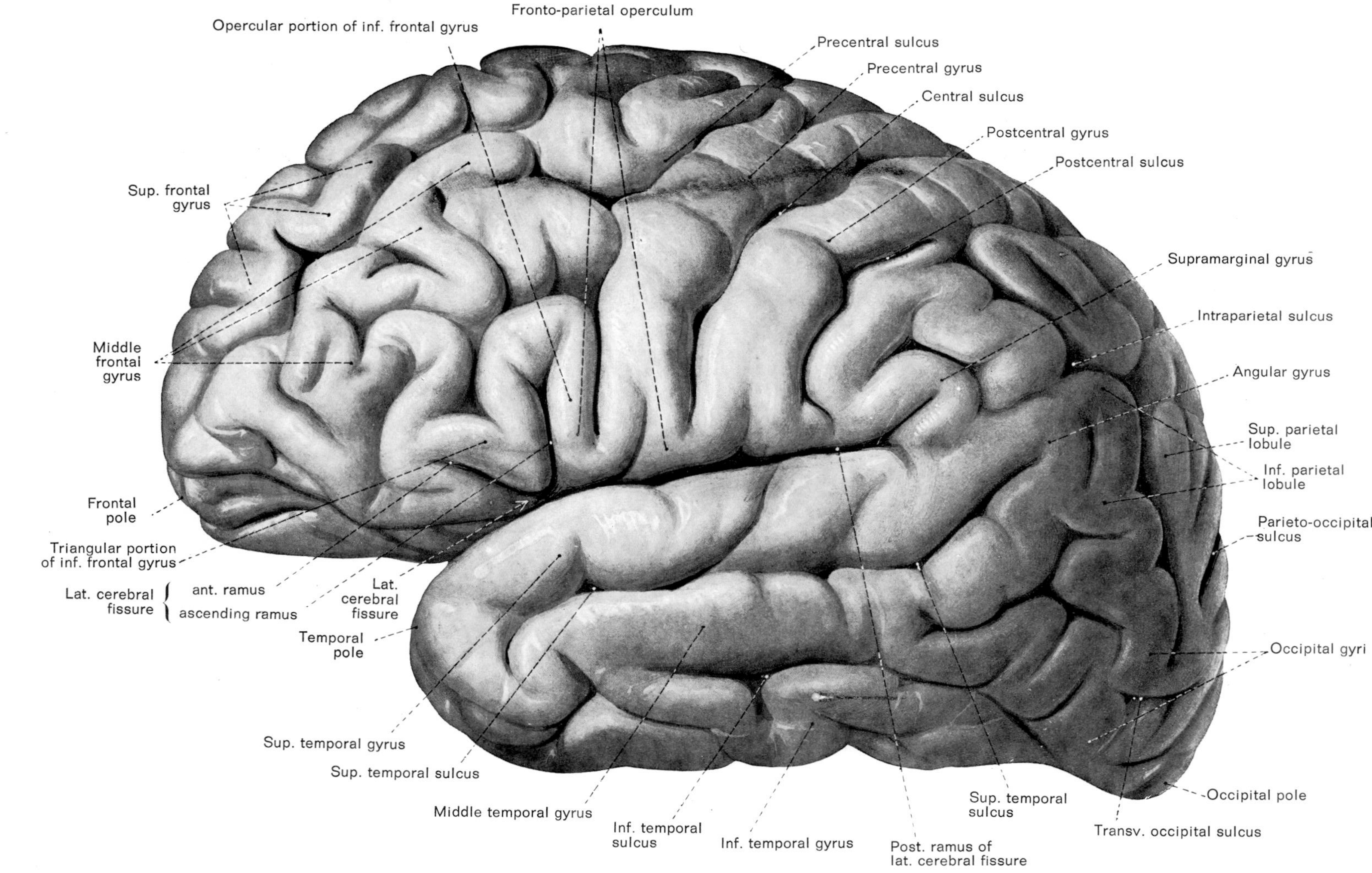
Fronto-parietal operculum
Opercular portion of inf. frontal gyrus
Precentral sulcus
Precentral gyrus
Central sulcus
Postcentral gyrus
Postcentral sulcus
Sup. frontal gyrus
Supramarginal gyrus
Intraparietal sulcus
Middle frontal gyrus
Angular gyrus
Sup. parietal lobule
Inf. parietal lobule
Frontal pole
Parieto-occipital sulcus
Triangular portion of inf. frontal gyrus
Lat. cerebral fissure
ant. ramus
ascending ramus
Lat. cerebral fissure
Temporal pole
Occipital gyri
Sup. temporal gyrus
Sup. temporal sulcus
Middle temporal gyrus
Inf. temporal sulcus
Inf. temporal gyrus
Post. ramus of lat. cerebral fissure
Sup. temporal sulcus
Occipital pole
Transv. occipital sulcus

Fig. 13. Sulci and Gyri of the left cerebral hemisphere. Lateral view.

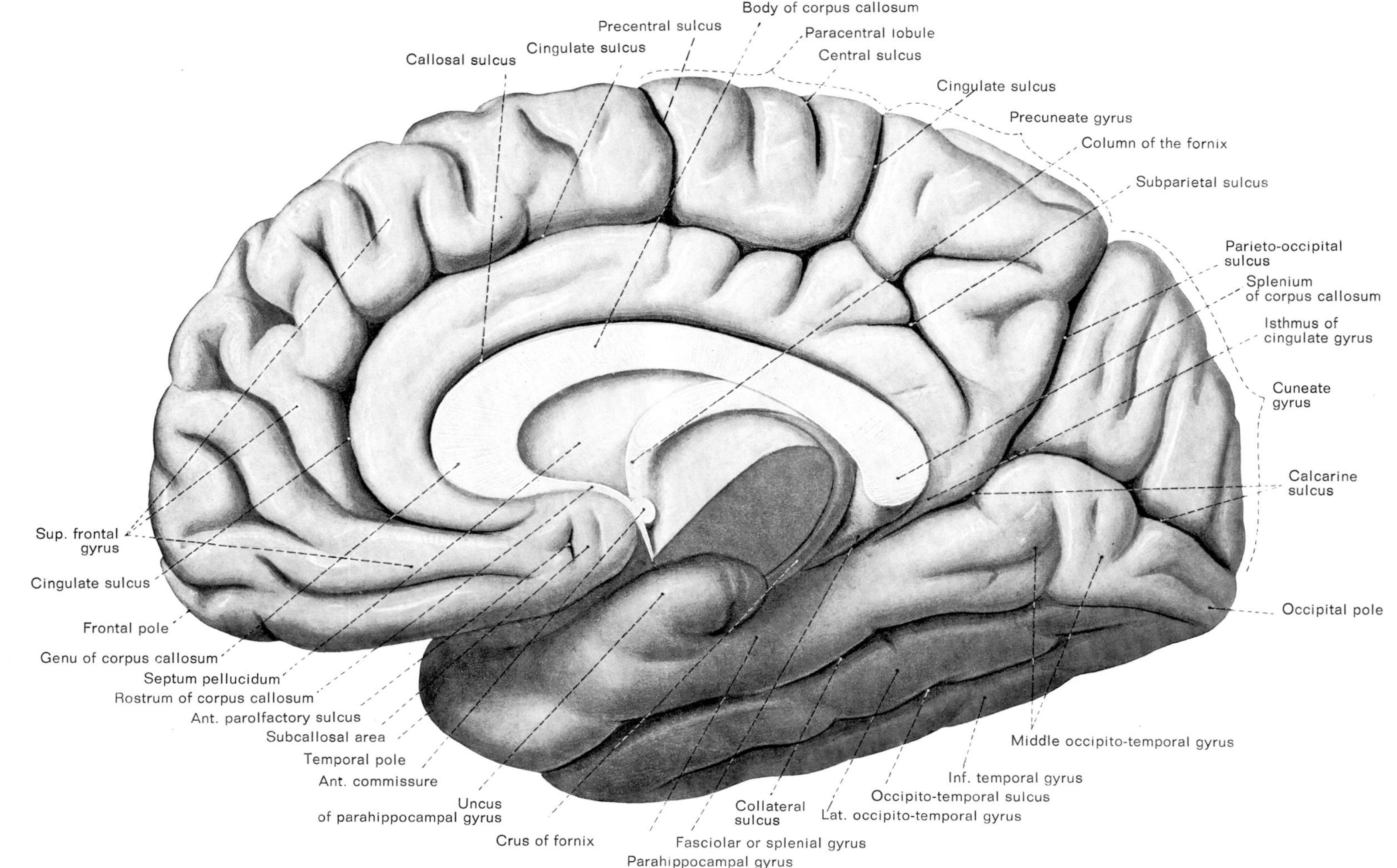

Body of corpus callosum
Precentral sulcus
Paracentral lobule
Cingulate sulcus
Callosal sulcus
Central sulcus
Cingulate sulcus
Precuneate gyrus
Column of the fornix
Subparietal sulcus
Parieto-occipital sulcus
Splenium of corpus callosum
Isthmus of cingulate gyrus
Cuneate gyrus
Calcarine sulcus
Sup. frontal gyrus
Cingulate sulcus
Occipital pole
Frontal pole
Genu of corpus callosum
Septum pellucidum
Rostrum of corpus callosum
Ant. parolfactory sulcus
Subcallosal area
Temporal pole
Ant. commissure
Middle occipito-temporal gyrus
Inf. temporal gyrus
Occipito-temporal sulcus
Uncus of parahippocampal gyrus
Collateral sulcus
Lat. occipito-temporal gyrus
Crus of fornix
Fasciolar or splenial gyrus
Parahippocampal gyrus

Fig. 14. Right cerebral hemisphere. The brain has been halved in the midline, the brain stem together with the cerebellum have been removed by an oblique section through the thalamus. View onto the medial and inferior surface of the hemisphere.

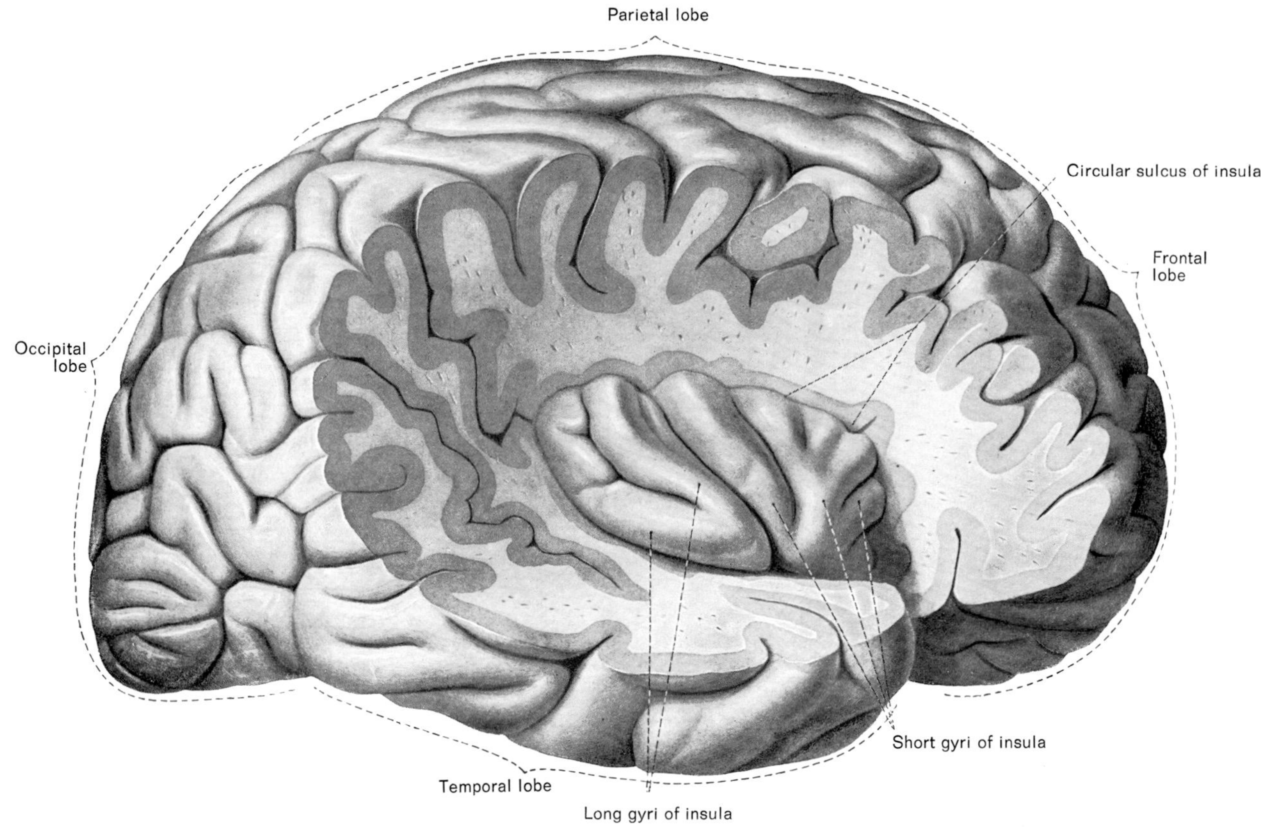
Parietal lobe
Circular sulcus of insula
Frontal lobe
Occipital lobe
Short gyri of insula
Temporal lobe
Long gyri of insula

Fig. 15. Right hemisphere. Lateral view. The insula is brought into view by removing the frontal, fronto-parietal and temporal opercular portions.

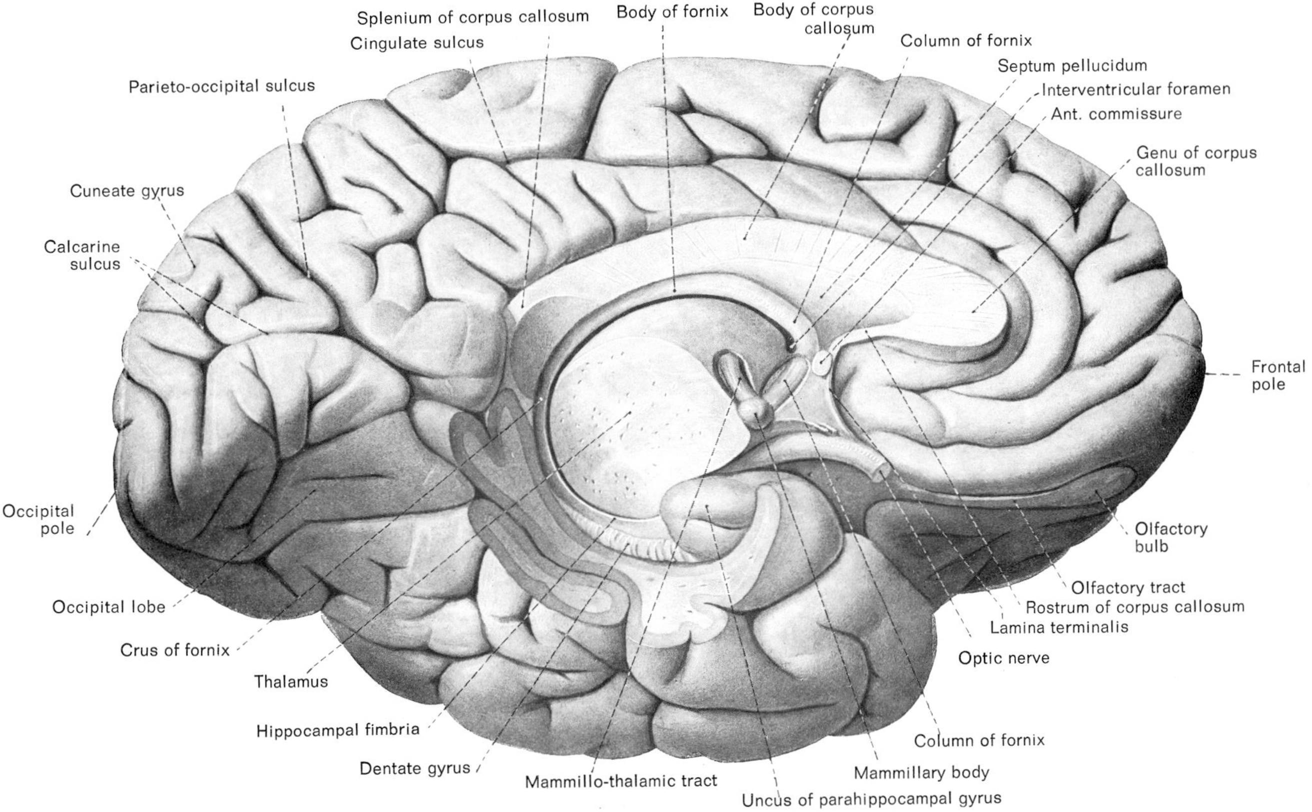
Splenium of corpus callosum
Cingulate sulcus
Body of fornix
Body of corpus callosum
Column of fornix
Septum pellucidum
Interventricular foramen
Ant. commissure
Parieto-occipital sulcus
Genu of corpus callosum
Cuneate gyrus
Calcarine sulcus
Frontal pole
Occipital pole
Olfactory bulb
Olfactory tract
Occipital lobe
Rostrum of corpus callosum
Lamina terminalis
Crus of fornix
Optic nerve
Thalamus
Hippocampal fimbria
Column of fornix
Dentate gyrus
Mammillo-thalamic tract
Mammillary body
Uncus of parahippocampal gyrus

Fig. 16. The fornix exposed in its entire extent and in its natural position. The brain has been halved in the midline, the brain stem together with the cerebellum has been removed by an oblique section through the thalamus. The parahippocampal gyrus has been removed to such an extent as to reveal the hippocampal fimbria and the dentate gyrus. After removal of the lateral wall of the third ventricle (hypothalamic area) the column of the fornix and the mammillo-thalamic tract have been dissected free down to the mammillary body. View from medial and below.

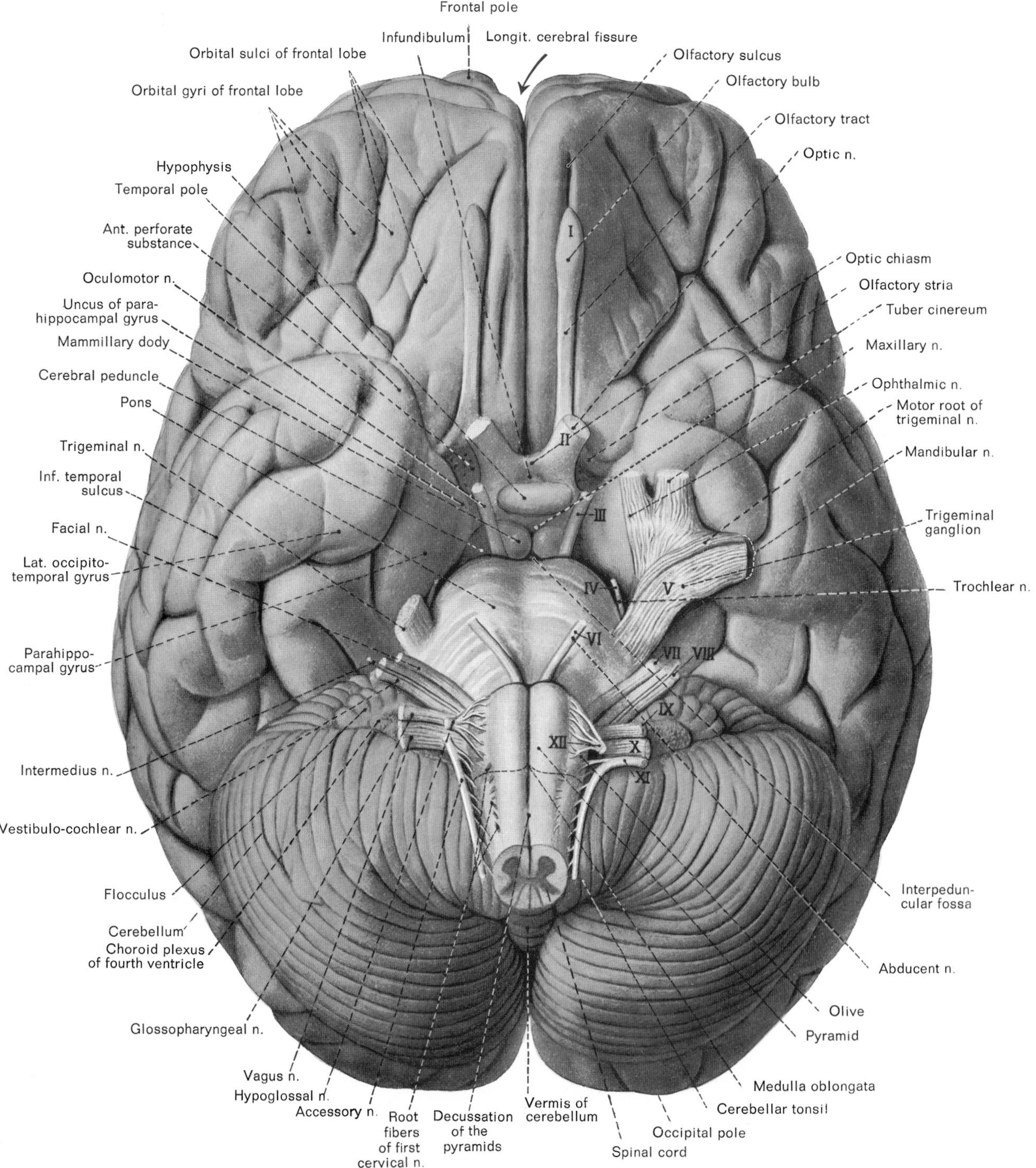
Frontal pole
Infundibulum
Longit. cerebral fissure
Orbital sulci of frontal lobe
Olfactory sulcus
Olfactory bulb
Orbital gyri of frontal lobe
Olfactory tract
Optic n.
Hypophysis
Temporal pole
Ant. perforate substance
Optic chiasm
Oculomotor n.
Olfactory stria
Uncus of parahippocampal gyrus
Tuber cinereum
Mammillary dody
Maxillary n.
Cerebral peduncle
Ophthalmic n.
Pons
Motor root of trigeminal n.
Trigeminal n.
Mandibular n.
Inf. temporal sulcus
Trigeminal ganglion
Facial n.
Lat. occipito-temporal gyrus
Trochlear n.
Parahippocampal gyrus
Intermedius n.
Vestibulo-cochlear n.
Interpeduncular fossa
Flocculus
Cerebellum
Choroid plexus of fourth ventricle
Abducent n.
Olive
Glossopharyngeal n.
Pyramid
Vagus n.
Medulla oblongata
Hypoglossal n.
Vermis of cerebellum
Cerebellar tonsil
Accessory n.
Root fibers of first cervical n.
Decussation of the pyramids
Occipital pole
Spinal cord
I
II
III
IV
V
VI
VII
VIII
IX
X
XI
XII

Fig. 17. Basal view of the brain revealing the sites of origin of the cranial nerves (I–XII). Telencephalon yellow, cerebellum orange, brain stem and cranial nerves white. The left trigeminal ganglion is preserved. The hypophysis is slightly deflected posteriorly in order to reveal the infundibulum.

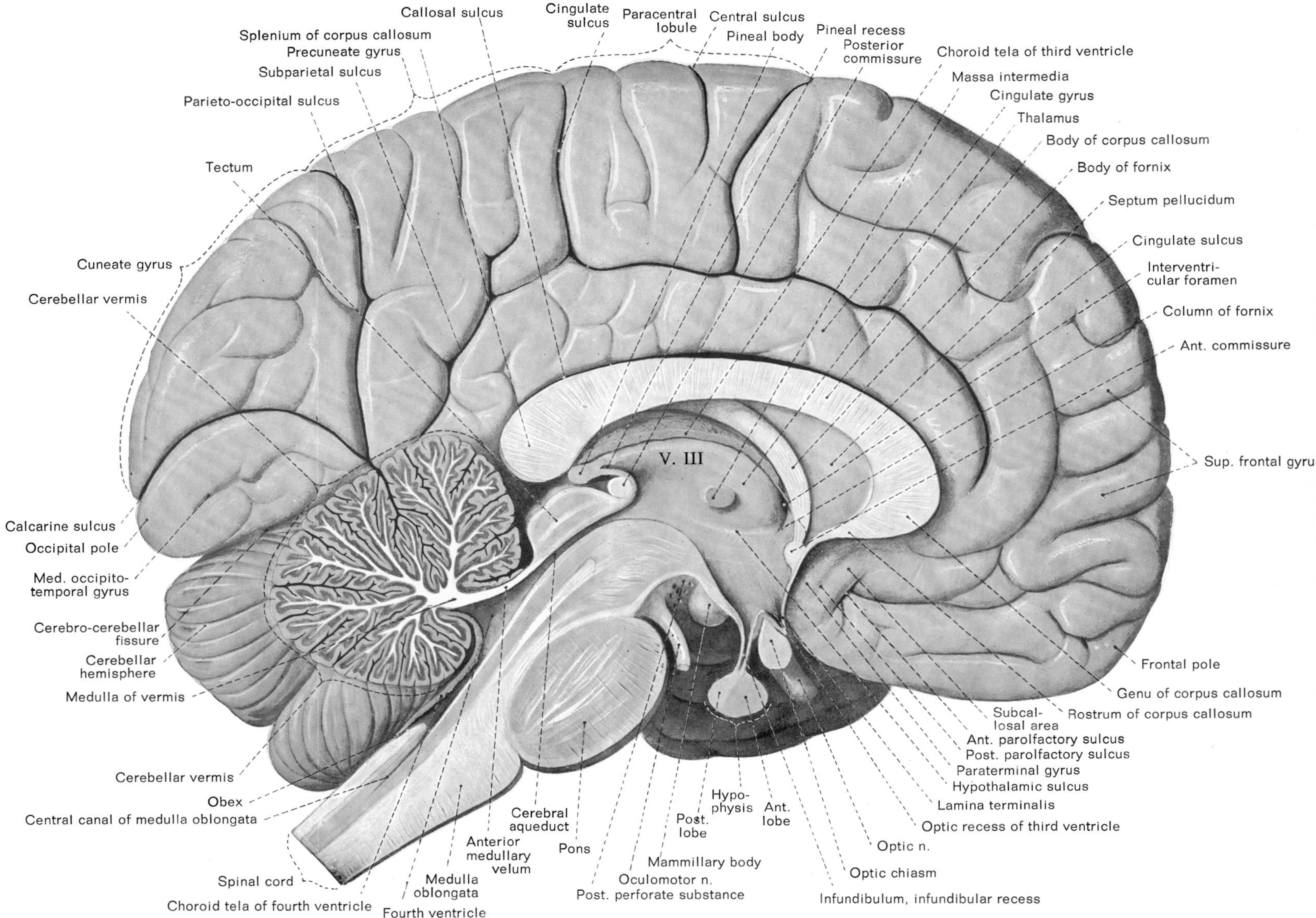
Callosal sulcus
Splenium of corpus callosum
Precuneate gyrus
Subparietal sulcus
Parieto-occipital sulcus
Tectum
Cuneate gyrus
Cerebellar vermis
Cingulate sulcus
Paracentral lobule
Central sulcus
Pineal body
Pineal recess
Posterior commissure
Choroid tela of third ventricle
Massa intermedia
Cingulate gyrus
Thalamus
Body of corpus callosum
Body of fornix
Septum pellucidum
Cingulate sulcus
Interventricular foramen
Column of fornix
Ant. commissure
Sup. frontal gyrus
V. III
Calcarine sulcus
Occipital pole
Med. occipito-temporal gyrus
Cerebro-cerebellar fissure
Cerebellar hemisphere
Medulla of vermis
Cerebellar vermis
Obex
Central canal of medulla oblongata
Spinal cord
Choroid tela of fourth ventricle
Fourth ventricle
Medulla oblongata
Anterior medullary velum
Cerebral aqueduct
Pons
Post. perforate substance
Oculomotor n.
Mammillary body
Post. lobe
Hypophysis
Ant. lobe
Infundibulum, infundibular recess
Optic chiasm
Optic n.
Optic recess of third ventricle
Lamina terminalis
Hypothalamic sulcus
Paraterminal gyrus
Post. parolfactory sulcus
Ant. parolfactory sulcus
Subcallosal area
Rostrum of corpus callosum
Genu of corpus callosum
Frontal pole

Fig. 18. Sagittal section through the brain. Medial aspect of the left half of the brain. V. III = third ventricle.

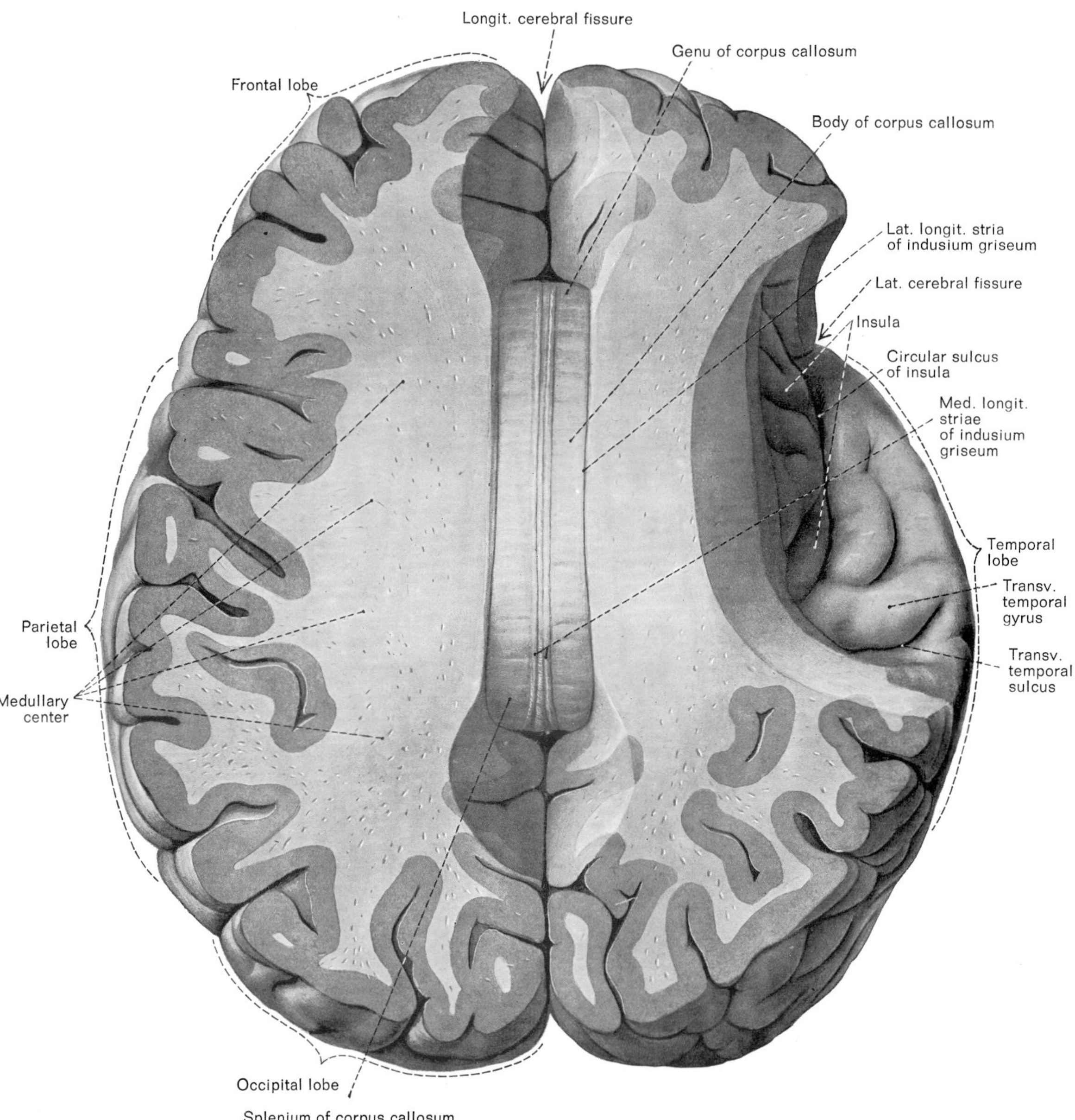

Longit. cerebral fissure
Genu of corpus callosum
Frontal lobe
Body of corpus callosum
Lat. longit. stria
of indusium griseum
Lat. cerebral fissure
Insula
Circular sulcus
of insula
Med. longit.
striae
of indusium
griseum
Temporal
lobe
Transv.
temporal
gyrus
Transv.
temporal
sulcus
Parietal
lobe
Medullary
center
Occipital lobe
Splenium of corpus callosum

Fig. 19. Horizontal section through both hemispheres. The corpus callosum is exposed. View from above. The insula is dissected free on the right side; anteriorly the genu and posteriorly the splenium of the corpus callosum have been exposed.

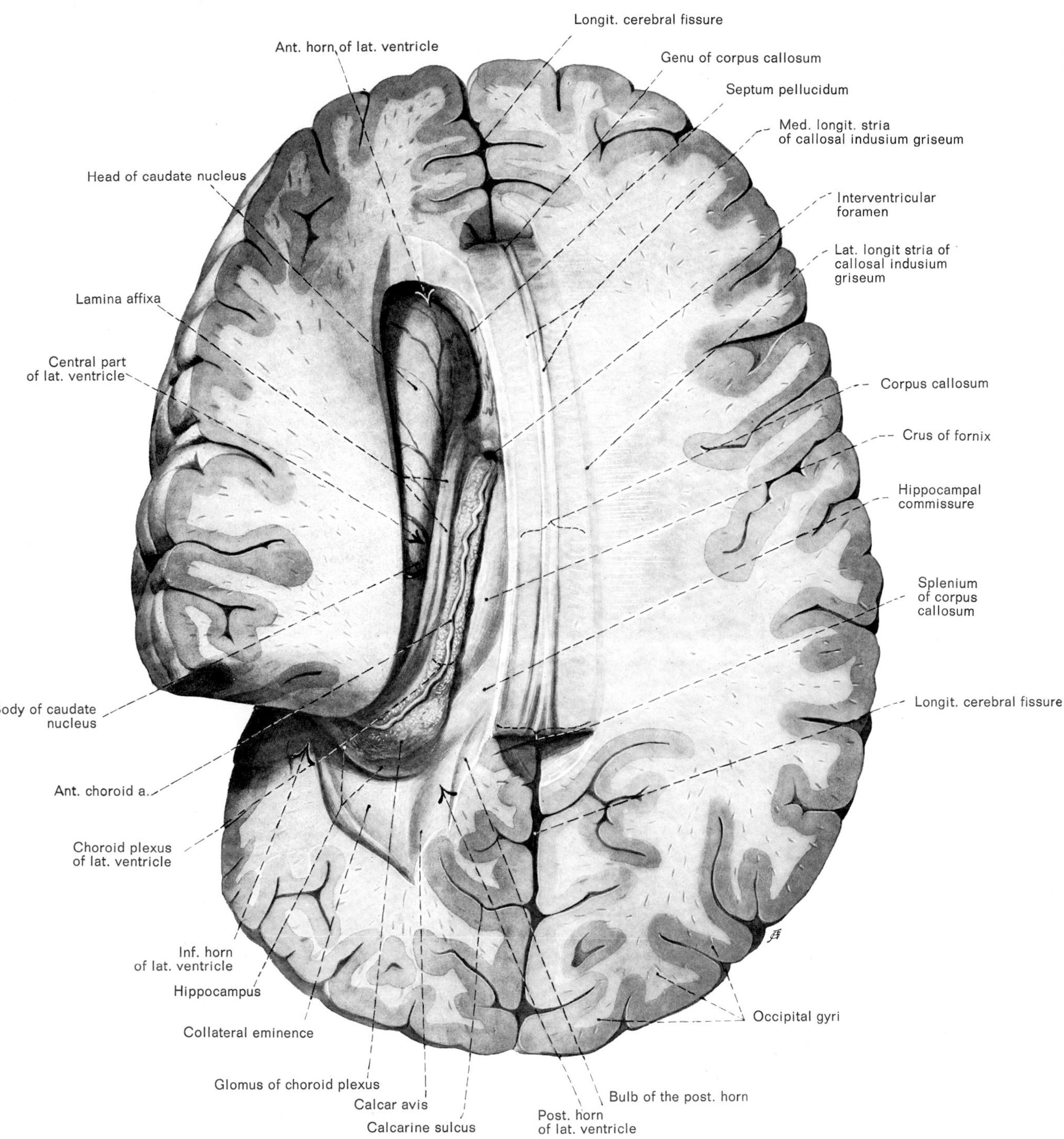
Longit. cerebral fissure
Ant. horn of lat. ventricle
Genu of corpus callosum
Septum pellucidum
Med. longit. stria
of callosal indusium griseum
Head of caudate nucleus
Interventricular
foramen
Lat. longit stria of
callosal indusium
griseum
Lamina affixa
Central part
of lat. ventricle
Corpus callosum
Crus of fornix
Hippocampal
commissure
Splenium
of corpus
callosum
Body of caudate
nucleus
Longit. cerebral fissure
Ant. choroid a.
Choroid plexus
of lat. ventricle
Inf. horn
of lat. ventricle
Hippocampus
Collateral eminence
Occipital gyri
Glomus of choroid plexus
Calcar avis
Calcarine sulcus
Bulb of the post. horn
Post. horn
of lat. ventricle

Fig. 20. Horizontal section through both hemispheres. The corpus callosum and the left lateral ventricle are seen from above and left. Preparation similar to the one in Fig. 19, but the roof of the left lateral ventricle has also been removed.

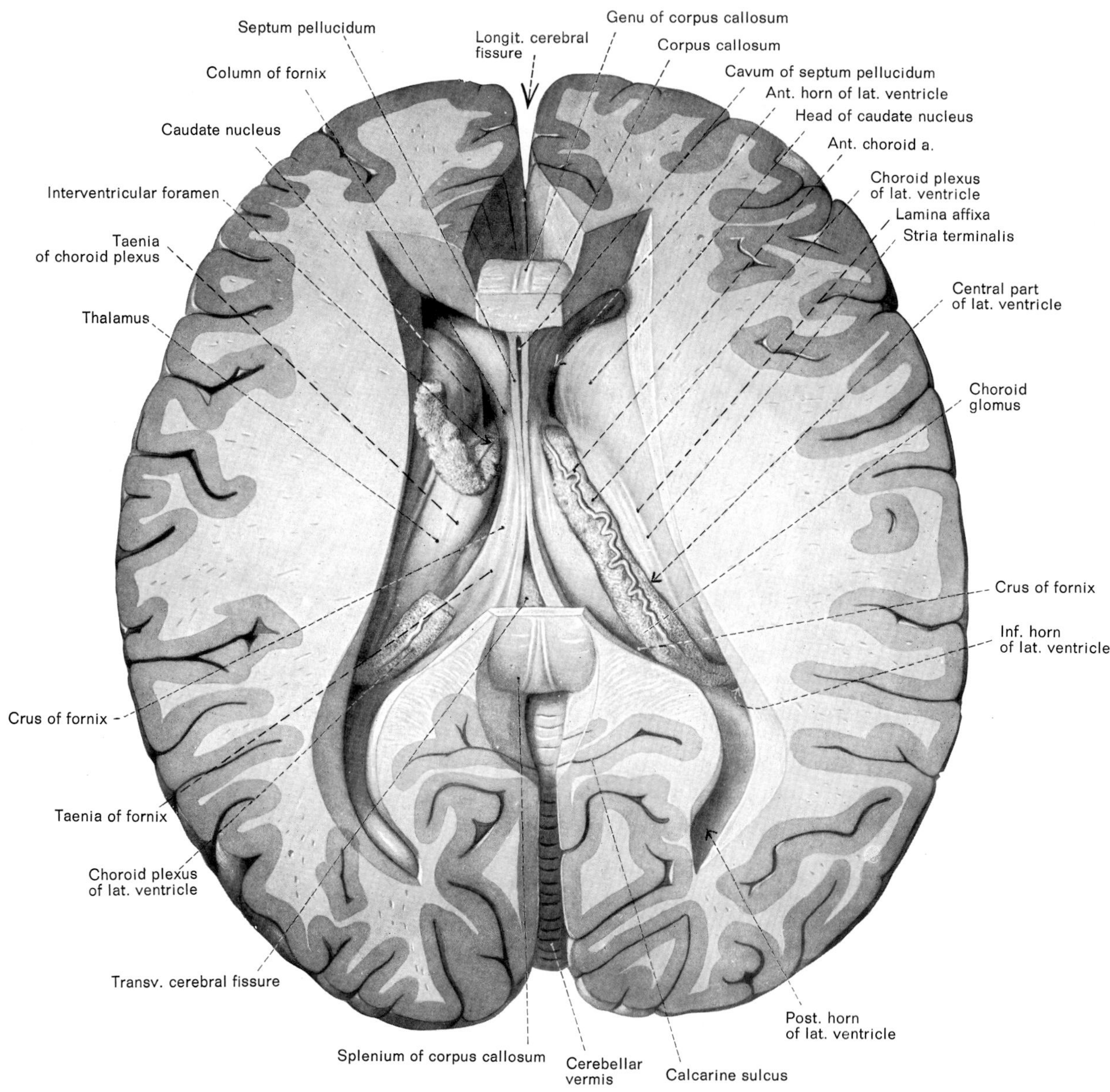

Septum pellucidum
Longit. cerebral fissure
Genu of corpus callosum
Corpus callosum
Column of fornix
Cavum of septum pellucidum
Ant. horn of lat. ventricle
Head of caudate nucleus
Caudate nucleus
Ant. choroid a.
Interventricular foramen
Choroid plexus of lat. ventricle
Lamina affixa
Stria terminalis
Taenia of choroid plexus
Central part of lat. ventricle
Thalamus
Choroid glomus
Crus of fornix
Inf. horn of lat. ventricle
Crus of fornix
Taenia of fornix
Choroid plexus of lat. ventricle
Transv. cerebral fissure
Post. horn of lat. ventricle
Splenium of corpus callosum
Cerebellar vermis
Calcarine sulcus

Fig. 21. Horizontal section through both hemispheres. The lateral ventricles are opened and seen from above. Fornix and septum pellucidum are visible following partial removal of the corpus callosum. On the left side the choroid plexus has been sectioned and reflected.

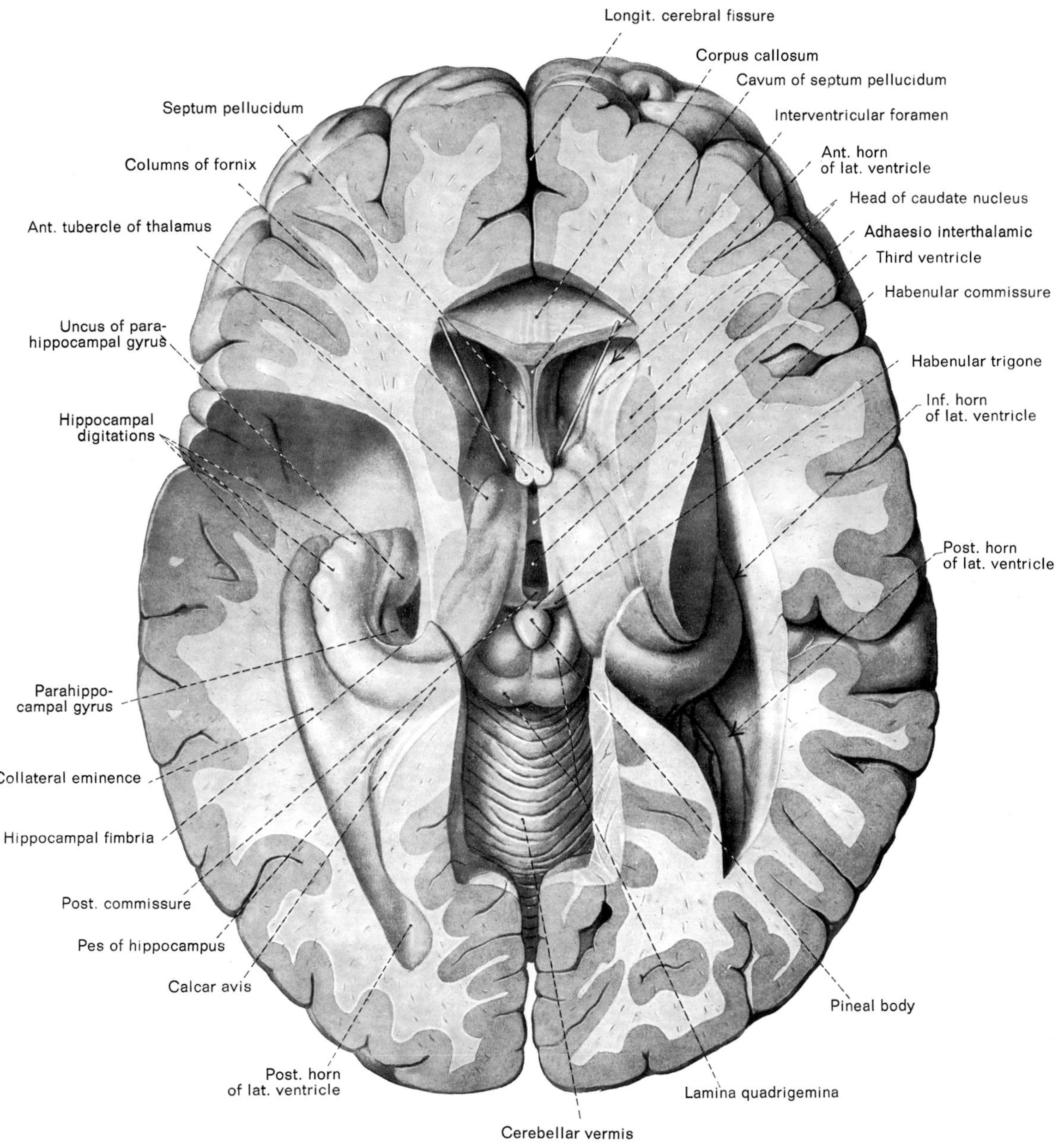
Longit. cerebral fissure
Corpus callosum
Cavum of septum pellucidum
Septum pellucidum
Interventricular foramen
Columns of fornix
Ant. horn
of lat. ventricle
Head of caudate nucleus
Ant. tubercle of thalamus
Adhaesio interthalamic
Third ventricle
Habenular commissure
Uncus of para-
hippocampal gyrus
Habenular trigone
Inf. horn
of lat. ventricle
Hippocampal
digitations
Post. horn
of lat. ventricle
Parahippo-
campal gyrus
Collateral eminence
Hippocampal fimbria
Post. commissure
Pes of hippocampus
Calcar avis
Pineal body
Post. horn
of lat. ventricle
Lamina quadrigemina
Cerebellar vermis

Fig. 22. Horizontal section through both hemispheres. Lateral ventricles and third ventricle are seen from above. The body and splenium of the corpus callosum as well as the columns of the fornix and the choroid tela of the third ventricle have been removed. The left temporal lobe has been excavated down to the inferior horn of the lateral ventricle. Probe in the interventricular foramen.

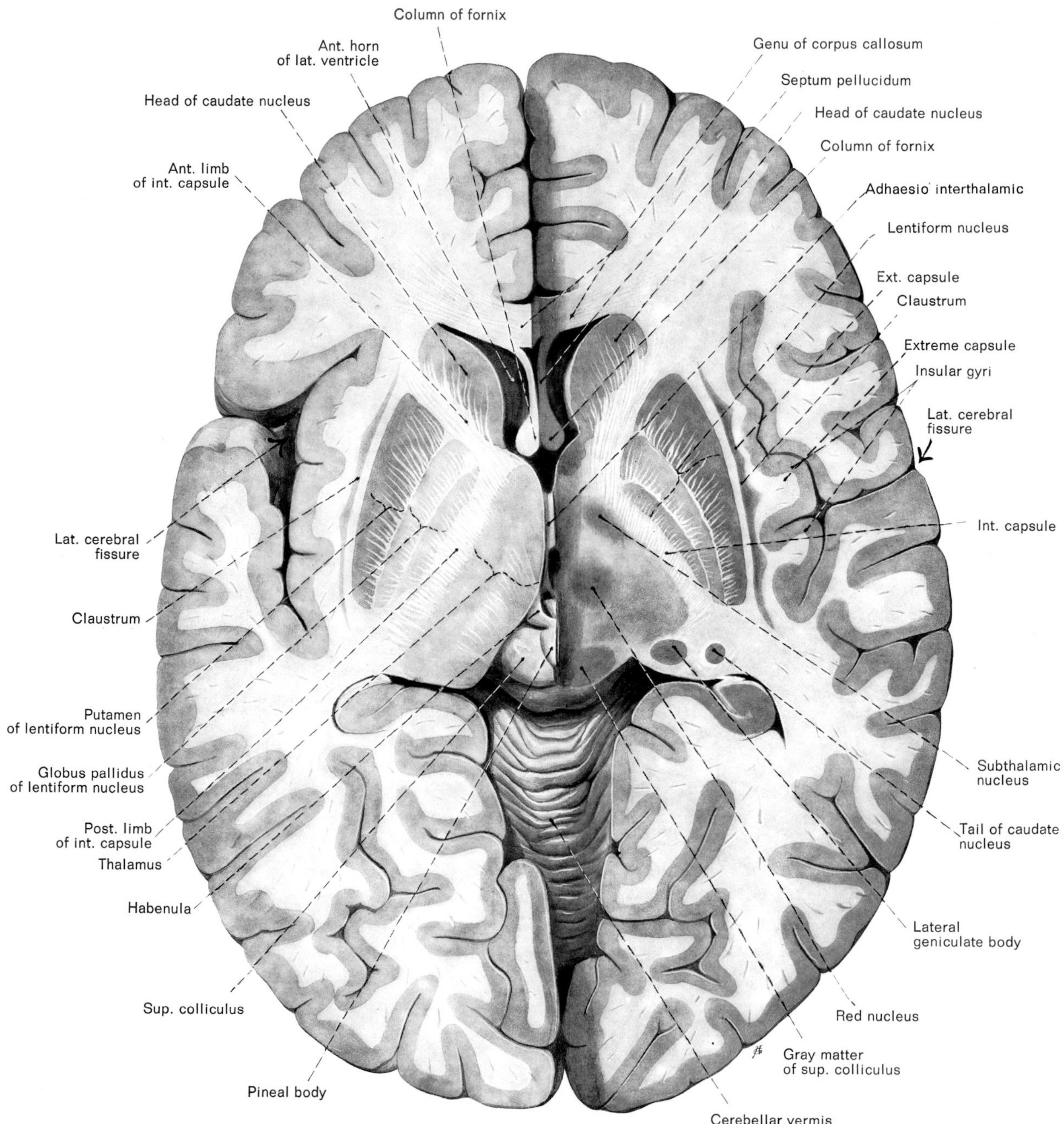
Column of fornix
Ant. horn
of lat. ventricle
Head of caudate nucleus
Ant. limb
of int. capsule
Genu of corpus callosum
Septum pellucidum
Head of caudate nucleus
Column of fornix
Adhaesio interthalamic
Lentiform nucleus
Ext. capsule
Claustrum
Extreme capsule
Insular gyri
Lat. cerebral
fissure
Int. capsule
Lat. cerebral
fissure
Claustrum
Putamen
of lentiform nucleus
Globus pallidus
of lentiform nucleus
Post. limb
of int. capsule
Thalamus
Habenula
Sup. colliculus
Pineal body
Subthalamic
nucleus
Tail of caudate
nucleus
Lateral
geniculate body
Red nucleus
Gray matter
of sup. colliculus
Cerebellar vermis

Fig. 23. Horizontal section through the telencephalon to show the basal ganglia (thalamus, lentiform nucleus, caudate nucleus) and the internal capsule. The plane of section on the left side is at the level of the thalamus; on the right side it is about 1 cm lower going through the lamina quadrigemina and the subthalamic nucleus.

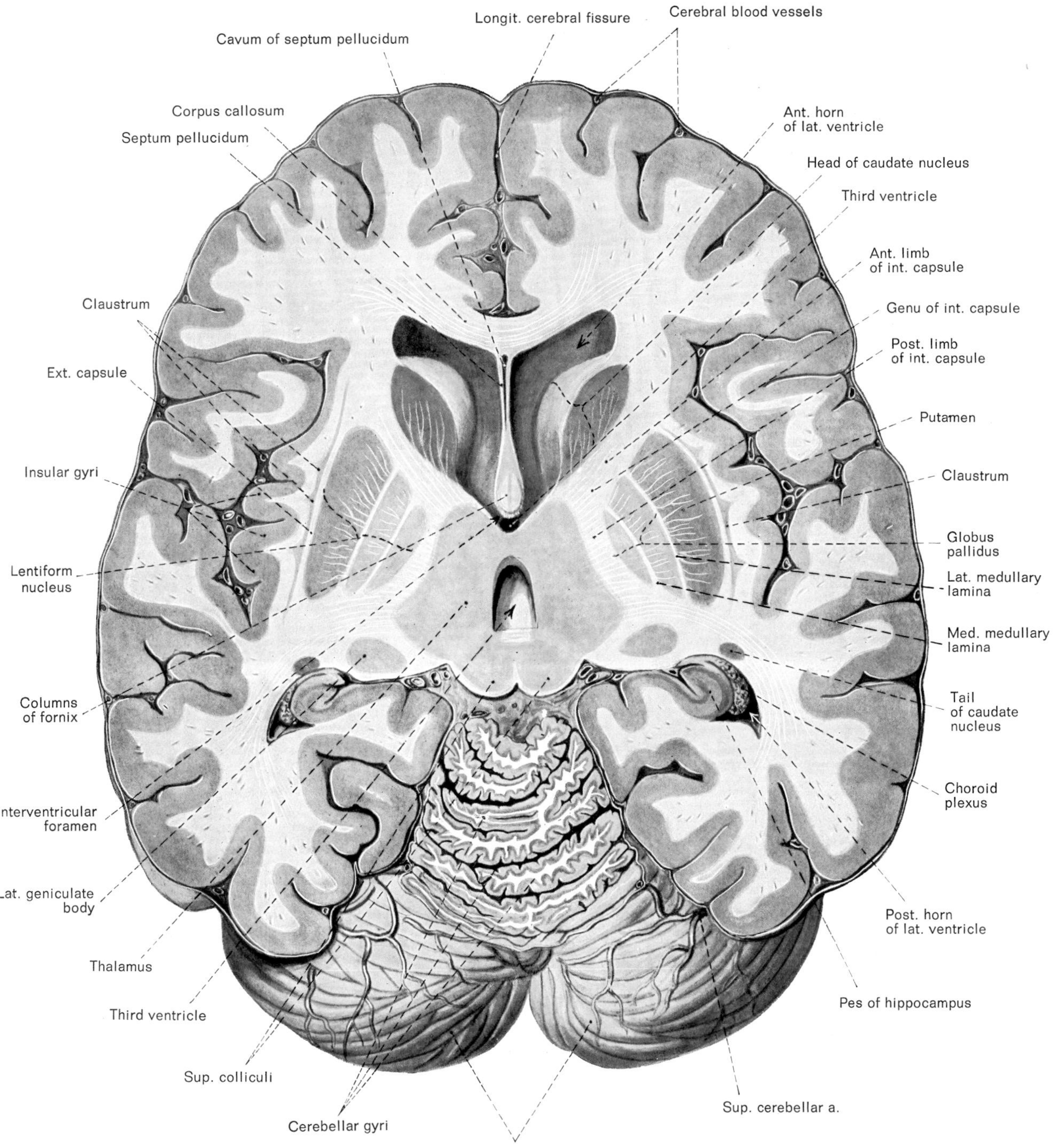
Cavum of septum pellucidum
Longit. cerebral fissure
Cerebral blood vessels
Corpus callosum
Septum pellucidum
Ant. horn of lat. ventricle
Head of caudate nucleus
Third ventricle
Ant. limb of int. capsule
Claustrum
Genu of int. capsule
Post. limb of int. capsule
Ext. capsule
Putamen
Insular gyri
Claustrum
Globus pallidus
Lentiform nucleus
Lat. medullary lamina
Med. medullary lamina
Columns of fornix
Tail of caudate nucleus
Choroid plexus
Interventricular foramen
Lat. geniculate body
Post. horn of lat. ventricle
Thalamus
Pes of hippocampus
Third ventricle
Sup. colliculi
Sup. cerebellar a.
Cerebellar gyri
Cerebellum

Fig. 24. Horizontal section through the telencephalon at the level of the basal ganglia and the internal capsule. The plane of section is somewhat lower than that in Fig. 23. Pia and arachnoid membrane are preserved.

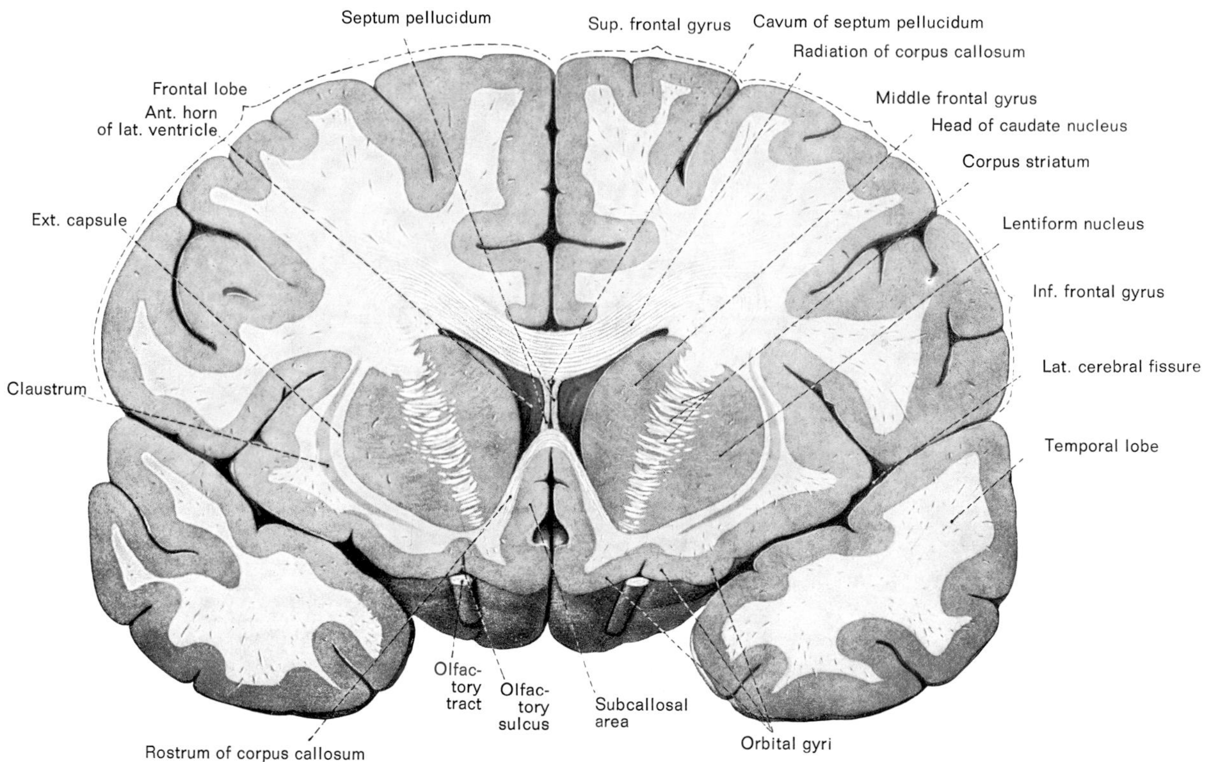
Septum pellucidum
Sup. frontal gyrus
Cavum of septum pellucidum
Radiation of corpus callosum
Frontal lobe
Ant. horn
of lat. ventricle
Middle frontal gyrus
Head of caudate nucleus
Corpus striatum
Ext. capsule
Lentiform nucleus
Inf. frontal gyrus
Lat. cerebral fissure
Claustrum
Temporal lobe
Olfac-
tory
tract
Olfac-
tory
sulcus
Subcallosal
area
Orbital gyri
Rostrum of corpus callosum

Fig. 25. Frontal section through the telencephalon, rostral to the thalamus at the plane of the anterior portion of the septum pellucidum.

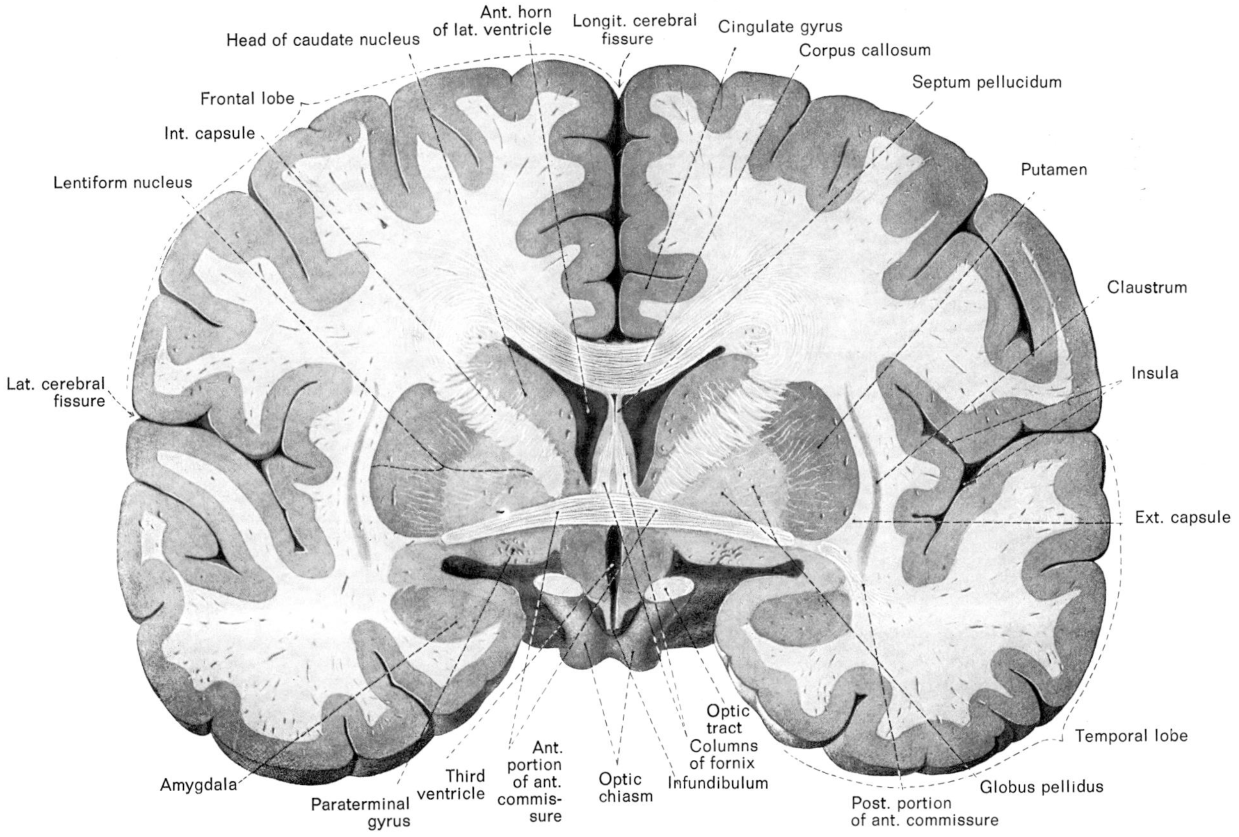
Head of caudate nucleus
Ant. horn of lat. ventricle
Longit. cerebral fissure
Cingulate gyrus
Corpus callosum
Septum pellucidum
Frontal lobe
Int. capsule
Lentiform nucleus
Putamen
Claustrum
Insula
Lat. cerebral fissure
Ext. capsule
Temporal lobe
Optic tract
Columns of fornix
Infundibulum
Globus pellidus
Post. portion of ant. commissure
Amygdala
Paraterminal gyrus
Third ventricle
Ant. portion of ant. commis-sure
Optic chiasm

Fig. 26. Frontal section through the telencephalon at the plane of the anterior commissure. Figg. 25 and 26 show the anterior plane of the section.

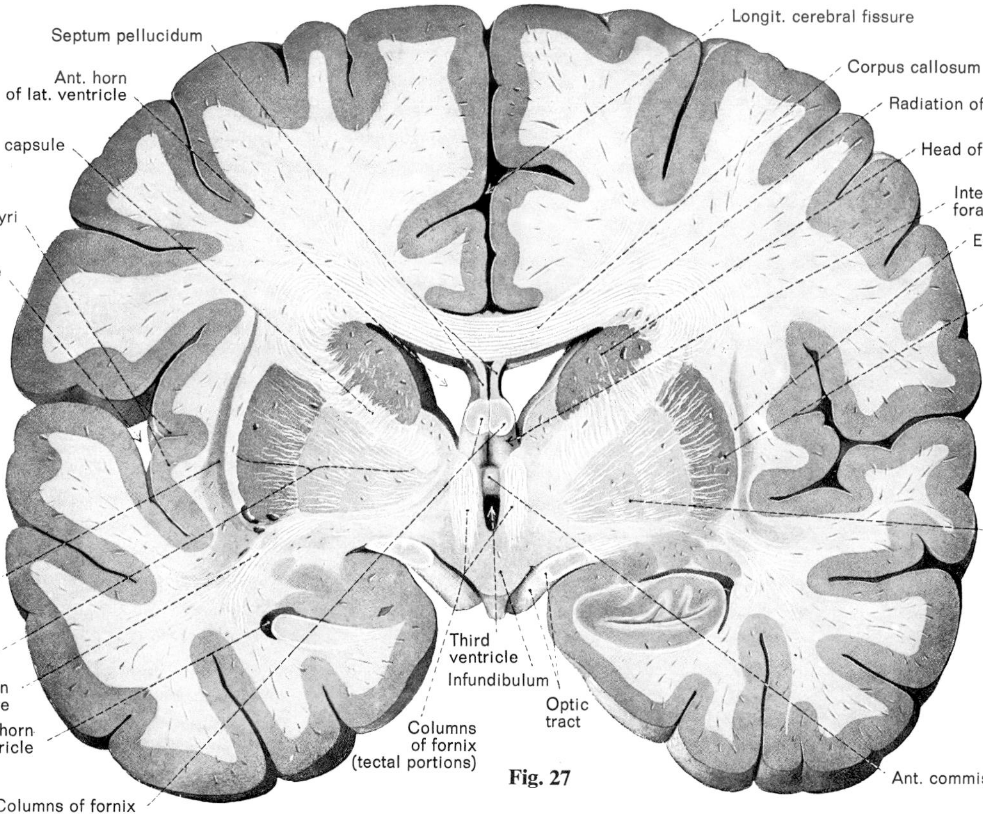

Longit. cerebral fissure
Septum pellucidum
Corpus callosum
Ant. horn of lat. ventricle
Radiation of corpus callosum
Int. capsule
Head of caudate nucleus
Interventricular foramen
Insular gyri
Ext. capsule
Lat. cerebral fissure
Putamen
Globus pallidus
Claustrum
Lentiform nucleus
Third ventricle
Infundibulum
Post. portion of ant. commissure
Optic tract
Inf. horn of. lat. ventricle
Columns of fornix (tectal portions)
Ant. commissure
Columns of fornix

Fig. 27

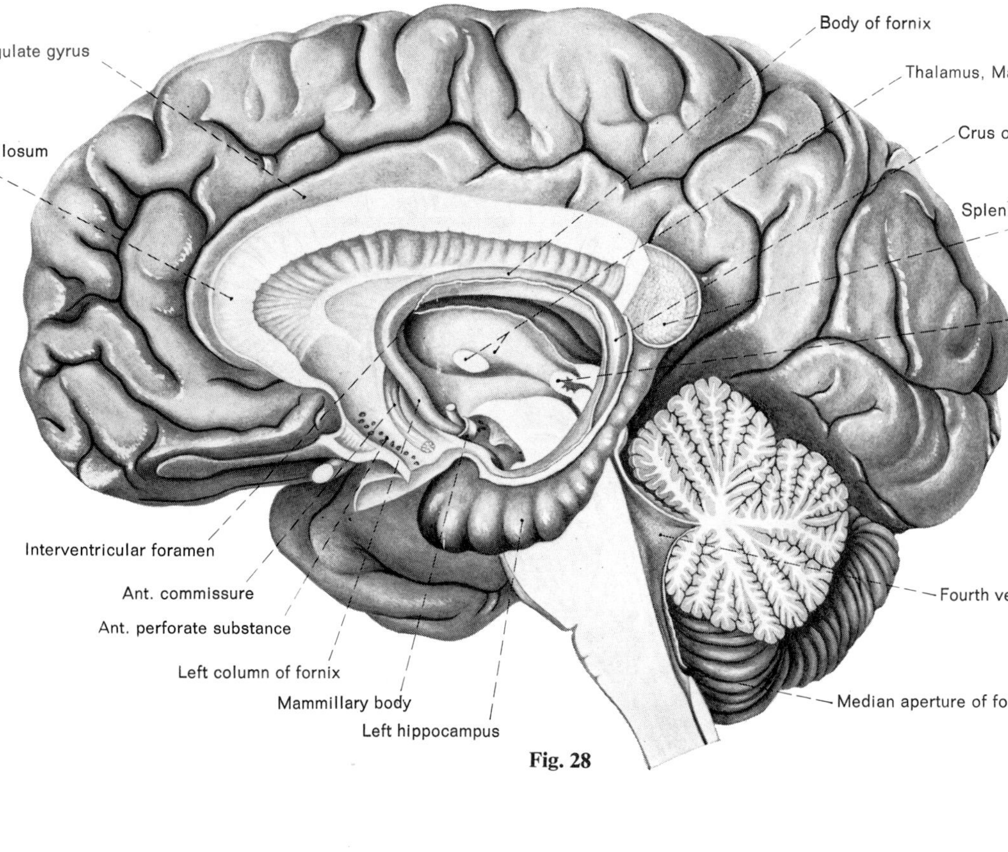

Body of fornix
Cingulate gyrus
Thalamus, Massa intermedia
Genu of corpus callosum
Crus of fornix
Splenium of corpus callosum
Post. commissure
Interventricular foramen
Fourth ventricle
Ant. commissure
Ant. perforate substance
Left column of fornix
Median aperture of fourth ventricle
Mammillary body
Left hippocampus

Fig. 28

Fig. 27. Frontal section through the telencephalon immediately behind the anterior commissure and rostral to the interventricular foramen (of *Monro*).

Fig. 28. Lateral view of the fornix of the left half of the brain. Hippocampus, anterior commissure, olfactory bulb and tract of the left side are also shown. The corpus callosum has been sectioned in a left parasagittal plane, the brain stem in the sagittal plane (from *Pernkopf/Ferner:* Atlas der topographischen und angewandten Anatomie des Menschen. Vol. 1. Urban & Schwarzenberg, München–Berlin 1963).

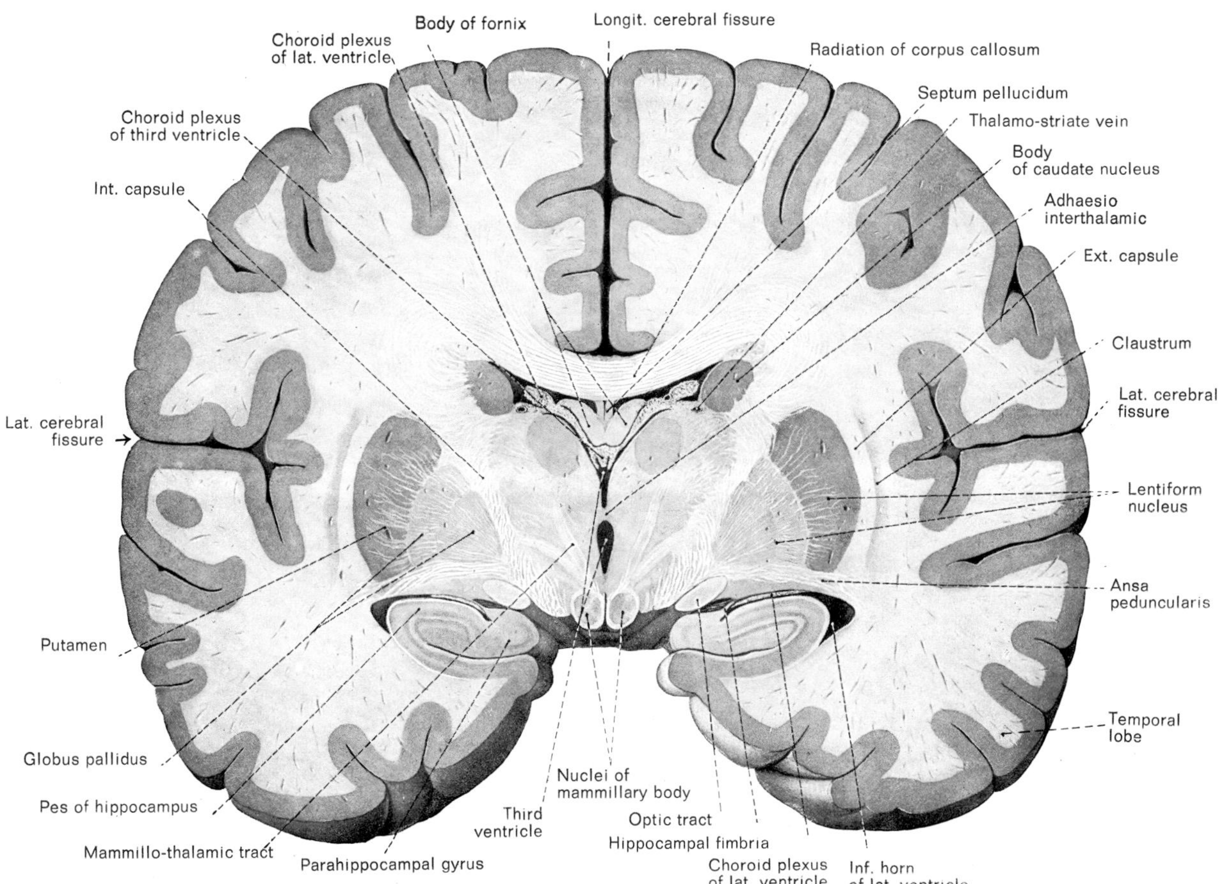
Body of fornix
Longit. cerebral fissure
Choroid plexus of lat. ventricle
Radiation of corpus callosum
Septum pellucidum
Choroid plexus of third ventricle
Thalamo-striate vein
Body of caudate nucleus
Int. capsule
Adhaesio interthalamic
Ext. capsule
Claustrum
Lat. cerebral fissure
Lat. cerebral fissure
Lentiform nucleus
Ansa peduncularis
Putamen
Temporal lobe
Globus pallidus
Nuclei of mammillary body
Pes of hippocampus
Third ventricle
Optic tract
Hippocampal fimbria
Mammillo-thalamic tract
Parahippocampal gyrus
Choroid plexus of lat. ventricle
Inf. horn of lat. ventricle

Fig. 29. Frontal section through the telencephalon at the plane of the mammillary bodies and the thalamus. Figg. 27 and 28 show the anterior plane of the section.

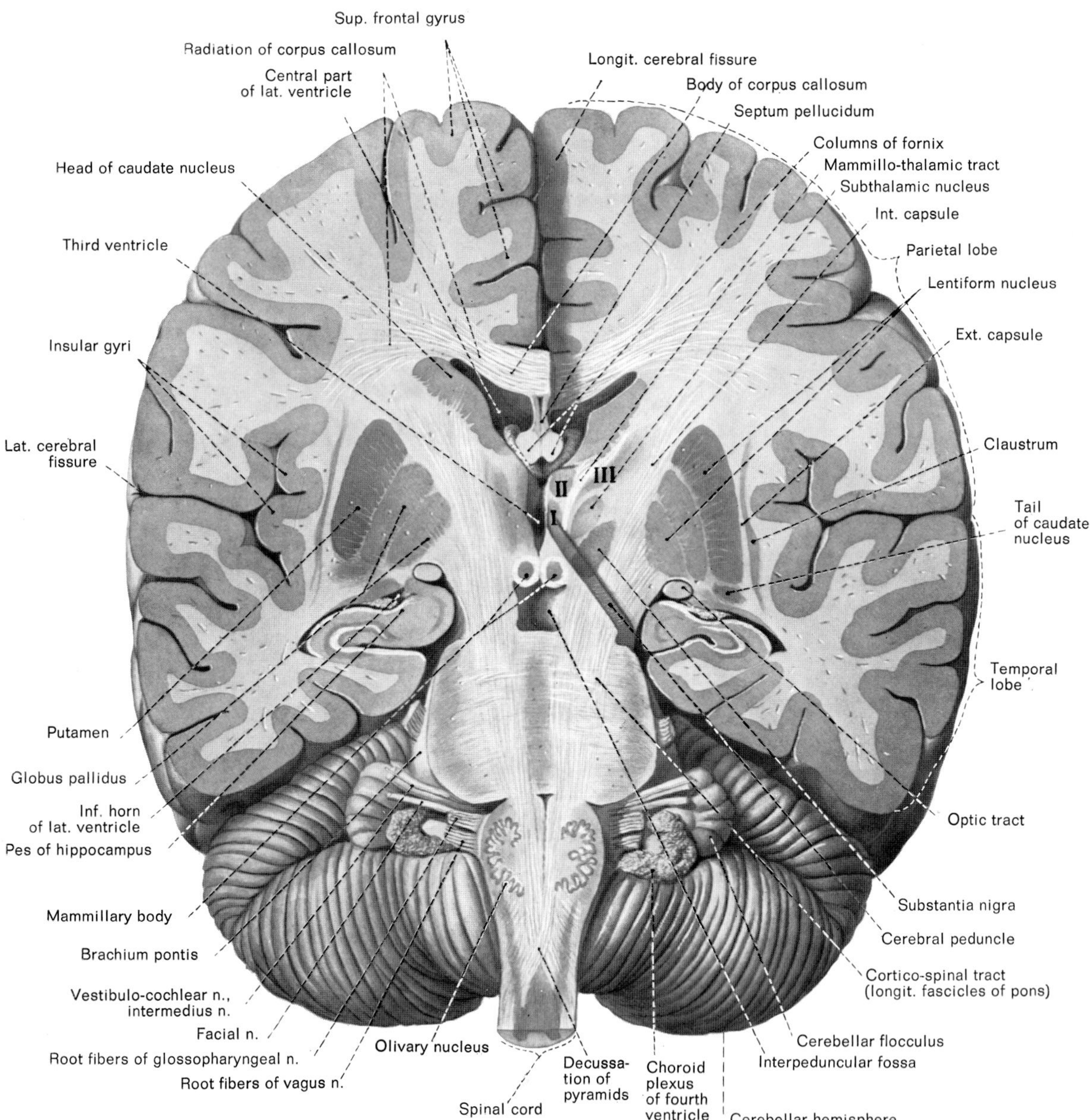
Sup. frontal gyrus
Radiation of corpus callosum
Central part of lat. ventricle
Longit. cerebral fissure
Body of corpus callosum
Septum pellucidum
Columns of fornix
Mammillo-thalamic tract
Subthalamic nucleus
Int. capsule
Parietal lobe
Lentiform nucleus
Ext. capsule
Head of caudate nucleus
Third ventricle
Insular gyri
Lat. cerebral fissure
II
III
I
Claustrum
Tail of caudate nucleus
Temporal lobe
Putamen
Globus pallidus
Inf. horn of lat. ventricle
Pes of hippocampus
Optic tract
Mammillary body
Brachium pontis
Vestibulo-cochlear n., intermedius n.
Facial n.
Root fibers of glossopharyngeal n.
Root fibers of vagus n.
Olivary nucleus
Spinal cord
Decussation of pyramids
Choroid plexus of fourth ventricle
Cerebellar hemisphere
Substantia nigra
Cerebral peduncle
Cortico-spinal tract (longit. fascicles of pons)
Cerebellar flocculus
Interpeduncular fossa

Fig. 30. Section through telencephalon and brain stem parallel to the cerebral peduncles. View of the posterior surface of the plane of sectioning. On the right side of the figure the section reaches back to about the middle of the cerebral peduncle (oblique section). I–III thalamic nuclei. I = medial nucleus, II = anterior nucleus, III = lateral nucleus.

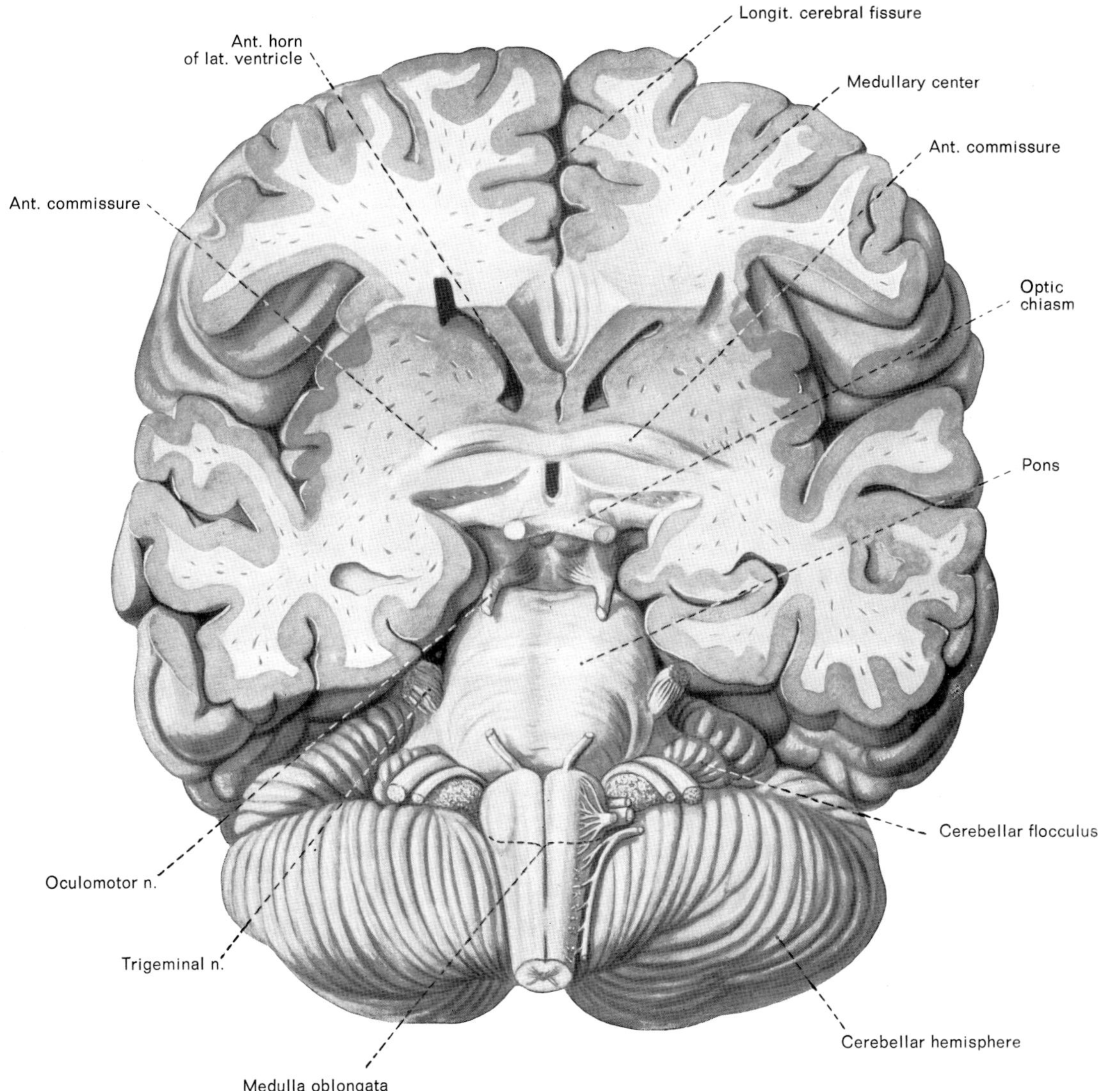
Longit. cerebral fissure
Ant. horn of lat. ventricle
Medullary center
Ant. commissure
Ant. commissure
Optic chiasm
Pons
Cerebellar flocculus
Oculomotor n.
Trigeminal n.
Cerebellar hemisphere
Medulla oblongata

Fig. 31. Anterior commissure exposed by a curved section from the base of the brain. The section shows only the middle portion of the commissure; its anterior and posterior radiations are not seen.

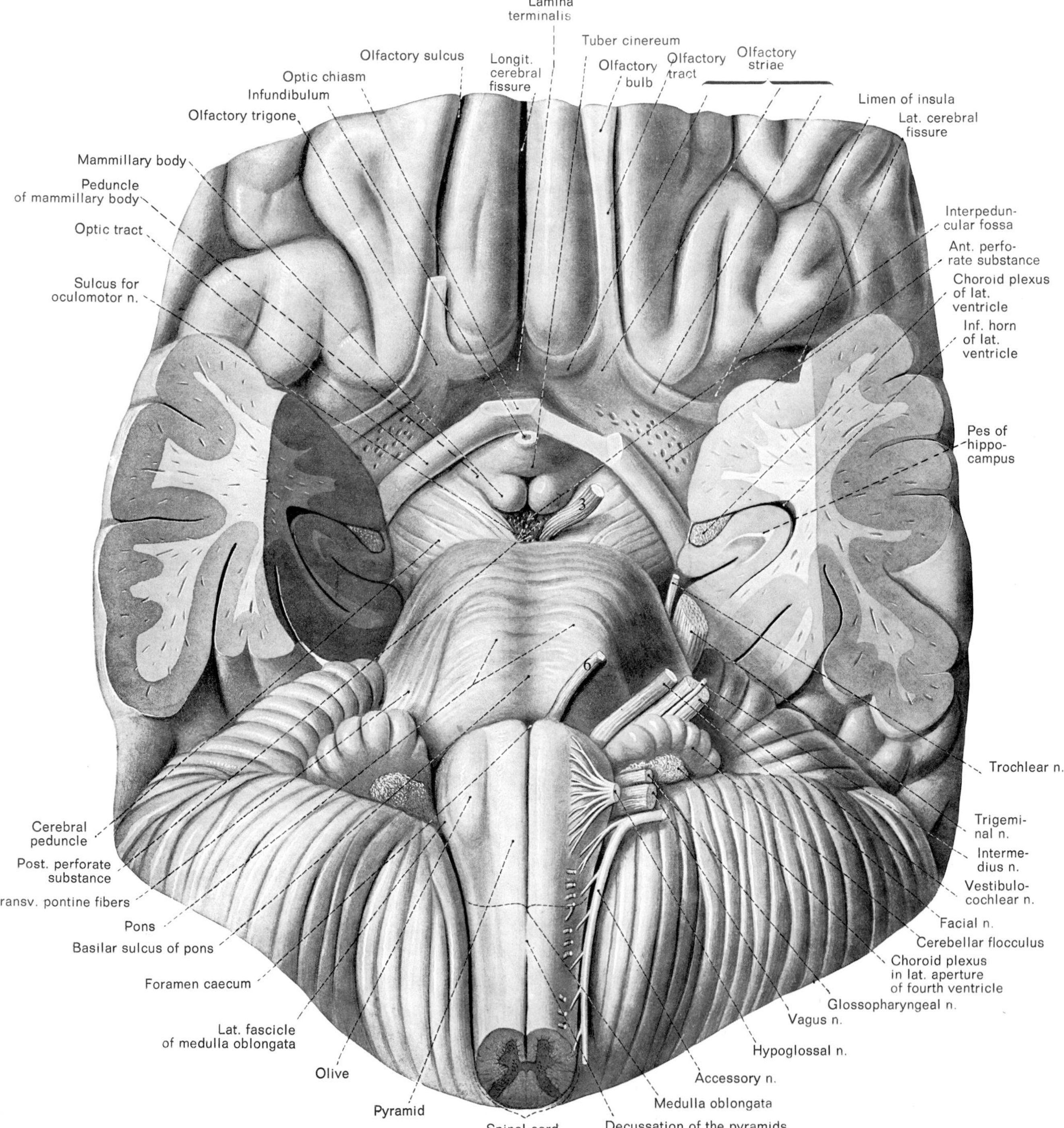

Lamina terminalis
Tuber cinereum
Olfactory sulcus
Longit. cerebral fissure
Olfactory bulb
Olfactory tract
Olfactory striae
Optic chiasm
Infundibulum
Olfactory trigone
Limen of insula
Lat. cerebral fissure
Mammillary body
Peduncle of mammillary body
Optic tract
Sulcus for oculomotor n.
Interpeduncular fossa
Ant. perforate substance
Choroid plexus of lat. ventricle
Inf. horn of lat. ventricle
Pes of hippocampus
3
6
Trochlear n.
Trigeminal n.
Intermedius n.
Vestibulocochlear n.
Facial n.
Cerebellar flocculus
Choroid plexus in lat. aperture of fourth ventricle
Glossopharyngeal n.
Vagus n.
Hypoglossal n.
Accessory n.
Medulla oblongata
Decussation of the pyramids
Spinal cord
Pyramid
Olive
Lat. fascicle of medulla oblongata
Foramen caecum
Basilar sulcus of pons
Pons
Transv. pontine fibers
Post. perforate substance
Cerebral peduncle

Fig. 32. Basal view of the brain stem with adjacent parts of the brain: diencephalon, midbrain, pons, medulla oblongata (bulbus). The temporal poles have been removed. The origins of the cranial nerves are preserved on the left side, on the right side they have been removed (3 = oculomotor nerve, 6 = abducent nerve). Somewhat enlarged over natural size.

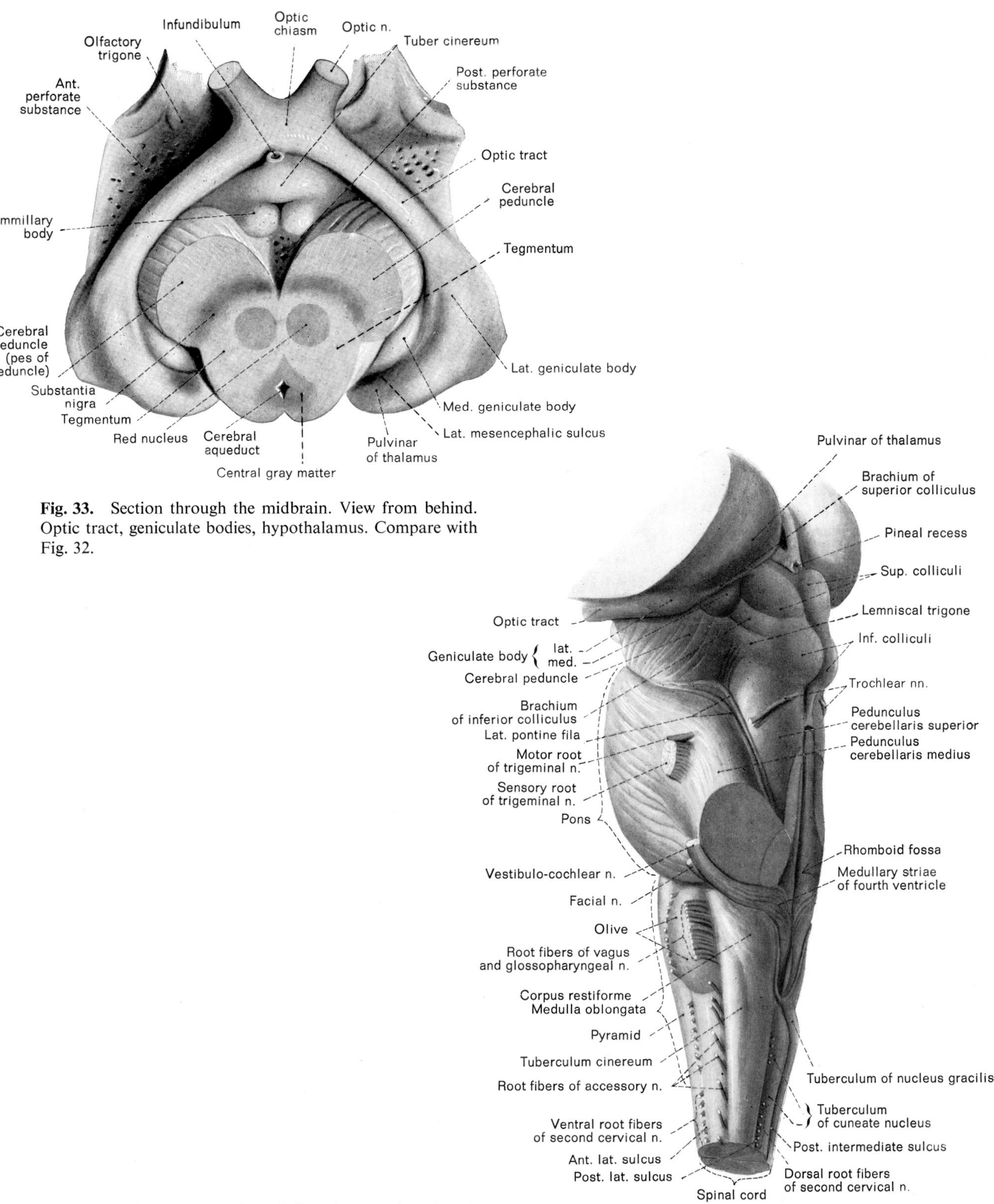
Infundibulum
Optic chiasm
Optic n.
Olfactory trigone
Tuber cinereum
Post. perforate substance
Ant. perforate substance
Optic tract
Cerebral peduncle
mmillary body
Tegmentum
Cerebral eduncle (pes of eduncle)
Lat. geniculate body
Substantia nigra
Tegmentum
Med. geniculate body
Red nucleus
Cerebral aqueduct
Pulvinar of thalamus
Lat. mesencephalic sulcus
Central gray matter
Pulvinar of thalamus
Brachium of superior colliculus
Pineal recess
Sup. colliculi
Optic tract
Lemniscal trigone
Geniculate body { lat. med.
Inf. colliculi
Cerebral peduncle
Trochlear nn.
Brachium of inferior colliculus
Pedunculus cerebellaris superior
Lat. pontine fila
Pedunculus cerebellaris medius
Motor root of trigeminal n.
Sensory root of trigeminal n.
Pons
Rhomboid fossa
Vestibulo-cochlear n.
Medullary striae of fourth ventricle
Facial n.
Olive
Root fibers of vagus and glossopharyngeal n.
Corpus restiforme
Medulla oblongata
Pyramid
Tuberculum cinereum
Tuberculum of nucleus gracilis
Root fibers of accessory n.
Tuberculum of cuneate nucleus
Ventral root fibers of second cervical n.
Post. intermediate sulcus
Ant. lat. sulcus
Post. lat. sulcus
Dorsal root fibers of second cervical n.
Spinal cord

Fig. 33. Section through the midbrain. View from behind. Optic tract, geniculate bodies, hypothalamus. Compare with Fig. 32.

Fig. 34. Brain stem seen from left and somewhat dorsal.

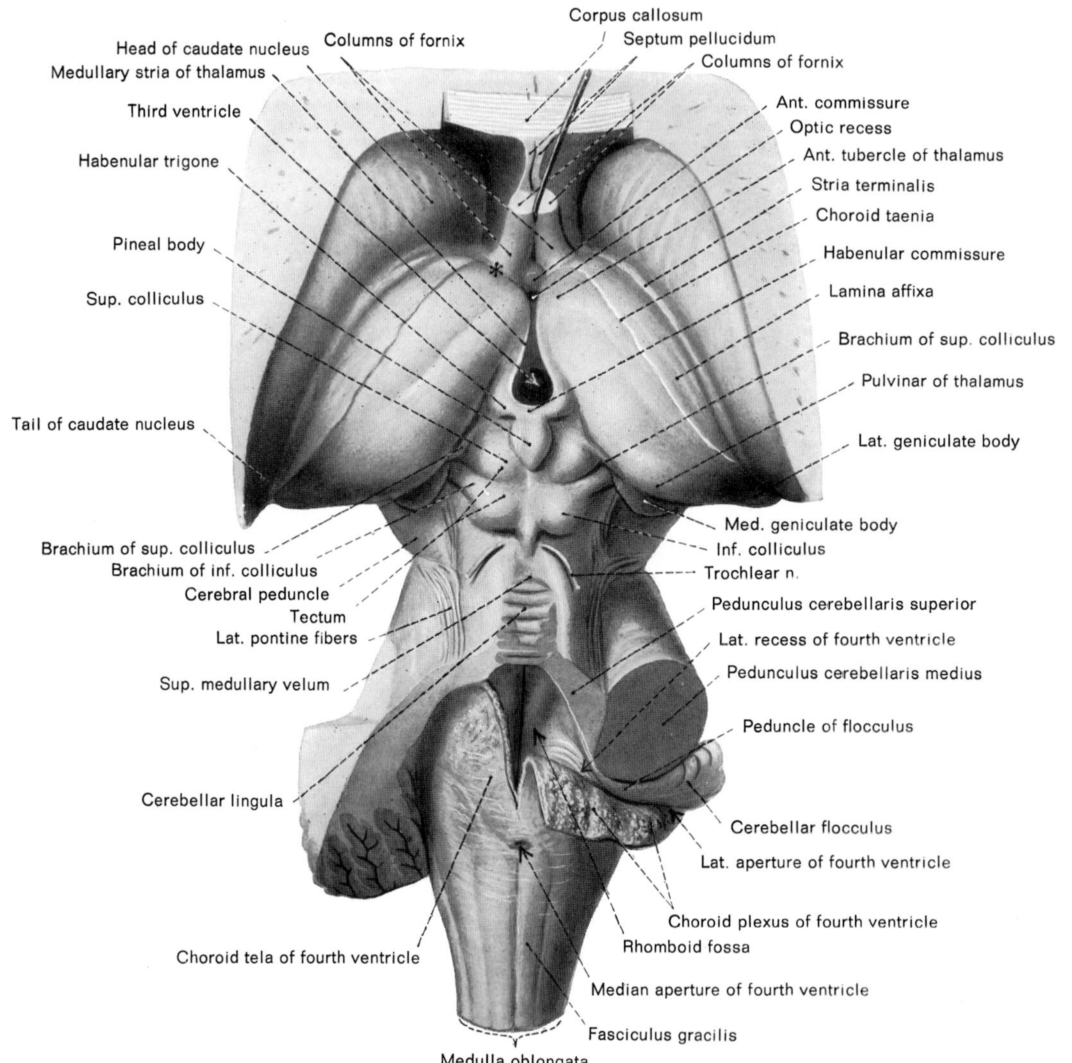
Corpus callosum
Head of caudate nucleus
Columns of fornix
Septum pellucidum
Medullary stria of thalamus
Columns of fornix
Third ventricle
Ant. commissure
Optic recess
Ant. tubercle of thalamus
Habenular trigone
Stria terminalis
Choroid taenia
Pineal body
Habenular commissure
Sup. colliculus
Lamina affixa
Brachium of sup. colliculus
Pulvinar of thalamus
Tail of caudate nucleus
Lat. geniculate body
Med. geniculate body
Brachium of sup. colliculus
Inf. colliculus
Brachium of inf. colliculus
Trochlear n.
Cerebral peduncle
Pedunculus cerebellaris superior
Tectum
Lat. pontine fibers
Lat. recess of fourth ventricle
Pedunculus cerebellaris medius
Sup. medullary velum
Peduncle of flocculus
Cerebellar lingula
Cerebellar flocculus
Lat. aperture of fourth ventricle
Choroid plexus of fourth ventricle
Rhomboid fossa
Choroid tela of fourth ventricle
Median aperture of fourth ventricle
Fasciculus gracilis
Medulla oblongata

Fig. 35. Brain stem seen from dorsal and above. The caudate nuclei, thalami and third ventricle have been made visible by removing the corpus callosum, the fornix and the choroid tela of the third ventricle. The cerebellum has been removed except the flocculus on the right side and a part of the hemisphere on the left side. The choroid tela of the fourth ventricle has been split in the midline and is reflected on the right side. * = interventricular foramen.

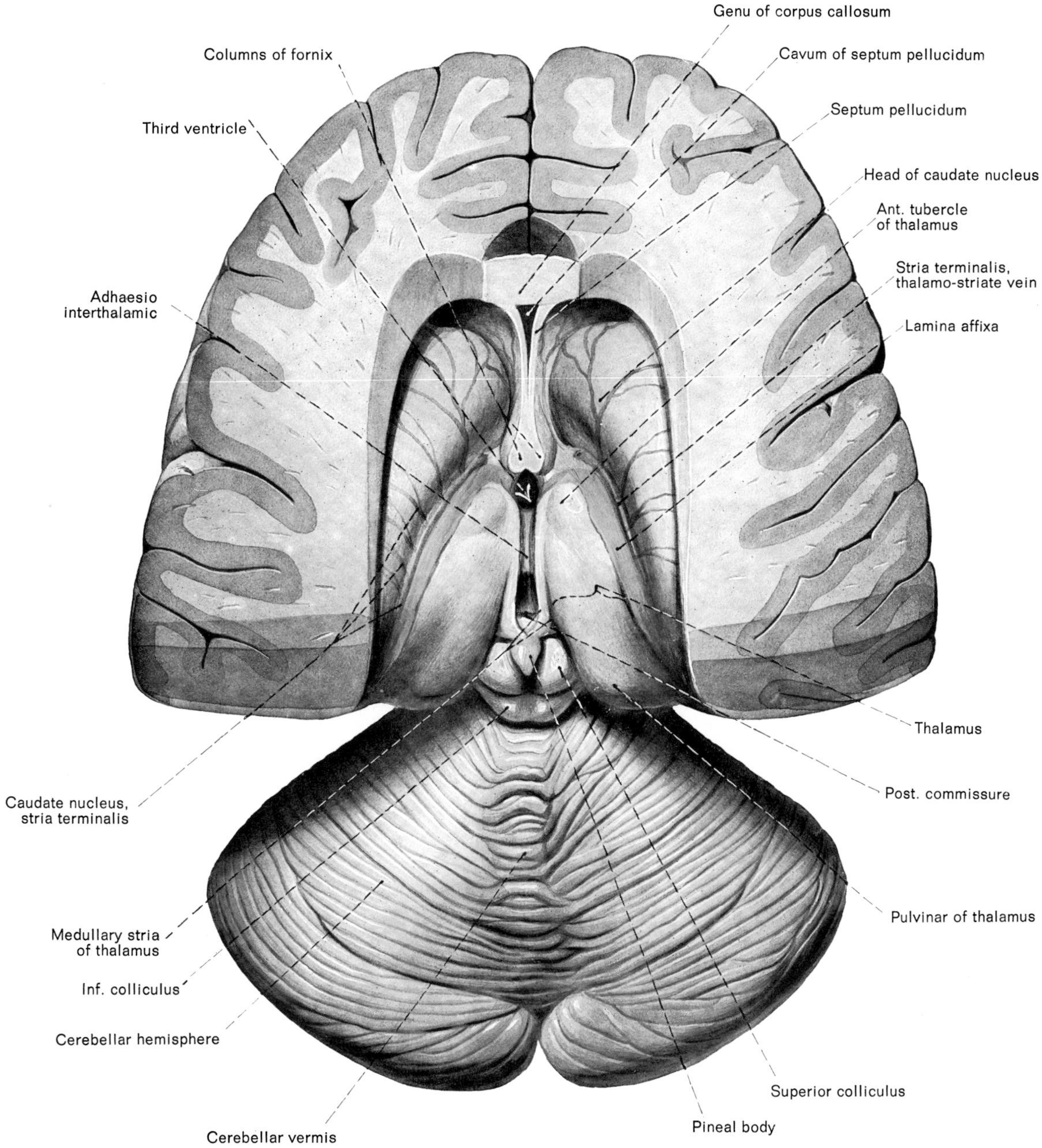
Genu of corpus callosum
Columns of fornix
Cavum of septum pellucidum
Third ventricle
Septum pellucidum
Head of caudate nucleus
Ant. tubercle of thalamus
Stria terminalis, thalamo-striate vein
Adhaesio interthalamic
Lamina affixa
Thalamus
Post. commissure
Caudate nucleus, stria terminalis
Pulvinar of thalamus
Medullary stria of thalamus
Inf. colliculus
Cerebellar hemisphere
Superior colliculus
Pineal body
Cerebellar vermis

Fig. 36. Basal ganglia of the forebrain (thalamus and caudate nucleus), third ventricle, lamina quadrigemina and cerebellum seen from above. The columns of the fornix, choroid plexus of the third ventricle as well as temporal and occipital lobes of the telencephalic hemispheres have been removed. The lamina affixa, that is the extremely thin portion of the telencephalic wall that abuts the thalamus, is shown in yellow.

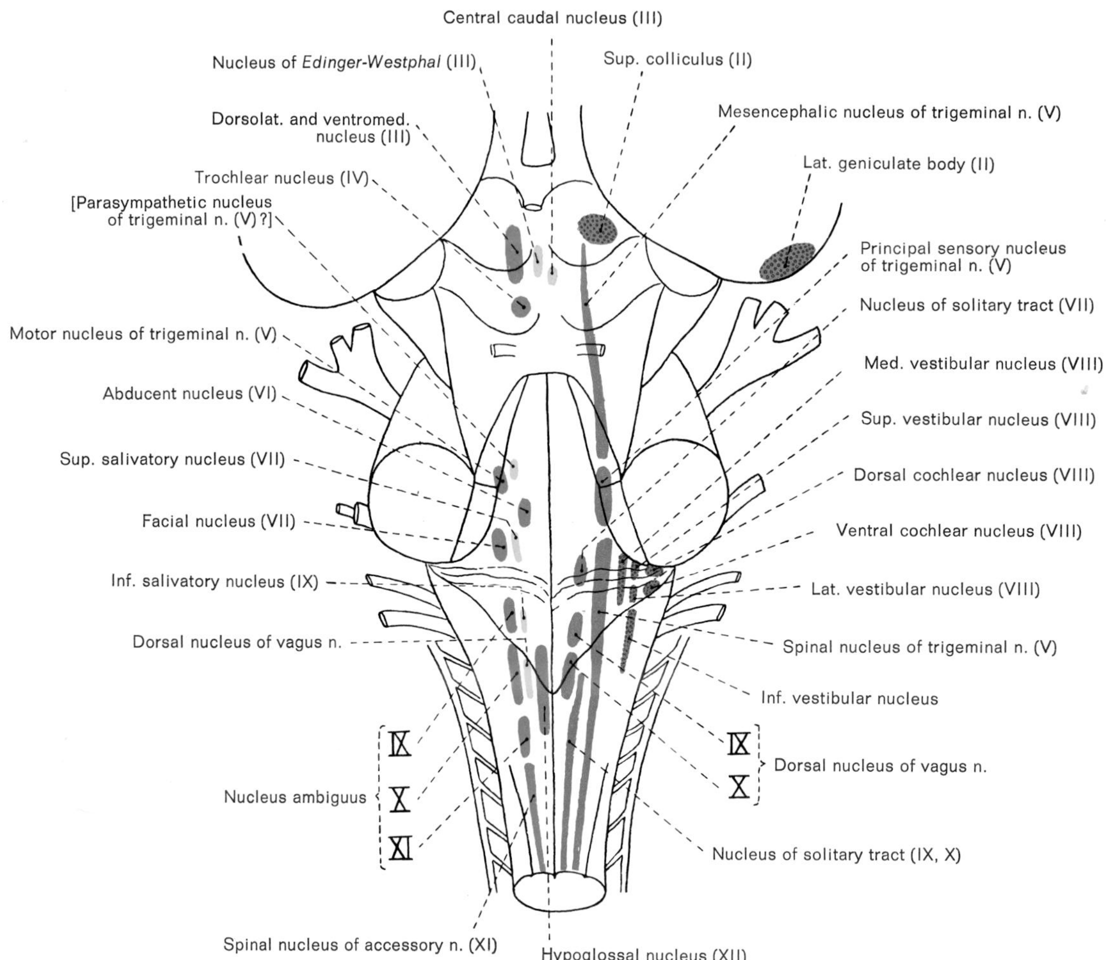
Central caudal nucleus (III)
Nucleus of Edinger-Westphal (III)
Sup. colliculus (II)
Dorsolat. and ventromed. nucleus (III)
Mesencephalic nucleus of trigeminal n. (V)
Lat. geniculate body (II)
Trochlear nucleus (IV)
[Parasympathetic nucleus of trigeminal n. (V)?]
Principal sensory nucleus of trigeminal n. (V)
Nucleus of solitary tract (VII)
Motor nucleus of trigeminal n. (V)
Med. vestibular nucleus (VIII)
Abducent nucleus (VI)
Sup. vestibular nucleus (VIII)
Sup. salivatory nucleus (VII)
Dorsal cochlear nucleus (VIII)
Facial nucleus (VII)
Ventral cochlear nucleus (VIII)
Inf. salivatory nucleus (IX)
Lat. vestibular nucleus (VIII)
Dorsal nucleus of vagus n.
Spinal nucleus of trigeminal n. (V)
Inf. vestibular nucleus
IX
X
XI
Nucleus ambiguus
IX
X
Dorsal nucleus of vagus n.
Nucleus of solitary tract (IX, X)
Spinal nucleus of accessory n. (XI)
Hypoglossal nucleus (XII)

Fig. 37. The nuclei of cranial nerves and of primary visual centers (schematically represented). Sensory terminal nuclei blue, motor nuclei red, parasympathetic nuclei yellow, terminal nuclei for vision, hearing and equilibrium stippled blue. The motor and parasympathetic nuclei are depicted on the left, the sensory nuclei on the right side.

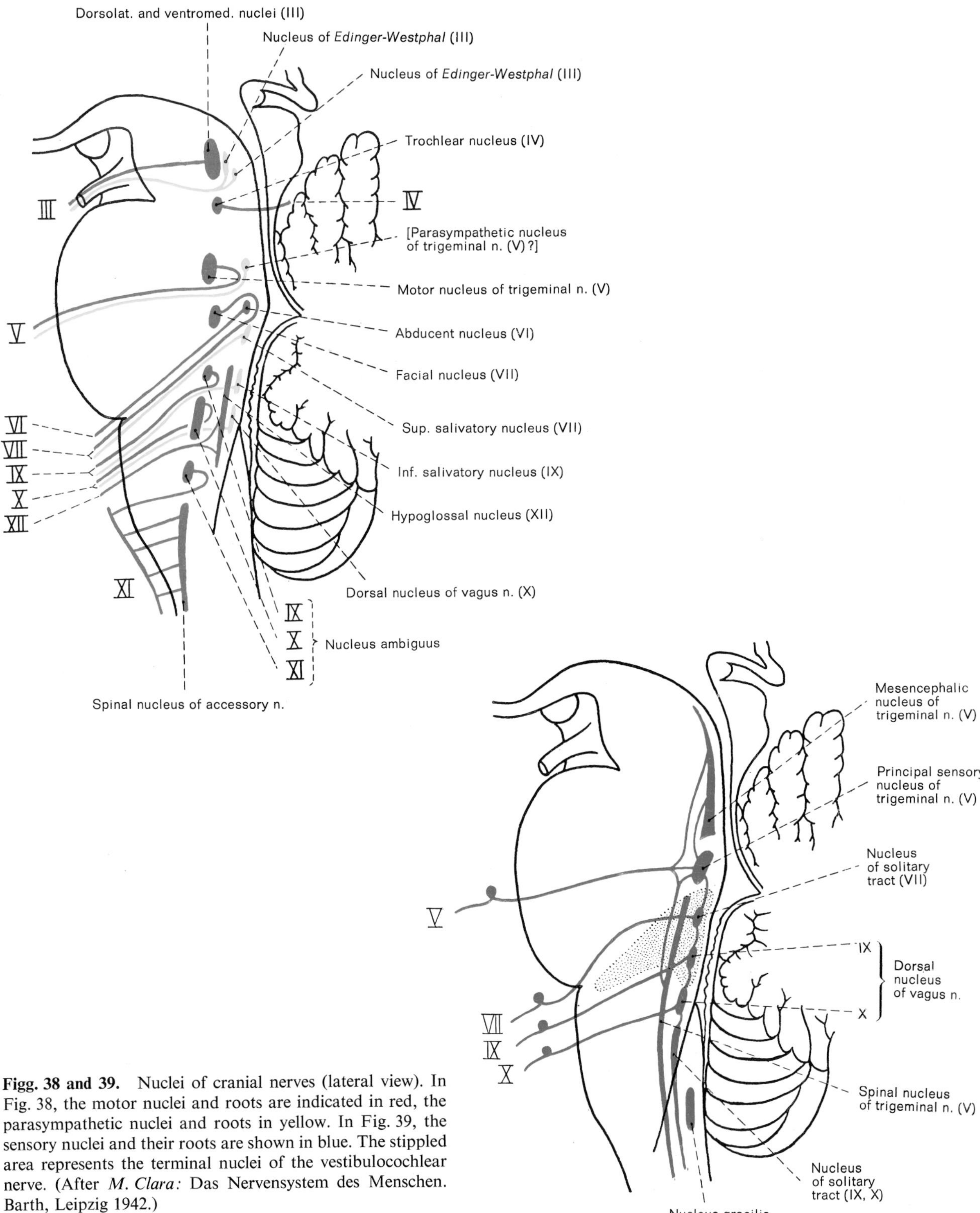
Dorsolat. and ventromed. nuclei (III)
Nucleus of Edinger-Westphal (III)
Nucleus of Edinger-Westphal (III)
Trochlear nucleus (IV)
III
IV
[Parasympathetic nucleus of trigeminal n. (V)?]
Motor nucleus of trigeminal n. (V)
V
Abducent nucleus (VI)
Facial nucleus (VII)
Sup. salivatory nucleus (VII)
VI
VII
IX
X
XII
Inf. salivatory nucleus (IX)
Hypoglossal nucleus (XII)
XI
Dorsal nucleus of vagus n. (X)
IX
X
XI
Nucleus ambiguus
Spinal nucleus of accessory n.
Mesencephalic nucleus of trigeminal n. (V)
Principal sensory nucleus of trigeminal n. (V)
Nucleus of solitary tract (VII)
V
IX
X
Dorsal nucleus of vagus n.
VII
IX
X
Spinal nucleus of trigeminal n. (V)
Nucleus of solitary tract (IX, X)
Nucleus gracilis

Figg. 38 and 39. Nuclei of cranial nerves (lateral view). In Fig. 38, the motor nuclei and roots are indicated in red, the parasympathetic nuclei and roots in yellow. In Fig. 39, the sensory nuclei and their roots are shown in blue. The stippled area represents the terminal nuclei of the vestibulocochlear nerve. (After *M. Clara:* Das Nervensystem des Menschen. Barth, Leipzig 1942.)

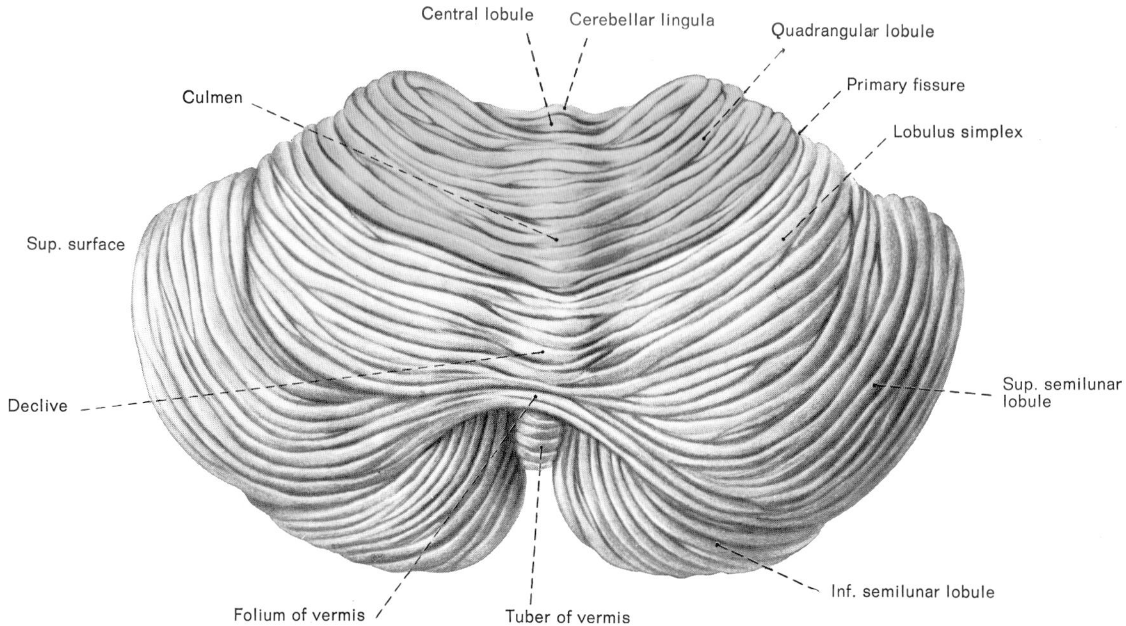
Central lobule
Cerebellar lingula
Quadrangular lobule
Culmen
Primary fissure
Lobulus simplex
Sup. surface
Declive
Sup. semilunar lobule
Inf. semilunar lobule
Folium of vermis
Tuber of vermis

Fig. 40. Cerebellum viewed from above and behind. Portions of the paleocerebellum are shown in yellow.

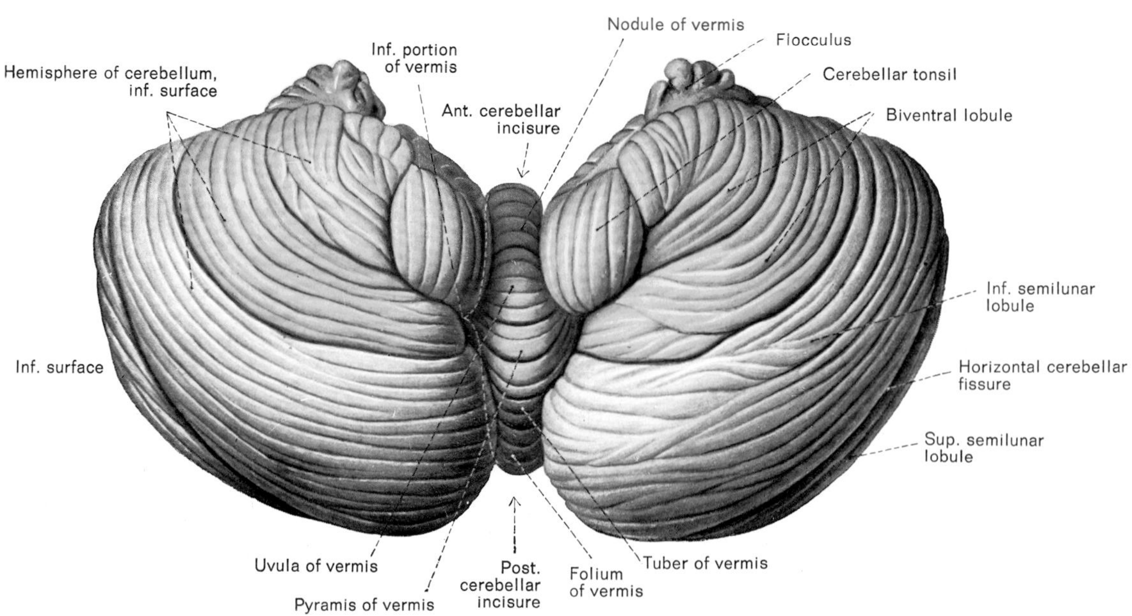
Nodule of vermis
Flocculus
Inf. portion of vermis
Hemisphere of cerebellum, inf. surface
Cerebellar tonsil
Ant. cerebellar incisure
Biventral lobule
Inf. semilunar lobule
Inf. surface
Horizontal cerebellar fissure
Sup. semilunar lobule
Uvula of vermis
Post. cerebellar incisure
Folium of vermis
Tuber of vermis
Pyramis of vermis

Fig. 41. Cerebellum seen from below. Portions of the paleocerebellum are shown in yellow.

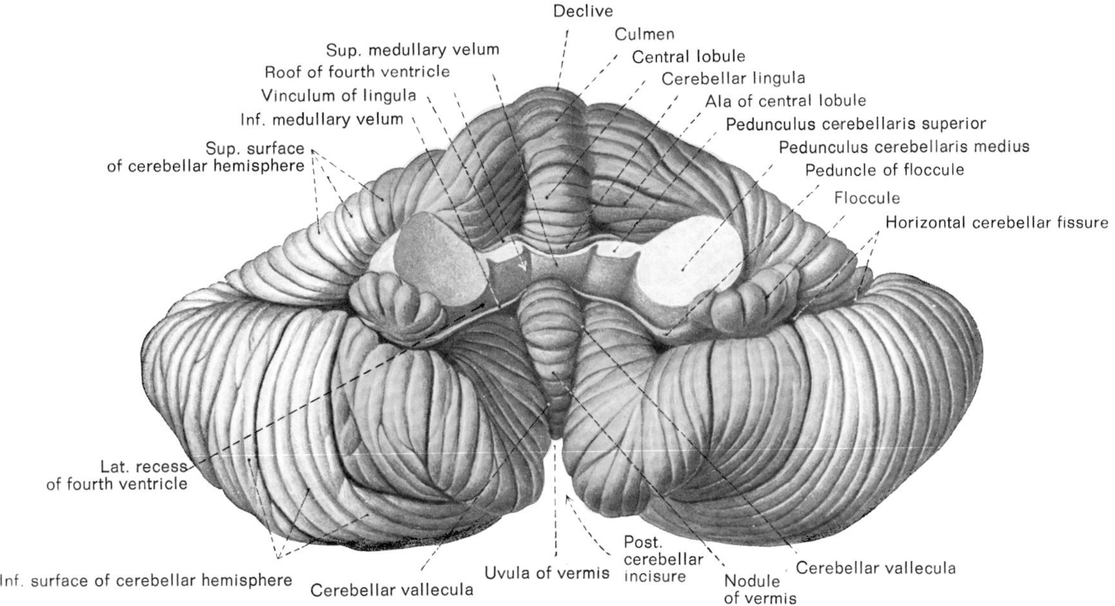
Declive
Culmen
Sup. medullary velum
Central lobule
Roof of fourth ventricle
Cerebellar lingula
Vinculum of lingula
Ala of central lobule
Inf. medullary velum
Pedunculus cerebellaris superior
Sup. surface of cerebellar hemisphere
Pedunculus cerebellaris medius
Peduncle of floccule
Floccule
Horizontal cerebellar fissure
Lat. recess of fourth ventricle
Post. cerebellar incisure
Cerebellar vallecula
Inf. surface of cerebellar hemisphere
Cerebellar vallecula
Uvula of vermis
Nodule of vermis

Fig. 42. Anterior view of cerebellum. Cerebral peduncles cut transversely.

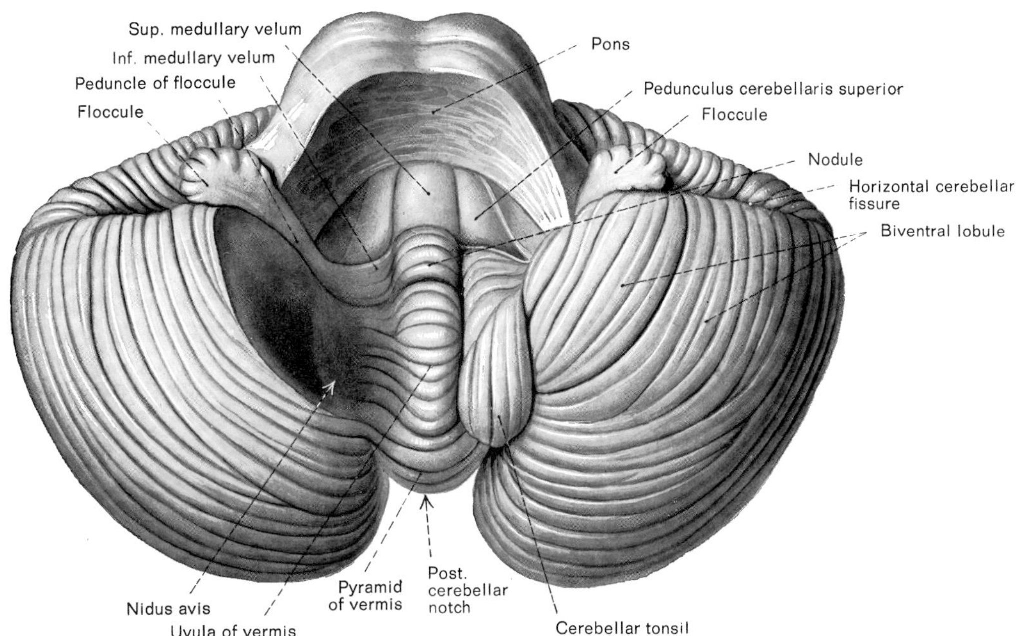
Sup. medullary velum
Inf. medullary velum
Pons
Peduncle of floccule
Pedunculus cerebellaris superior
Floccule
Floccule
Nodule
Horizontal cerebellar fissure
Biventral lobule
Post. cerebellar notch
Pyramid of vermis
Nidus avis
Uvula of vermis
Cerebellar tonsil

Fig. 43. Inferior cerebellar surface after removal of the right tonsil and a part of the biventral lobule. Pons sectioned transversely. View from below onto the roof of the fourth ventricle.

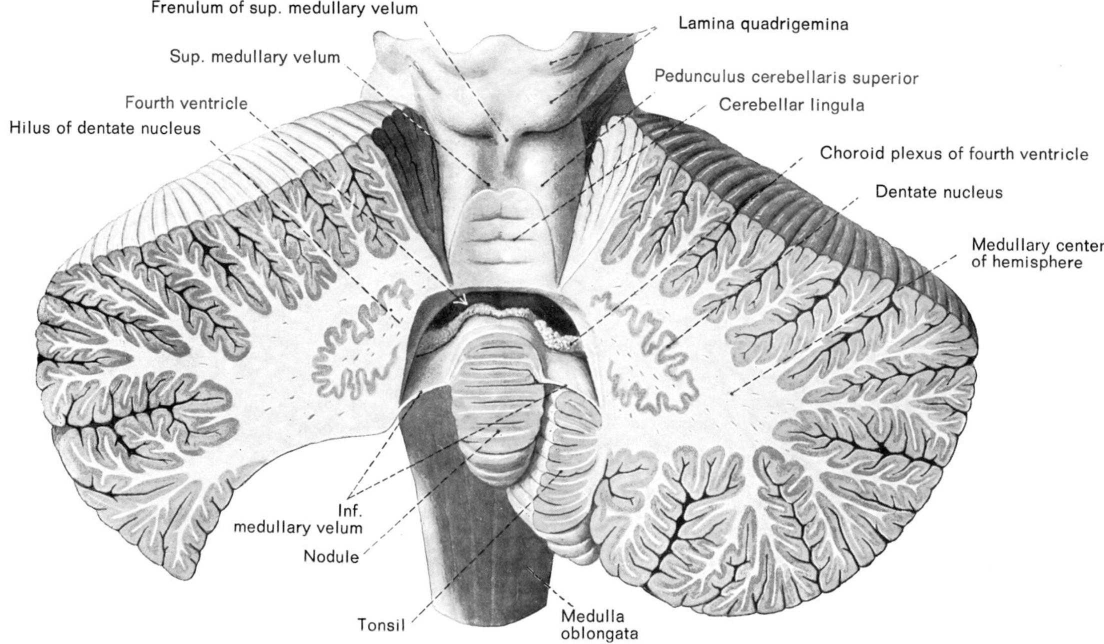
Frenulum of sup. medullary velum
Lamina quadrigemina
Sup. medullary velum
Pedunculus cerebellaris superior
Fourth ventricle
Cerebellar lingula
Hilus of dentate nucleus
Choroid plexus of fourth ventricle
Dentate nucleus
Medullary center of hemisphere
Inf. medullary velum
Nodule
Tonsil
Medulla oblongata

Fig. 44. Transverse section through the cerebellum exposing the fourth ventricle.

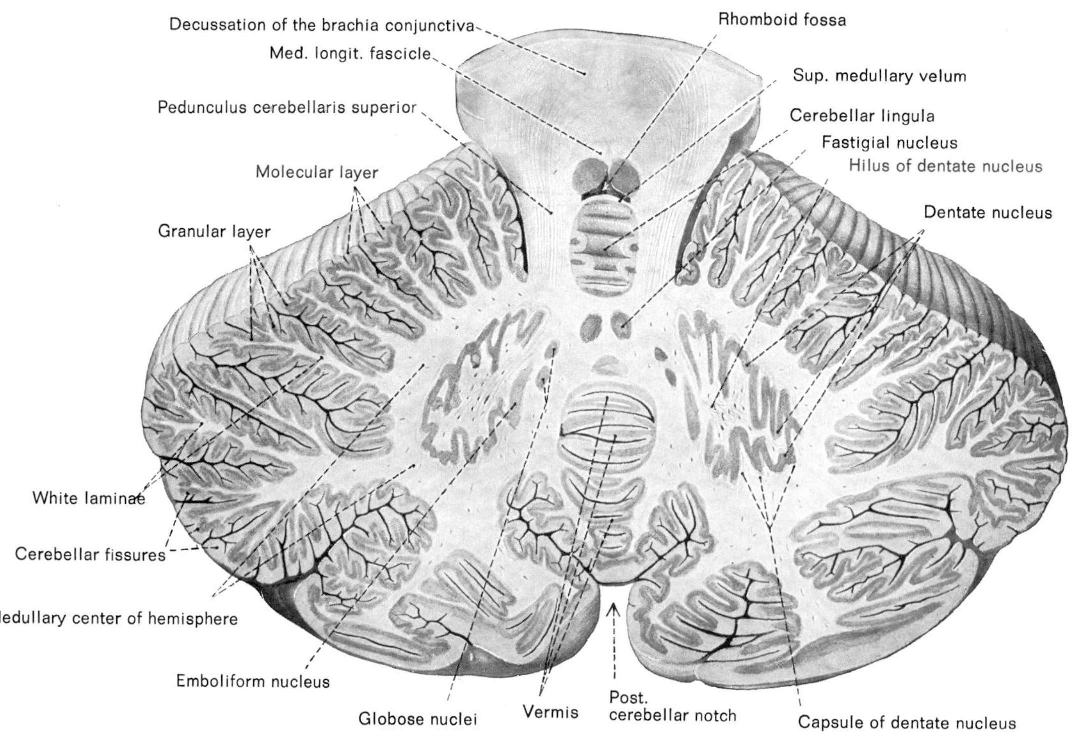
Decussation of the brachia conjunctiva
Rhomboid fossa
Med. longit. fascicle
Sup. medullary velum
Pedunculus cerebellaris superior
Cerebellar lingula
Fastigial nucleus
Hilus of dentate nucleus
Molecular layer
Dentate nucleus
Granular layer
White laminae
Cerebellar fissures
Medullary center of hemisphere
Emboliform nucleus
Globose nuclei
Vermis
Post. cerebellar notch
Capsule of dentate nucleus

Fig. 45. Section through the cerebellum parallel to the brachium conjunctivum. Cerebellar nuclei.

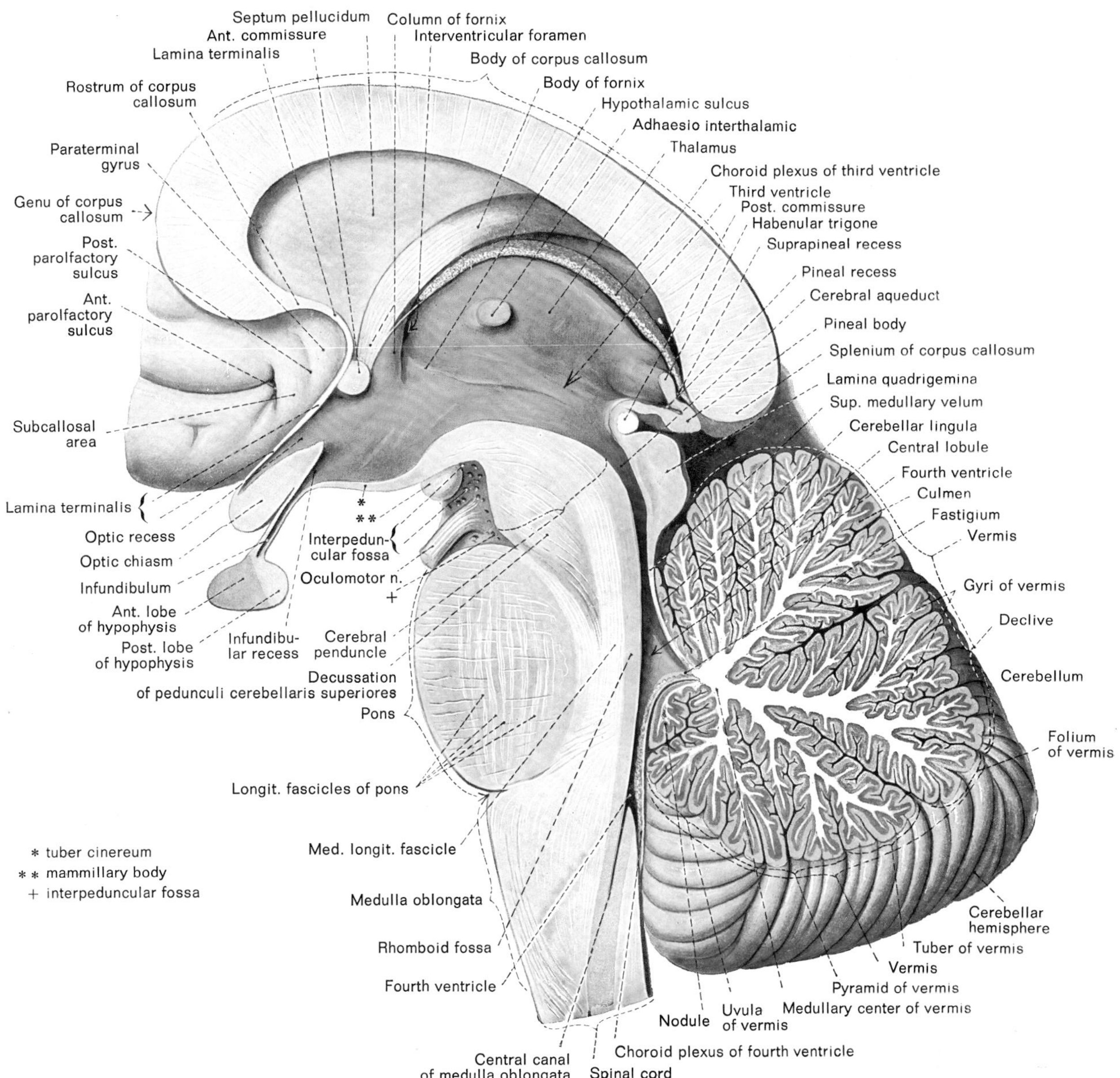
Septum pellucidum
Column of fornix
Ant. commissure
Interventricular foramen
Lamina terminalis
Body of corpus callosum
Rostrum of corpus callosum
Body of fornix
Hypothalamic sulcus
Adhaesio interthalamic
Paraterminal gyrus
Thalamus
Choroid plexus of third ventricle
Genu of corpus callosum
Third ventricle
Post. commissure
Habenular trigone
Post. parolfactory sulcus
Suprapineal recess
Pineal recess
Ant. parolfactory sulcus
Cerebral aqueduct
Pineal body
Splenium of corpus callosum
Lamina quadrigemina
Subcallosal area
Sup. medullary velum
Cerebellar lingula
Central lobule
Fourth ventricle
Culmen
Lamina terminalis
*
**
Fastigium
Vermis
Optic recess
Interpedun-cular fossa
Optic chiasm
Oculomotor n.
Gyri of vermis
Infundibulum
+
Ant. lobe of hypophysis
Declive
Post. lobe of hypophysis
Infundibu-lar recess
Cerebral peduncle
Cerebellum
Decussation of pedunculi cerebellaris superiores
Pons
Folium of vermis
Longit. fascicles of pons
* tuber cinereum
** mammillary body
+ interpeduncular fossa
Med. longit. fascicle
Medulla oblongata
Cerebellar hemisphere
Rhomboid fossa
Tuber of vermis
Vermis
Fourth ventricle
Pyramid of vermis
Uvula of vermis
Medullary center of vermis
Nodule
Central canal of medulla oblongata
Choroid plexus of fourth ventricle
Spinal cord

Fig. 46. Sagittal section through the brain stem. Cut surface of the right half. Walls of the third and fourth ventricle as well as of the cerebral aqueduct are shown in yellow.

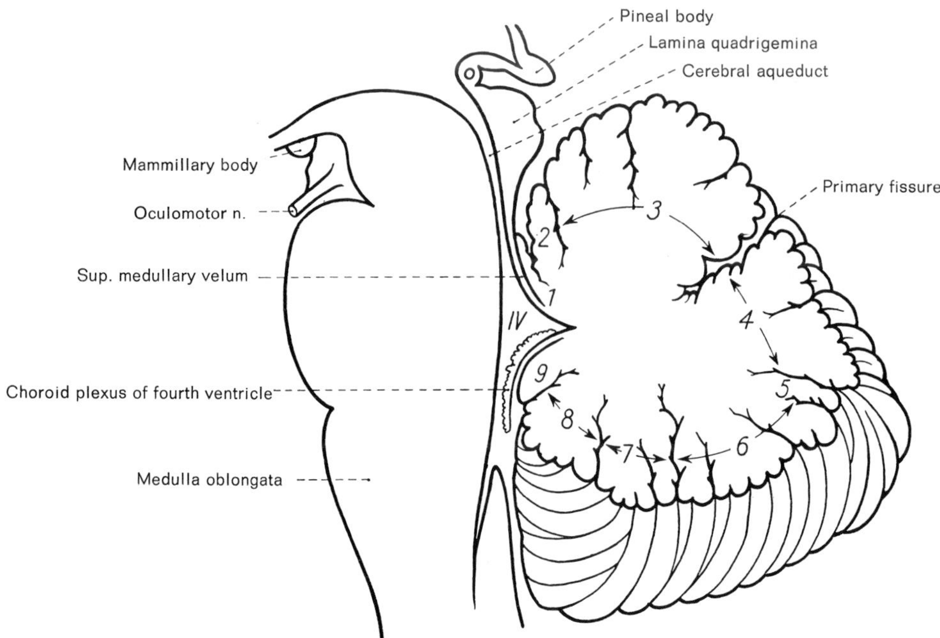
Pineal body
Lamina quadrigemina
Cerebral aqueduct
Mammillary body
Oculomotor n.
Primary fissure
Sup. medullary velum
IV
Choroid plexus of fourth ventricle
Medulla oblongata
1
2
3
4
5
6
7
8
9

Fig. 47. Sagittal section through brain stem with cerebellum. IV = fourth ventricle. The numerals within the cerebellum indicate the subdivisions of the vermis. 1 lingula, 2 central lobe, 3 culmen, 4 declive, 5 folium, 6 tuber, 7 pyramid, 8 uvula, 9 nodule.

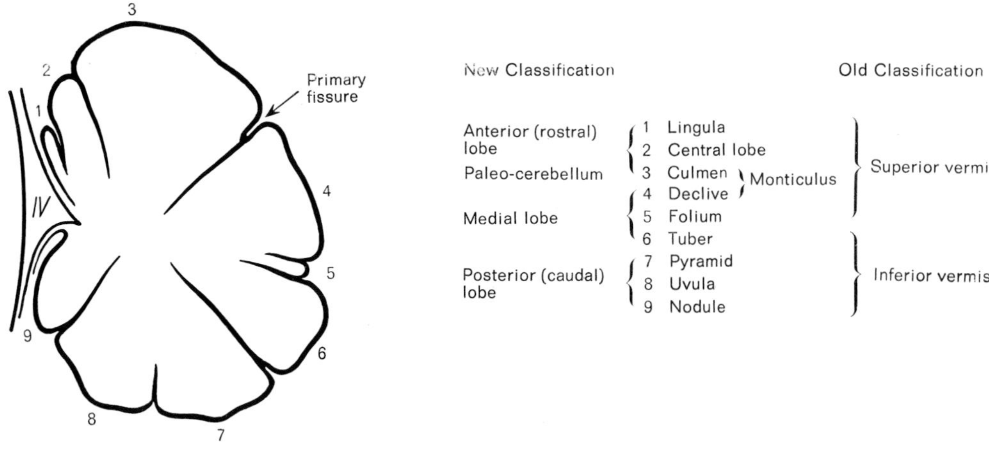
3
2
1
Primary fissure
4
IV
5
9
6
8
7
New Classification
Old Classification
Anterior (rostral) lobe
Paleo-cerebellum
1 Lingula
2 Central lobe
3 Culmen
Monticulus
4 Declive
Medial lobe
5 Folium
6 Tuber
Superior vermis
Posterior (caudal) lobe
7 Pyramid
8 Uvula
9 Nodule
Inferior vermis

Fig. 48. Sagittal section through the cerebellum indicating the subdivisions of the vermis and a comparison of the old and new classifications.

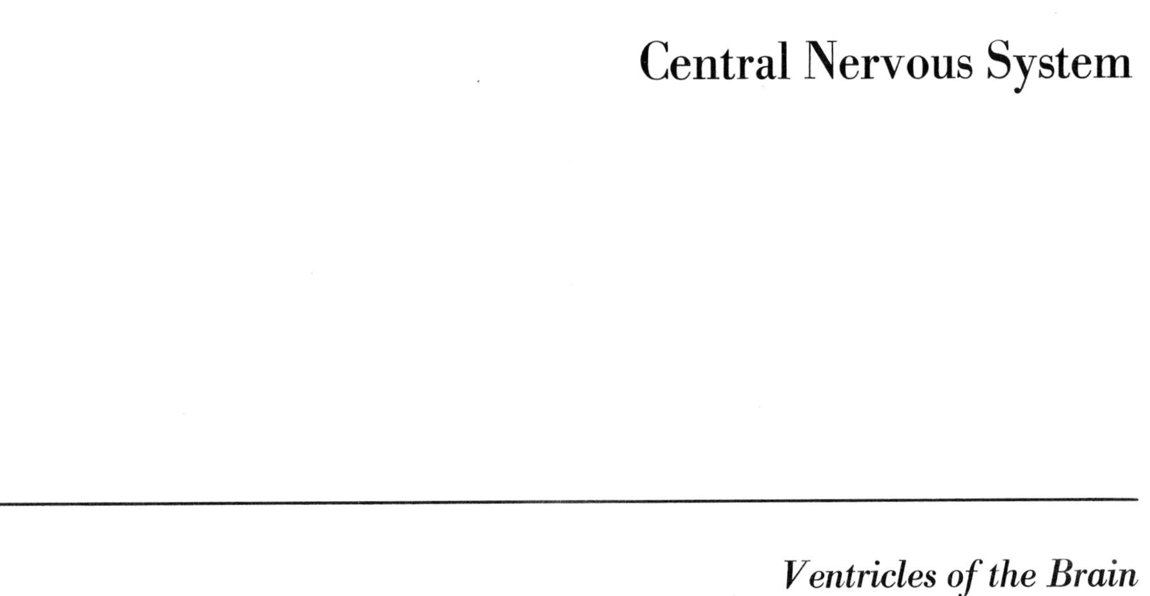

Central Nervous System

Ventricles of the Brain

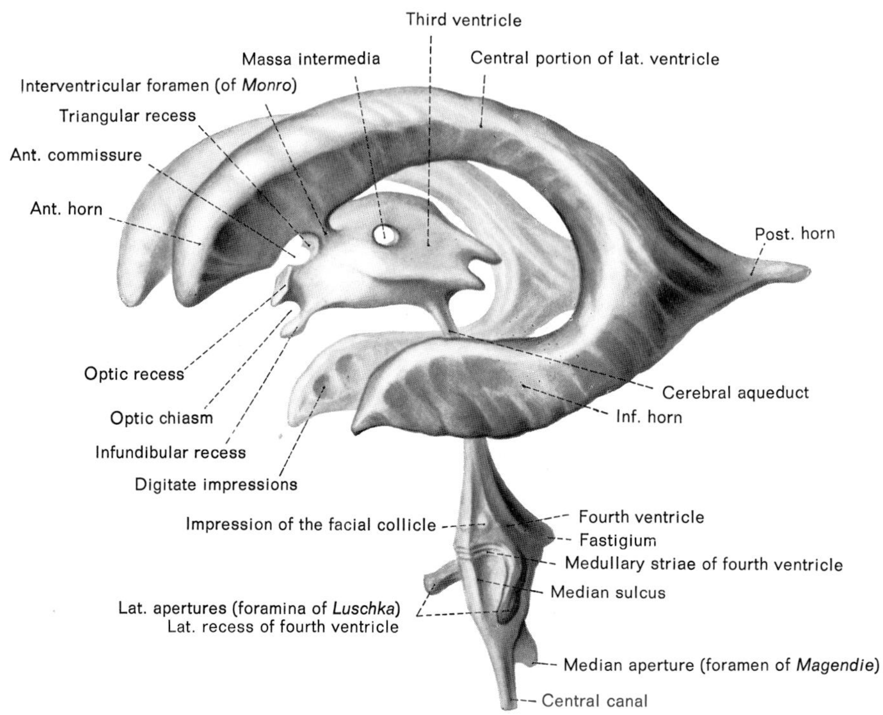
Third ventricle
Massa intermedia
Central portion of lat. ventricle
Interventricular foramen (of Monro)
Triangular recess
Ant. commissure
Ant. horn
Post. horn
Optic recess
Optic chiasm
Infundibular recess
Digitate impressions
Cerebral aqueduct
Inf. horn
Impression of the facial collicle
Fourth ventricle
Fastigium
Medullary striae of fourth ventricle
Median sulcus
Lat. apertures (foramina of Luschka)
Lat. recess of fourth ventricle
Median aperture (foramen of Magendie)
Central canal

Fig. 49. Cast of the ventricular system of the adult human brain viewed from the left side.

Note: Obstruction of the narrow passages of the ventricular system, i.e., cerebral aqueduct and median and lateral apertures of the fourth ventricle may lead to the condition called internal obstructive hydrocephalus.

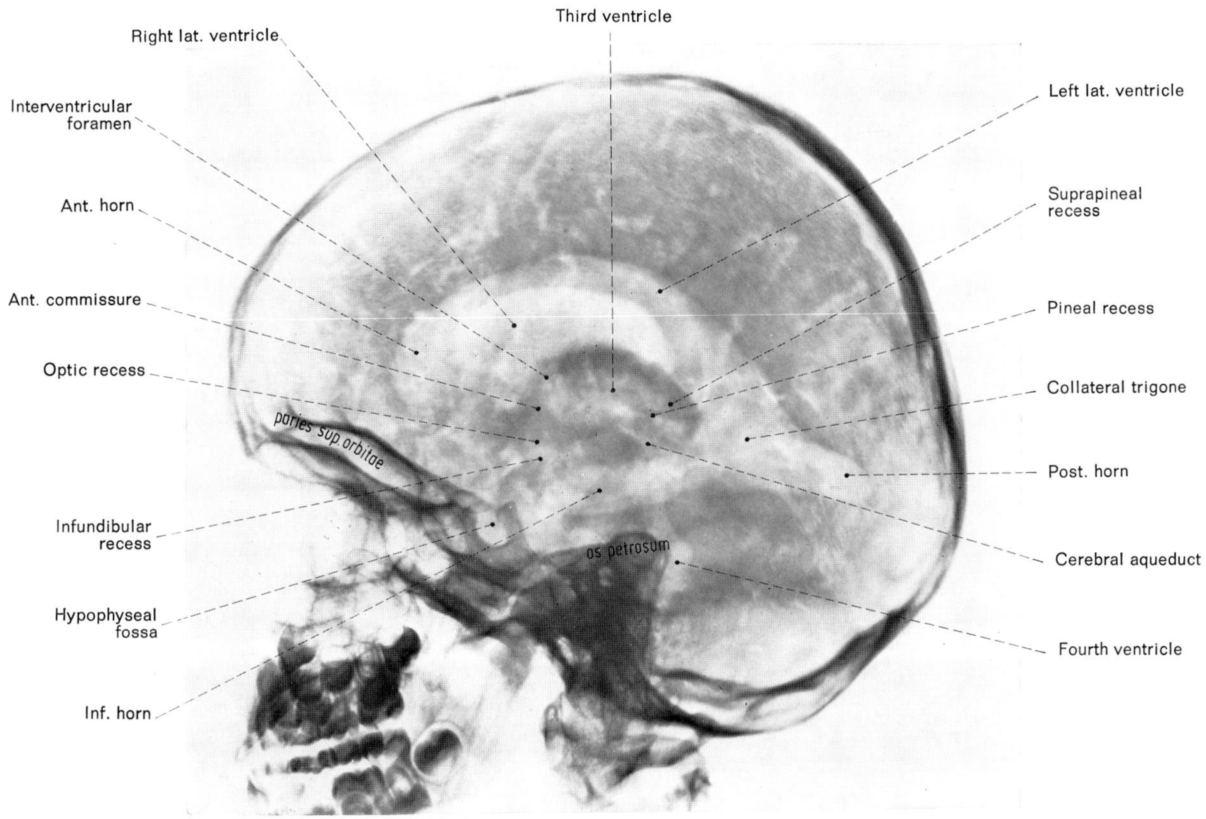

Third ventricle
Right lat. ventricle
Interventricular foramen
Ant. horn
Ant. commissure
Optic recess
Infundibular recess
Hypophyseal fossa
Inf. horn
Left lat. ventricle
Suprapineal recess
Pineal recess
Collateral trigone
Post. horn
Cerebral aqueduct
Fourth ventricle
paries sup. orbitae
os petrosum

Fig. 50. Ventriculogram after filling the ventricles with air by direct injection. Compare with Fig. 49.

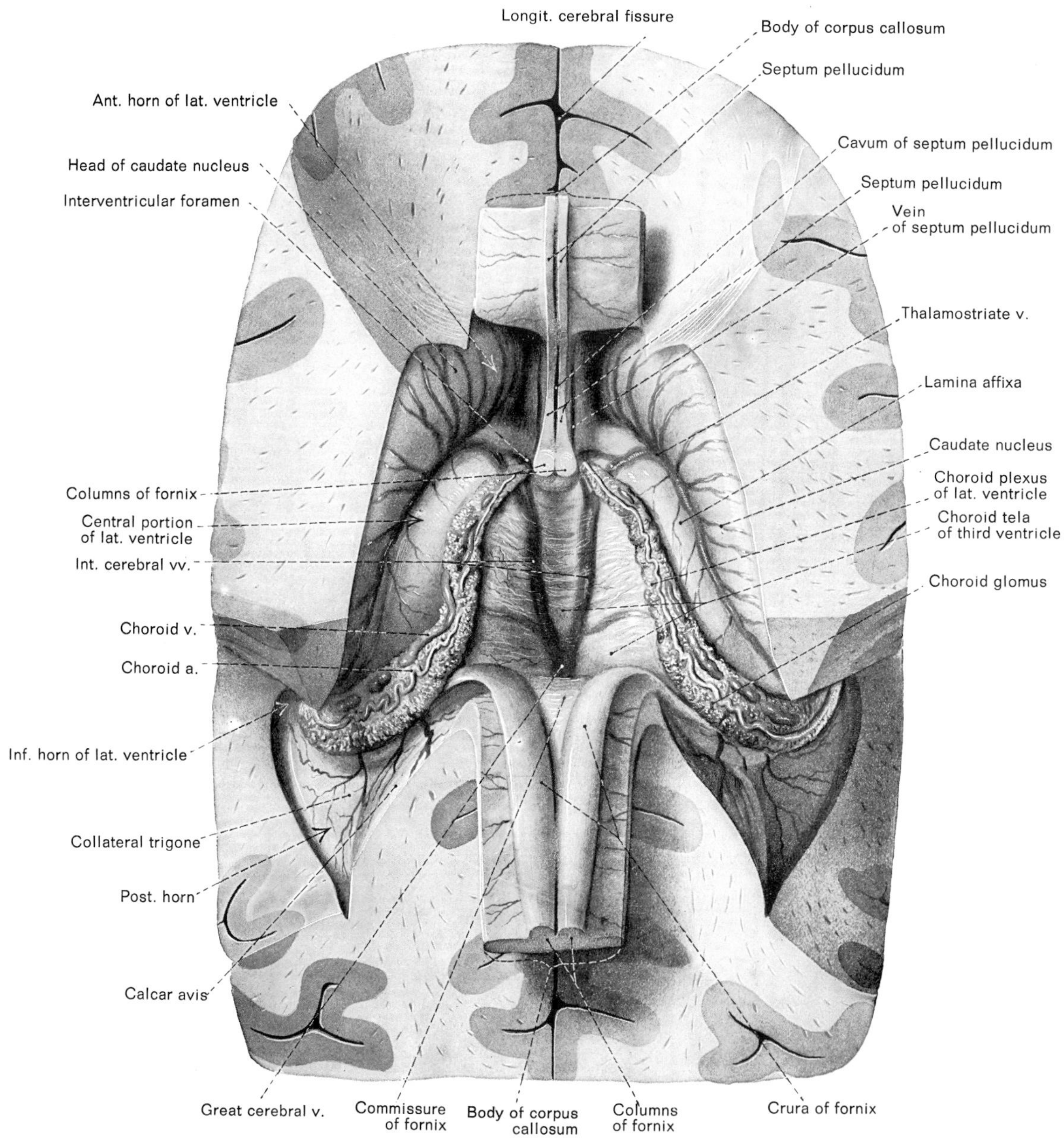
Longit. cerebral fissure
Body of corpus callosum
Septum pellucidum
Ant. horn of lat. ventricle
Cavum of septum pellucidum
Head of caudate nucleus
Septum pellucidum
Interventricular foramen
Vein of septum pellucidum
Thalamostriate v.
Lamina affixa
Caudate nucleus
Choroid plexus of lat. ventricle
Columns of fornix
Central portion of lat. ventricle
Choroid tela of third ventricle
Int. cerebral vv.
Choroid glomus
Choroid v.
Choroid a.
Inf. horn of lat. ventricle
Collateral trigone
Post. horn
Calcar avis
Great cerebral v.
Commissure of fornix
Body of corpus callosum
Columns of fornix
Crura of fornix

Fig. 51. Lateral ventricles opened from above to expose the choroid tela of the prosencephalon. Corpus callosum and fornix are transected and deflected forward and backward.

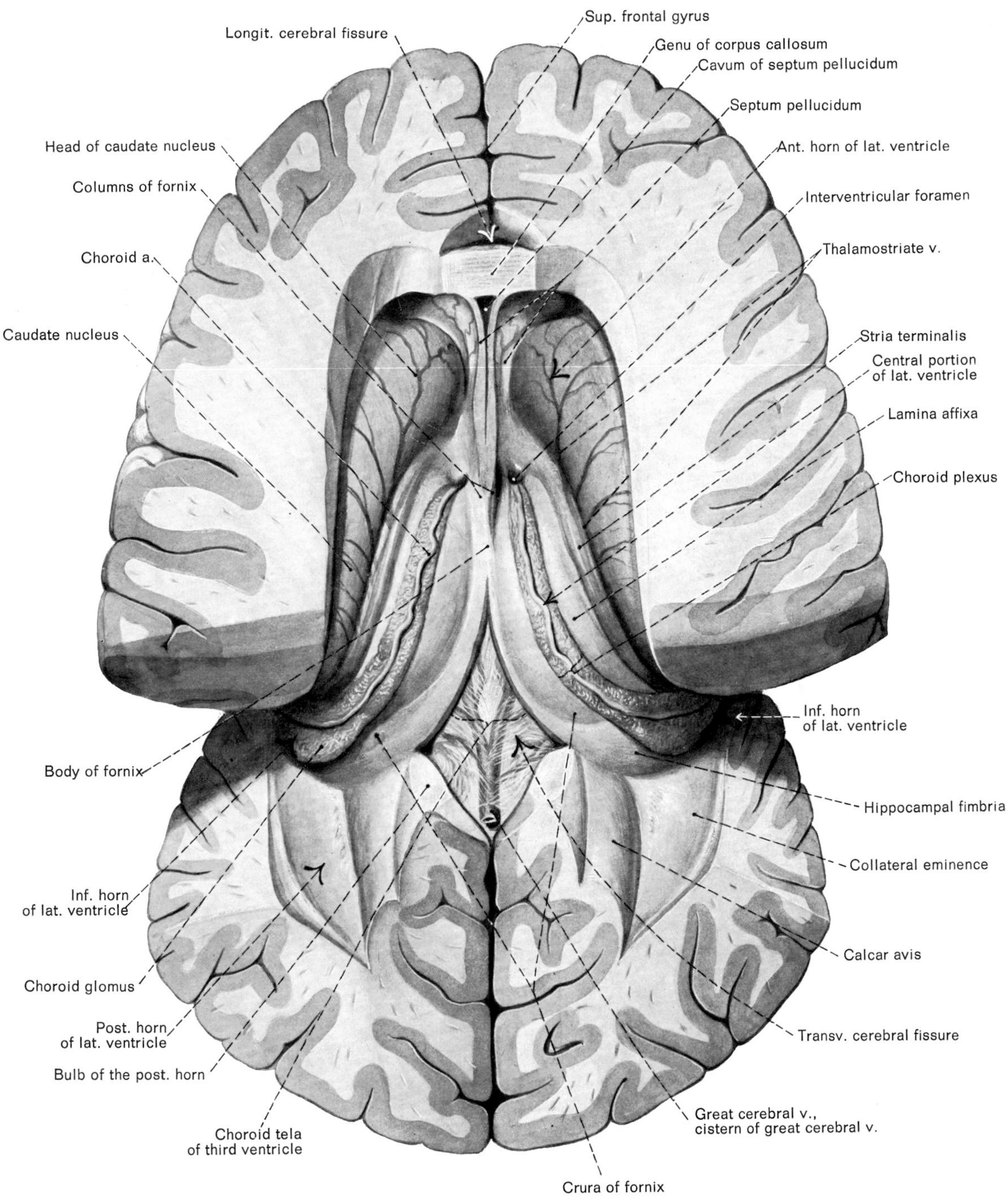

Sup. frontal gyrus
Longit. cerebral fissure
Genu of corpus callosum
Cavum of septum pellucidum
Septum pellucidum
Head of caudate nucleus
Ant. horn of lat. ventricle
Columns of fornix
Interventricular foramen
Choroid a.
Thalamostriate v.
Caudate nucleus
Stria terminalis
Central portion of lat. ventricle
Lamina affixa
Choroid plexus
Inf. horn of lat. ventricle
Body of fornix
Hippocampal fimbria
Collateral eminence
Inf. horn of lat. ventricle
Calcar avis
Choroid glomus
Post. horn of lat. ventricle
Transv. cerebral fissure
Bulb of the post. horn
Great cerebral v., cistern of great cerebral v.
Choroid tela of third ventricle
Crura of fornix

Fig. 52. Lateral ventricles opened from above. The major portion of the corpus callosum has been removed. The posterior horns of both lateral ventricles have been exposed.

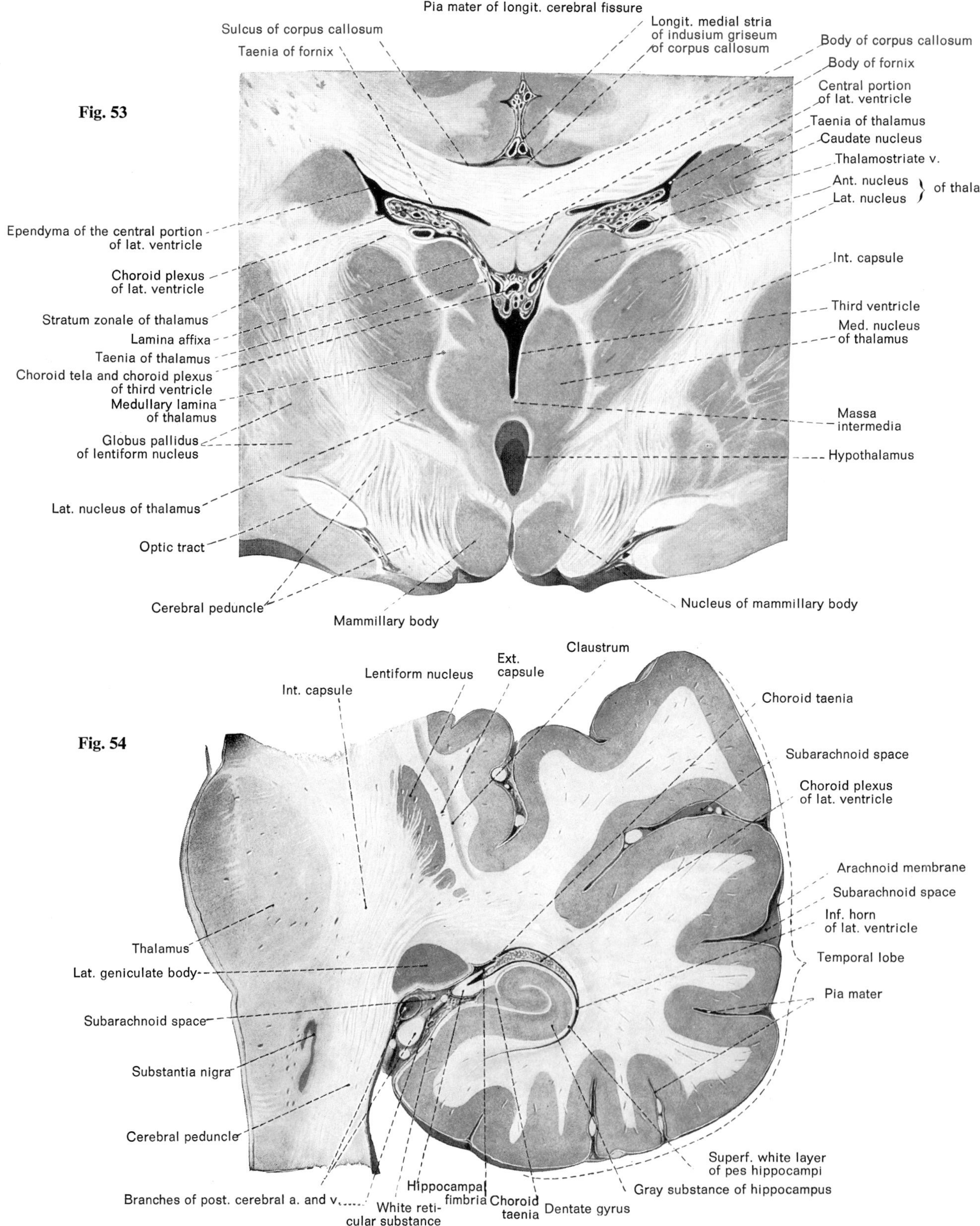
Fig. 53
Pia mater of longit. cerebral fissure
Sulcus of corpus callosum
Taenia of fornix
Longit. medial stria of indusium griseum of corpus callosum
Body of corpus callosum
Body of fornix
Central portion of lat. ventricle
Taenia of thalamus
Caudate nucleus
Thalamostriate v.
Ant. nucleus
Lat. nucleus
of thalamus
Ependyma of the central portion of lat. ventricle
Choroid plexus of lat. ventricle
Int. capsule
Stratum zonale of thalamus
Third ventricle
Lamina affixa
Med. nucleus of thalamus
Taenia of thalamus
Choroid tela and choroid plexus of third ventricle
Medullary lamina of thalamus
Massa intermedia
Globus pallidus of lentiform nucleus
Hypothalamus
Lat. nucleus of thalamus
Optic tract
Cerebral peduncle
Nucleus of mammillary body
Mammillary body
Fig. 54
Claustrum
Ext. capsule
Lentiform nucleus
Int. capsule
Choroid taenia
Subarachnoid space
Choroid plexus of lat. ventricle
Arachnoid membrane
Subarachnoid space
Inf. horn of lat. ventricle
Thalamus
Temporal lobe
Lat. geniculate body
Pia mater
Subarachnoid space
Substantia nigra
Cerebral peduncle
Superf. white layer of pes hippocampi
Gray substance of hippocampus
Branches of post. cerebral a. and v.
Hippocampal fimbria
White reticular substance
Choroid taenia
Dentate gyrus

Fig. 53. Frontal section through lateral ventricles, third ventricle, corpus callosum, fornix and hypothalamus at the plane of the mammillary bodies.

Fig. 54. Frontal section through the temporal lobe. Boundaries of the inferior horn of the lateral ventricle.

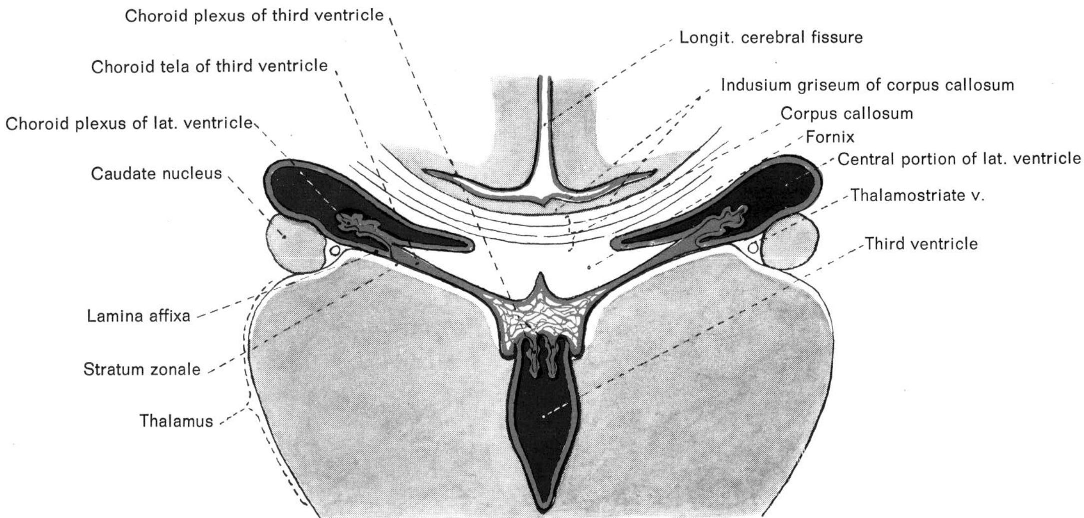
Choroid plexus of third ventricle
Choroid tela of third ventricle
Choroid plexus of lat. ventricle
Caudate nucleus
Lamina affixa
Stratum zonale
Thalamus
Longit. cerebral fissure
Indusium griseum of corpus callosum
Corpus callosum
Fornix
Central portion of lat. ventricle
Thalamostriate v.
Third ventricle

Fig. 55. Schematic representation of a transverse section through the central portion of the lateral ventricle. Roof of the third ventricle, choroid tela of the third ventricle, pia mater and arachnoid membrane are shown in red, the ependyma and the epithelium of the choroid plexus in blue. Compare with Fig. 53.

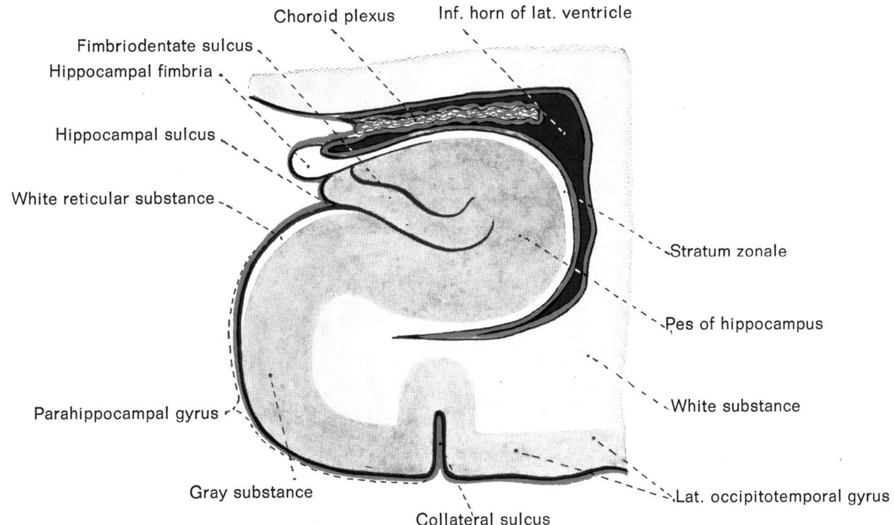
Choroid plexus
Inf. horn of lat. ventricle
Fimbriodentate sulcus
Hippocampal fimbria
Hippocampal sulcus
White reticular substance
Stratum zonale
Pes of hippocampus
White substance
Parahippocampal gyrus
Gray substance
Collateral sulcus
Lat. occipitotemporal gyrus

Fig. 56. Schematic representation of a frontal section through the inferior horn of the lateral ventricle. The pia mater is shown in red, the ependyma and epithelium of the choroid plexus in blue. Compare with Fig. 54.

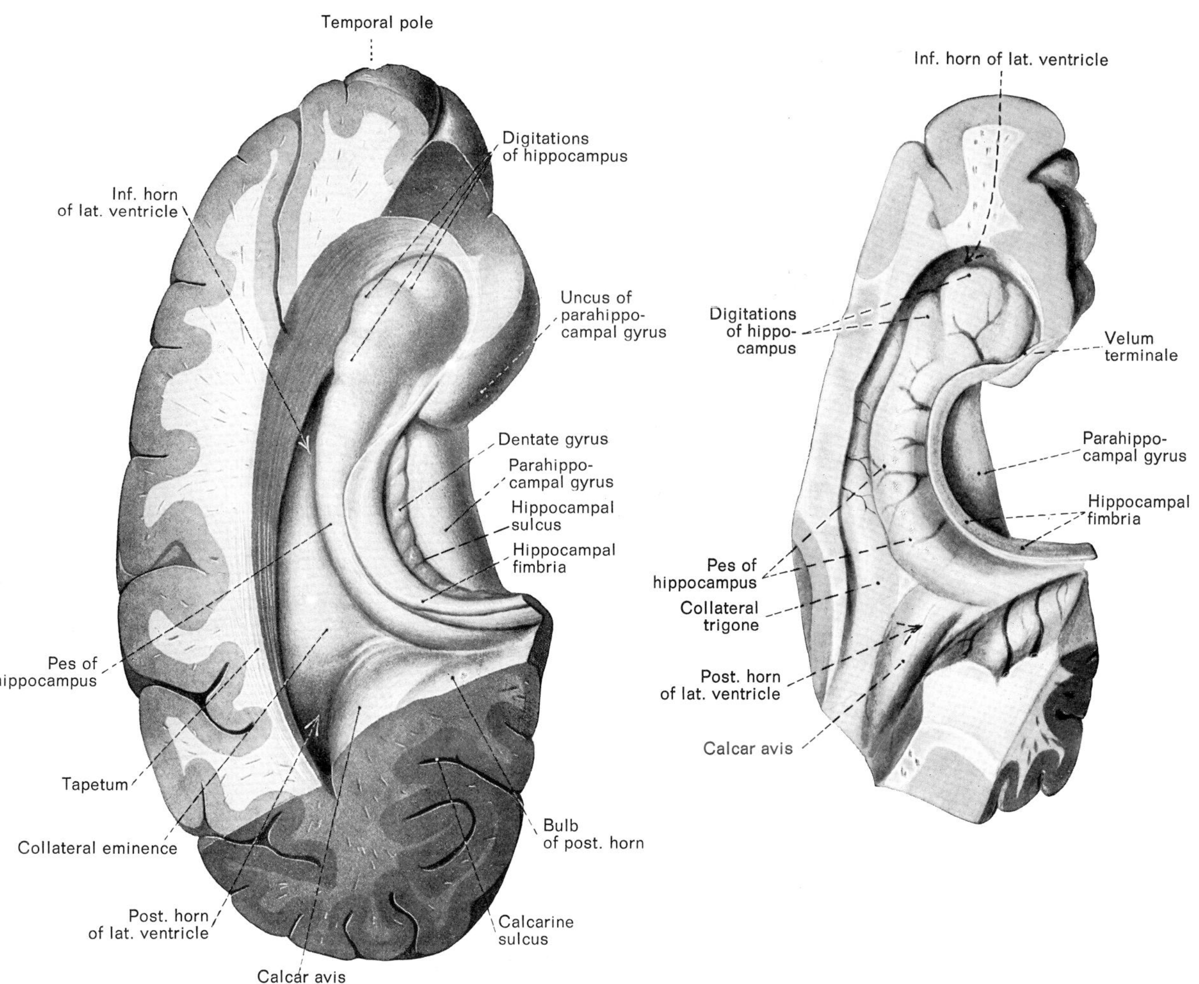
Temporal pole
Digitations of hippocampus
Inf. horn of lat. ventricle
Uncus of parahippo-campal gyrus
Dentate gyrus
Parahippo-campal gyrus
Hippocampal sulcus
Hippocampal fimbria
Pes of hippocampus
Tapetum
Collateral eminence
Post. horn of lat. ventricle
Calcar avis
Bulb of post. horn
Calcarine sulcus
Inf. horn of lat. ventricle
Digitations of hippo-campus
Velum terminale
Parahippo-campal gyrus
Hippocampal fimbria
Pes of hippocampus
Collateral trigone
Post. horn of lat. ventricle
Calcar avis

Fig. 57. Posterior and inferior horns of the left lateral ventricle, opened from lateral.

Fig. 58. Floor of the inferior horn of the lateral ventricle with pes of hippocampus, parahippocampal gyrus and hippocampal fimbria. The dentate gyrus has been removed. Compare with Fig. 57.

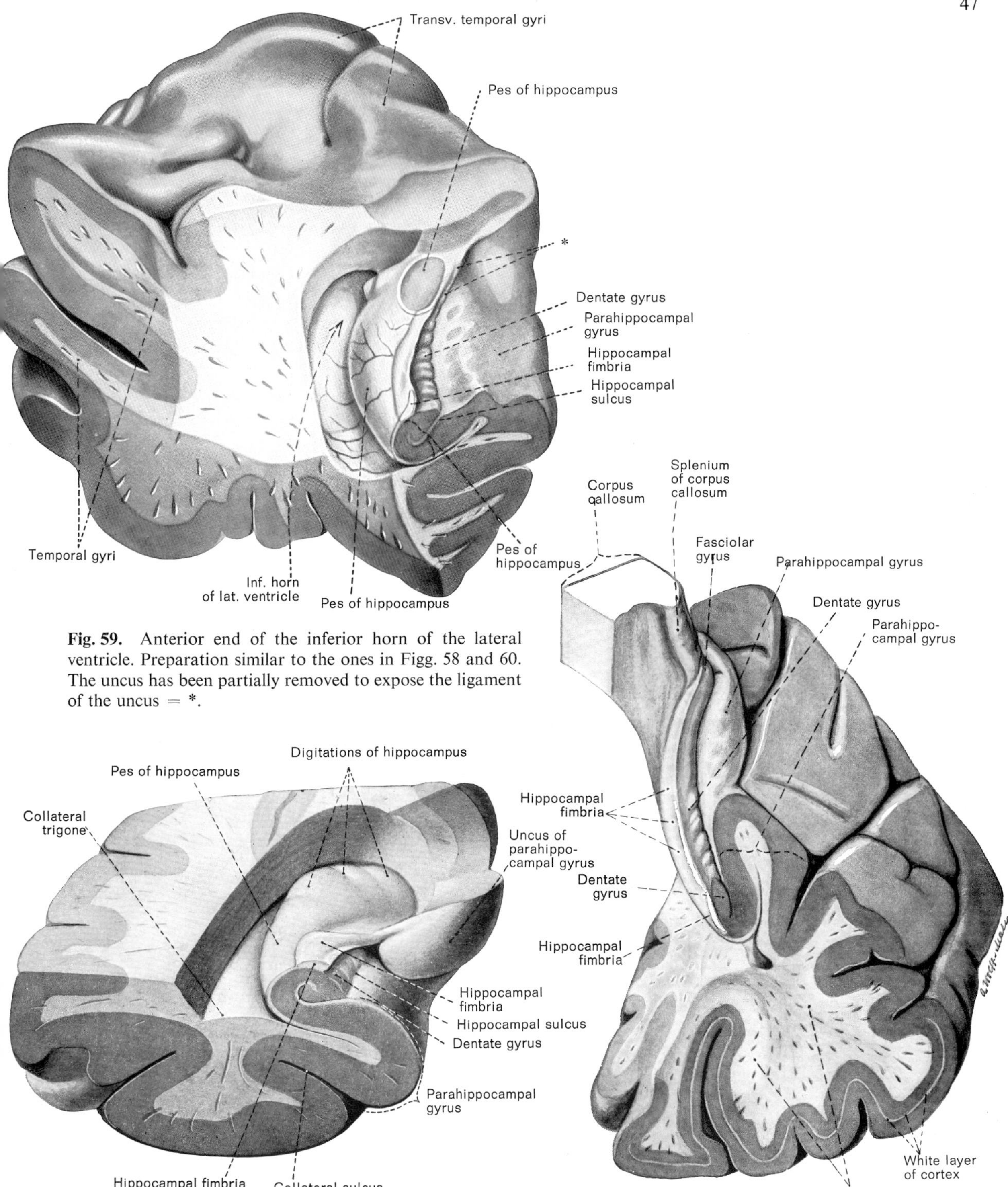

Transv. temporal gyri
Pes of hippocampus
*
Dentate gyrus
Parahippocampal gyrus
Hippocampal fimbria
Hippocampal sulcus
Temporal gyri
Inf. horn of lat. ventricle
Pes of hippocampus
Pes of hippocampus
Corpus callosum
Splenium of corpus callosum
Fasciolar gyrus
Parahippocampal gyrus
Dentate gyrus
Parahippocampal gyrus
Digitations of hippocampus
Pes of hippocampus
Collateral trigone
Hippocampal fimbria
Uncus of parahippocampal gyrus
Dentate gyrus
Hippocampal fimbria
Hippocampal fimbria
Hippocampal sulcus
Dentate gyrus
Parahippocampal gyrus
Hippocampal fimbria
Collateral sulcus
White layer of cortex
White substance

Fig. 59. Anterior end of the inferior horn of the lateral ventricle. Preparation similar to the ones in Figg. 58 and 60. The uncus has been partially removed to expose the ligament of the uncus = *.

Fig. 60. Anterior end of the temporal lobe after opening the inferior horn of the lateral ventricle by frontal section. View from behind and above.

Fig. 61. Anterior end of the temporal lobe with the splenium of the corpus callosum. View from behind and below. The transition of the dentate gyrus into the fasciolar gyrus is visible.

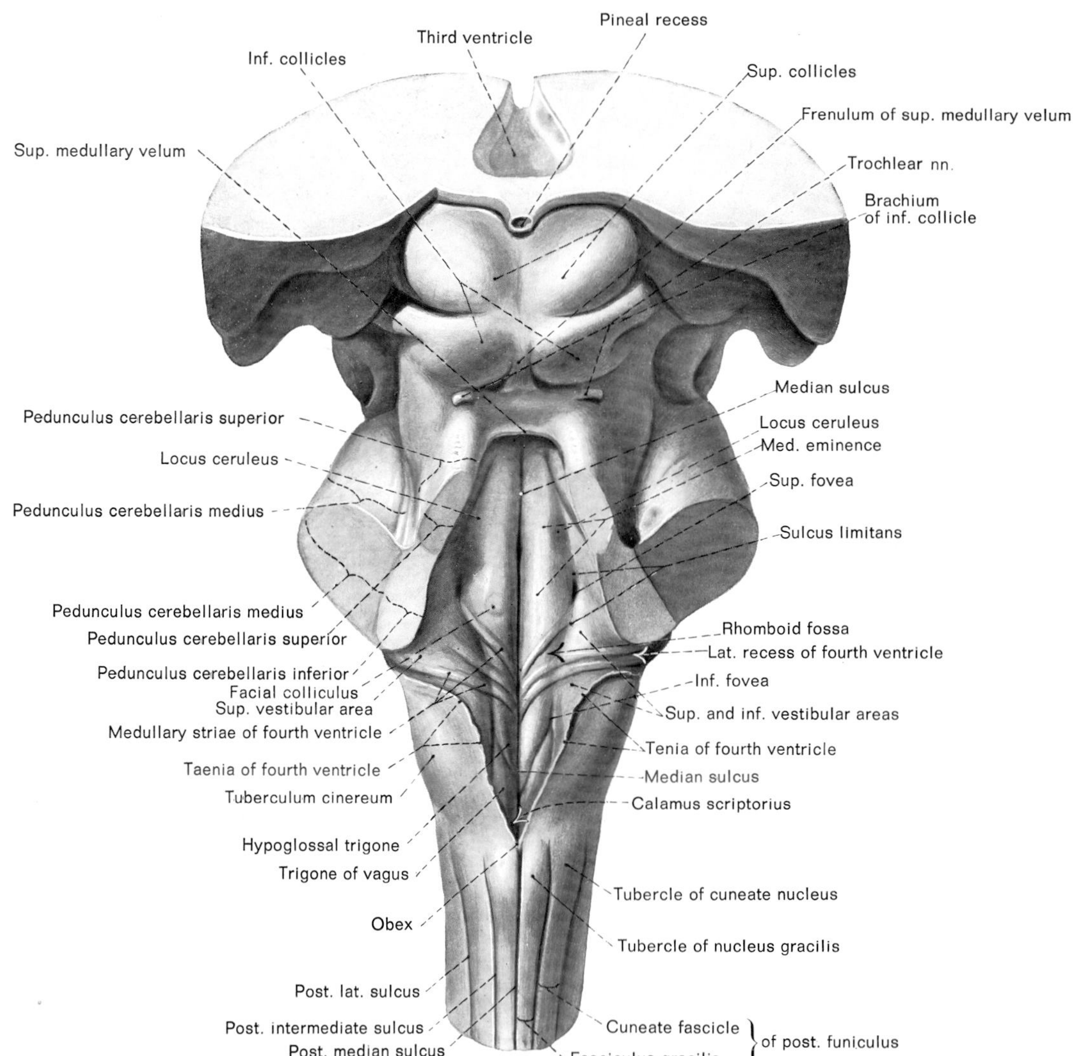
Pineal recess
Third ventricle
Inf. colliculus
Sup. colliculus
Frenulum of sup. medullary velum
Sup. medullary velum
Trochlear nn.
Brachium of inf. collicle
Median sulcus
Pedunculus cerebellaris superior
Locus ceruleus
Locus ceruleus
Med. eminence
Sup. fovea
Pedunculus cerebellaris medius
Sulcus limitans
Pedunculus cerebellaris medius
Pedunculus cerebellaris superior
Rhomboid fossa
Lat. recess of fourth ventricle
Pedunculus cerebellaris inferior
Facial colliculus
Sup. vestibular area
Inf. fovea
Sup. and inf. vestibular areas
Medullary striae of fourth ventricle
Tenia of fourth ventricle
Taenia of fourth ventricle
Median sulcus
Tuberculum cinereum
Calamus scriptorius
Hypoglossal trigone
Trigone of vagus
Tubercle of cuneate nucleus
Obex
Tubercle of nucleus gracilis
Post. lat. sulcus
Post. intermediate sulcus
Cuneate fascicle
of post. funiculus
Post. median sulcus
Fasciculus gracilis

Fig. 62. Floor of the fourth ventricle (rhomboid fossa). Dorsal view of the lamina **tecti** (quadrigemina). Cerebellum and pineal body have been removed.

Central Nervous System

Meninges, Cerebral Blood Vessels, Hypophysis

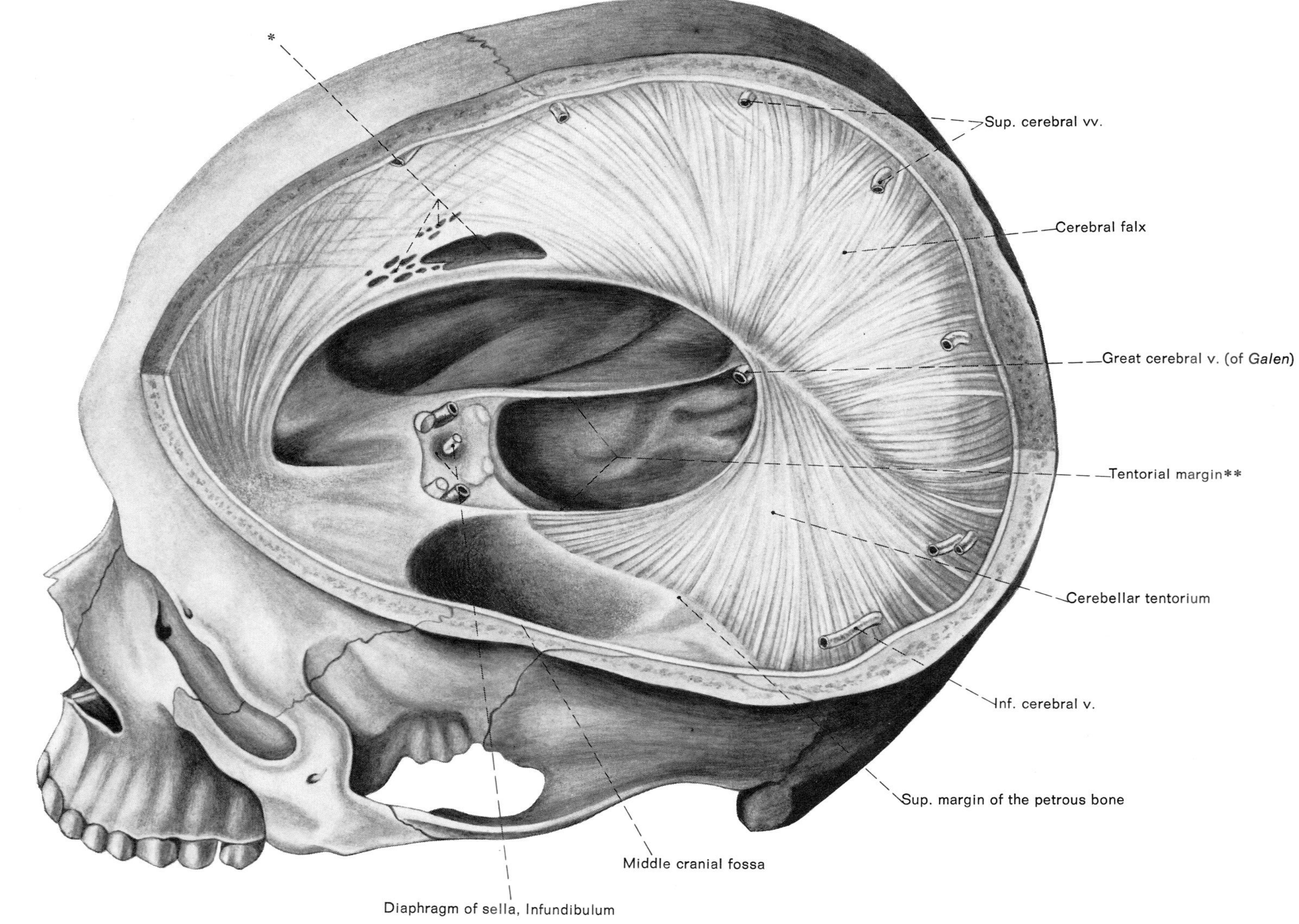
*
Sup. cerebral vv.
Cerebral falx
Great cerebral v. (of *Galen*)
Tentorial margin**
Cerebellar tentorium
Inf. cerebral v.
Sup. margin of the petrous bone
Middle cranial fossa
Diaphragm of sella, Infundibulum

Fig. 63. Cerebral falx and cerebellar tentorium. After removal of the brain the three partitions of the cranial cavity are readily seen. View from left and above (from *Ferner/Kautzky:* Angewandte Anatomie des Gehirns und seiner Hüllen. In *H. Olivecrona, W. Tönnis* [ed.]: Handbuch der Neurochirurgie I/1. Springer, Berlin–Göttingen–Heidelberg 1959). * = voids in the substance of the falx. ** Boundary of the tentorial notch.

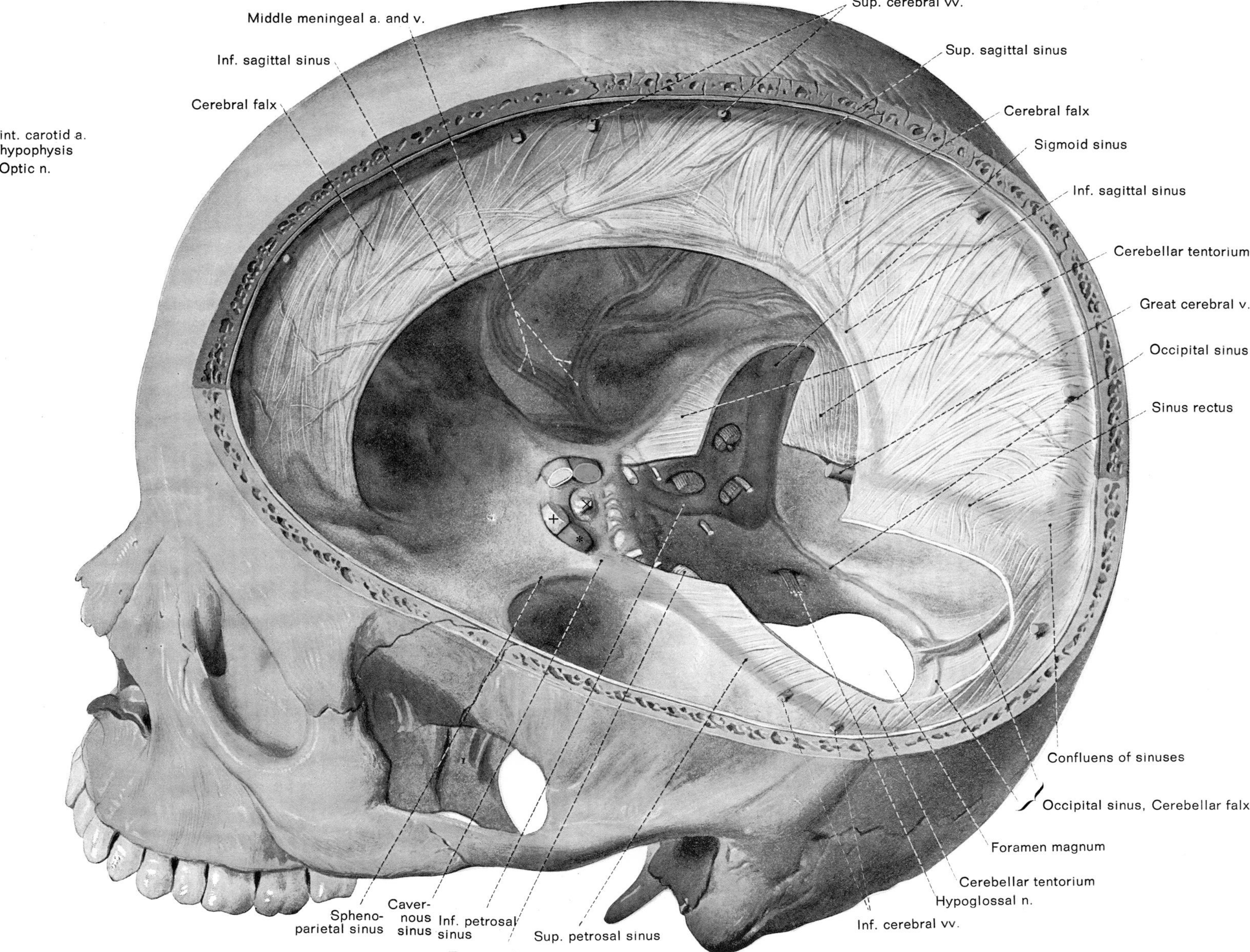
Middle meningeal a. and v.
Inf. sagittal sinus
Cerebral falx
* int. carotid a.
× hypophysis
+ Optic n.
Sup. cerebral vv.
Sup. sagittal sinus
Cerebral falx
Sigmoid sinus
Inf. sagittal sinus
Cerebellar tentorium
Great cerebral v.
Occipital sinus
Sinus rectus
Confluens of sinuses
Occipital sinus, Cerebellar falx
Foramen magnum
Cerebellar tentorium
Hypoglossal n.
Inf. cerebral vv.
Sup. petrosal sinus
Trigeminal n.
Inf. petrosal sinus
Cavernous sinus
Sphenoparietal sinus

Fig. 64. Dura mater and its sinuses seen from above and left. A large portion has been removed from the left side of the tentorium and a narrow strip from the right side.

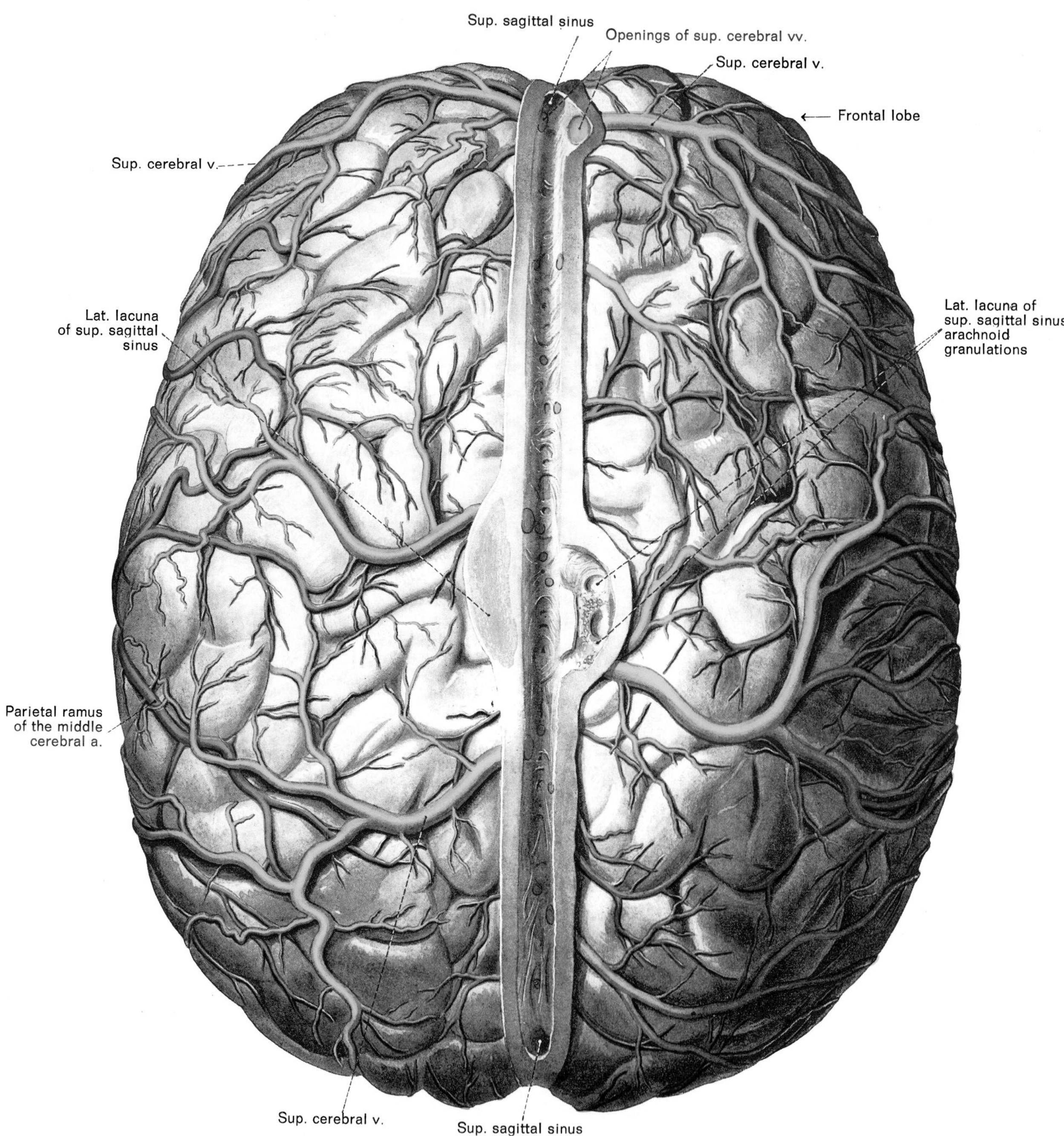
Sup. sagittal sinus
Openings of sup. cerebral vv.
Sup. cerebral v.
Frontal lobe
Sup. cerebral v.
Lat. lacuna of sup. sagittal sinus
Lat. lacuna of sup. sagittal sinus, arachnoid granulations
Parietal ramus of the middle cerebral a.
Sup. cerebral v.
Sup. sagittal sinus

Fig. 65. Superior sagittal sinus, lateral lacunae, veins and arteries of the brain seen from above. A strip of dura mater has been maintained alongside the superior sagittal sinus, the sinus itself as well as a lateral lacuna on the right side have been opened.

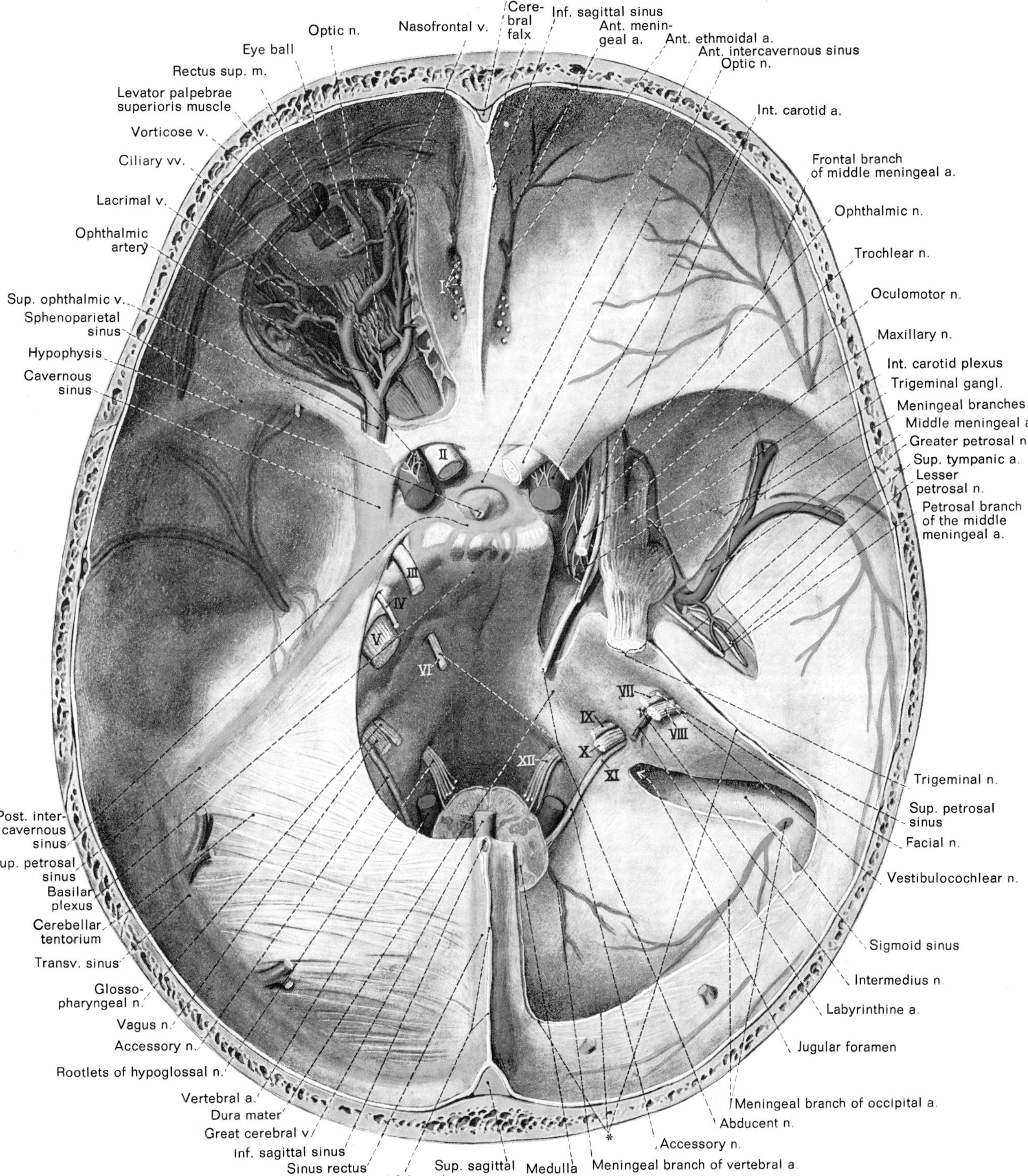
Sup. sagittal sinus
Cerebral falx
Inf. sagittal sinus
Nasofrontal v.
Optic n.
Ant. meningeal a.
Ant. ethmoidal a.
Ant. intercavernous sinus
Optic n.
Eye ball
Rectus sup. m.
Levator palpebrae superioris muscle
Vorticose v.
Ciliary vv.
Lacrimal v.
Ophthalmic artery
Sup. ophthalmic v.
Sphenoparietal sinus
Hypophysis
Cavernous sinus
Int. carotid a.
Frontal branch of middle meningeal a.
Ophthalmic n.
Trochlear n.
Oculomotor n.
Maxillary n.
Int. carotid plexus
Trigeminal gangl.
Meningeal branches
Middle meningeal a.
Greater petrosal n.
Sup. tympanic a.
Lesser petrosal n.
Petrosal branch of the middle meningeal a.
I
II
III
IV
V
VI
VII
VIII
IX
X
XI
XII
Post. intercavernous sinus
Sup. petrosal sinus
Basilar plexus
Cerebellar tentorium
Transv. sinus
Glossopharyngeal n.
Vagus n.
Accessory n.
Rootlets of hypoglossal n.
Vertebral a.
Dura mater
Great cerebral v.
Inf. sagittal sinus
Sinus rectus
Cerebral falx
Sup. sagittal sinus
Medulla oblongata
Trigeminal n.
Sup. petrosal sinus
Facial n.
Vestibulocochlear n.
Sigmoid sinus
Intermedius n.
Labyrinthine a.
Jugular foramen
Meningeal branch of occipital a.
Abducent n.
*
Accessory n.
Meningeal branch of vertebral a.

Fig. 66. Dura mater with its arteries and sinuses; arteries and veins of the orbit; cranial nerves (I = XII) in the floor of the cranial cavity exiting through the dura mater. The roof of the left orbit is removed, sigmoid and cavernous sinus on the right side are opened, the right trigeminal ganglion and middle meningeal artery are exposed. Concerning the position of the internal carotid artery within the cavernous sinus compare Fig. 86. * cerebellar tentorium.

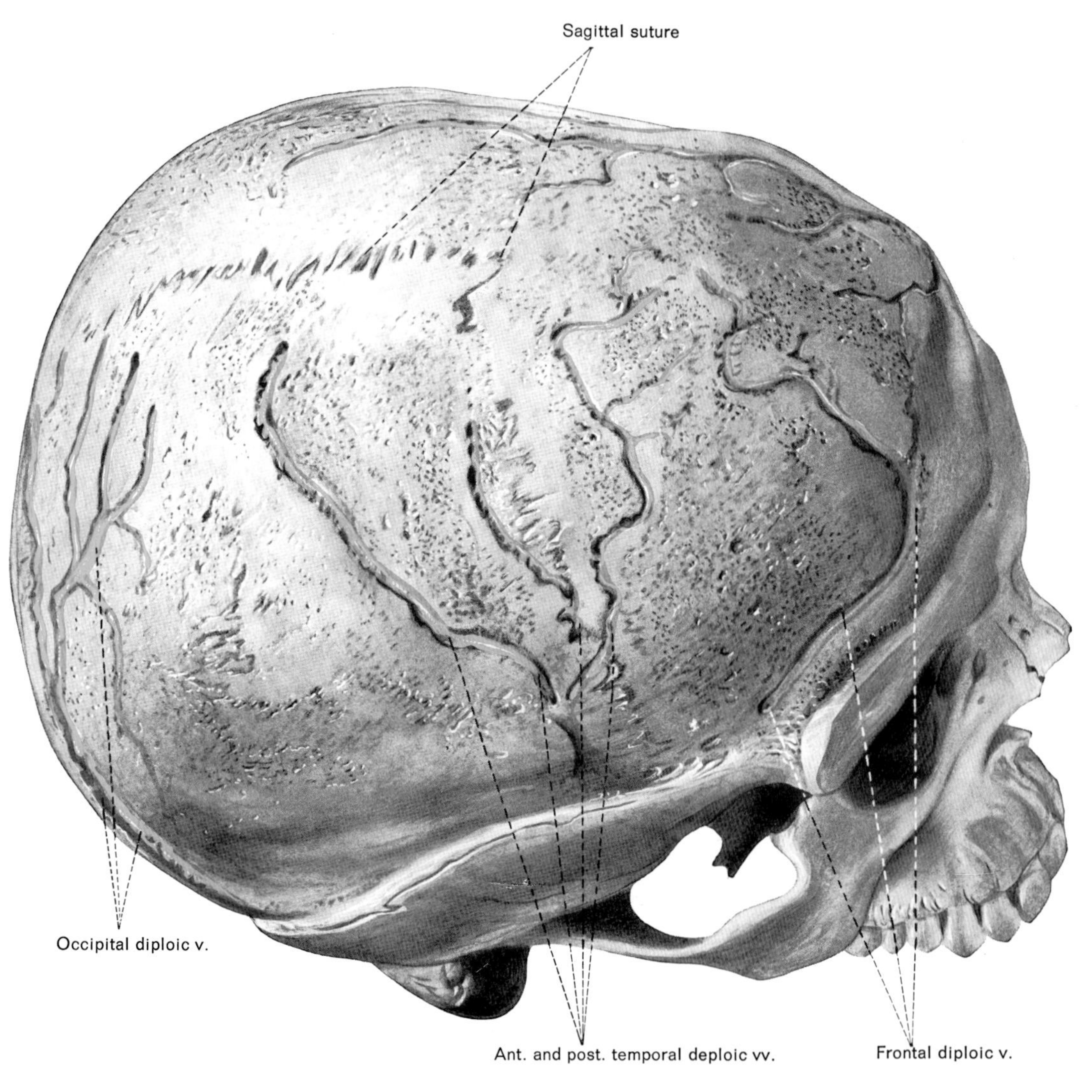
Sagittal suture
Occipital diploic v.
Ant. and post. temporal deploic vv.
Frontal diploic v.

Fig. 67. Diploic veins of the cranial vault exposed by removing the external lamina of the flat cranial bones. Compare with Fig. 305.

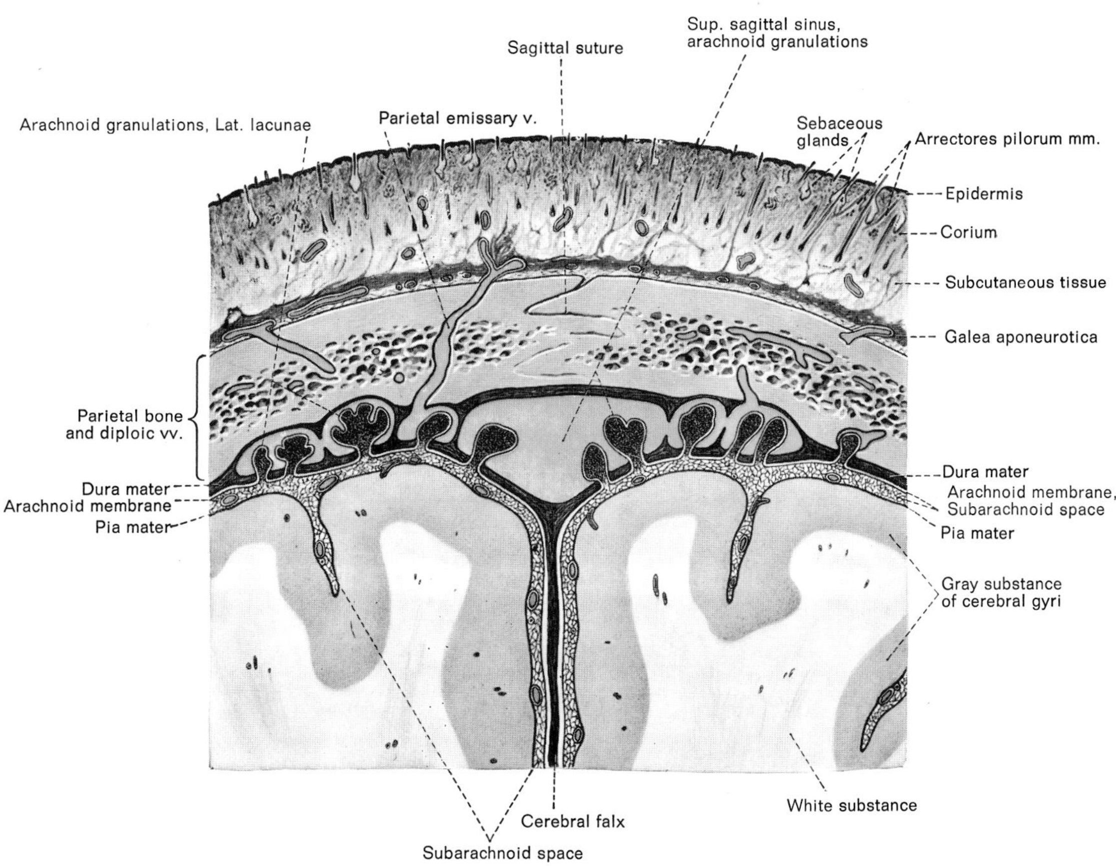
Sup. sagittal sinus,
arachnoid granulations
Sagittal suture
Arachnoid granulations, Lat. lacunae
Parietal emissary v.
Sebaceous
glands
Arrectores pilorum mm.
Epidermis
Corium
Subcutaneous tissue
Galea aponeurotica
Parietal bone
and diploic vv.
Dura mater
Arachnoid membrane
Pia mater
Dura mater
Arachnoid membrane,
Subarachnoid space
Pia mater
Gray substance
of cerebral gyri
White substance
Cerebral falx
Subarachnoid space

Fig. 68. Schematic representation of the meninges and the subarachnoid space. Frontal section through the cranial vault with superior sagittal sinus and cerebral falx. Veins and sinuses blue.

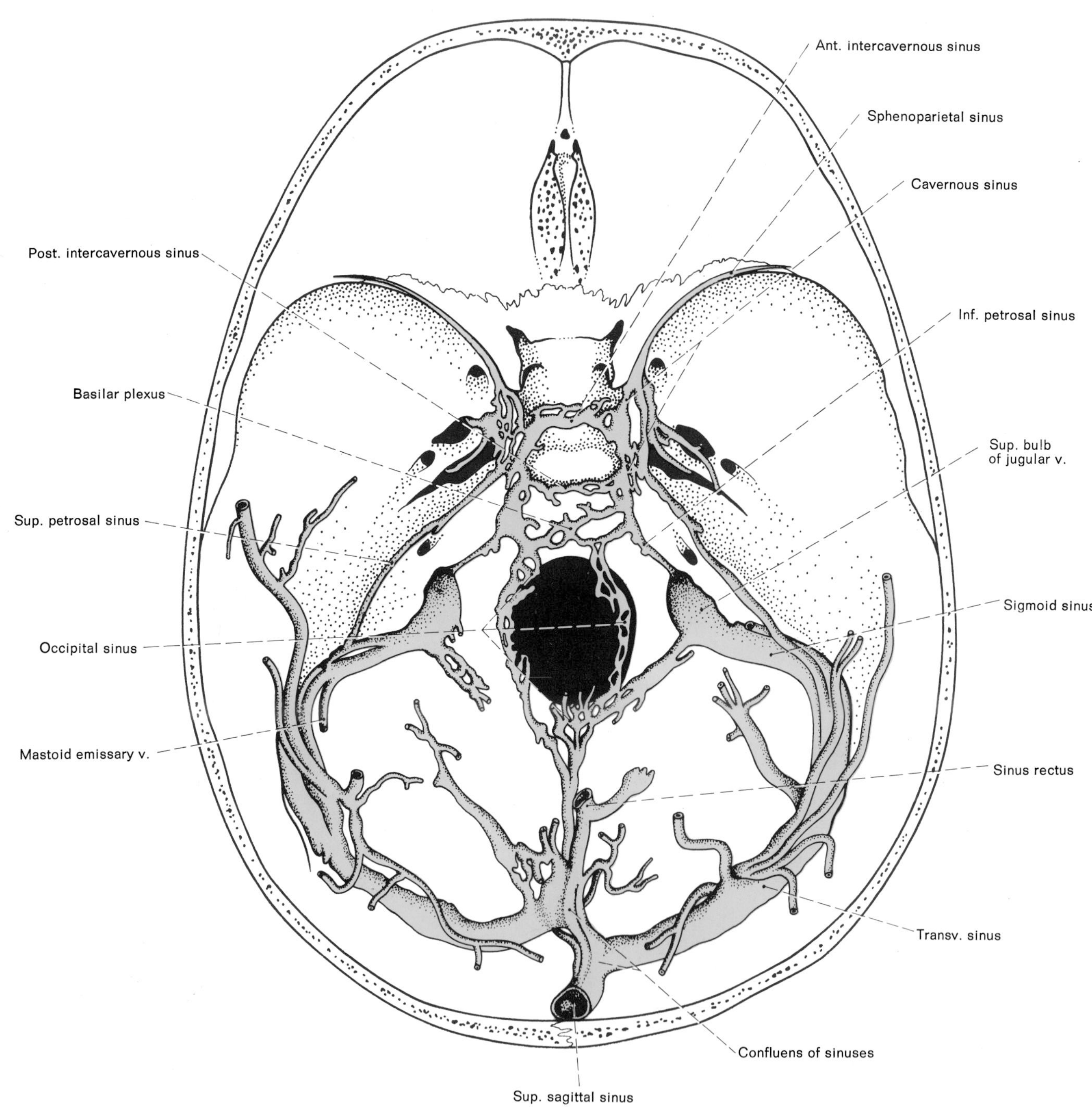
Ant. intercavernous sinus
Sphenoparietal sinus
Cavernous sinus
Post. intercavernous sinus
Inf. petrosal sinus
Basilar plexus
Sup. bulb
of jugular v.
Sup. petrosal sinus
Sigmoid sinus
Occipital sinus
Mastoid emissary v.
Sinus rectus
Transv. sinus
Confluens of sinuses
Sup. sagittal sinus

Fig. 69. Sinuses of the dura mater at the base of the skull.

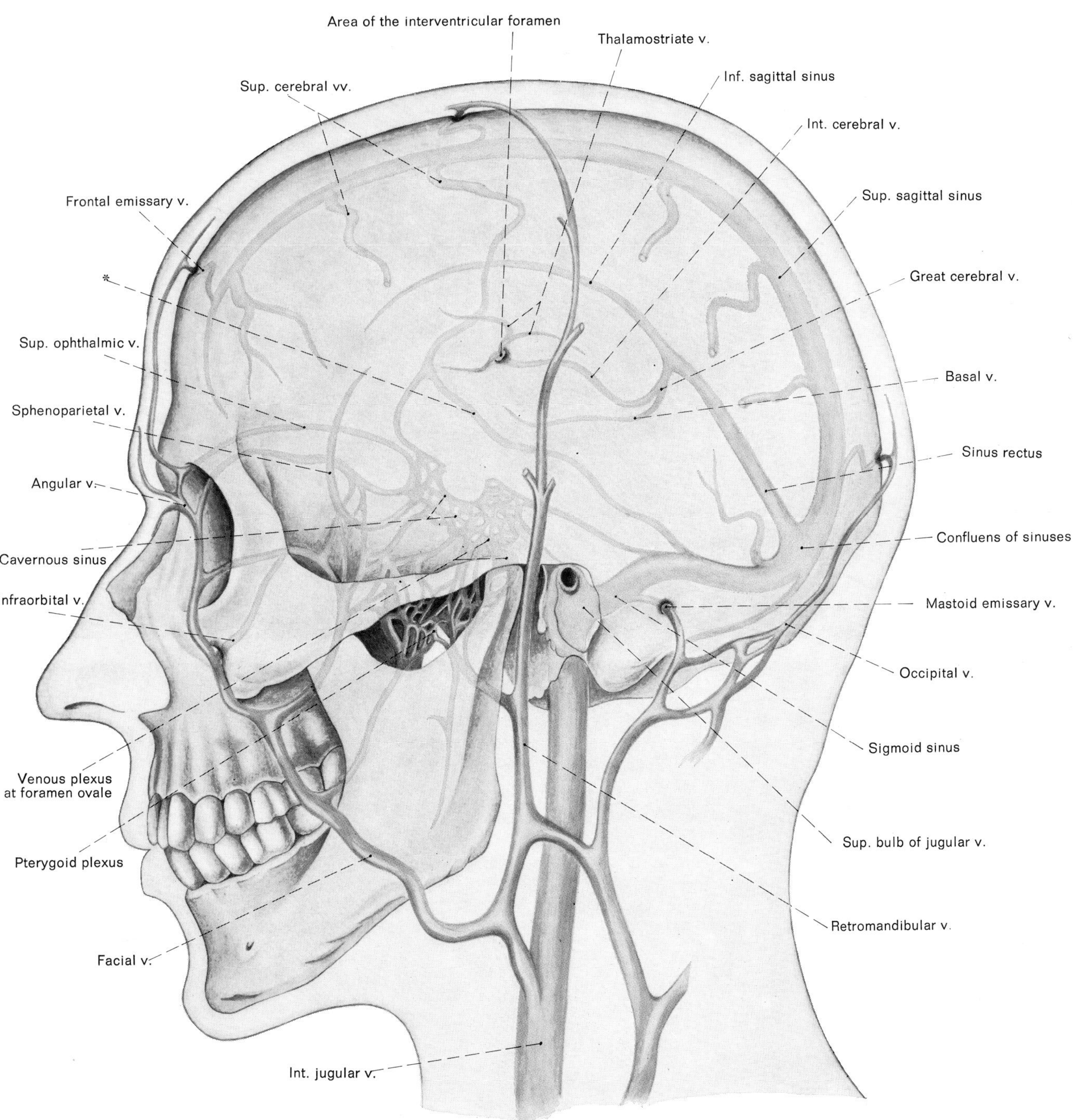
Area of the interventricular foramen
Thalamostriate v.
Inf. sagittal sinus
Sup. cerebral vv.
Int. cerebral v.
Sup. sagittal sinus
Frontal emissary v.
Great cerebral v.
*
Sup. ophthalmic v.
Basal v.
Sphenoparietal v.
Sinus rectus
Angular v.
Confluens of sinuses
Cavernous sinus
Infraorbital v.
Mastoid emissary v.
Occipital v.
Sigmoid sinus
Venous plexus
at foramen ovale
Sup. bulb of jugular v.
Pterygoid plexus
Retromandibular v.
Facial v.
Int. jugular v.

Fig. 70. Larger venous channels of the head, sinuses of the dura mater and the connections of the two systems. (From *Ferner/Kautzky:* Angewandte Anatomie des Gehirns und seiner Hüllen. In: *H. Olivecrona, W. Tönnis* [ed.]: Handbuch der Neurochirurgie I/1. Springer, Berlin–Göttingen–Heidelberg 1959.) * so-called anastomosis of *Labbé*.

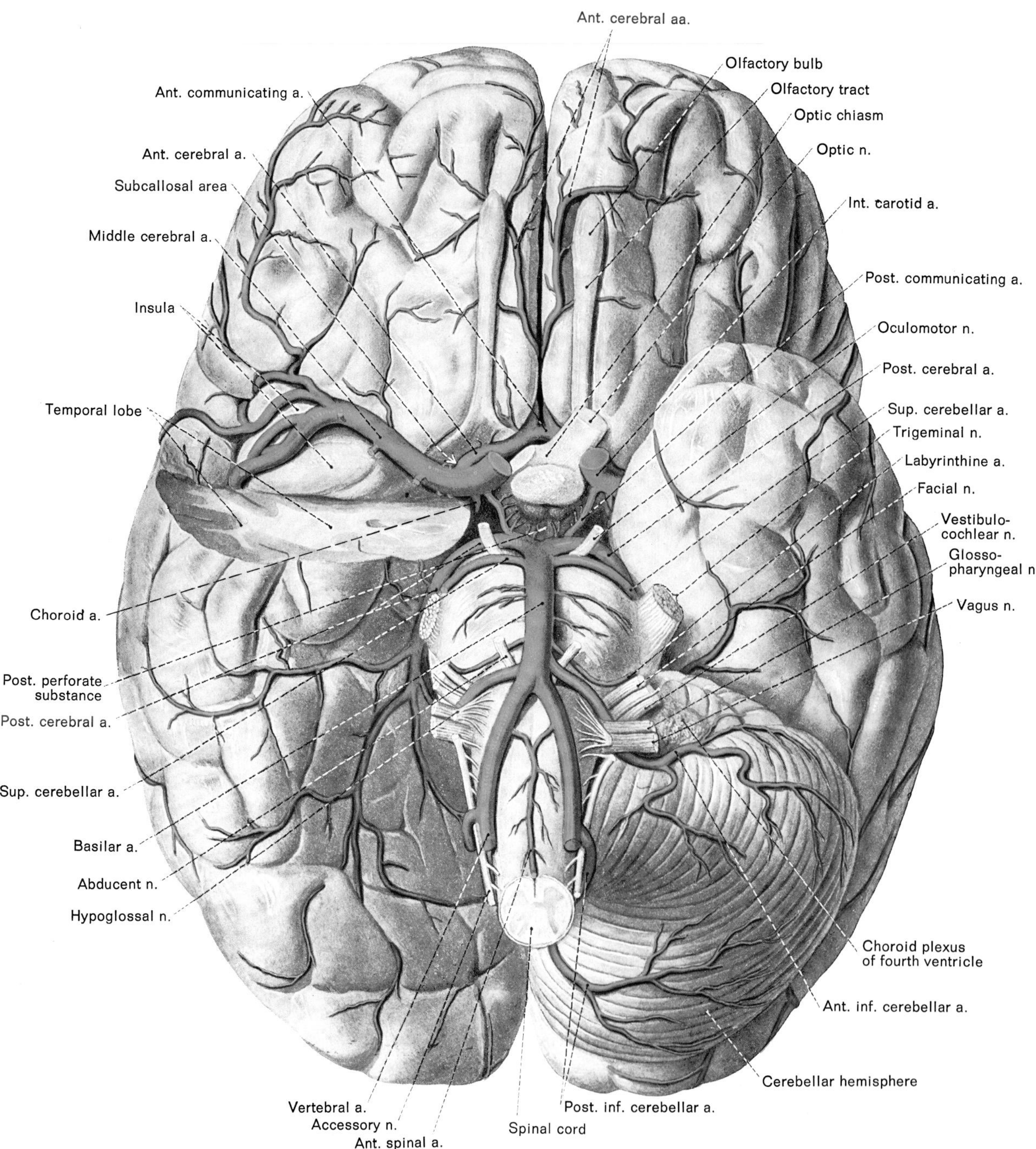

Ant. cerebral aa.
Olfactory bulb
Olfactory tract
Optic chiasm
Optic n.
Int. carotid a.
Post. communicating a.
Oculomotor n.
Post. cerebral a.
Sup. cerebellar a.
Trigeminal n.
Labyrinthine a.
Facial n.
Vestibulo-
cochlear n.
Glosso-
pharyngeal n.
Vagus n.
Choroid plexus
of fourth ventricle
Ant. inf. cerebellar a.
Cerebellar hemisphere
Post. inf. cerebellar a.
Spinal cord
Ant. spinal a.
Accessory n.
Vertebral a.
Hypoglossal n.
Abducent n.
Basilar a.
Sup. cerebellar a.
Post. cerebral a.
Post. perforate
substance
Choroid a.
Temporal lobe
Insula
Middle cerebral a.
Subcallosal area
Ant. cerebral a.
Ant. communicating a.

Fig. 71. Arteries at the base of the brain, arterial circle of *Willis*. The optic nerve, the anterior portion of the temporal lobe and the cerebellar hemisphere of the right side have been removed.

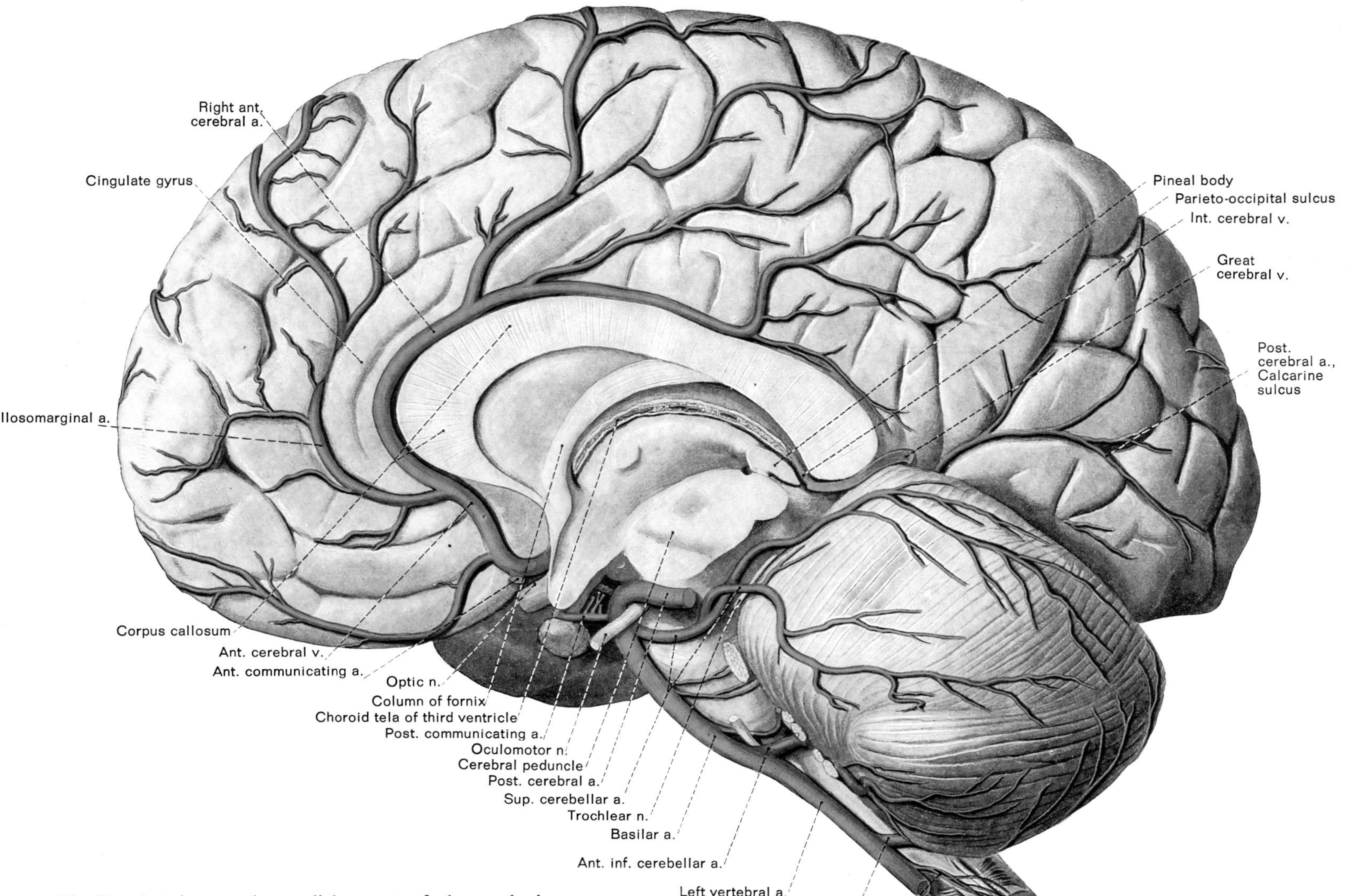
Right ant. cerebral a.
Cingulate gyrus
Callosomarginal a.
Corpus callosum
Ant. cerebral v.
Ant. communicating a.
Optic n.
Column of fornix
Choroid tela of third ventricle
Post. communicating a.
Oculomotor n.
Cerebral peduncle
Post. cerebral a.
Sup. cerebellar a.
Trochlear n.
Basilar a.
Ant. inf. cerebellar a.
Left vertebral a.
Post. inf. cerebellar a.
Post. spinal a.
Ant. spinal a.
Pineal body
Parieto-occipital sulcus
Int. cerebral v.
Great cerebral v.
Post. cerebral a., Calcarine sulcus

Fig. 72. Arteries on the medial aspect of the cerebral hemisphere and on the surface of the cerebellum. The left hemisphere has been removed. Medial view.

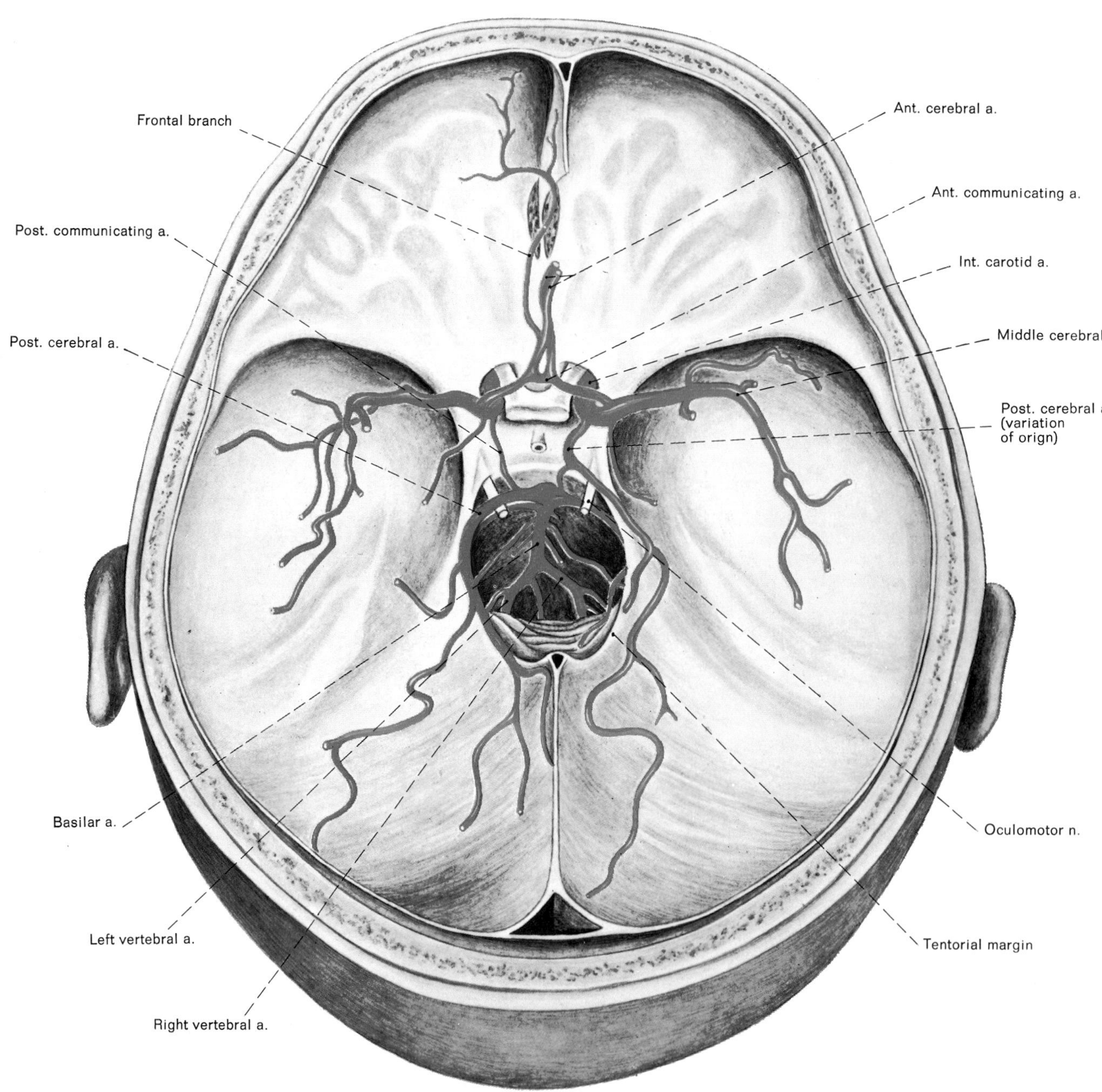

Frontal branch
Ant. cerebral a.
Ant. communicating a.
Post. communicating a.
Int. carotid a.
Post. cerebral a.
Middle cerebral
Post. cerebral
(variation
of orign)
Basilar a.
Oculomotor n.
Left vertebral a.
Tentorial margin
Right vertebral a.

Fig. 73. Cerebral arteries projected onto the base of the skull. Basilar artery and vertebral arteries are seen through the tentorial incisure (from *Ferner/Kautzky:* Angewandte Anatomie des Gehirns und seiner Hüllen. In: *H. Olivecrona, W. Tönnis* [ed.]: Handbuch der Neurochirurgie I/1. Springer, Berlin–Göttingen–Heidelberg 1959.)

Fig. 74. Basal vein (of *Rosenthal*) and great cerebral vein (of *Galen*) after *Toldt/Hochstetter:* Anatomischer Atlas. Vol. 2. Urban & Schwarzenberg, Wien–Innsbruck 1961.

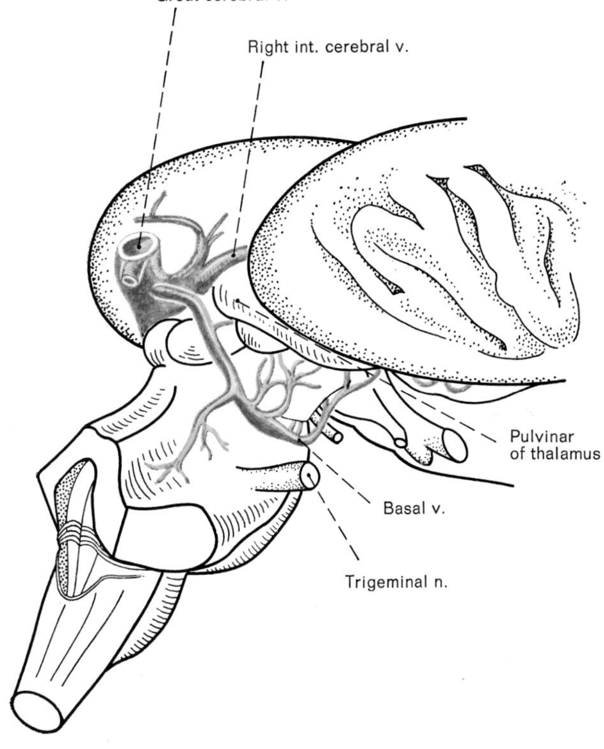
Great cerebral v.
Right int. cerebral v.
Pulvinar of thalamus
Basal v.
Trigeminal n.

Fig. 75. Vascular supply of the cerebrum. In this schematized frontal section the veins are shown on the left side, the arteries on the right (after corrosion preparations by *H. Ferner*). th = thalamus, nl = lentiform nucleus, III = third ventricle.

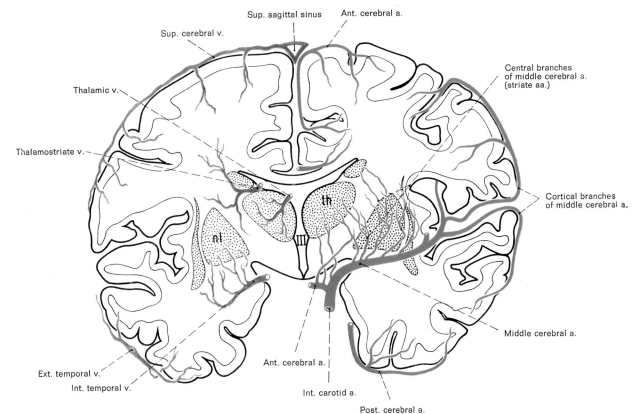

Sup. sagittal sinus
Ant. cerebral a.
Sup. cerebral v.
Central branches of middle cerebral a. (striate aa.)
Thalamic v.
Thalamostriate v.
Cortical branches of middle cerebral a.
th
nl
III
Middle cerebral a.
Ant. cerebral a.
Ext. temporal v.
Int. temporal v.
Int. carotid a.
Post. cerebral a.

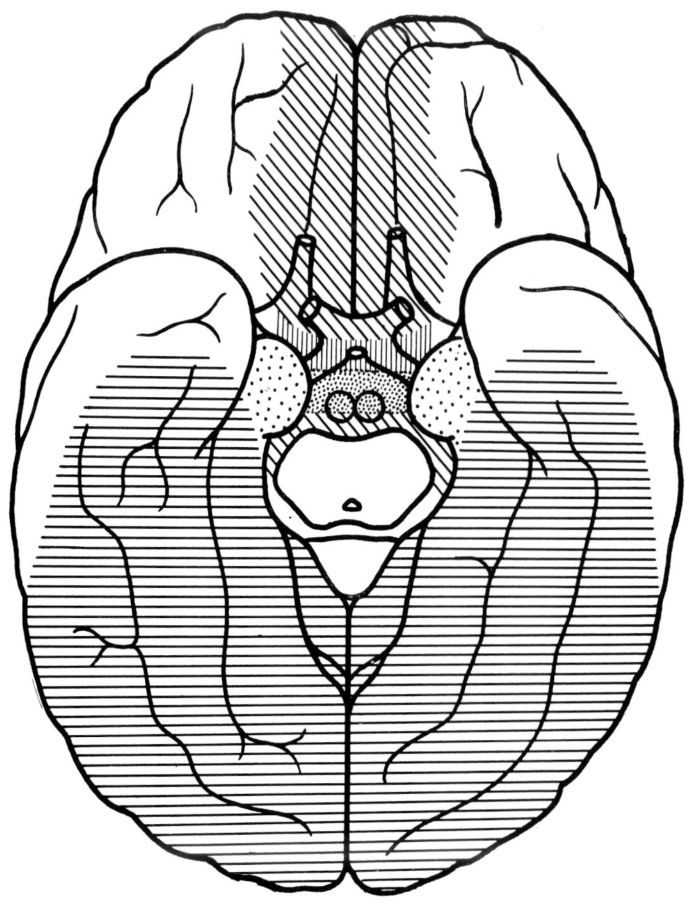

Fig. 76. Supply areas of the cerebral arteries. (Figg. 76–78 after *Töndury:* Angewandte und topographische Anatomie, 4th edition. Thieme, Stuttgart 1970.)

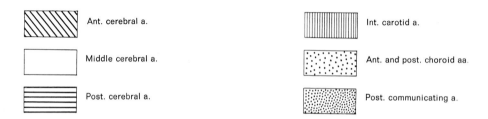

Ant. cerebral a.
Middle cerebral a.
Post. cerebral a.
Int. carotid a.
Ant. and post. choroid aa.
Post. communicating a.

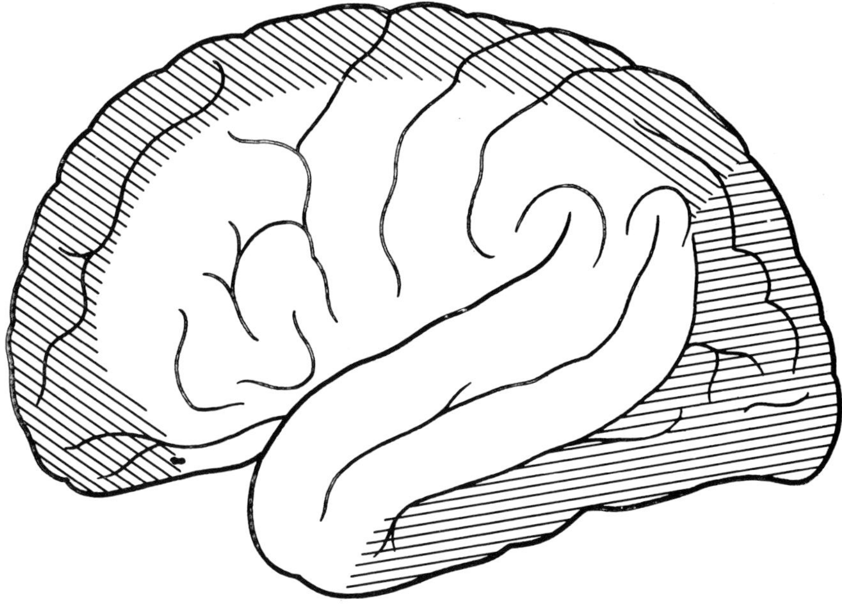

Fig. 77. Supply areas of the cerebral arteries. Lateral aspect. For key see Fig. 76.

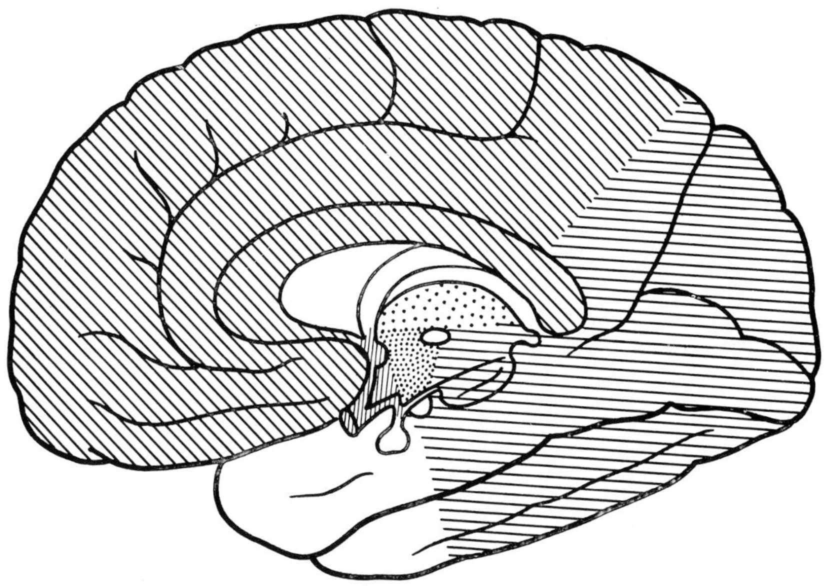

Fig. 78. Supply areas of the cerebral arteries. Medial aspect. For key see Fig. 76.

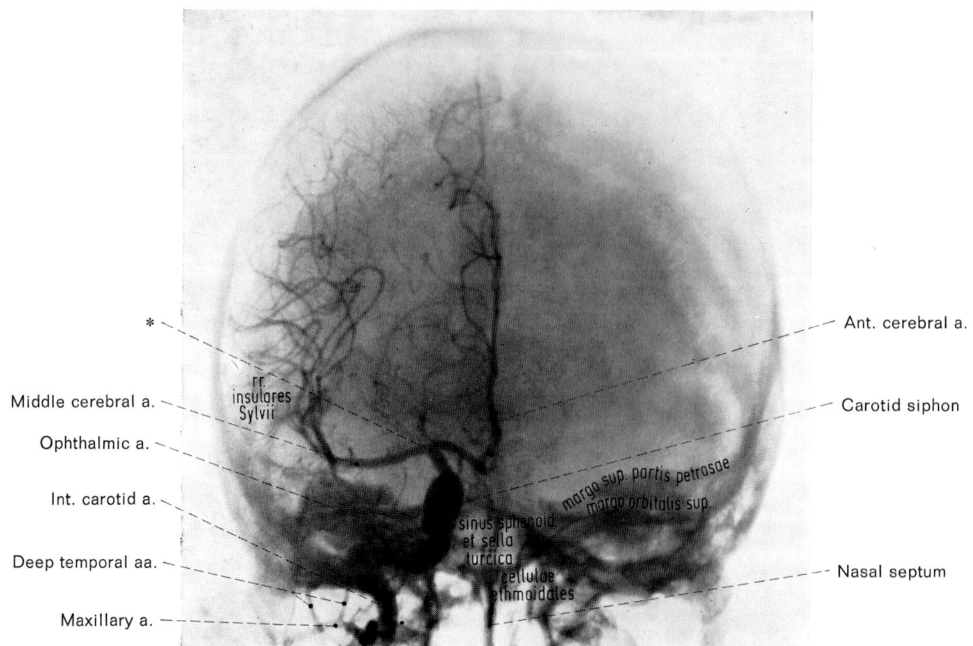
*
Middle cerebral a.
Ophthalmic a.
Int. carotid a.
Deep temporal aa.
Maxillary a.
rr. insulares Sylvii
sinus sphenoid. et sella turcica
cellulae ethmoidales
margo sup. partis petrosae
margo orbitalis sup.
Ant. cerebral a.
Carotid siphon
Nasal septum

Fig. 79. Fronto-occipital arteriogram of the right internal carotid artery and its branches. Note the T-shaped division of the internal carotid into the anterior and middle cerebral arteries. * Bifurcation of the carotid artery.

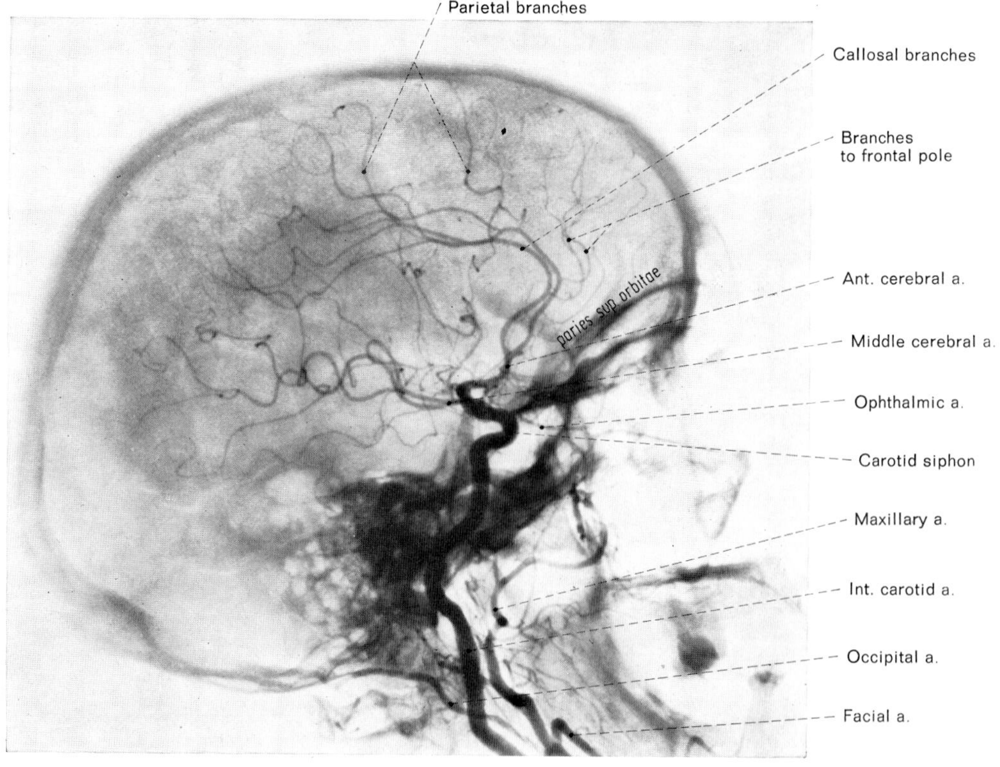
Parietal branches
Callosal branches
Branches to frontal pole
paries sup. orbitae
Ant. cerebral a.
Middle cerebral a.
Ophthalmic a.
Carotid siphon
Maxillary a.
Int. carotid a.
Occipital a.
Facial a.

Fig. 80. Right lateral arteriogram of internal and external carotid arteries.

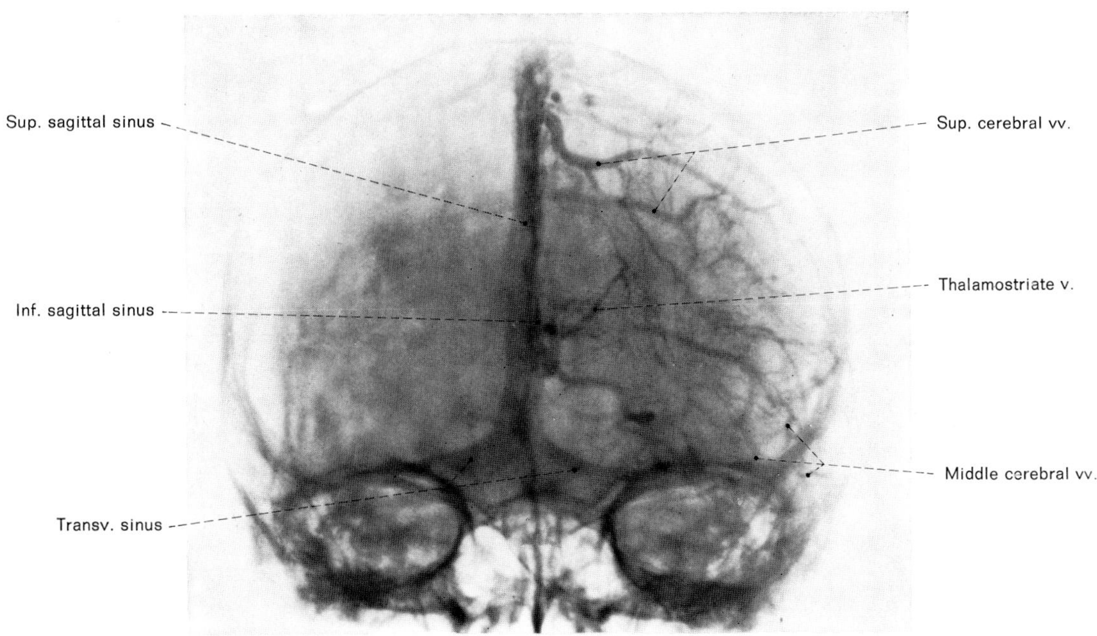
Sup. sagittal sinus
Sup. cerebral vv.
Thalamostriate v.
Inf. sagittal sinus
Middle cerebral vv.
Transv. sinus

Fig. 81. Fronto-occipital phlebogram and sinogram. The superior cerebral veins as well as the superior sagittal sinus and the transverse sinus can be recognized.

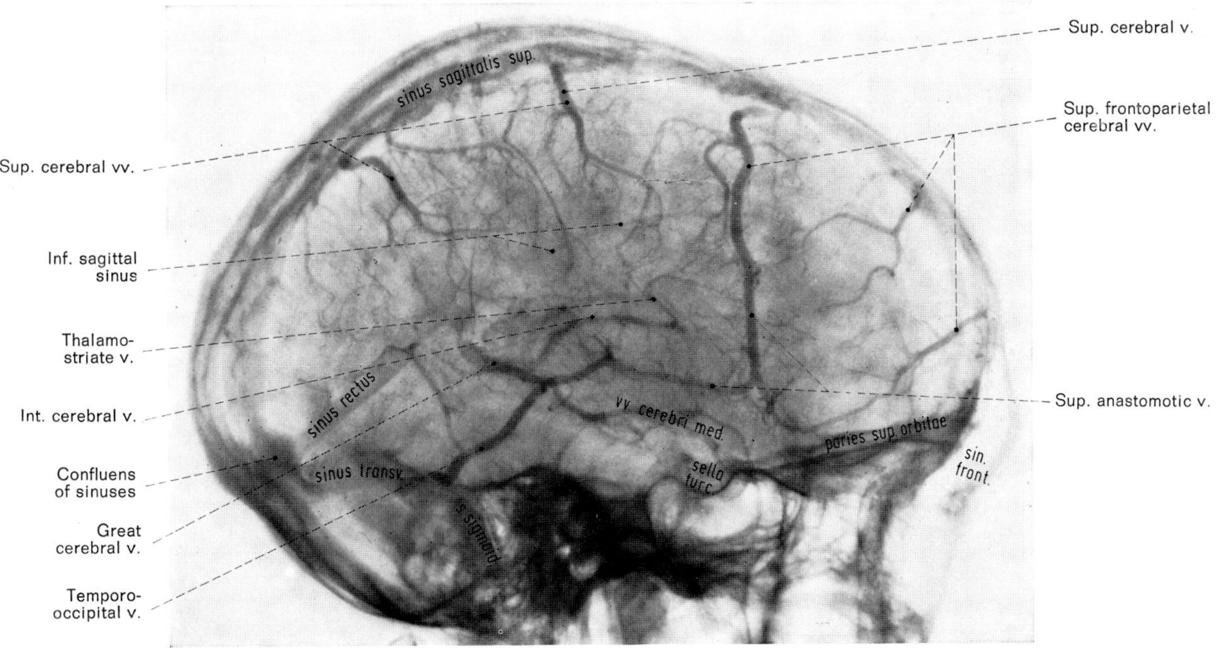
Sup. cerebral v.
sinus sagittalis sup.
Sup. frontoparietal cerebral vv.
Sup. cerebral vv.
Inf. sagittal sinus
Thalamo-striate v.
Sup. anastomotic v.
sinus rectus
vv. cerebri med.
Int. cerebral v.
paries sup. orbitae
sin. front.
Confluens of sinuses
sinus transv.
sella turc.
Great cerebral v.
Temporo-occipital v.

Fig. 82. Right lateral phlebogram and sinogram. Cerebral veins and sinuses of the dura mater.

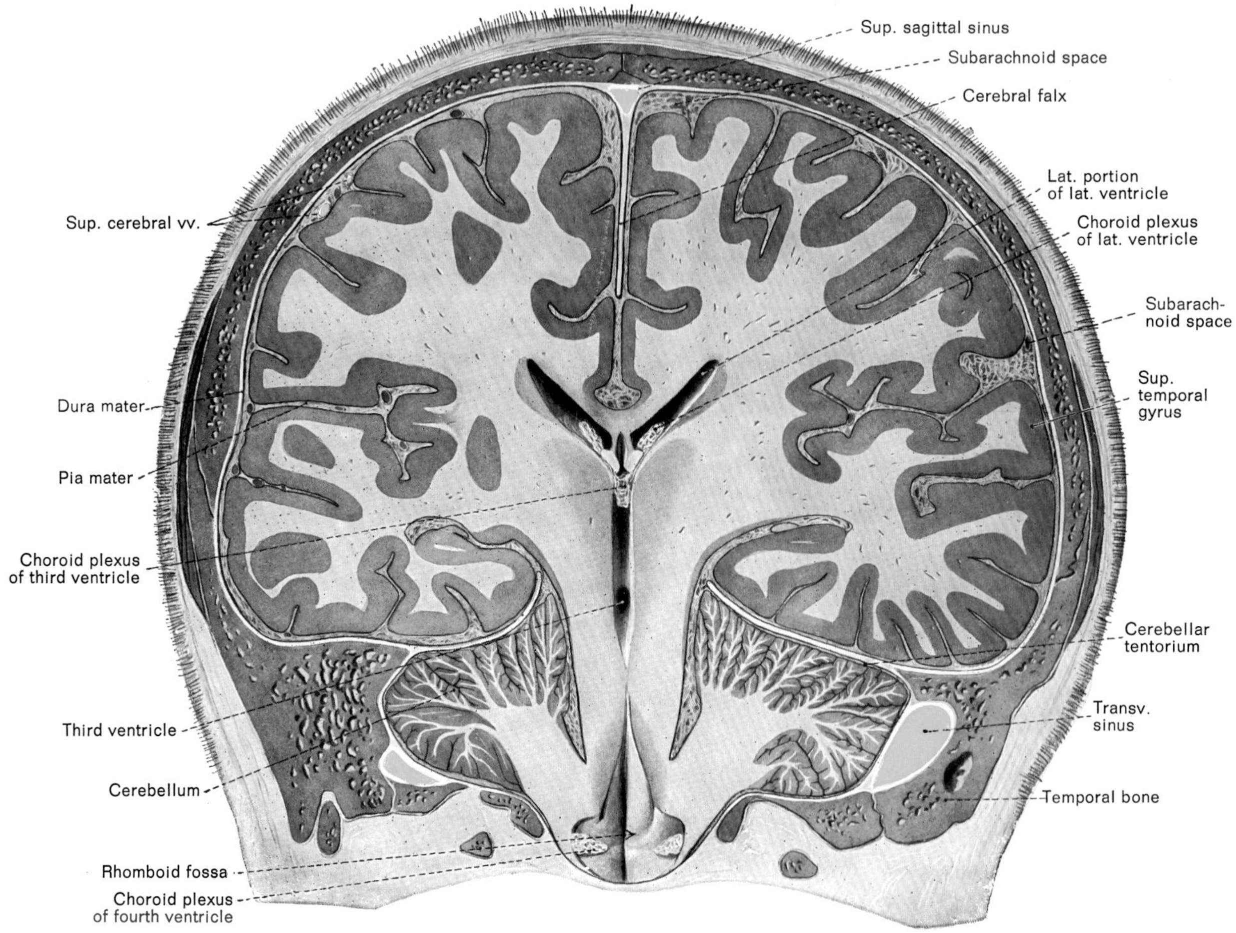

Sup. sagittal sinus
Subarachnoid space
Cerebral falx
Lat. portion of lat. ventricle
Choroid plexus of lat. ventricle
Subarachnoid space
Sup. temporal gyrus
Cerebellar tentorium
Transv. sinus
Temporal bone
Sup. cerebral vv.
Dura mater
Pia mater
Choroid plexus of third ventricle
Third ventricle
Cerebellum
Rhomboid fossa
Choroid plexus of fourth ventricle

Fig. 83. Frontal section through the neurocranium at the plane of the third ventricle. Dura mater white, arachnoid membrane and pia mater red, contents of sinuses and veins blue.

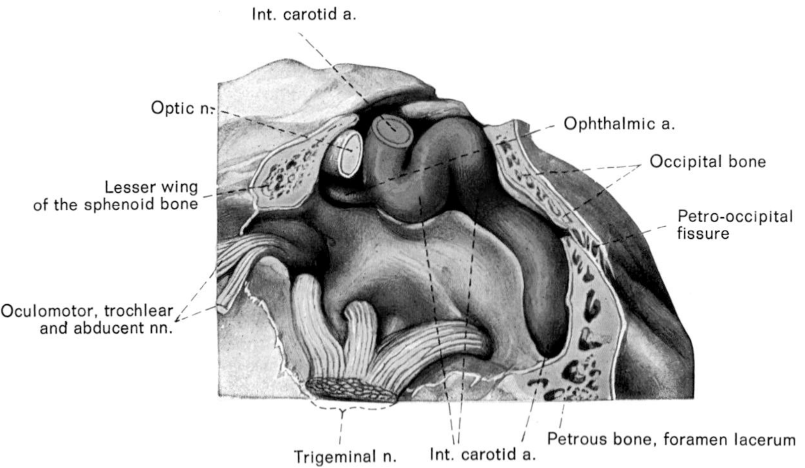
Int. carotid a.
Optic n.
Ophthalmic a.
Occipital bone
Lesser wing of the sphenoid bone
Petro-occipital fissure
Oculomotor, trochlear and abducent nn.
Petrous bone, foramen lacerum
Trigeminal n.
Int. carotid a.

Fig. 84. Intracranial course of the left internal carotid artery. The artery lies in a furrow of the lateral wall of the body of the sphenoid bone. Note the origin of the ophthalmic artery from the "carotid knee" and the S-shaped curve ("carotid siphon") of the carotid artery within the carotid sulcus next to the sella turcica. Trigeminal, oculomotor, trochlear and abducent nerves have been deflected laterally.

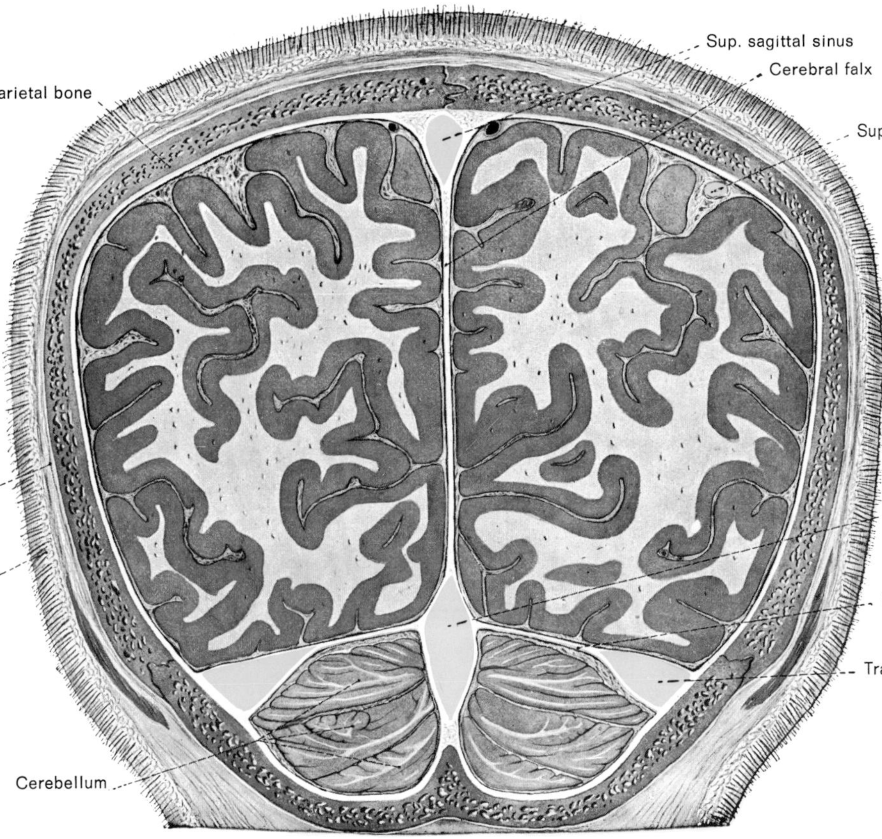

Sup. sagittal sinus
Cerebral falx
Parietal bone
Sup. cerebral v.
Galea aponeurotica
Confluens of the sinuses
Skin
Cerebellar tentorium
Transv. sinus
Cerebellum

Fig. 85. Frontal section through the neurocranium at the plane of the confluens of the sinuses. Color key as in Fig. 83.

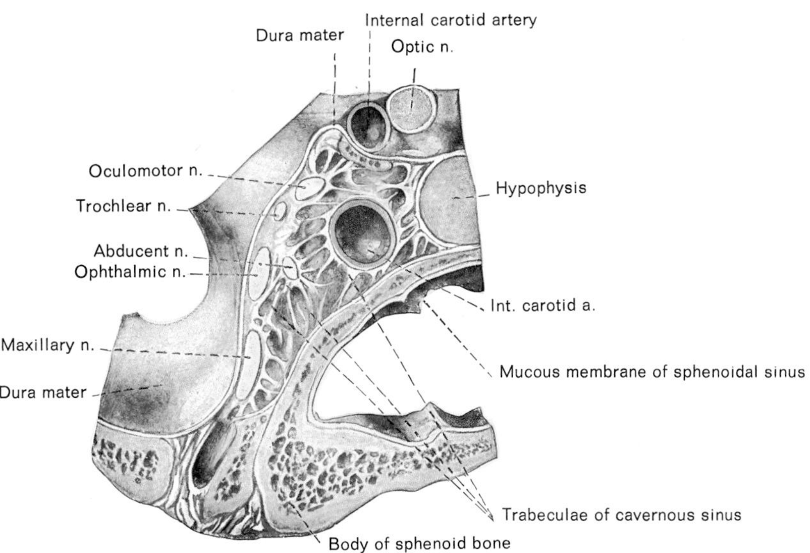
Internal carotid artery
Dura mater
Optic n.
Oculomotor n.
Hypophysis
Trochlear n.
Abducent n.
Ophthalmic n.
Int. carotid a.
Maxillary n.
Mucous membrane of sphenoidal sinus
Dura mater
Trabeculae of cavernous sinus
Body of sphenoid bone

Fig. 86. Frontal section through the left cavernous sinus at the plane of the hypophysis. The internal carotid artery (lower cross section) is surrounded by the venous chambers of the sinus. After forming the "carotid knee", from which the ophthalmic artery arises, the carotid artery penetrates the dura mater and appears below the optic nerve where it enters the optic canal (upper cross section). This segment of the artery is surrounded by cerebrospinal fluid ("cisternal segment"). The carotid cross sections have different diameters because of the origin of the ophthalmic artery.

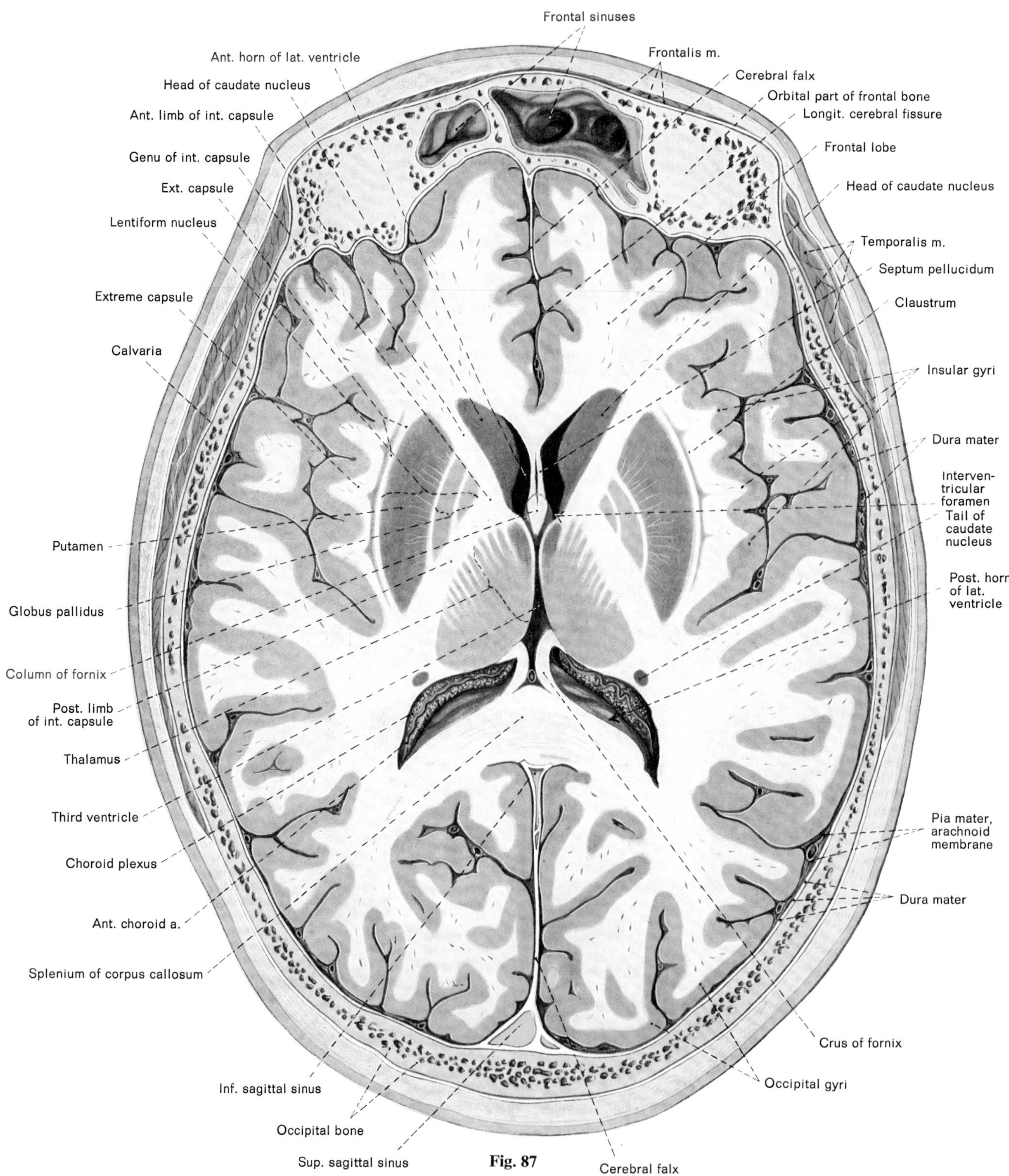

Frontal sinuses
Ant. horn of lat. ventricle
Frontalis m.
Cerebral falx
Head of caudate nucleus
Orbital part of frontal bone
Ant. limb of int. capsule
Longit. cerebral fissure
Frontal lobe
Genu of int. capsule
Ext. capsule
Head of caudate nucleus
Lentiform nucleus
Temporalis m.
Septum pellucidum
Extreme capsule
Claustrum
Calvaria
Insular gyri
Dura mater
Interven-
tricular
foramen
Tail of
caudate
nucleus
Putamen
Post. horn
of lat.
ventricle
Globus pallidus
Column of fornix
Post. limb
of int. capsule
Thalamus
Third ventricle
Pia mater,
arachnoid
membrane
Choroid plexus
Dura mater
Ant. choroid a.
Splenium of corpus callosum
Crus of fornix
Occipital gyri
Inf. sagittal sinus
Occipital bone
Sup. sagittal sinus
Cerebral falx

Fig. 87

Post. commissure, Pineal recess
Choroid plexus of third ventricle, Fornix
Choroid tela of prosencephalon, Diploie of parietal bone
Cerebral falx, Sup. sagittal sinus
Granular foveola
Subarachnoid space, med. aspect
Arachnoid granulations
Suprapineal recess, Cistern of corpus callosum
Dura mater
Ant. commissure
Inf. sagittal sinus
Third ventricle, Interventricular foramen
Sinus rectus
Optic recess
Chiasmatic cistern
Hypophysis
Interpeduncular cistern, Infundibular recess
Great cerebral v., Pineal body, Cerebral aqueduct
Basilar a.
Arbor vitae
Fourth ventricle
Choroid plexus of fourth ventricle, Median aperture
Cerebello-medullary cistern
Central canal

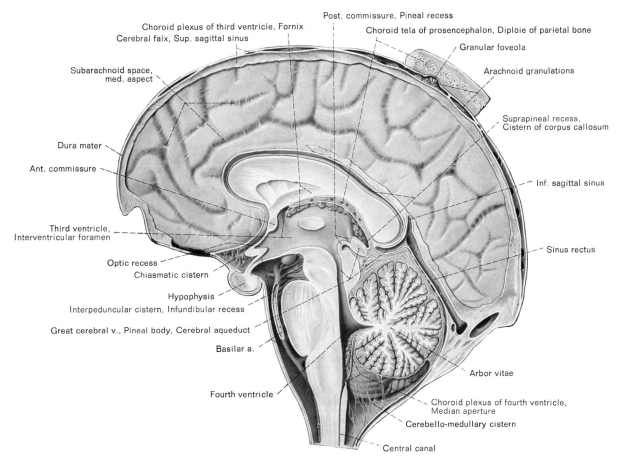

Fig. 88. Paramedian section through the neurocranium. Situs of the brain in the cranial cavity. The cerebrospinal fluid spaces are shown in blue. (From *Pernkopf/Ferner:* Atlas der topographischen und angewandten Anatomie des Menschen, vol. 1, Urban & Schwarzenberg, München–Berlin 1964.)

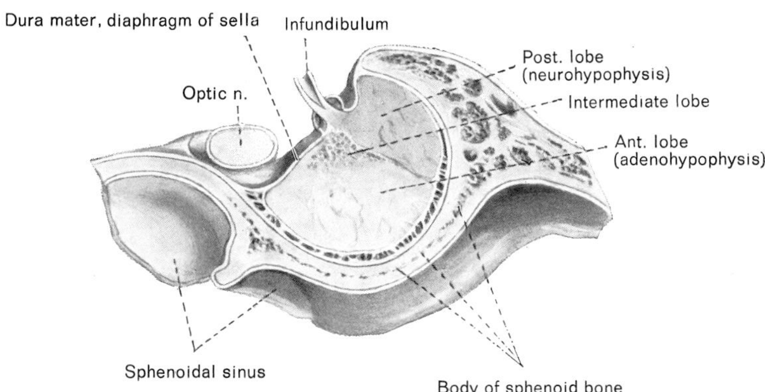
Dura mater, diaphragm of sella
Infundibulum
Post. lobe (neurohypophysis)
Optic n.
Intermediate lobe
Ant. lobe (adenohypophysis)
Sphenoidal sinus
Body of sphenoid bone

Fig. 87. Horizontal section through the neurocranium at the level of the basal ganglia. Situs of the brain in the cranial cavity.

Fig. 89. Paramedian section through the hypophysis. Situs of the hypophysis in the sella turcica.

Central Nervous System

Spinal Cord, Spinal Nerves

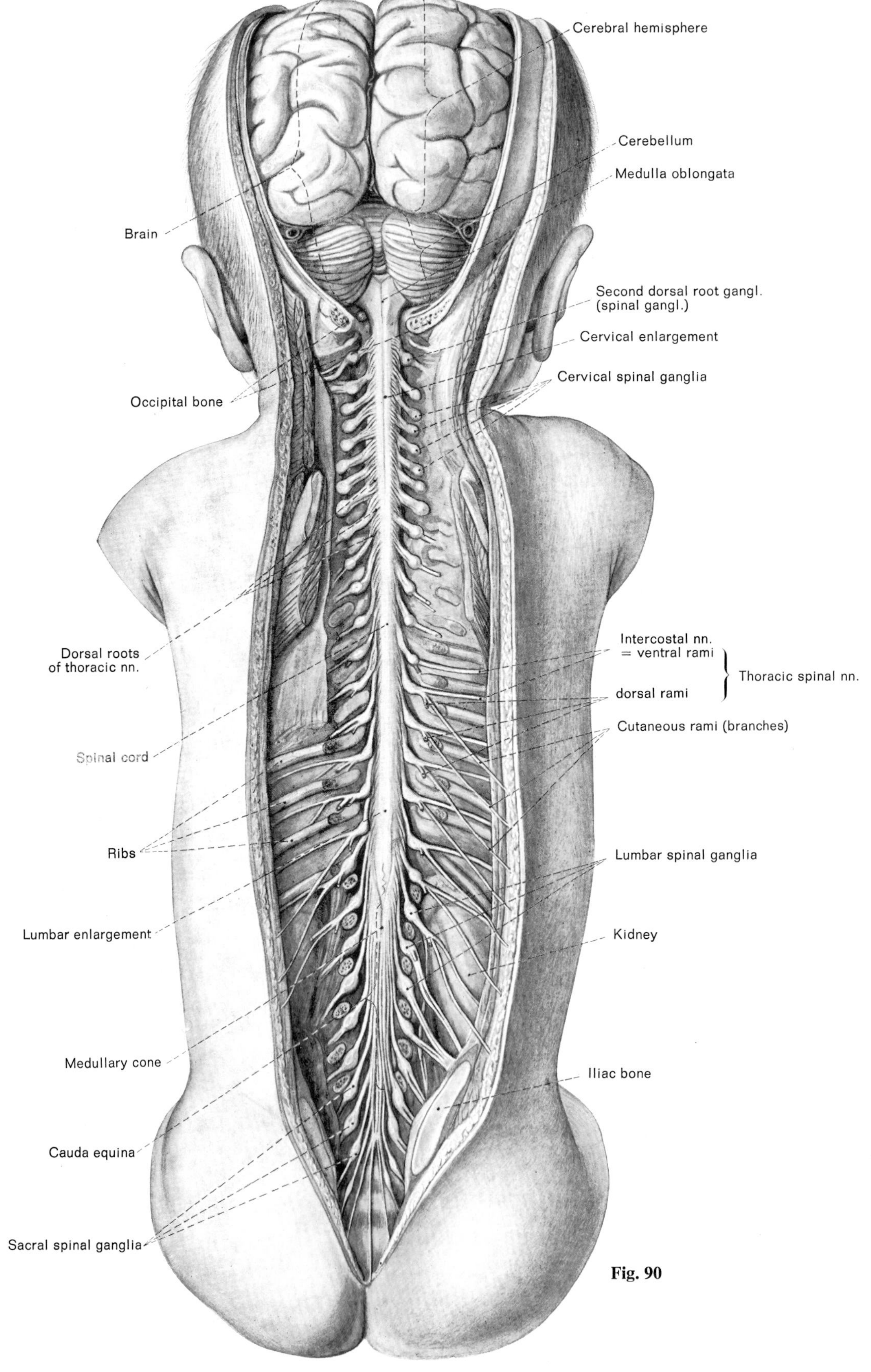

Cerebral hemisphere
Cerebellum
Medulla oblongata
Brain
Second dorsal root gangl. (spinal gangl.)
Cervical enlargement
Cervical spinal ganglia
Occipital bone
Dorsal roots of thoracic nn.
Intercostal nn. = ventral rami
dorsal rami
Thoracic spinal nn.
Cutaneous rami (branches)
Spinal cord
Ribs
Lumbar spinal ganglia
Lumbar enlargement
Kidney
Medullary cone
Iliac bone
Cauda equina
Sacral spinal ganglia

Fig. 90

Fig. 90. Central nervous system of a newborn. Dorsal view. Skin and musculature of the back, neural arches of the vertebrae and cranial vault partially removed. Dura mater completely removed.

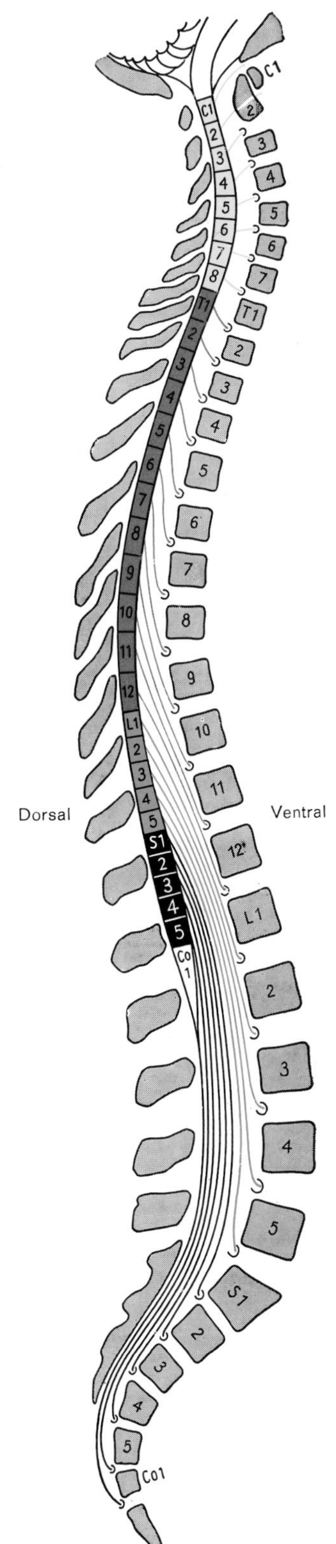

Dorsal
Ventral
C1

Fig. 91. Situs of the spinal cord in the vertebral canal and the origin of nerve roots (lateral view). Various segments are marked by transverse lines. Note the shifting of the origins of spinal nerve roots from their segments relative to their exiting points through the intervertebral foramina. Shift of the vertebral against the neural segments. The spinal cord of the adult terminates at the level of the second lumbar vertebra. Yellow: cervical segments C 1–8; red: thoracic segments T 1–12; blue: lumbar segments L 1–5; black: sacral segments S 1–5; white: coccygeal segment Co 1.

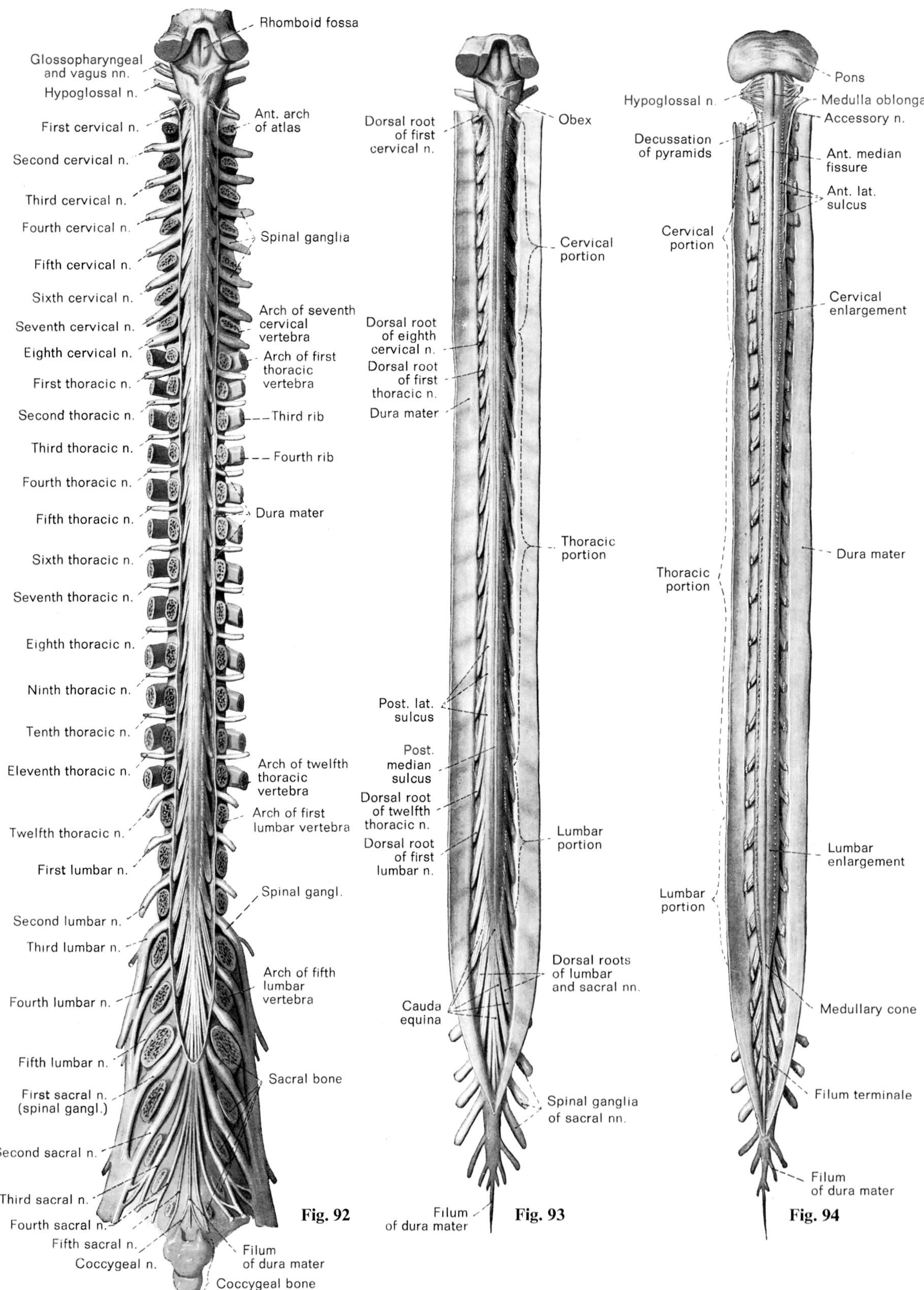

Rhomboid fossa
Glossopharyngeal and vagus nn.
Hypoglossal n.
First cervical n.
Ant. arch of atlas
Second cervical n.
Third cervical n.
Fourth cervical n.
Spinal ganglia
Fifth cervical n.
Sixth cervical n.
Arch of seventh cervical vertebra
Seventh cervical n.
Eighth cervical n.
Arch of first thoracic vertebra
First thoracic n.
Second thoracic n.
Third rib
Third thoracic n.
Fourth rib
Fourth thoracic n.
Fifth thoracic n.
Dura mater
Sixth thoracic n.
Seventh thoracic n.
Eighth thoracic n.
Ninth thoracic n.
Tenth thoracic n.
Eleventh thoracic n.
Arch of twelfth thoracic vertebra
Twelfth thoracic n.
Arch of first lumbar vertebra
First lumbar n.
Spinal gangl.
Second lumbar n.
Third lumbar n.
Fourth lumbar n.
Arch of fifth lumbar vertebra
Fifth lumbar n.
Sacral bone
First sacral n. (spinal gangl.)
Second sacral n.
Third sacral n.
Fourth sacral n.
Fifth sacral n.
Coccygeal n.
Filum of dura mater
Coccygeal bone
Dorsal root of first cervical n.
Obex
Cervical portion
Dorsal root of eighth cervical n.
Dorsal root of first thoracic n.
Dura mater
Thoracic portion
Post. lat. sulcus
Post. median sulcus
Dorsal root of twelfth thoracic n.
Dorsal root of first lumbar n.
Lumbar portion
Dorsal roots of lumbar and sacral nn.
Cauda equina
Spinal ganglia of sacral nn.
Filum of dura mater
Pons
Hypoglossal n.
Medulla oblongata
Accessory n.
Decussation of pyramids
Ant. median fissure
Ant. lat. sulcus
Cervical portion
Cervical enlargement
Dura mater
Thoracic portion
Lumbar enlargement
Lumbar portion
Medullary cone
Filum terminale
Filum of dura mater

Fig. 92

Fig. 93

Fig. 94

Fig. 92. Spinal cord within the vertebral canal, dorsal view. Neural arches and dura mater have been partially removed. Bones shown in yellow.

Fig. 93. Spinal cord and root of spinal nerves, dorsal view. Dura mater split longitudinally and reflected.

Fig. 94. Spinal cord, ventral view. Dura mater split longitudinally. The anterior roots of spinal nerves are severed at their origin from the spinal cord; the dorsal roots are seen from ventral.

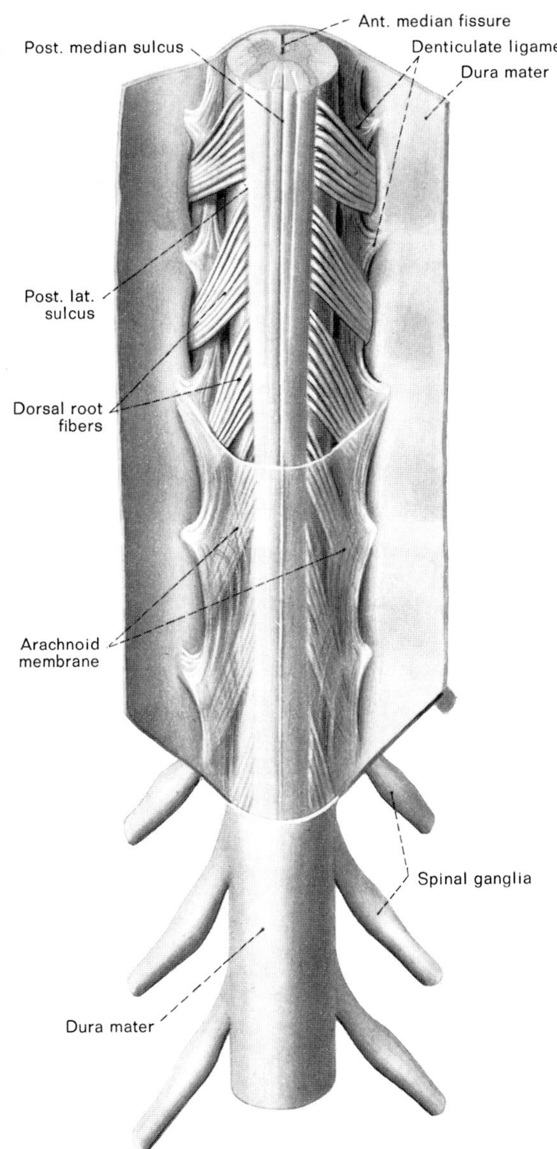
Ant. median fissure
Post. median sulcus
Denticulate ligament
Dura mater
Post. lat. sulcus
Dorsal root fibers
Arachnoid membrane
Spinal ganglia
Dura mater

Fig. 95. Spinal cord and meninges, dorsal view. In the lower third the dura mater is shown in its normal configuration; in the upper third the arachnoid membrane has been removed.

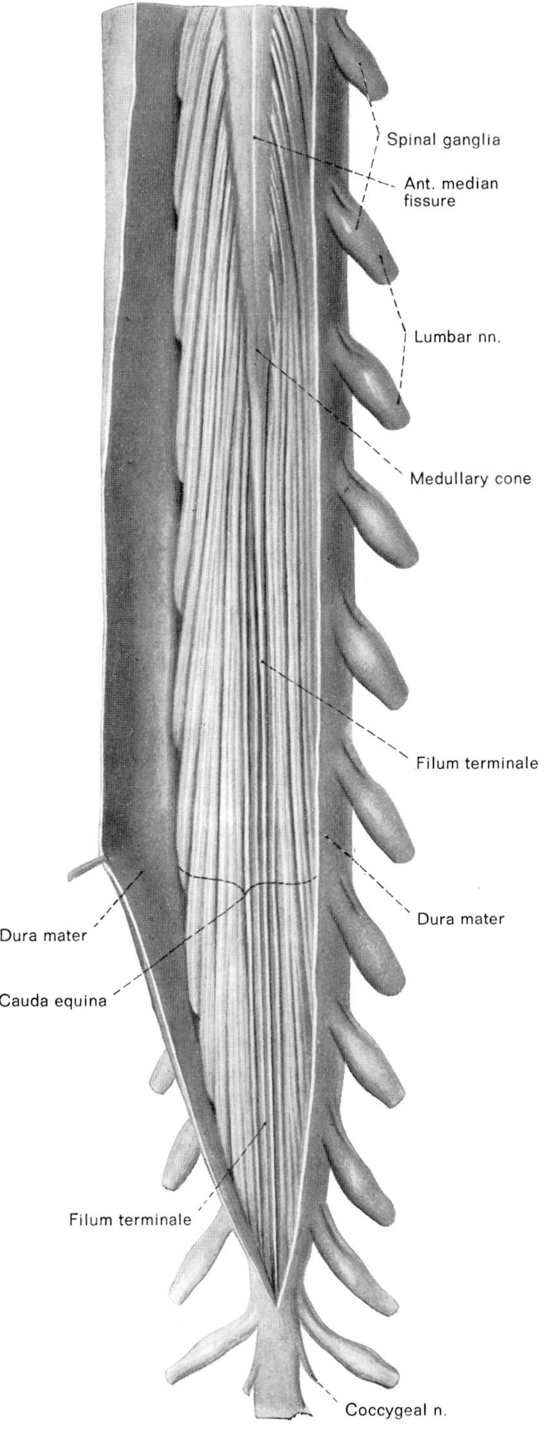
Spinal ganglia
Ant. median fissure
Lumbar nn.
Medullary cone
Filum terminale
Dura mater
Dura mater
Cauda equina
Filum terminale
Coccygeal n.

Fig. 96. Caudal portion of the spinal cord, ventral view. Dura mater opened longitudinally. Cauda equina = ventral and dorsal root fibers of the lumbar and sacral spinal nerves.

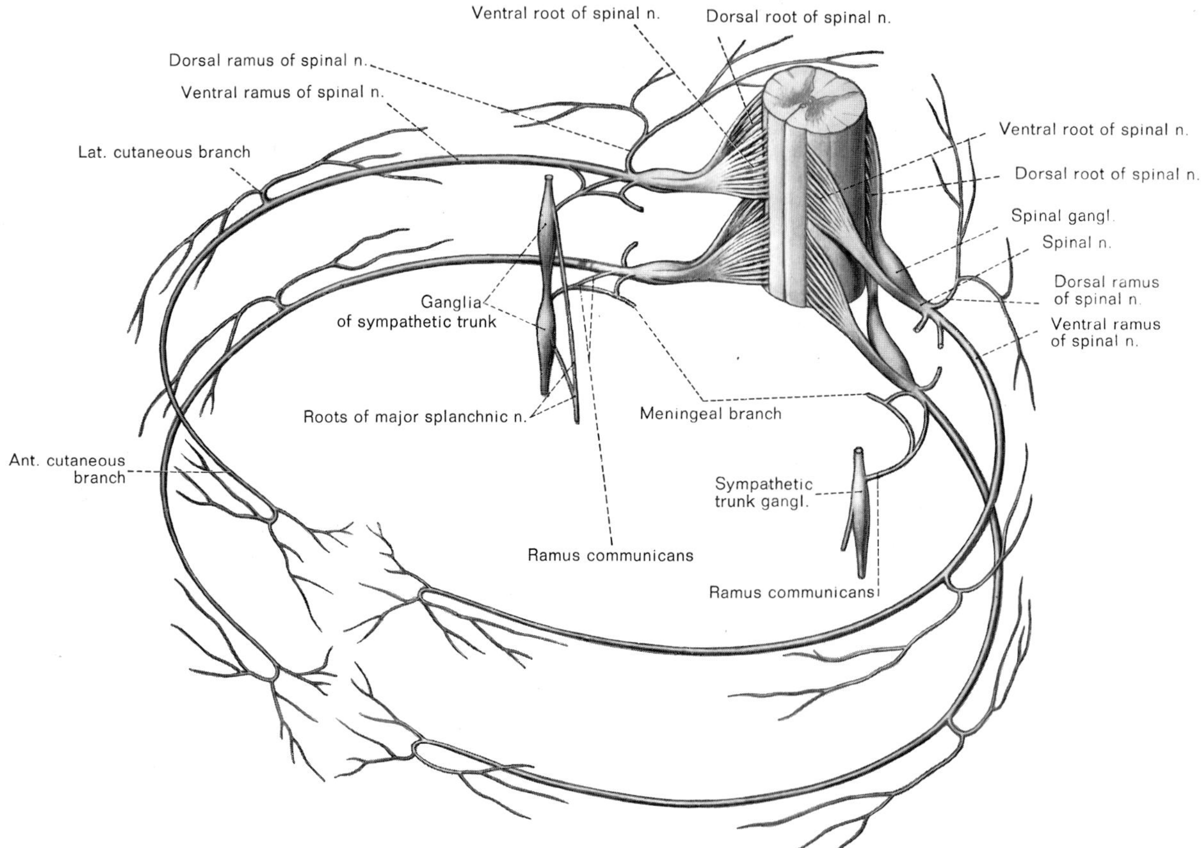
Ventral root of spinal n.
Dorsal root of spinal n.
Dorsal ramus of spinal n.
Ventral ramus of spinal n.
Lat. cutaneous branch
Ventral root of spinal n.
Dorsal root of spinal n.
Spinal gangl.
Spinal n.
Dorsal ramus of spinal n.
Ventral ramus of spinal n.
Ganglia of sympathetic trunk
Roots of major splanchnic n.
Meningeal branch
Ant. cutaneous branch
Sympathetic trunk gangl.
Ramus communicans
Ramus communicans

Fig. 97. Formation and ramification of spinal nerves in the thoracic region (Th 1–Th 12) and their connections with the sympathetic trunk, exemplified with two spinal cord segments. One spinal nerve is formed by the union of a ventral motor root with a dorsal sensory root. The roots are composed of radicular fibers. The perikarya of the ventral roots are located in the anterior horns of the spinal cord, those of the dorsal roots in the spinal ganglia.

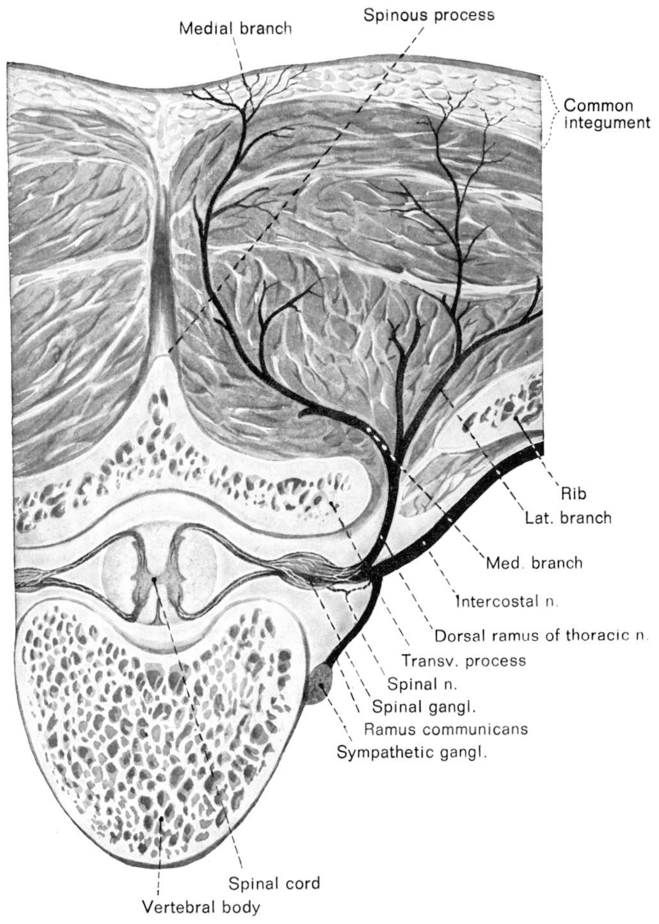
Medial branch
Spinous process
Common integument
Rib
Lat. branch
Med. branch
Intercostal n.
Dorsal ramus of thoracic n.
Transv. process
Spinal n.
Spinal gangl.
Ramus communicans
Sympathetic gangl.
Spinal cord
Vertebral body

Fig. 98. Schematic representation of a spinal nerve and its branches in the thoracic region.

Note: The mixed spinal nerve containing motor and sensory fibers gives rise to a ventral and dorsal ramus. The dorsal ramus supplies the antochthonous musculature and skin of the back. The ventral ramus, in the thoracic area, is identical with the intercostal nerve. It supplies the intercostal muscles and sends sensory fibers to the lateral and anterior thoracic wall in segmental arrangements (dermatomes; compare Figs. 99 and 100). Due to the inclination of the ribs the dermatomes are inclined from dorsal to ventral. For example, the dermatome of the tenth intercostal nerve reaches to the umbilical area. The ventral rami of the cervical, lumbar and sacral segments form plexuses (compare Figs. 105 and 106), so that here the peripheral innervation does not correspond any more to the segmental origin of nerve roots.

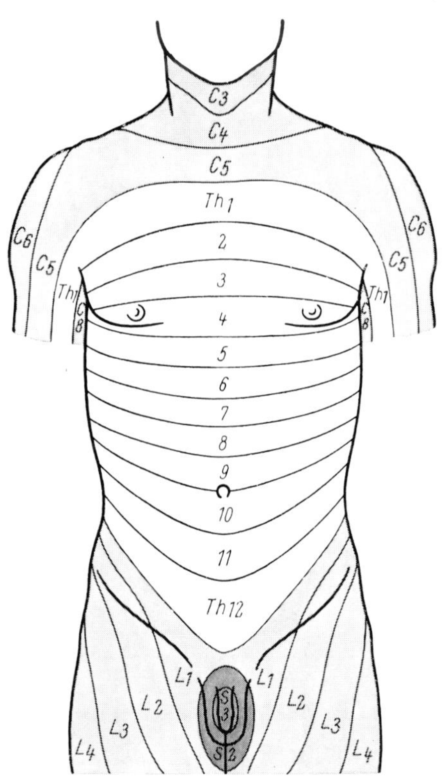
C3
C4
C5
Th1
2
3
4
5
6
7
8
9
10
11
Th12
C6
C5
Th1
C8
L1
L2
L3
L4
S3
S2

Fig. 99. Segmental distribution of dermatomes on the anterior body wall.

Fig. 101. Segmental distribution of dermatomes on the upper extremity. Palmar view.

Fig. 102. Segmental distribution of dermatomes on the upper extremity. Dorsal view.

Fig. 100. Segmental distribution of dermatomes on the dorsal body wall.

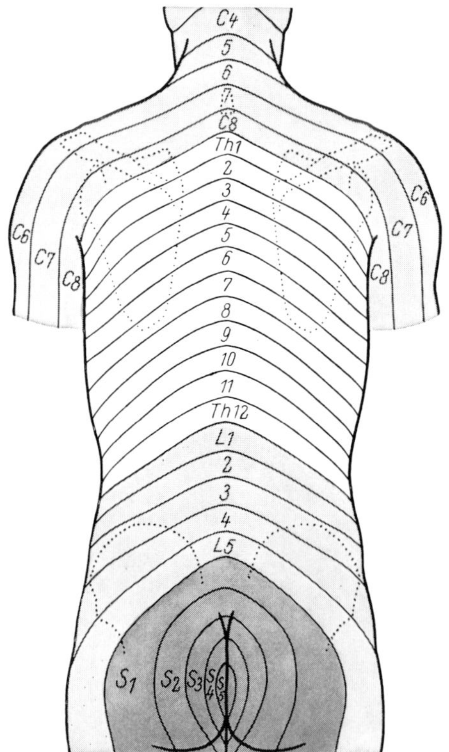
C4
5
6
7
C8
Th1
2
3
4
5
6
7
8
9
10
11
Th12
L1
2
3
4
L5
C6
C7
C8
S1
S2
S3
S4
S5

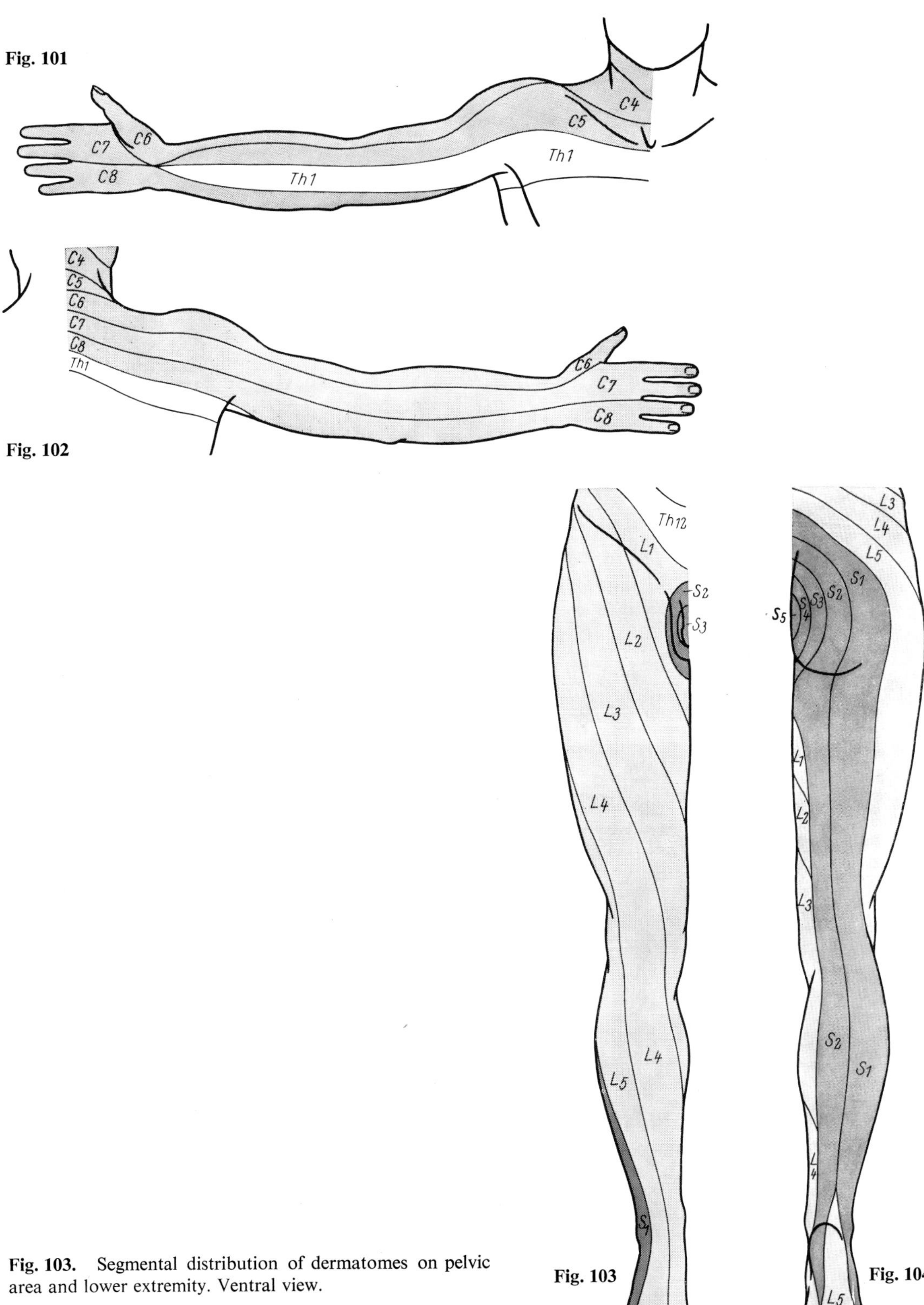
Fig. 101
C4
C5
C6
C7
C8
Th1
Th1
Fig. 102
C4
C5
C6
C7
C8
Th1
C6
C7
C8
Th12
L1
S2
S3
L2
L3
L4
L4
L5
S1
Fig. 103
L3
L4
L5
S1
S2
S3
S4
S5
L1
L2
L3
S2
S1
L4
L5
L4
Fig. 104

Fig. 103. Segmental distribution of dermatomes on pelvic area and lower extremity. Ventral view.

Fig. 104. Segmental distribution of dermatomes on pelvic area and lower extremity. Dorsal view.

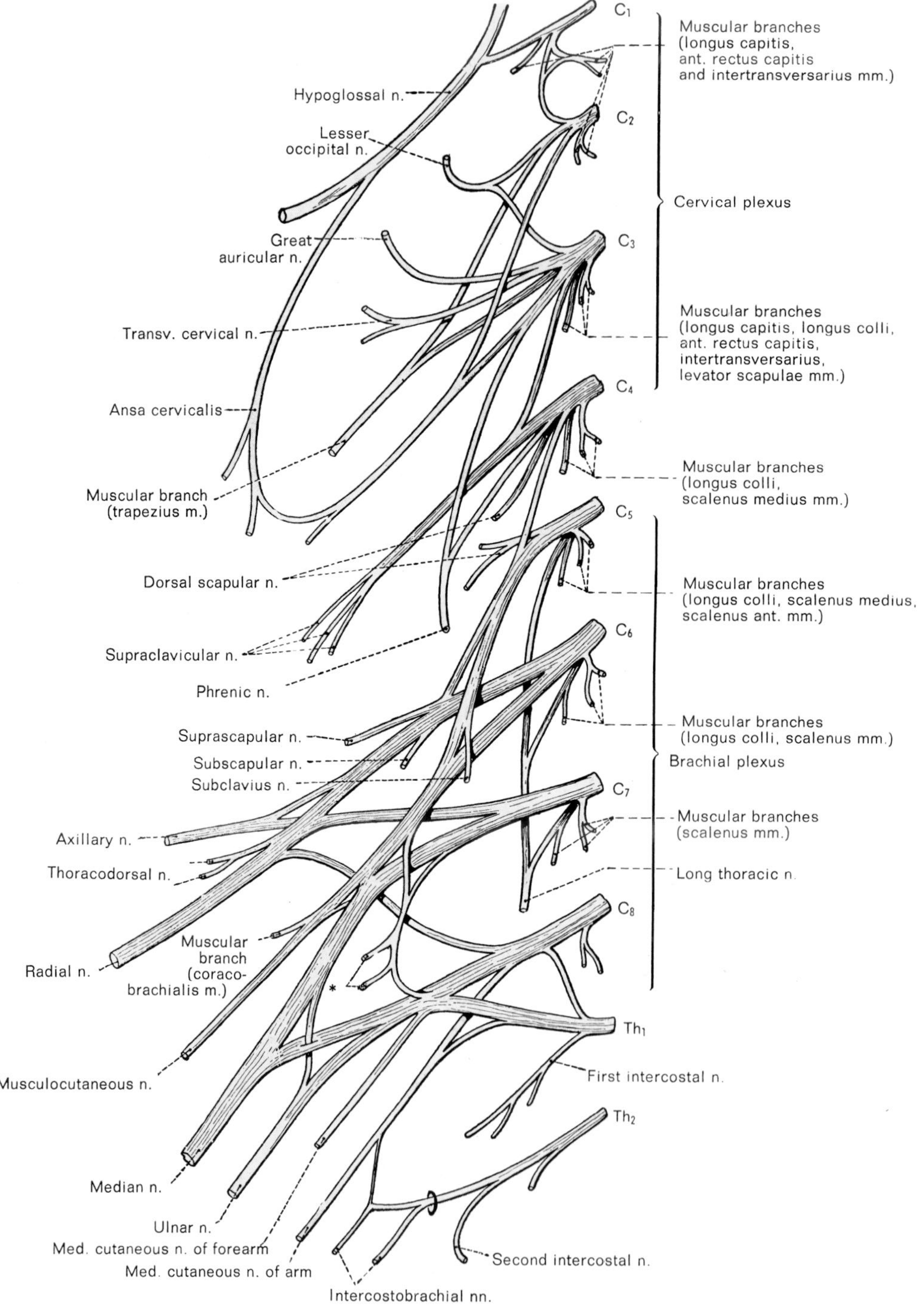
C1
Muscular branches
(longus capitis,
ant. rectus capitis
and intertransversarius mm.)
Hypoglossal n.
C2
Lesser
occipital n.
Cervical plexus
Great
auricular n.
C3
Muscular branches
(longus capitis, longus colli,
ant. rectus capitis,
intertransversarius,
levator scapulae mm.)
Transv. cervical n.
C4
Ansa cervicalis
Muscular branches
(longus colli,
scalenus medius mm.)
Muscular branch
(trapezius m.)
C5
Dorsal scapular n.
Muscular branches
(longus colli, scalenus medius,
scalenus ant. mm.)
C6
Supraclavicular n.
Phrenic n.
Muscular branches
(longus colli, scalenus mm.)
Suprascapular n.
Brachial plexus
Subscapular n.
Subclavius n.
C7
Muscular branches
(scalenus mm.)
Axillary n.
Thoracodorsal n.
Long thoracic n.
C8
Muscular
branch
(coraco-
brachialis m.)
Radial n.
*
Th1
Musculocutaneous n.
First intercostal n.
Th2
Median n.
Ulnar n.
Med. cutaneous n. of forearm
Med. cutaneous n. of arm
Second intercostal n.
Intercostobrachial nn.

Fig. 105. Schematic representation of the cervical and brachial plexuses (after *P. Eisler*). The cervical, brachial and lumbosacral nerve plexuses are formed by the union of the anterior rami of the spinal nerves. They subserve especially the motor and sensory innervation of the limbs. * Muscular branches (pectoralis major muscle).

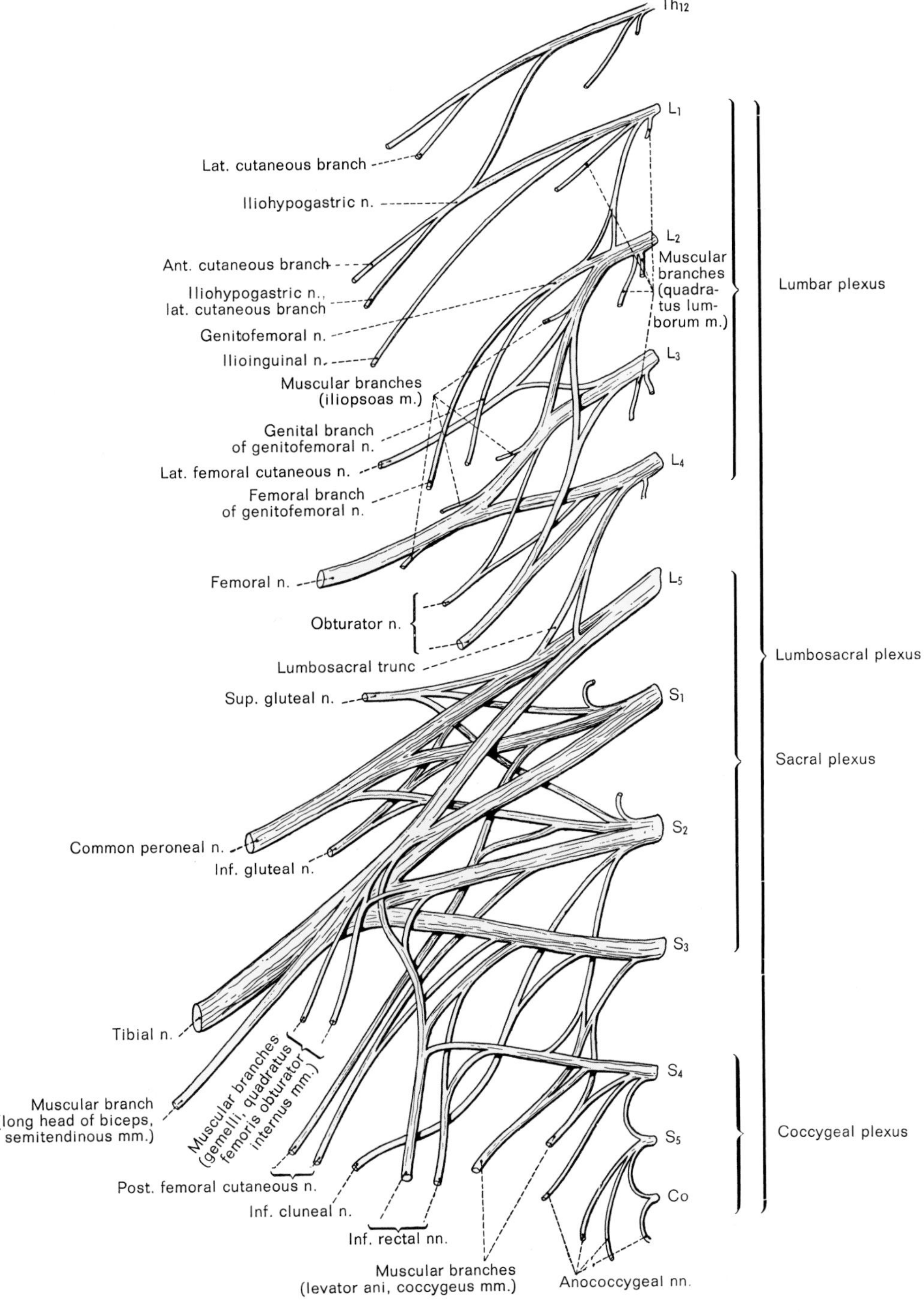

Th12
L1
L2
L3
L4
L5
S1
S2
S3
S4
S5
Co
Lat. cutaneous branch
Iliohypogastric n.
Ant. cutaneous branch
Iliohypogastric n., lat. cutaneous branch
Genitofemoral n.
Ilioinguinal n.
Muscular branches (iliopsoas m.)
Genital branch of genitofemoral n.
Lat. femoral cutaneous n.
Femoral branch of genitofemoral n.
Femoral n.
Obturator n.
Lumbosacral trunc
Sup. gluteal n.
Common peroneal n.
Inf. gluteal n.
Tibial n.
Muscular branch (long head of biceps, semitendinous mm.)
Muscular branches (gemelli, quadratus femoris obturator internus mm.)
Post. femoral cutaneous n.
Inf. cluneal n.
Inf. rectal nn.
Muscular branches (levator ani, coccygeus mm.)
Anococcygeal nn.
Muscular branches (quadratus lumborum m.)
Lumbar plexus
Lumbosacral plexus
Sacral plexus
Coccygeal plexus

Fig. 106. Schematic representation of lumbar, sacral and coccygeal plexuses (after *P. Eisler*).

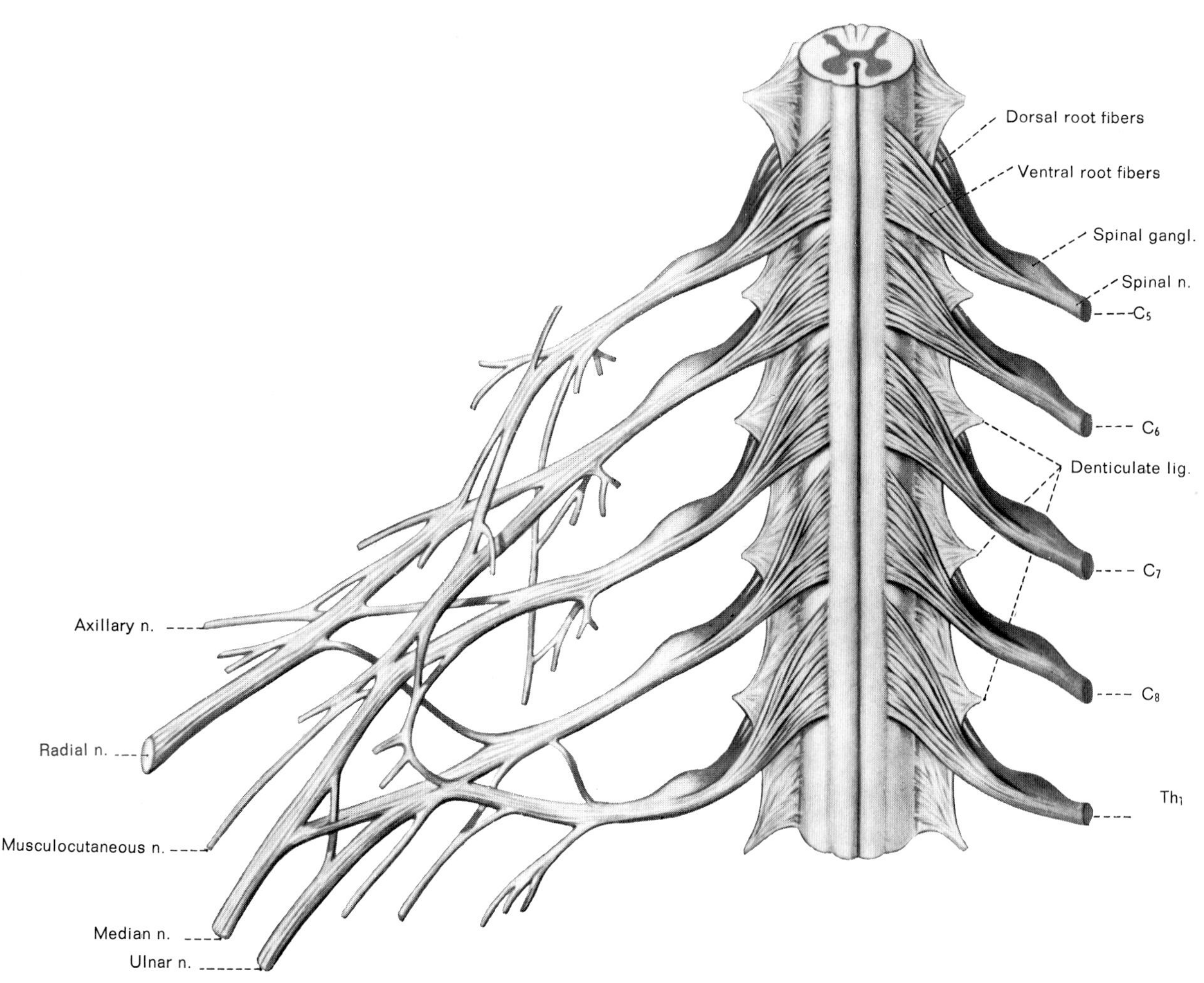
Dorsal root fibers
Ventral root fibers
Spinal gangl.
Spinal n.
C5
C6
Denticulate lig.
C7
C8
Th1
Axillary n.
Radial n.
Musculocutaneous n.
Median n.
Ulnar n.

Fig. 107. Formation of plexuses of spinal nerves, exemplified by the brachial plexus from C 5–Th 1. Ventral view. C = cervical segments; Th = thoracic segment.

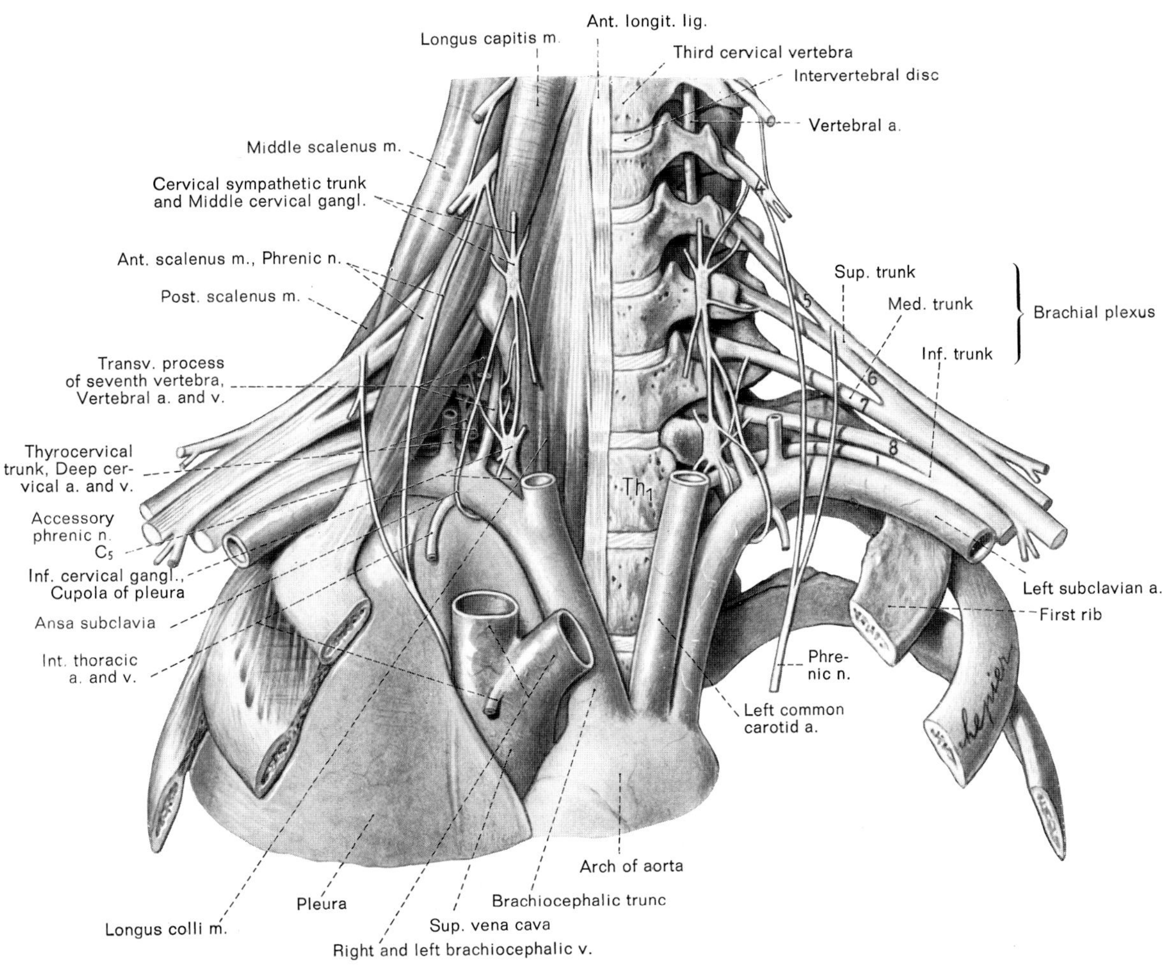
Ant. longit. lig.
Longus capitis m.
Third cervical vertebra
Intervertebral disc
Vertebral a.
Middle scalenus m.
Cervical sympathetic trunk and Middle cervical gangl.
Ant. scalenus m., Phrenic n.
Post. scalenus m.
Sup. trunk
Med. trunk
Inf. trunk
Brachial plexus
Transv. process of seventh vertebra, Vertebral a. and v.
Thyrocervical trunk, Deep cervical a. and v.
Accessory phrenic n.
C_5
Th$_1$
Inf. cervical gangl., Cupola of pleura
Ansa subclavia
Int. thoracic a. and v.
Left subclavian a.
First rib
Phrenic n.
Left common carotid a.
Arch of aorta
Brachiocephalic trunc
Pleura
Longus colli m.
Sup. vena cava
Right and left brachiocephalic v.

Fig. 108. Brachial and cervical plexuses and their relationships to the vertebral column (left), to the regional musculature (right), to structures in the upper thoracic aperture and to the sympathetic trunc.

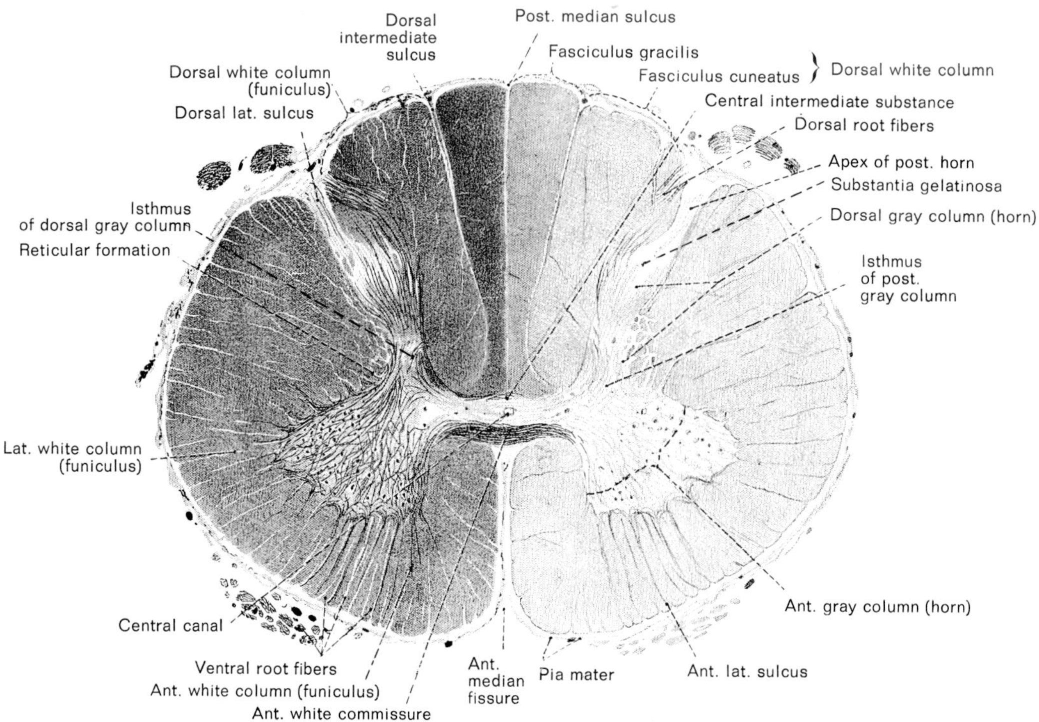
Dorsal
intermediate
sulcus
Post. median sulcus
Fasciculus gracilis
Fasciculus cuneatus
Dorsal white column
Dorsal white column
(funiculus)
Dorsal lat. sulcus
Central intermediate substance
Dorsal root fibers
Apex of post. horn
Substantia gelatinosa
Isthmus
of dorsal gray column
Dorsal gray column (horn)
Reticular formation
Isthmus
of post.
gray column
Lat. white column
(funiculus)
Ant. gray column (horn)
Central canal
Ventral root fibers
Ant. white column (funiculus)
Ant. white commissure
Ant.
median
fissure
Pia mater
Ant. lat. sulcus

Fig. 109. Cross section through the spinal cord at the level of the cervical enlargement.

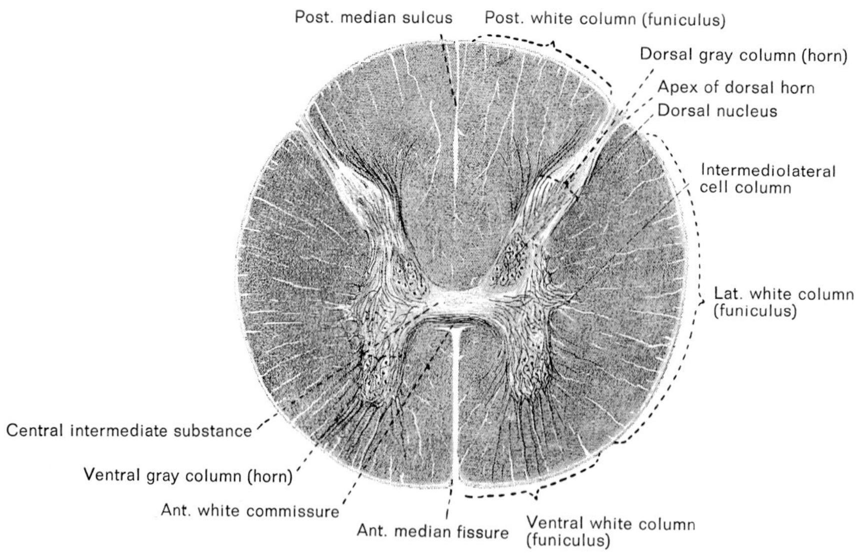
Post. median sulcus
Post. white column (funiculus)
Dorsal gray column (horn)
Apex of dorsal horn
Dorsal nucleus
Intermediolateral
cell column
Lat. white column
(funiculus)
Central intermediate substance
Ventral gray column (horn)
Ant. white commissure
Ant. median fissure
Ventral white column
(funiculus)

Fig. 110. Cross section through the spinal cord, thoracic region.

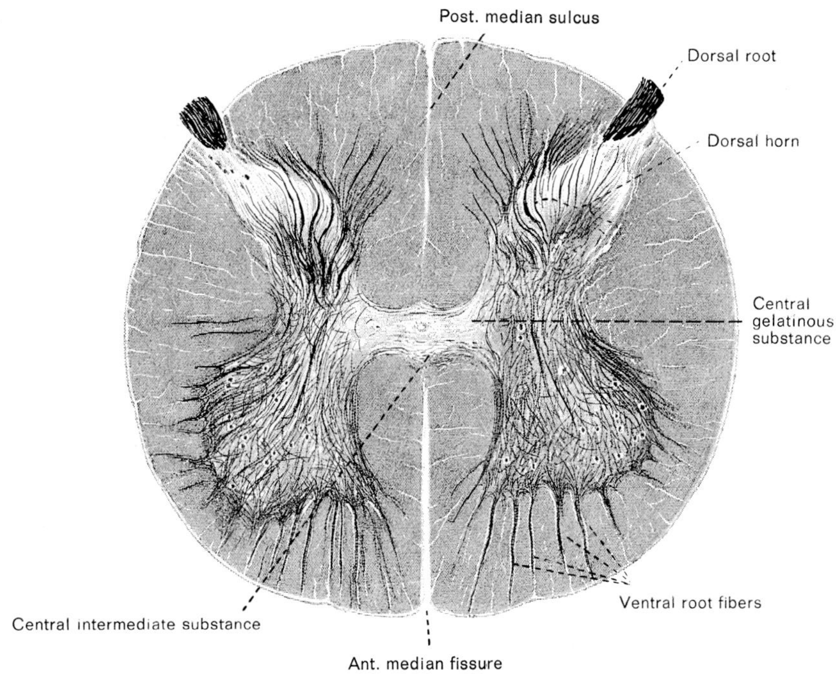
Post. median sulcus
Dorsal root
Dorsal horn
Central gelatinous substance
Ventral root fibers
Central intermediate substance
Ant. median fissure

Fig. 111. Cross section through the spinal cord at the level of the lumbar enlargement.

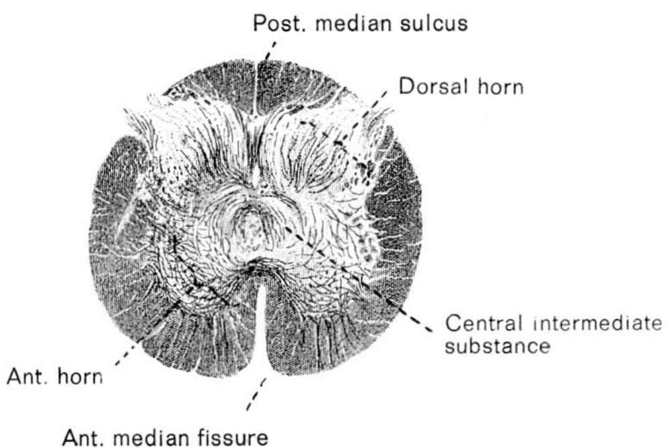
Post. median sulcus
Dorsal horn
Central intermediate substance
Ant. horn
Ant. median fissure

Fig. 112. Cross section through the spinal cord at the level of the medullary cone.

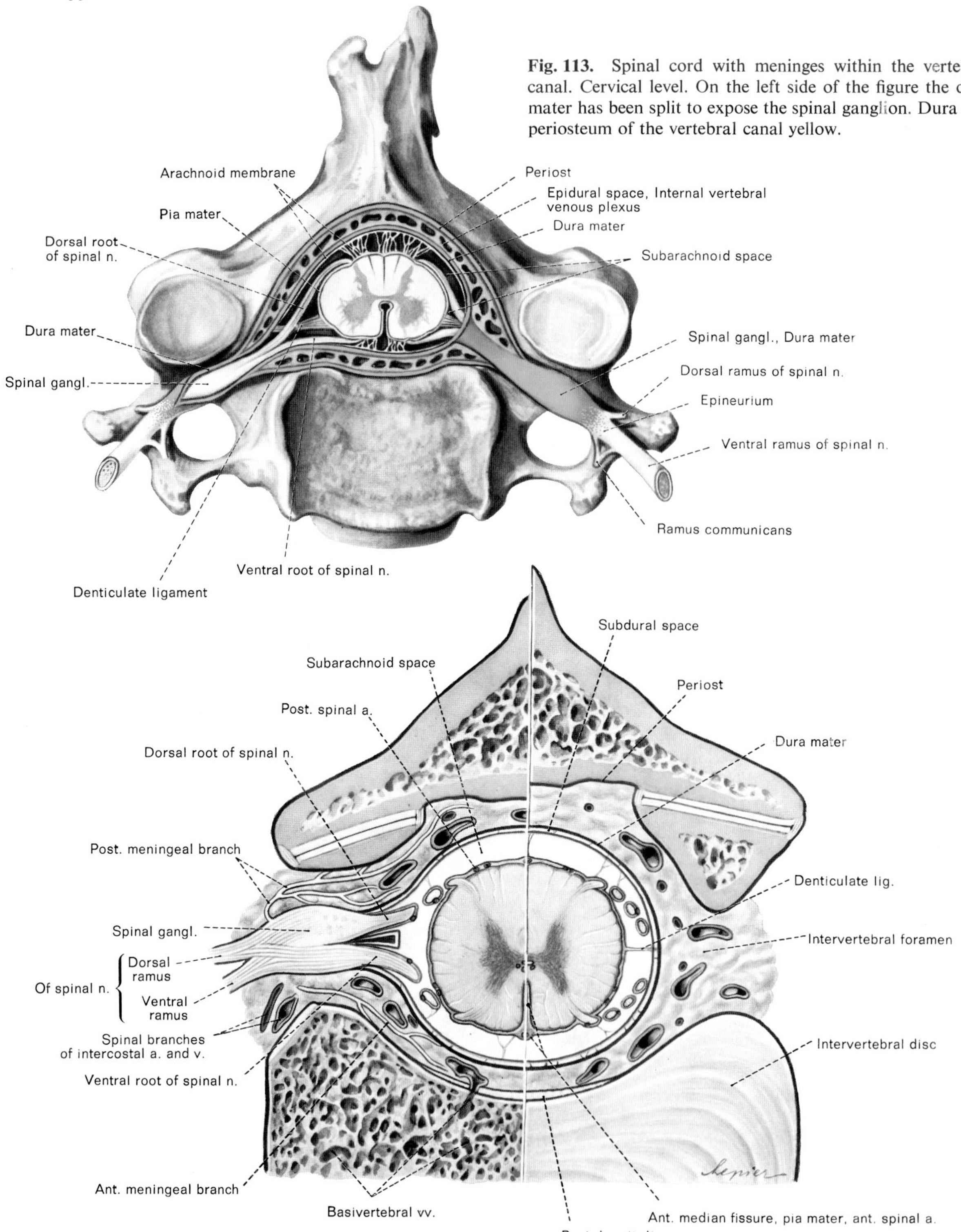
Arachnoid membrane
Pia mater
Dorsal root of spinal n.
Dura mater
Spinal gangl.
Periost
Epidural space, Internal vertebral venous plexus
Dura mater
Subarachnoid space
Spinal gangl., Dura mater
Dorsal ramus of spinal n.
Epineurium
Ventral ramus of spinal n.
Ramus communicans
Ventral root of spinal n.
Denticulate ligament
Subdural space
Subarachnoid space
Periost
Post. spinal a.
Dura mater
Dorsal root of spinal n.
Post. meningeal branch
Denticulate lig.
Spinal gangl.
Intervertebral foramen
Of spinal n.
Dorsal ramus
Ventral ramus
Spinal branches of intercostal a. and v.
Intervertebral disc
Ventral root of spinal n.
Ant. meningeal branch
Basivertebral vv.
Ant. median fissure, pia mater, ant. spinal a.
Post. longit. lig.

Fig. 113. Spinal cord with meninges within the vertebral canal. Cervical level. On the left side of the figure the dura mater has been split to expose the spinal ganglion. Dura and periosteum of the vertebral canal yellow.

Fig. 114. Contents of the vertebral canal at a thoracic level. On the right side the cross section passes through an intervertebral disc, on the left through a vertebral body. Dura mater black, arachnoid membrane red, pia mater light blue, arteries red, veins blue. (After *Pernkopf/Ferner:* Atlas der topographischen und angewandten Anatomie des Menschen, vol. 2. Urban & Schwarzenberg, München–Berlin 1964.)

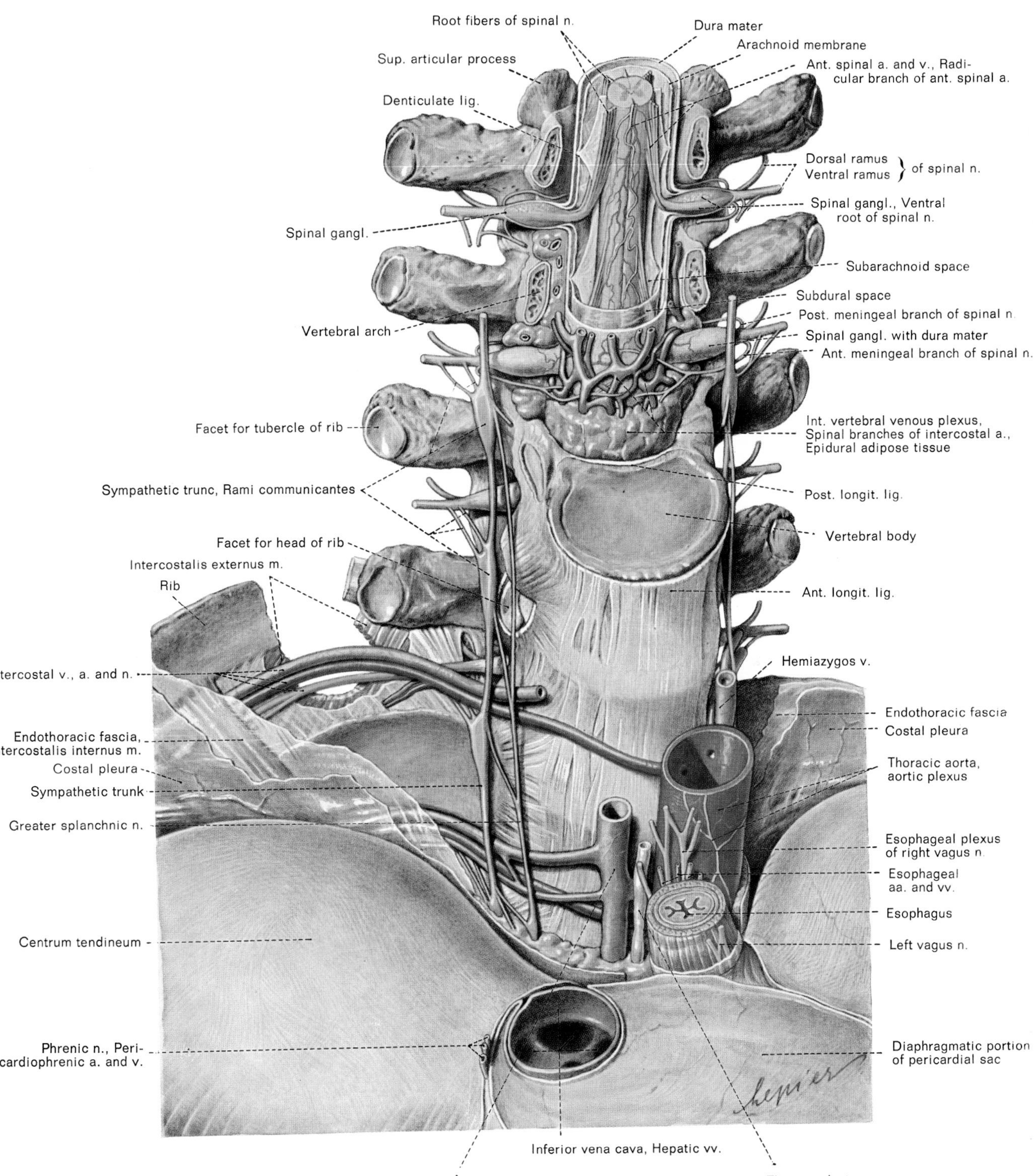
Root fibers of spinal n.
Dura mater
Arachnoid membrane
Sup. articular process
Ant. spinal a. and v., Radicular branch of ant. spinal a.
Denticulate lig.
Dorsal ramus
Ventral ramus
of spinal n.
Spinal gangl., Ventral root of spinal n.
Spinal gangl.
Subarachnoid space
Subdural space
Post. meningeal branch of spinal n.
Vertebral arch
Spinal gangl. with dura mater
Ant. meningeal branch of spinal n.
Int. vertebral venous plexus, Spinal branches of intercostal a., Epidural adipose tissue
Facet for tubercle of rib
Sympathetic trunc, Rami communicantes
Post. longit. lig.
Vertebral body
Facet for head of rib
Intercostalis externus m.
Rib
Ant. longit. lig.
Hemiazygos v.
Intercostal v., a. and n.
Endothoracic fascia
Costal pleura
Endothoracic fascia, Intercostalis internus m.
Costal pleura
Thoracic aorta, aortic plexus
Sympathetic trunk
Greater splanchnic n.
Esophageal plexus of right vagus n.
Esophageal aa. and vv.
Esophagus
Centrum tendineum
Left vagus n.
Phrenic n., Pericardiophrenic a. and v.
Diaphragmatic portion of pericardial sac
Inferior vena cava, Hepatic vv.
Azygos v.
Thoracic duct

Fig. 115. Spinal cord, meninges and other contents of the vertebral canal in the thoracic region. Stepwise dissection of various layers. View from ventral and above.

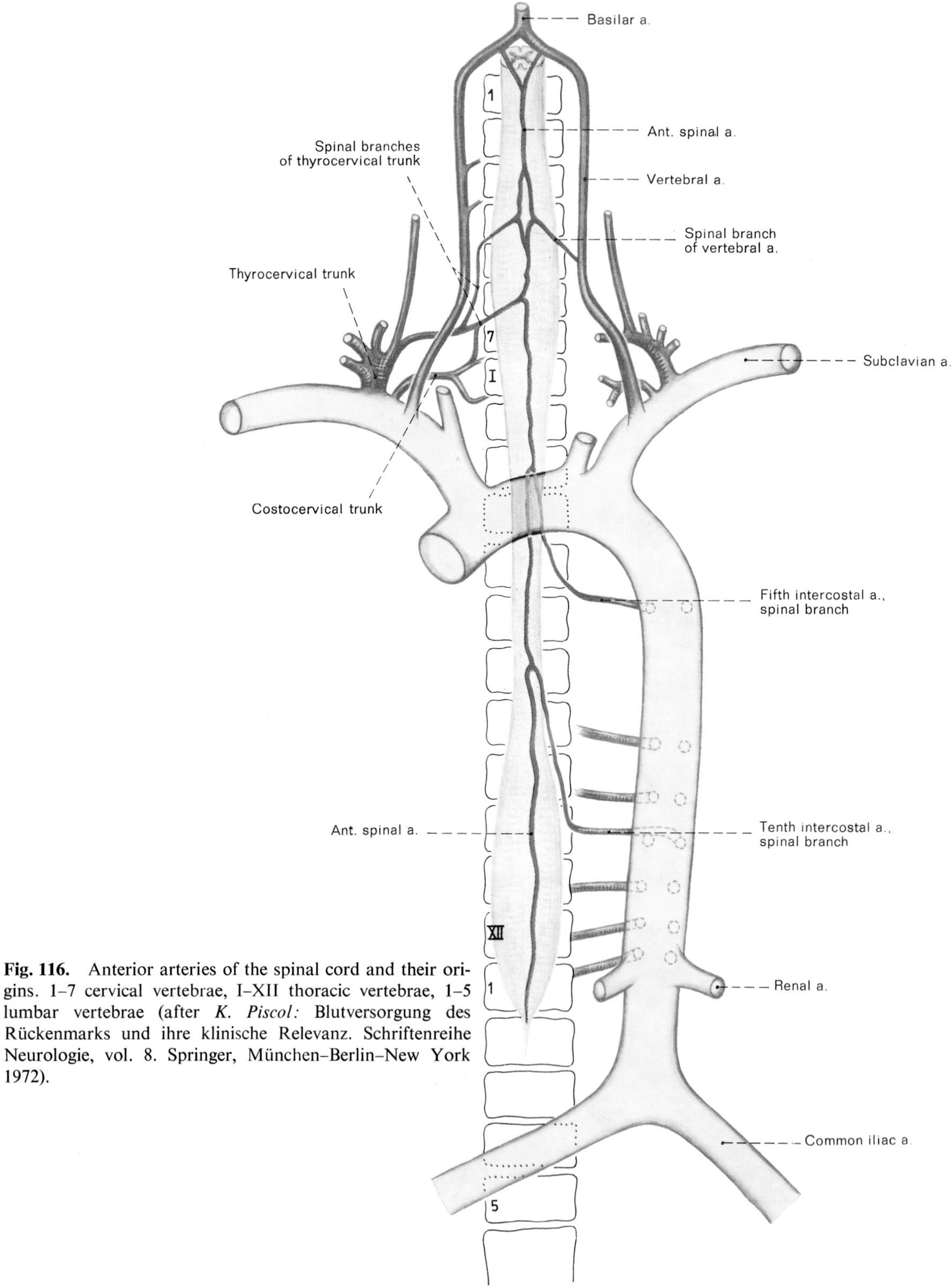
Basilar a.
Ant. spinal a.
Vertebral a.
Spinal branches of thyrocervical trunk
Spinal branch of vertebral a.
Thyrocervical trunk
Subclavian a.
Costocervical trunk
Fifth intercostal a., spinal branch
Ant. spinal a.
Tenth intercostal a., spinal branch
Renal a.
Common iliac a.
1
7
I
XII
1
5

Fig. 116. Anterior arteries of the spinal cord and their origins. 1–7 cervical vertebrae, I–XII thoracic vertebrae, 1–5 lumbar vertebrae (after *K. Piscol:* Blutversorgung des Rückenmarks und ihre klinische Relevanz. Schriftenreihe Neurologie, vol. 8. Springer, München–Berlin–New York 1972).

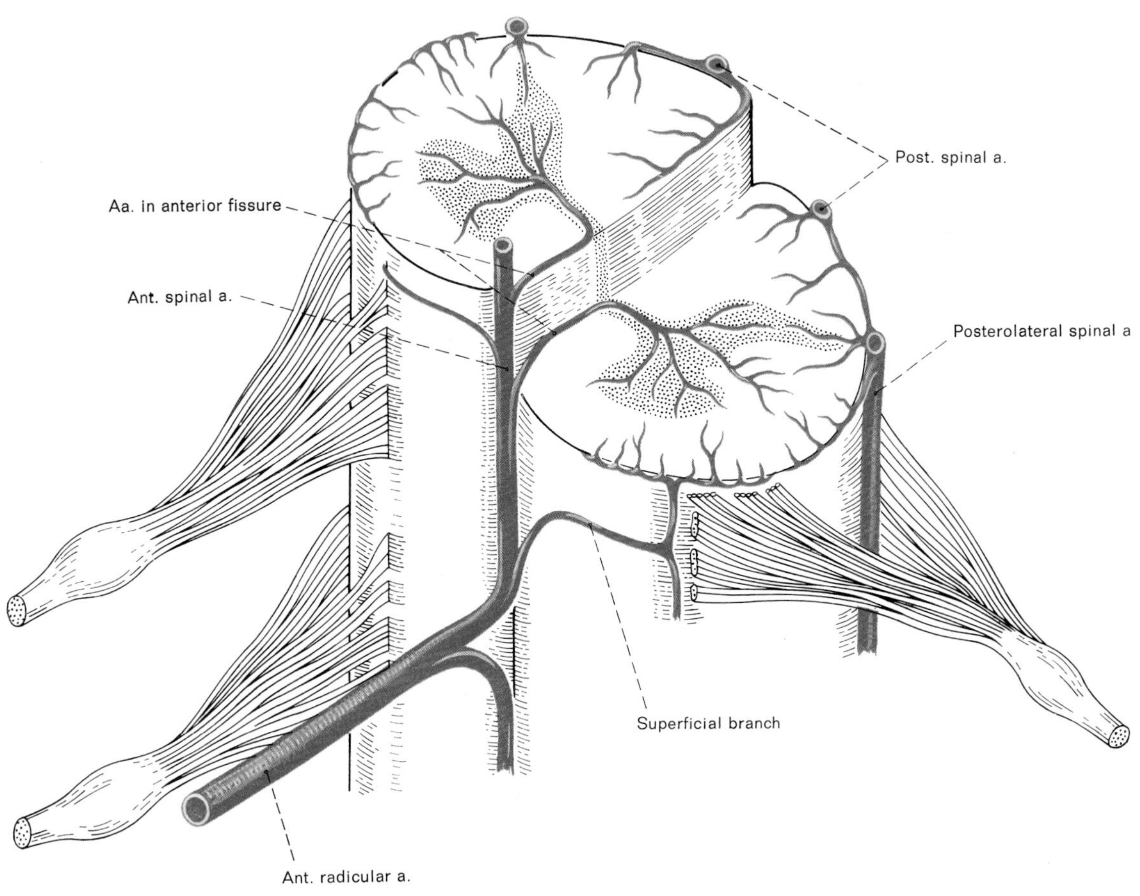
Post. spinal a.
Aa. in anterior fissure
Ant. spinal a.
Posterolateral spinal a
Superficial branch
Ant. radicular a.

Fig. 117. Arterial supply of the spinal cord (after *K. Piscol:* Blutversorgung des Rückenmarks und ihre klinische Relevanz. Schriftenreihe Neurologie, vol. 8. Springer, München–Berlin–New York 1972).

Central Nervous System

Pathways

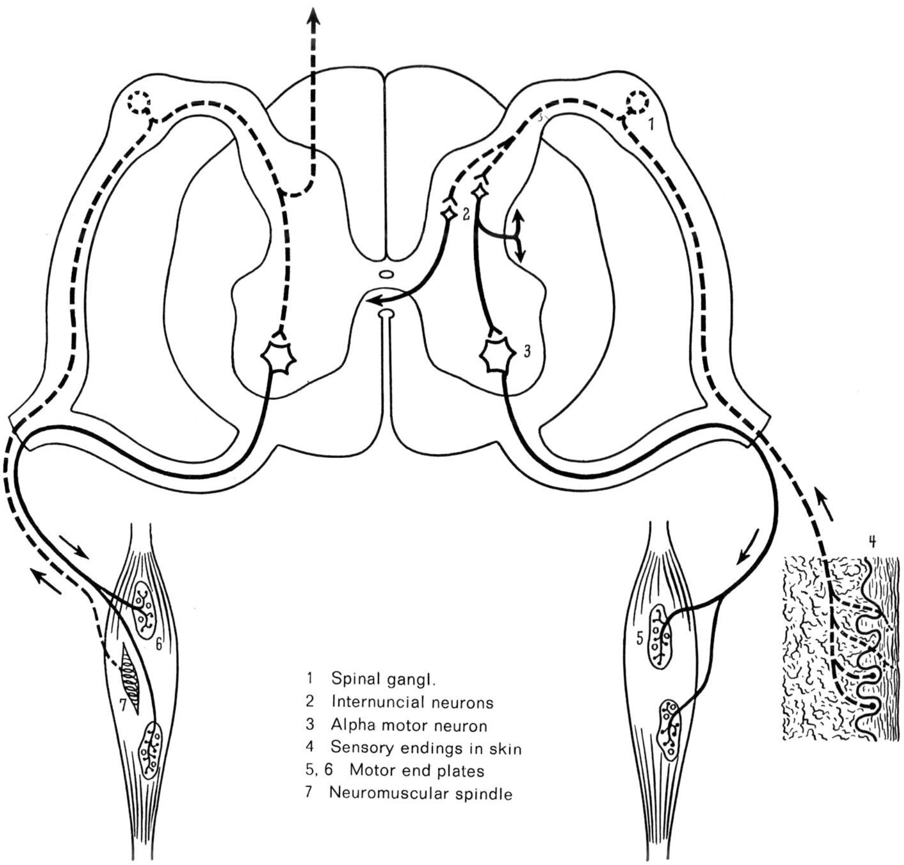
1 Spinal gangl.
2 Internuncial neurons
3 Alpha motor neuron
4 Sensory endings in skin
5, 6 Motor end plates
7 Neuromuscular spindle
1
2
3
4
5
6
7

Fig. 118. Diagram of a monosynaptic (left) and a polysynaptic (right) reflex are of the spinal cord. Dashed line = afferent limb, solid line = efferent limb.

Included among the basic mechanisms of the spinal cord are the following:

1. The direct bineuronal monosynaptic proprioceptive reflex arc (e.g. knee jerk reflex).
2. The indirect pleurineuronal polysynaptic reflex arc in which several neurons of the ipsilateral or contralateral side are involved (e.g. plantar reflex, cremasteric reflex, abdominal reflex, mucous membrane reflex).
3. The medial longitudinal fasciculus, descending branches of dorsal funicular fibers and others.

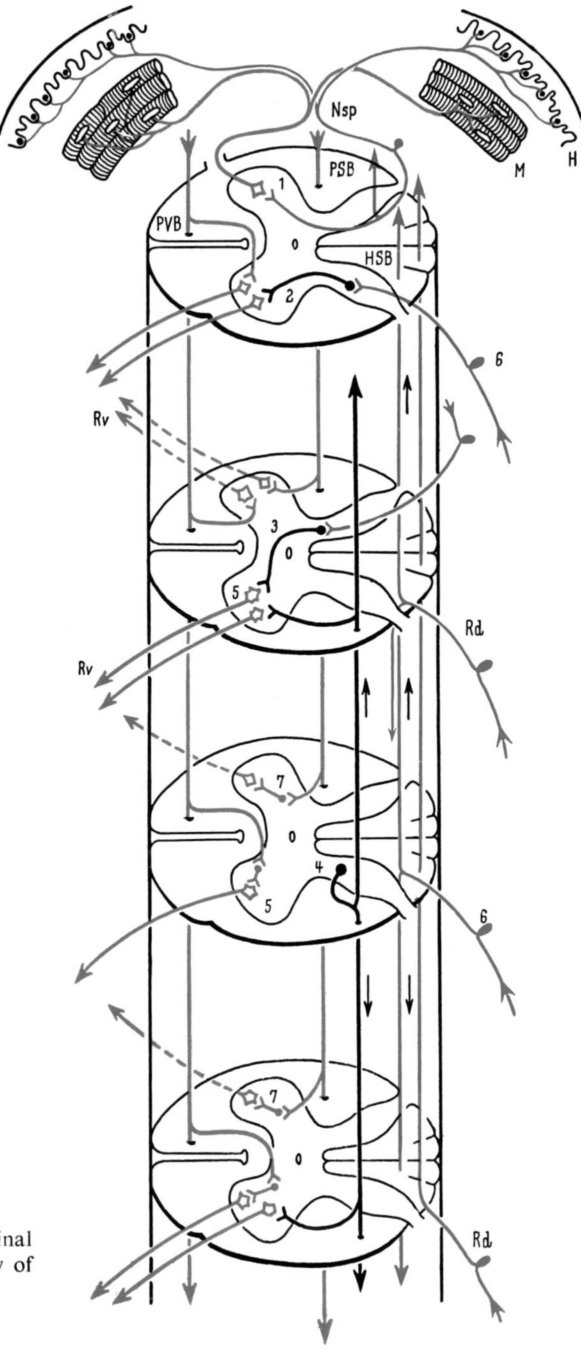
Nsp
PSB
PVB
HSB
M
H
1
2
3
4
5
6
7
0
Rv
Rd

Fig. 119. Reflex and association apparatuses in the spinal cord. Lateral view of the spinal cord with oblique view of four cross-sectional planes.

Red: motor pathway (centrifugal)
Blue: sensory pathways (centripetal)
Black: associative, comissural and funicular neurons

1 synapse of the direct reflex arc
2 relay neuron of the indirect reflex arc
3 commissural neuron
4 funicular neuron, indirect reflex arc
5 multipolar, motor anterior horn neuron
6 pseudounipolar, sensory spinal ganglion neuron
7 motor relay neuron

Rd dorsal root
Rv ventral root
PSB lateral corticospinal tract
PVB ventral corticospinal tract
HSB dorsal funiculi
Nsp spinal nerve
H skin
M muscle

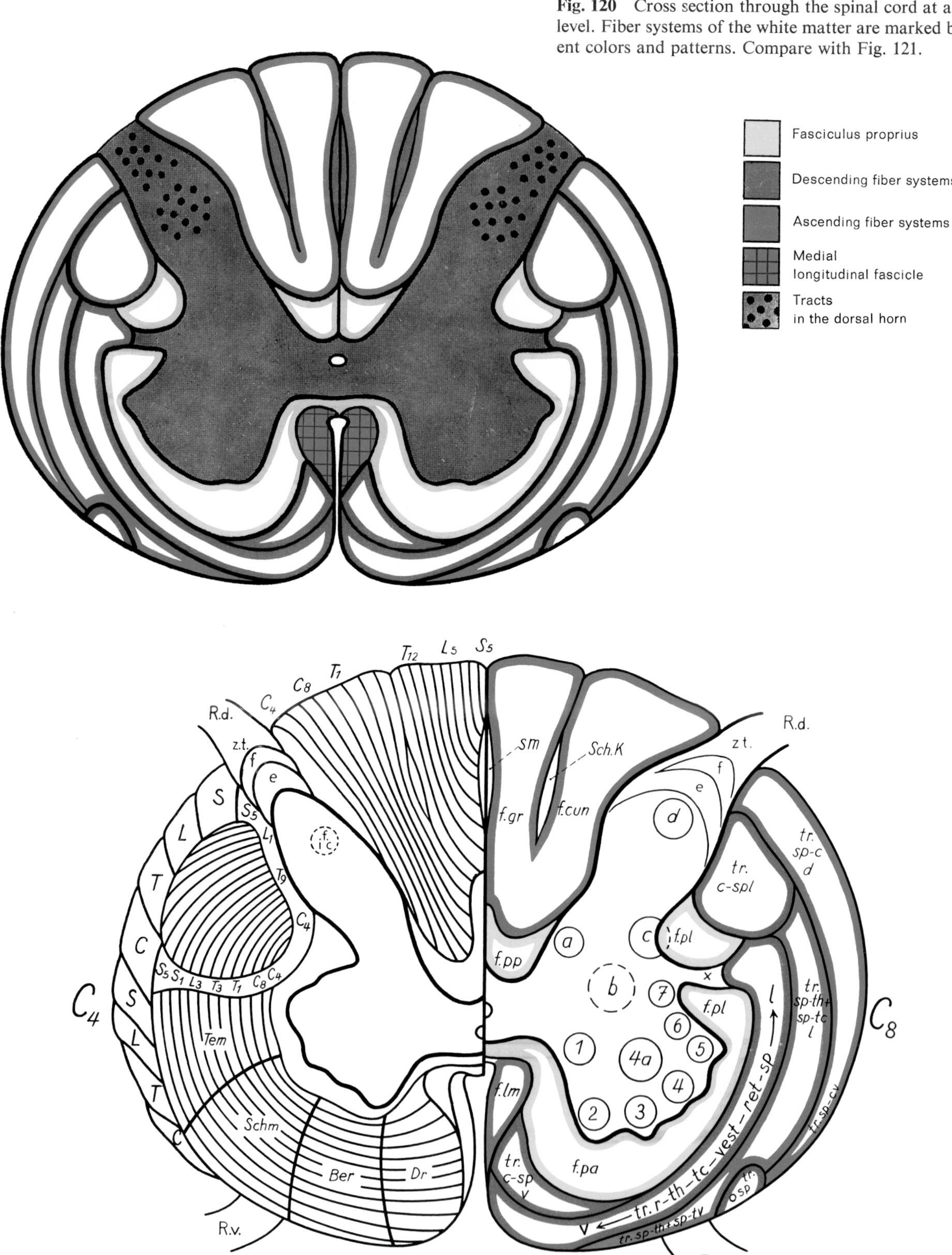
Fasciculus proprius
Descending fiber systems
Ascending fiber systems
Medial longitudinal fascicle
Tracts in the dorsal horn
T_{12} L_5 S_5
T_1
C_8
C_4
R.d.
z.t.
f
e
S
S_5
L_1
L
f.ic
T_9
T
C_4
C
S_5 S_1 L_3 T_3 T_1 C_8 C_4
C_4
S
L
Tem
T
C
Schm
Ber
Dr
R.v.
sm
Sch.K
R.d.
z t.
f
e
f.gr
f.cun
d
tr. sp-c d
tr. c-spl
a
c
f.pl
f.pp
b
x
7
f.pl
l
tr. sp-th+ sp-tc l
C_8
6
5
1
4a
4
f.lm
2
3
tr. c-sp v
f.pa
tr. r-th-tc-vest-ret-sp
tr. sp-cv
tr. osp
v
tr. r-th-tc-vest-ret-sp
tr. sp-th+sp-tv
R.v.

Fig. 120 Cross section through the spinal cord at a cervical level. Fiber systems of the white matter are marked by different colors and patterns. Compare with Fig. 121.

Fig. 121. Cross section of the spinal cord. Two different levels are represented, and various structures are indicated in the two halves. Markings in the left half after *O. Foerster:* Symptomatologie der Erkrankungen des Rückenmarks und seiner Wurzeln. In *Bumke/Foerster* (ed.): Rückenmark – Hirnstamm – Kleinhirn. Handbuch der Neurologie, vol. 5. Springer, Berlin 1936. The right side shows the nuclear areas of the gray matter, after *Benninghoff/Goerttler:* Lehrbuch der Anatomie des Menschen. vol. 3. Urban & Schwarzenberg, München–Berlin 1960.

Left half at the level of the fourth cervical segment

R.d.	dorsal root
R.v.	ventral root
z.t.	terminal zone with fasc. term.
f	zona spongiosa
e	zona gelatinosa
f.ic.	posterior intercolumnar fasc.

Dorsal funiculus

Laminar arrangement of the afferent fiber systems in that fibers from more cranial segments are superimposed upon fibers from more caudal segments. S 5–L 5–T 12–I 1–C 8–C 4 epicritic sensibilities of touch, position, movement, vibration, pressure.

Ventrolateral funiculus

In the lateral marginal zone are located the dorsal spinocerebellar tract *(Flechsig)* and the ventral spinocerebellar tract *(Gowers)*. Medial to the dorsal spinocerebellar tract runs the lateral corticospinal tract with the following laminar arrangement (from outside in) S 5–L 1–T 9–C 4.

In the narrow zone between the lateral corticospinal tract there run descending autonomic fibers in segmental lamination. The ventrolateral funiculus shows a laminar segmental arrangement (from outside in) S 5–S 1–L 3–T 3–T 1–C 8–C 4 as well as an arrangement according to the quality of the sensibilities: protopathic sensibility.

Tem	fibers for temperature
Schm	fibers for pain
Ber	fibers for touch
Dr	fibers for pressure

Right half at the level of the eighth cervical segment

R.d.	dorsal root
R.v.	ventral root
z.t.	terminal zone with terminal fasciculus
f.pp	dorsal fasciculus proprius
f.pl	lateral fasciculus proprius
f.pa	ventral fasciculus proprius
f.gr	fasciculus gracilis *(Goll)*
f.cun	fasciculus cuneatus *(Burdach)*
sm	septomarginal fasciculus
Sch.K.	fasciculus interfascicularis
tr.c–spl	lateral corticospinal tract
tr.c–spv	ventral corticospinal tract
v←tr. r–th–tc–vest–ret–→l	ventral and lateral rubrothalamotectovestibulo-reticulospinal tract
tr. sp–th + sp–tc l tr. sp–th + sp–tv	ventral and lateral spinothalamic and spinotectal tract
tr. sp–cd	dorsal spinocerebellar tract
tr. sp–cv	ventral spinocerebellar tract
tr. o sp	olivospinal and spinoolivary tract
f. lm	medial longitudinal fascicle
×	descending autonomic fibers

Gray Substance

Nuclei for:

1, 2	dorsal muscles of trunk
3	ventral muscles of trunk
4	girdle muscles of trunk
4a	girdle muscles of extremities
5	muscles of arm and thigh
6	muscles of forearm and leg
7	muscles of hand and foot

a	dorsal nucleus
b	intermediomedial nucleus (uncertain boundaries, parasympathetic root cells)
c	intermediolateral nucleus (sympathetic root cells)
d	central nucleus of dorsal horn
e	nucleus of substantia gelatinosa (parvicellular)
f	apical nucleus of dorsal horn (magnocellular, zona spongiosa)

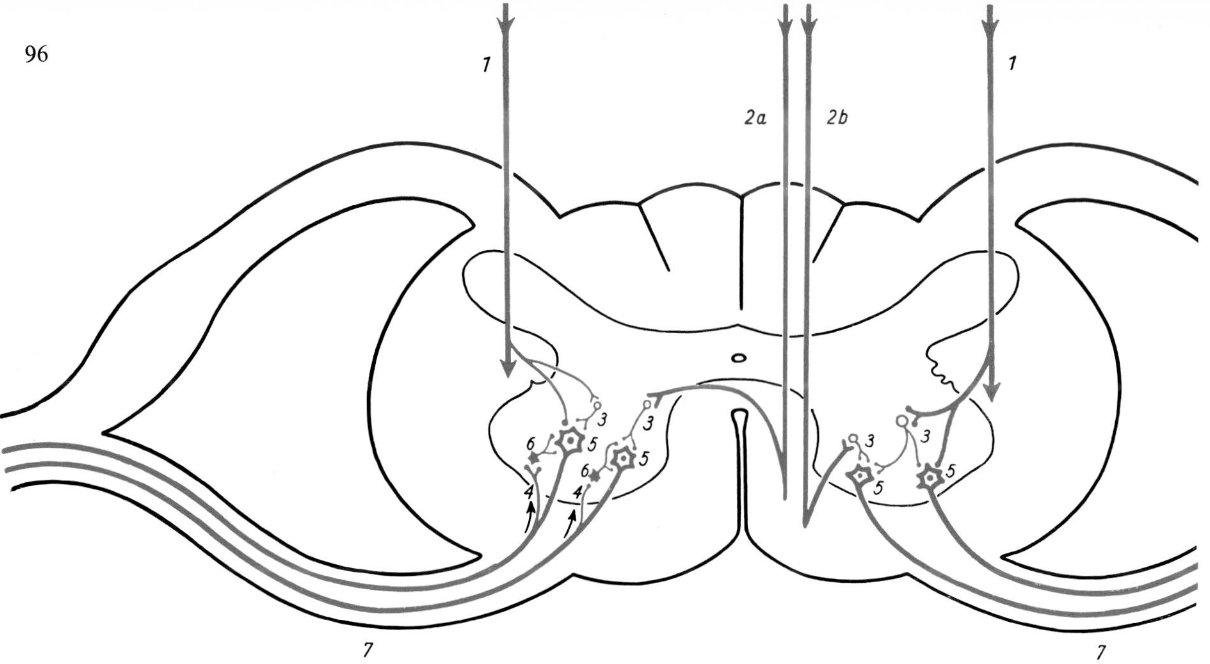
1
2a
2b
1
3
3
3
3
6
5
5
6
5
5
5
4
4
7
7

Fig. 122. Corticospinal tract in the spinal cord. Left and right: 1, lateral corticospinal tract (crossed in the decussation of the pyramids); right: 2, ventral corticospinal tract (2a, majority of fibers crossed in the anterior commissure; 2b, minority of fibers uncrossed). 3, small relay neurons subserve the conduction of the impulse from the first neuron in the precentral gyrus to the multipolar motor neuron in the ventral horn. 4, recurrent collaterals from the initial unmyelinated segment of the neurite of the ventral horn motor neuron (5) accomplish, via interneurons called Renshaw cells (6), inhibition of the motor neuron. 7, ventral root of spinal nerve.

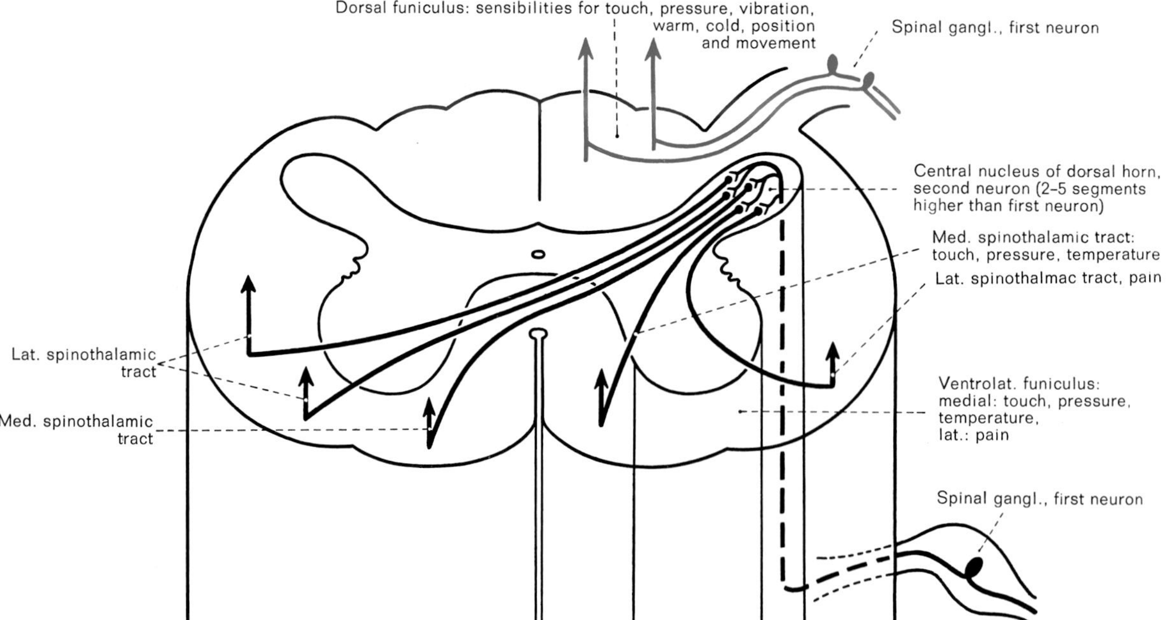
Dorsal funiculus: sensibilities for touch, pressure, vibration, warm, cold, position and movement
Spinal gangl., first neuron
Central nucleus of dorsal horn, second neuron (2–5 segments higher than first neuron)
Med. spinothalamic tract: touch, pressure, temperature
Lat. spinothalmac tract, pain
Lat. spinothalamic tract
Med. spinothalamic tract
Ventrolat. funiculus: medial: touch, pressure, temperature, lat.: pain
Spinal gangl., first neuron

Fig. 123. Tracts in the ventrolateral and dorsal funiculi of the spinal cord. Dorsal funiculi: medial spinobulbar tract *(Goll)* and lateral spinobulbar tract *(Burdach)*; these cross in the medial lemniscus, subserve epicritical sensibility, and are shown in blue. Ventrolateral funiculi: medial and lateral spinothalamic tracts; these are crossed or uncrossed in the spinal cord, subserve protopathic and visceral sensibility, and are shown in black.

Pathways of the spinal cord

Exact localization of various pathways in spinal cord cross sections is impossible because they do not form well defined bundles. Therefore, schematic representations are valuable only for general understanding but are not absolutely correct. The following is a summary of the main pathways in the three funiculi.

I. Ventral funiculus

1. *Ventral fasciculus proprius;* neurites from propriospinal neurons ending on ventral horn neurons.
2. *Medial longitudinal fasciculus;* reaches from the midbrain to the lower thoracic cord and ends upon ventral horn neurons.
3. *Sulcomarginal tract;* neurites from dorsal propriospinal neurons coursing close to the anterior median fissure and ending upon ventral horn cells.
4. *Tectospinal tract;* originating from contralateral anterior colliculi and ending upon ventral horn cells via interneurons.
5. *Reticulospinal tract;* collective name for various pathways which formerly have been named separately (e.g. thalamo-rubro-tecto-vestibulo-spinal tract). Its fibers are widely scattered throughout the ventral funiculus and are either crossed or uncrossed. The motor reticular nucleus is located in the tegmentum, the fibers end upon ventral horn cells.
6. *Ventral corticospinal tract;* originates in the precentral gyrus and ends upon ipsilateral and contralateral ventral horn neurons via interneurons.
7. *Olivospinal tract;* present only in the cervical spinal cord.

II. Lateral funiculus

1. *Lateral fasciculus proprius;* neurites from propriospinal neurons of the dorsal horn and dorsal part of the substantia gelatinosa ending upon ventral horn neurons.
2. *Reticulospinal tract;* fibers from the lateral vestibular nucleus and red nucleus ending upon ventral horn neurons via interneurons.
3. *Spinothalamic tract;* from the thalamus to ventral horn neurons via interneurons.
4. *Spinotectal and spinothalamic tracts;* crossed and uncrossed. Fibers ending upon neurons in the anterior colliculi, ventral thalamic nuclei, and reticular formation of brain stem (spinoreticular tract).
5. *Ventral spinocerebellar tract;* crossed pathway.
6. *Dorsal spinocerebellar tract;* uncrossed pathway. Axons from nucleus dorsalis neurons ending in the cerebellar vermis.
7. *Lateral corticospinal tract;* originating in the precentral gyrus. 80% of the fibers cross in the decussation of the pyramids, ending upon ventral horn neurons via interneurons.

III. Dorsal funiculus

1. *Dorsal fasciculus proprius;* neurites from propriospinal neurons of dorsal horn and substantia gelatinosa ending upon ventral horn neurons.
2. *Fasciculus gracilis and cuneatus;* dorsal root fibers ending upon neurons of the nucleus gracilis and nucleus cuneatus in the medulla oblongata. These neurons represent the second neuron of the pathway. The fasciculus gracilis contains fibers from coccygeal to the fourth thoracic segments, the fasciculus cuneatus contains fibers from segments Th 5–C 1. The fibers which enter from lower segments are thrust medially by fibers entering from higher segments. The fibers of the second neuron cross in the medial lemniscus of the medulla oblongata and end in the thalamus where the third neuron of the pathway begins. These fibers course through the posterior limb of the internal capsule and terminate in the postcentral cortex.

Descending branches of dorsal funicular fibers, in some places, are bundled together thus forming the comma bundle of Schultze, the oval field of Flechsig, and the triangle of Philippe-Gombault (Fig. 126).

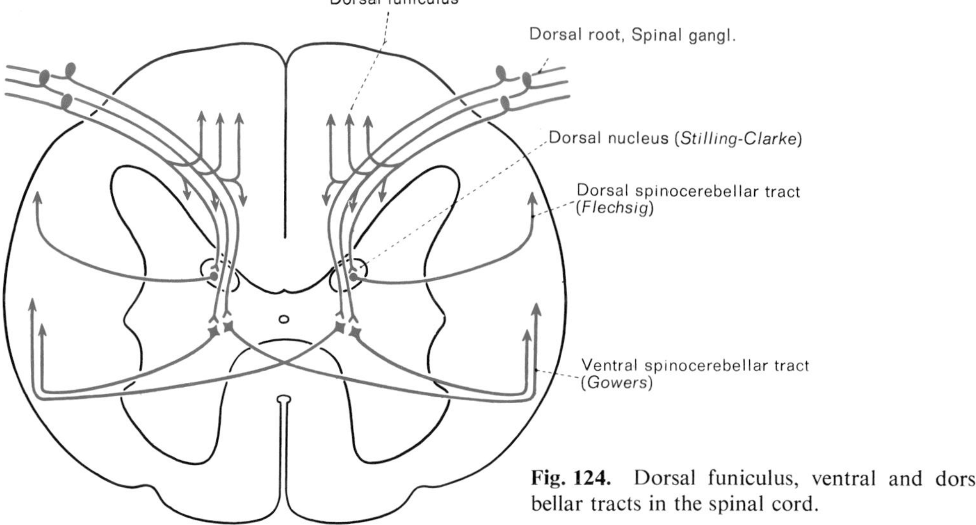
Dorsal funiculus
Dorsal root, Spinal gangl.
Dorsal nucleus (*Stilling-Clarke*)
Dorsal spinocerebellar tract
(*Flechsig*)
Ventral spinocerebellar tract
(*Gowers*)

Fig. 124. Dorsal funiculus, ventral and dorsal spinocerebellar tracts in the spinal cord.

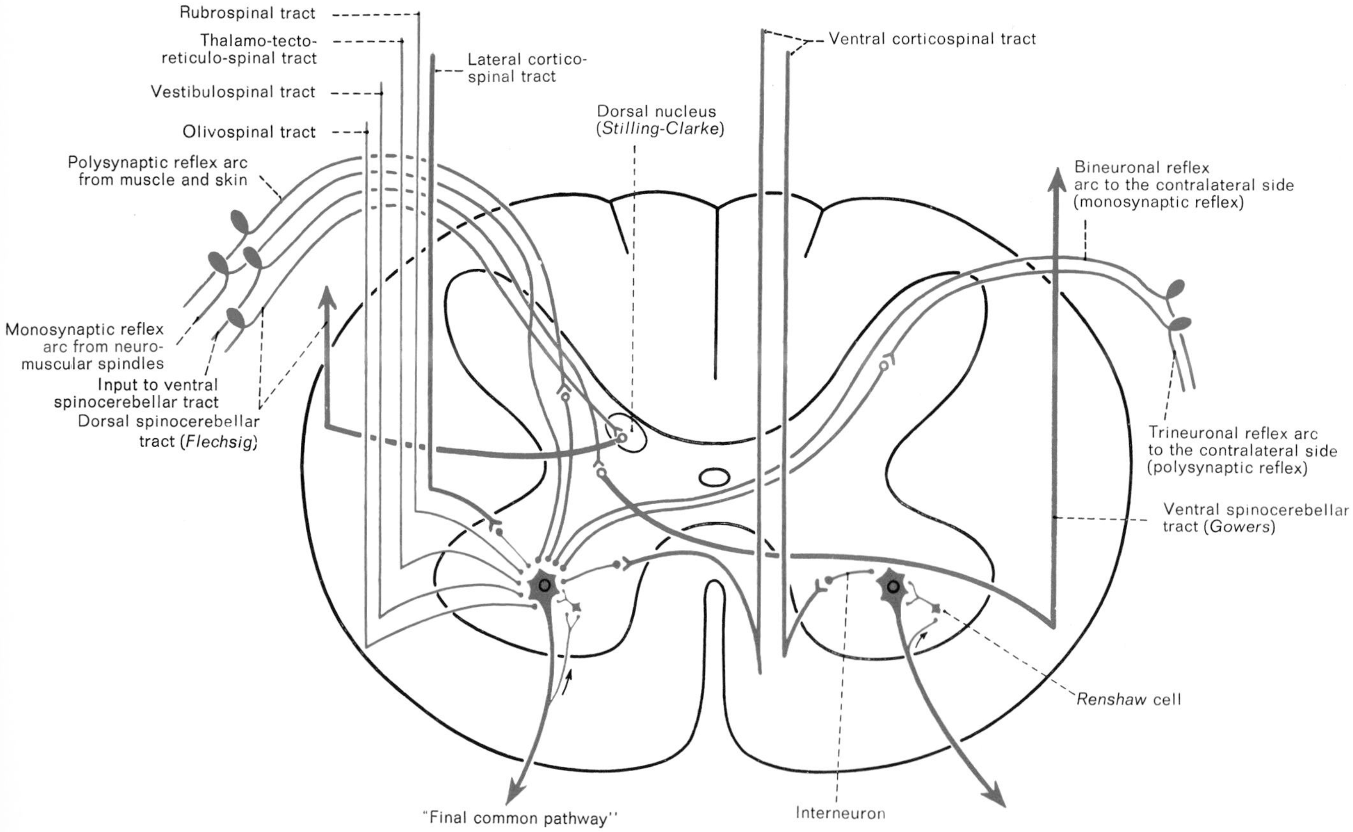

Rubrospinal tract
Thalamo-tecto-reticulo-spinal tract
Vestibulospinal tract
Olivospinal tract
Polysynaptic reflex arc from muscle and skin
Monosynaptic reflex arc from neuro-muscular spindles
Input to ventral spinocerebellar tract
Dorsal spinocerebellar tract (*Flechsig*)
Lateral cortico-spinal tract
Dorsal nucleus (*Stilling-Clarke*)
Ventral corticospinal tract
Bineuronal reflex arc to the contralateral side (monosynaptic reflex)
Trineuronal reflex arc to the contralateral side (polysynaptic reflex)
Ventral spinocerebellar tract (*Gowers*)
Renshaw cell
"Final common pathway"
Interneuron

Fig. 125. The ventral horn motor neurons as "final common pathway" for numerous conduction pathways. Red: motor pathways; heavy line: ventral and lateral corticospinal tract; thin lines: extrapyramidal tracts; blue: thin lines: reflex connections of the dorsal roots; heavy lines: dorsal and ventral spinocerebellar tracts. Note the inhibitory pathway via recurrent collaterals from the initial segment of the axon and *Renshaw* cells. Black arrows: recurrent collaterals from the unmyelinated initial axon segment of the ventral horn motor neurons.

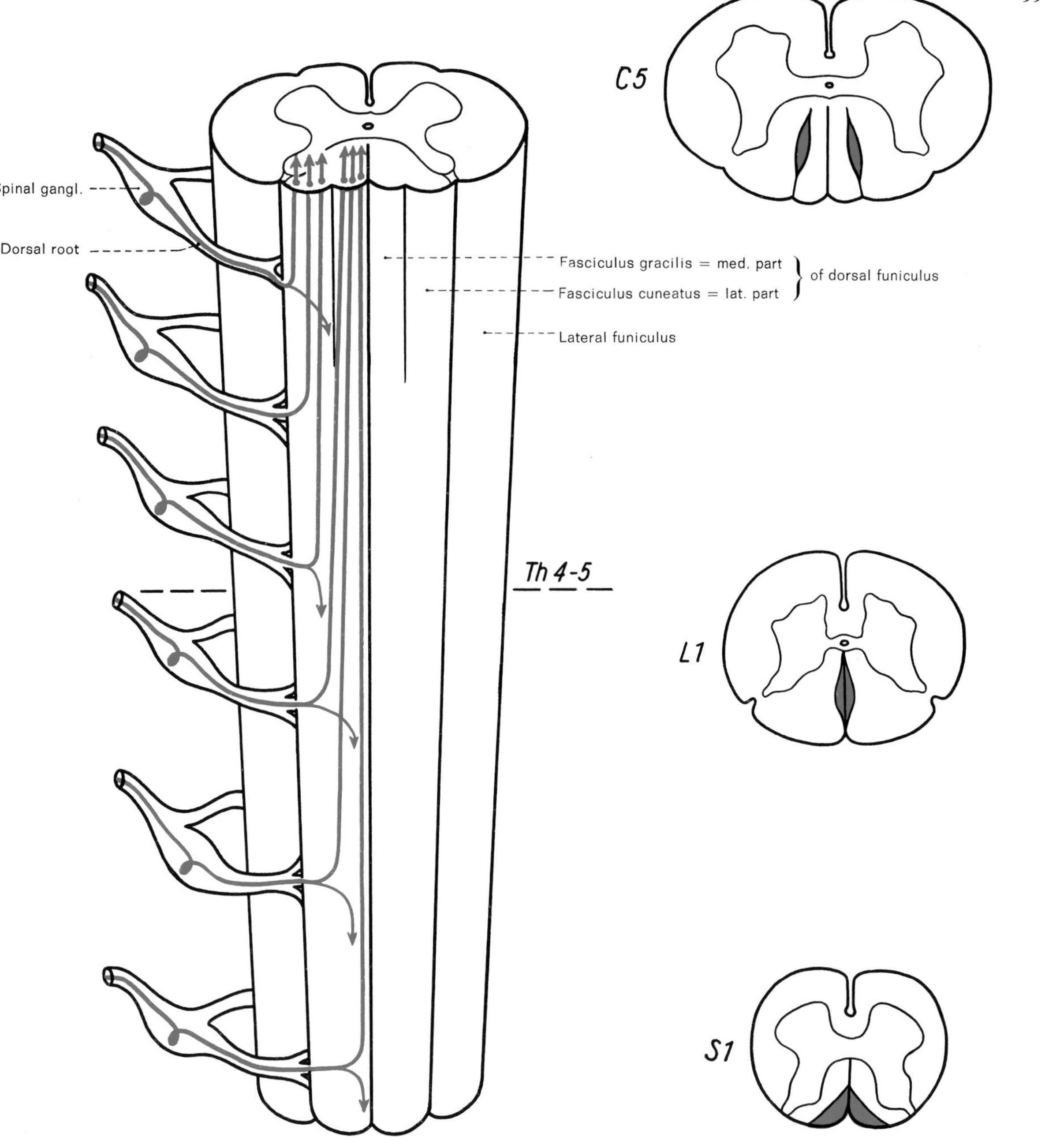
C5
Spinal gangl.
Dorsal root
Fasciculus gracilis = med. part
Fasciculus cuneatus = lat. part
of dorsal funiculus
Lateral funiculus
Th 4-5
L1
S1

Fig. 126. Arrangement of the spinobulbar tract in the spinal cord. Dorsal view. Fibers entering through the dorsal roots divide close to their place of entry into a larger ascending branch and a smaller descending branch. The ascending fibers in the dorsal funiculus are arranged in such a manner that fibers from each higher segment are layered upon those from each lower segment. Thus, ascending fibers from the coccygeo-sacral, lumbar and lower thoracic segments (Co–Th 5) form the medial portion (fasciculus gracilis), while fibers from the upper thoracic and cervical segments (Th 4–C 1) form the lateral portion (fasciculus cuneatus) of the dorsal funiculus. The approximate border line between the two is at the level of Th 4–Th 5. The descending fibers of the dorsal funiculus are found in different locations as shown in cross sections through the segments C 5, L 1, and S 1: in the cervical and upper thoracic region they form the comma tract of *Schultze,* also known as the semilunar tract or the interfascicular fasciculus; in the lower thoracic and lumbar region they form the "oval field of *Flechsig*" and in the medullary cone the "triangular field of *Gombault* and *Philippe*".

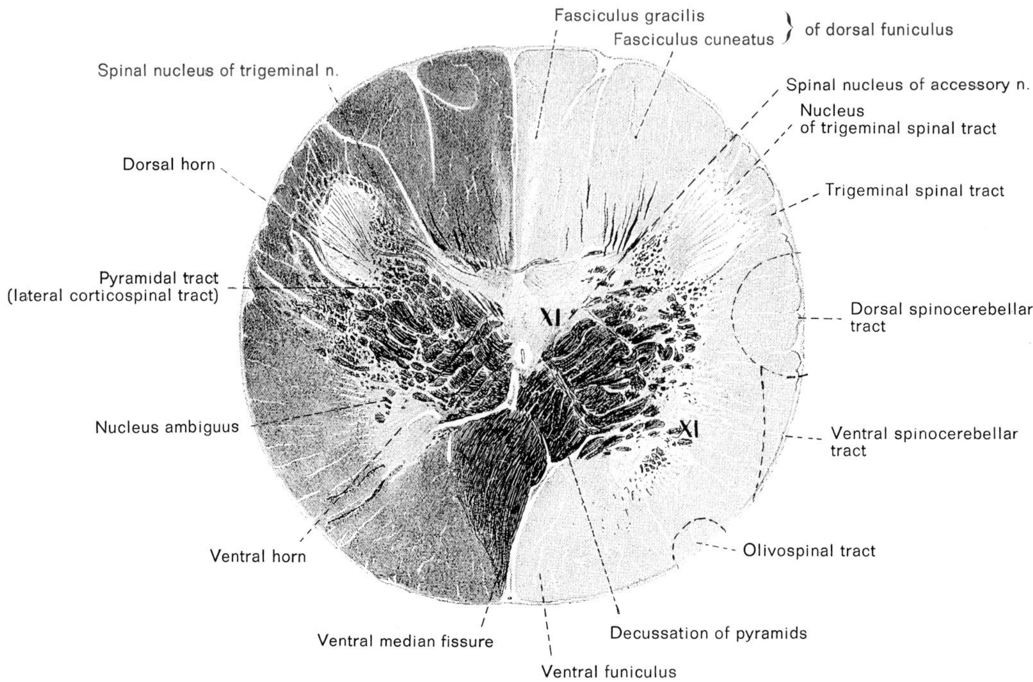
Fasciculus gracilis
Fasciculus cuneatus
} of dorsal funiculus
Spinal nucleus of trigeminal n.
Spinal nucleus of accessory n.
Nucleus
of trigeminal spinal tract
Dorsal horn
Trigeminal spinal tract
Pyramidal tract
(lateral corticospinal tract)
XI
Dorsal spinocerebellar
tract
Nucleus ambiguus
XI
Ventral spinocerebellar
tract
Ventral horn
Olivospinal tract
Ventral median fissure
Decussation of pyramids
Ventral funiculus

Fig. 127. Cross section through the medulla oblongata at the level of the lower pole of the decussation of the pyramids.

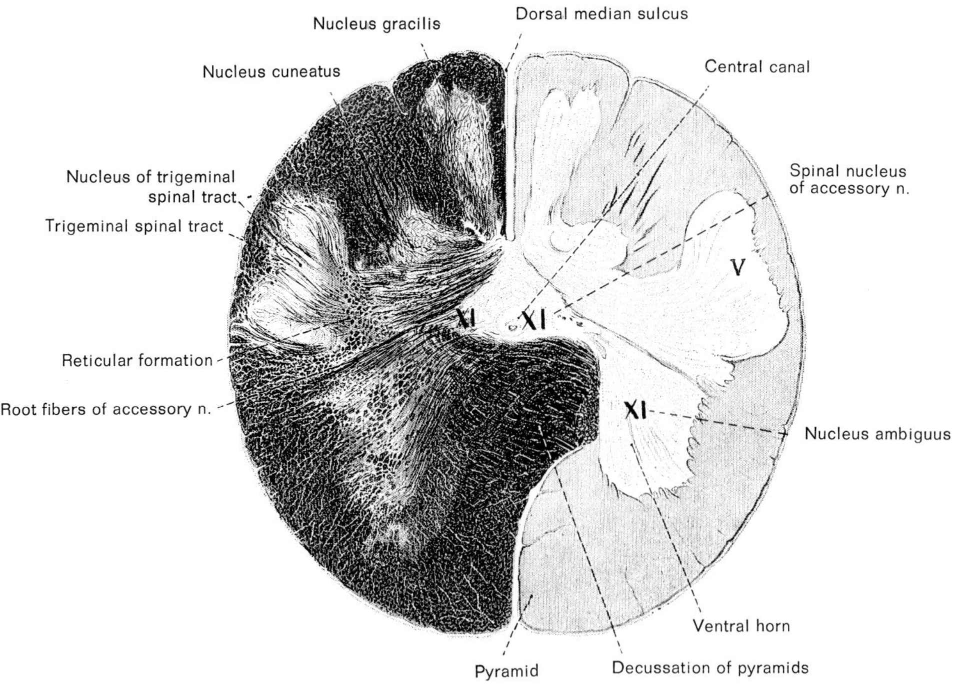
Nucleus gracilis
Dorsal median sulcus
Nucleus cuneatus
Central canal
Nucleus of trigeminal
spinal tract
Spinal nucleus
of accessory n.
Trigeminal spinal tract
V
XI
XI
Reticular formation
Root fibers of accessory n.
XI
Nucleus ambiguus
Ventral horn
Pyramid
Decussation of pyramids

Fig. 128. Cross section through the medulla oblongata at the level of the upper pole of the decussation of the pyramids. The Roman numerals indicate the position of the corresponding cranial nerve nuclei.

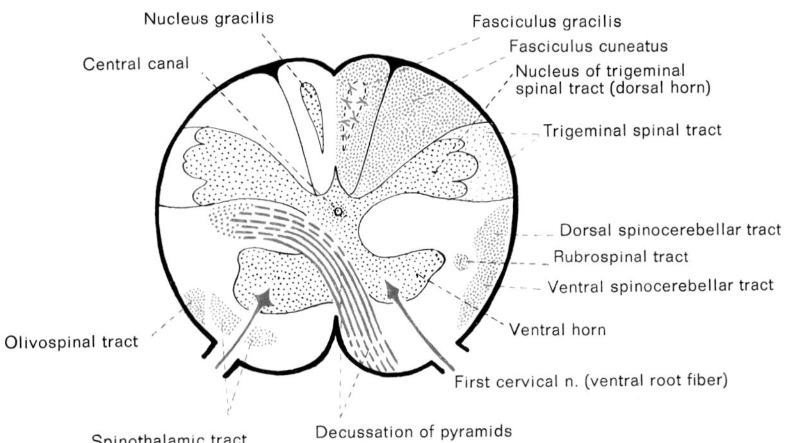
Nucleus gracilis
Central canal
Fasciculus gracilis
Fasciculus cuneatus
Nucleus of trigeminal spinal tract (dorsal horn)
Trigeminal spinal tract
Dorsal spinocerebellar tract
Rubrospinal tract
Ventral spinocerebellar tract
Ventral horn
Olivospinal tract
First cervical n. (ventral root fiber)
Spinothalamic tract
Decussation of pyramids

Fig. 129. Architecture of the medulla oblongata at the level of the decussation of the pyramids. Schematic cross section.*

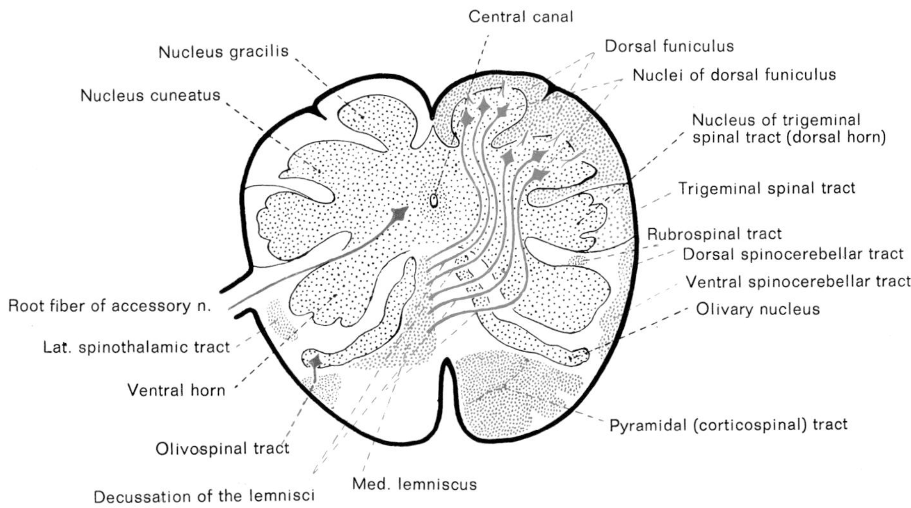
Central canal
Nucleus gracilis
Dorsal funiculus
Nuclei of dorsal funiculus
Nucleus cuneatus
Nucleus of trigeminal spinal tract (dorsal horn)
Trigeminal spinal tract
Rubrospinal tract
Dorsal spinocerebellar tract
Ventral spinocerebellar tract
Root fiber of accessory n.
Olivary nucleus
Lat. spinothalamic tract
Ventral horn
Pyramidal (corticospinal) tract
Olivospinal tract
Med. lemniscus
Decussation of the lemnisci

Fig. 130. Architecture of the medulla oblongata at the level of the decussation of the lemnisci. Schematic cross section.*

* Red: descending pathways, blue: ascending pathways.

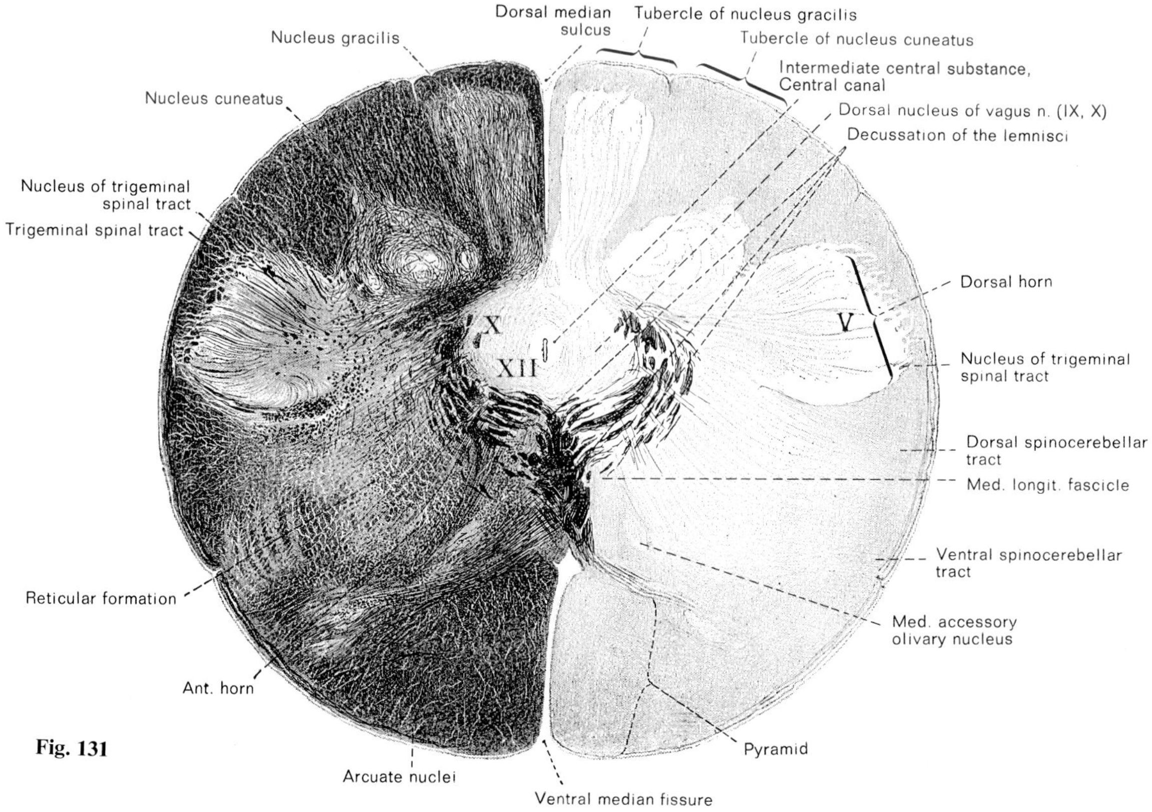

Dorsal median sulcus
Tubercle of nucleus gracilis
Nucleus gracilis
Tubercle of nucleus cuneatus
Intermediate central substance, Central canal
Nucleus cuneatus
Dorsal nucleus of vagus n. (IX, X)
Decussation of the lemnisci
Nucleus of trigeminal spinal tract
Trigeminal spinal tract
Dorsal horn
X
XII
V
Nucleus of trigeminal spinal tract
Dorsal spinocerebellar tract
Med. longit. fascicle
Ventral spinocerebellar tract
Reticular formation
Med. accessory olivary nucleus
Ant. horn
Pyramid
Arcuate nuclei
Ventral median fissure

Fig. 131

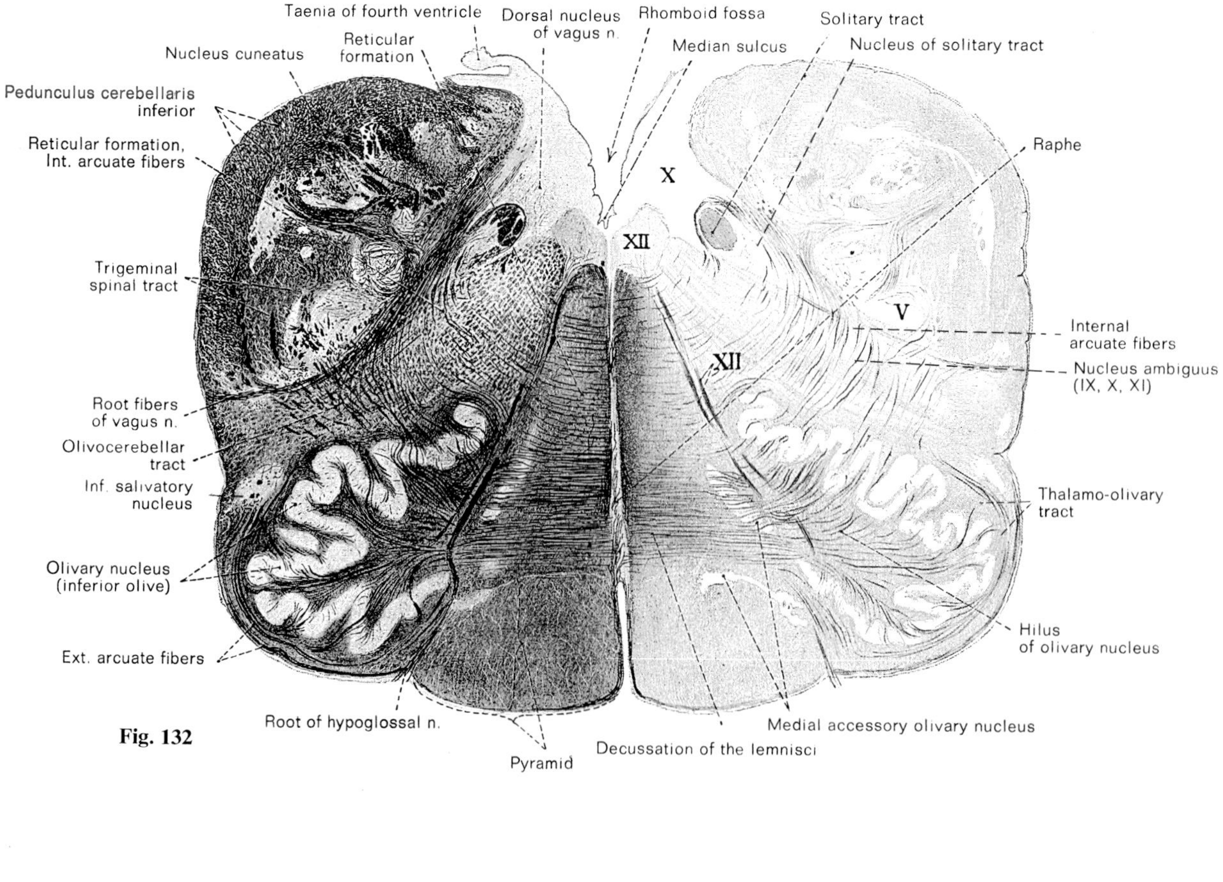

Taenia of fourth ventricle
Dorsal nucleus of vagus n.
Rhomboid fossa
Solitary tract
Reticular formation
Median sulcus
Nucleus of solitary tract
Nucleus cuneatus
Pedunculus cerebellaris inferior
Raphe
Reticular formation, Int. arcuate fibers
X
XII
Trigeminal spinal tract
V
Internal arcuate fibers
XII
Nucleus ambiguus (IX, X, XI)
Root fibers of vagus n.
Olivocerebellar tract
Inf. salivatory nucleus
Thalamo-olivary tract
Olivary nucleus (inferior olive)
Hilus of olivary nucleus
Ext. arcuate fibers
Root of hypoglossal n.
Medial accessory olivary nucleus
Decussation of the lemnisci
Pyramid

Fig. 132

◀ **Fig. 131.** Cross section through the medulla oblongata at the level of the decussation of the lemnisci.
Fig. 132. Cross section through the medulla oblongata at the level of the obex.

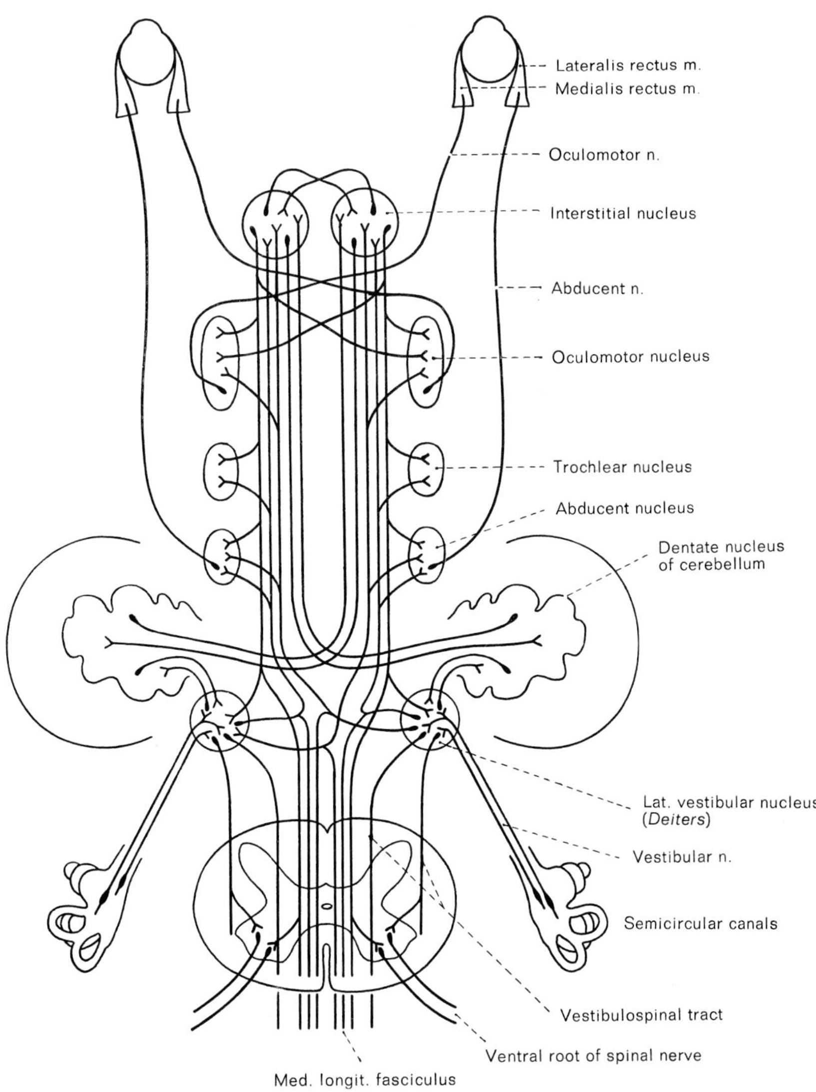

Lateralis rectus m.
Medialis rectus m.
Oculomotor n.
Interstitial nucleus
Abducent n.
Oculomotor nucleus
Trochlear nucleus
Abducent nucleus
Dentate nucleus of cerebellum
Lat. vestibular nucleus (Deiters)
Vestibular n.
Semicircular canals
Vestibulospinal tract
Ventral root of spinal nerve
Med. longit. fasciculus

Fig. 133. Connections of the medial longitudinal fasciculus. Schematic representation of the brain stem (modified after *Villiger/Ludwig:* Gehirn und Rückenmark. Schwabe, Basel 1946).

Nucleus intercalatus
Med. vestibular nucleus
Reticular formation
Dorsal nucleus of vagus n.
Solitary tract
Root of vestibular n.
Ala cinerea
Nucleus of solitary tract
Raphe
Med. longit. fasciculus
b
Dorsal cochlear nucleus
Pedunculus cerebellaris inferior
IX
VIII a
XII
X
Nucleus of trigeminal spinal tract
X
Root fibers of accessory n.
V
XI
Olivocerebellar tract
Root fibers of vagus n.
Root fibers of vagus n.
Dorsal accessory olivary nucleus
Root fibers of accessory n.
Olivary nucleus
Reticular formation
XII
Hilus of olivary nucleus
Nucleus ambiguus
Olivary nucleus (inf. olive)
Root fibers of hypoglossal n.
Med. accessory olivary nucleus
Pyramid
Ext. arcuate fibers
Med. lemniscus
Arcuate nucleus

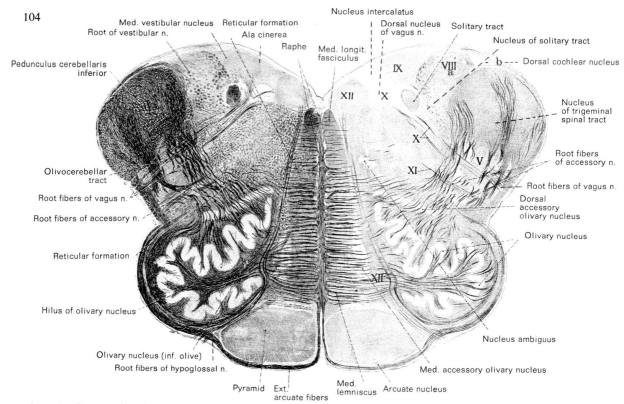

Fig. 134. Cross section through the medulla oblongata at the level of the caudal part of the rhomboid fossa and the hilus of the olivary nucleus. The Roman numerals indicate the location of the nuclei of the corresponding cranial nerves. VIII a = vestibular nucleus, b = cochlear nucleus.

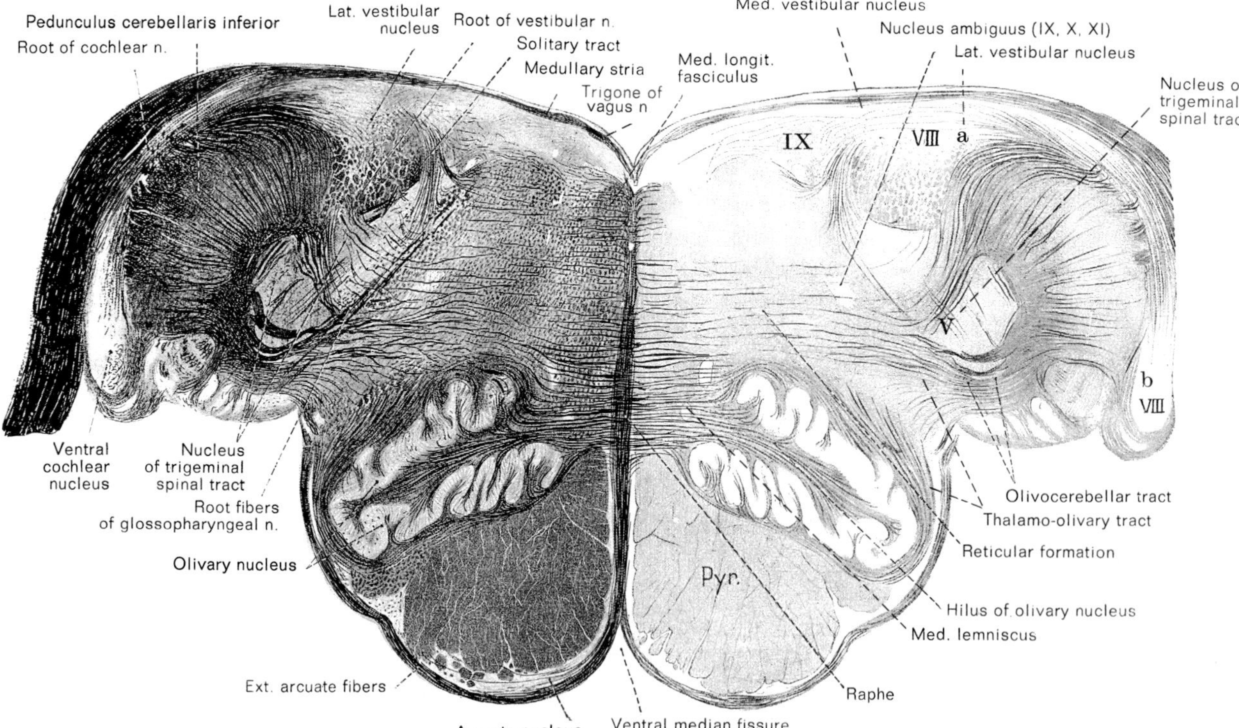

Pedunculus cerebellaris inferior
Lat. vestibular nucleus
Root of vestibular n.
Med. vestibular nucleus
Nucleus ambiguus (IX, X, XI)
Root of cochlear n.
Solitary tract
Lat. vestibular nucleus
Medullary stria
Med. longit. fasciculus
Trigone of vagus n
Nucleus of trigeminal spinal tract
IX
VIII a
V
b
VIII
Ventral cochlear nucleus
Nucleus of trigeminal spinal tract
Root fibers of glossopharyngeal n.
Olivocerebellar tract
Thalamo-olivary tract
Reticular formation
Olivary nucleus
Pyr.
Hilus of olivary nucleus
Med. lemniscus
Ext. arcuate fibers
Raphe
Arcuate nucleus
Ventral median fissure

Fig. 135. Cross section through the medulla oblongata in the middle area of the rhomboid fossa and at the level of the root of the cochlear nerve. The Roman numerals indicate the nuclei of the corresponding cranial nerves. VIII a = vestibular nucleus, VIII b = cochlear nucleus.

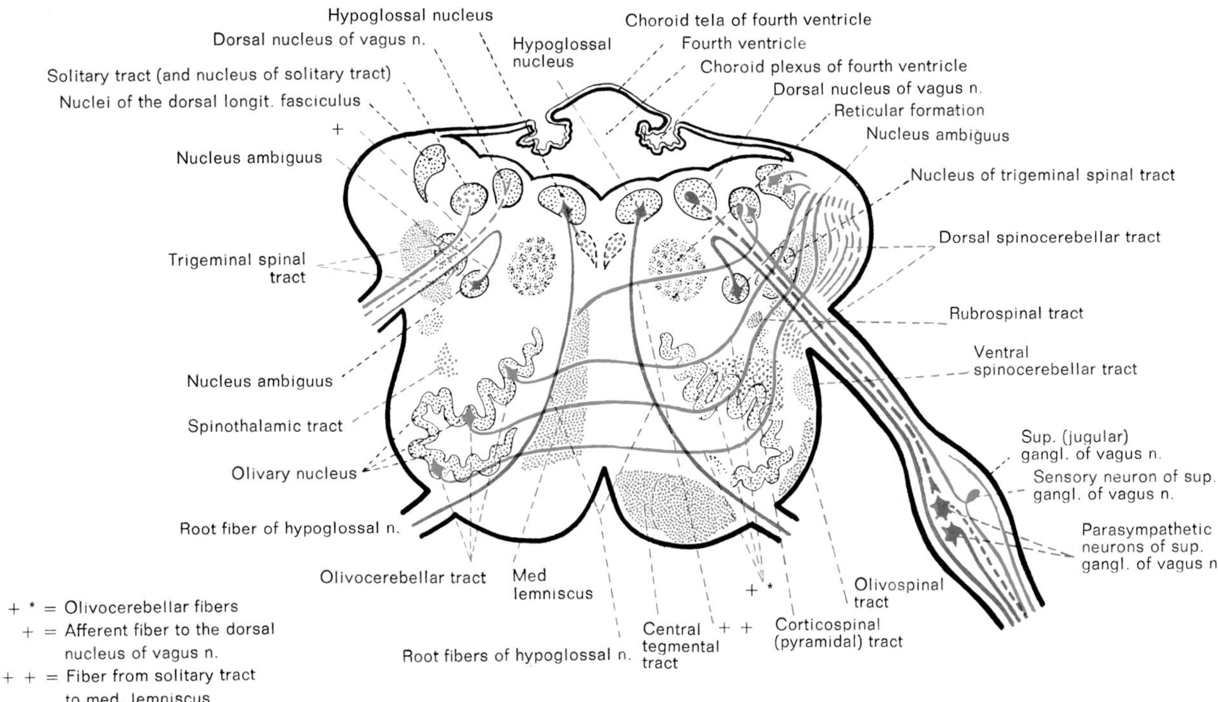
Hypoglossal nucleus
Dorsal nucleus of vagus n.
Solitary tract (and nucleus of solitary tract)
Nuclei of the dorsal longit. fasciculus
Nucleus ambiguus
Trigeminal spinal tract
Nucleus ambiguus
Spinothalamic tract
Olivary nucleus
Root fiber of hypoglossal n.
Olivocerebellar tract
Med lemniscus
Root fibers of hypoglossal n.
Central tegmental tract
Corticospinal (pyramidal) tract
Olivospinal tract
Hypoglossal nucleus
Choroid tela of fourth ventricle
Fourth ventricle
Choroid plexus of fourth ventricle
Dorsal nucleus of vagus n.
Reticular formation
Nucleus ambiguus
Nucleus of trigeminal spinal tract
Dorsal spinocerebellar tract
Rubrospinal tract
Ventral spinocerebellar tract
Sup. (jugular) gangl. of vagus n.
Sensory neuron of sup. gangl. of vagus n.
Parasympathetic neurons of sup. gangl. of vagus n.
+ * = Olivocerebellar fibers
+ = Afferent fiber to the dorsal nucleus of vagus n.
+ + = Fiber from solitary tract to med. lemniscus

Fig. 136. Architecture of the medulla oblongata in the region of the caudal part of the rhomboid fossa. Schematic cross section; compare with Fig. 134. Red: descending pathways, blue: ascending pathways.

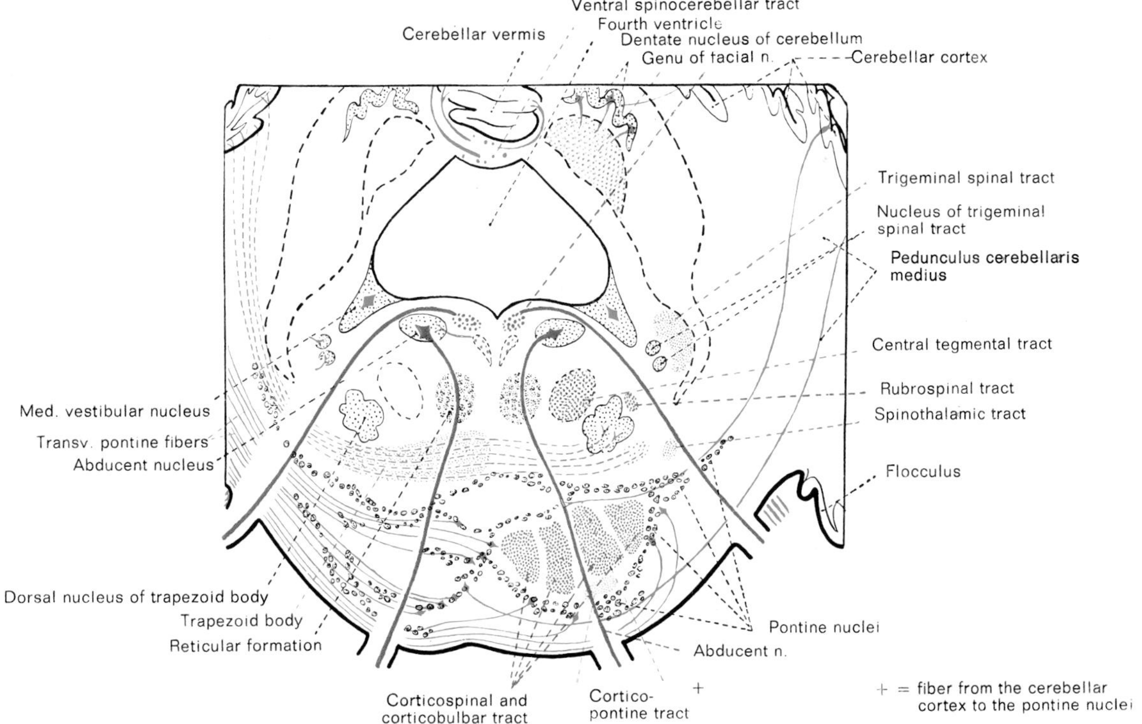
Ventral spinocerebellar tract
Cerebellar vermis
Fourth ventricle
Dentate nucleus of cerebellum
Genu of facial n.
Cerebellar cortex
Trigeminal spinal tract
Nucleus of trigeminal spinal tract
Pedunculus cerebellaris medius
Central tegmental tract
Rubrospinal tract
Spinothalamic tract
Flocculus
Med. vestibular nucleus
Transv. pontine fibers
Abducent nucleus
Dorsal nucleus of trapezoid body
Trapezoid body
Reticular formation
Pontine nuclei
Abducent n.
Corticospinal and corticobulbar tract
Cortico-pontine tract
+ = fiber from the cerebellar cortex to the pontine nuclei

Fig. 137. Architecture of the caudal portion of the pons. Schematic cross section. Red and yellow: descending pathways; blue: ascending pathways.

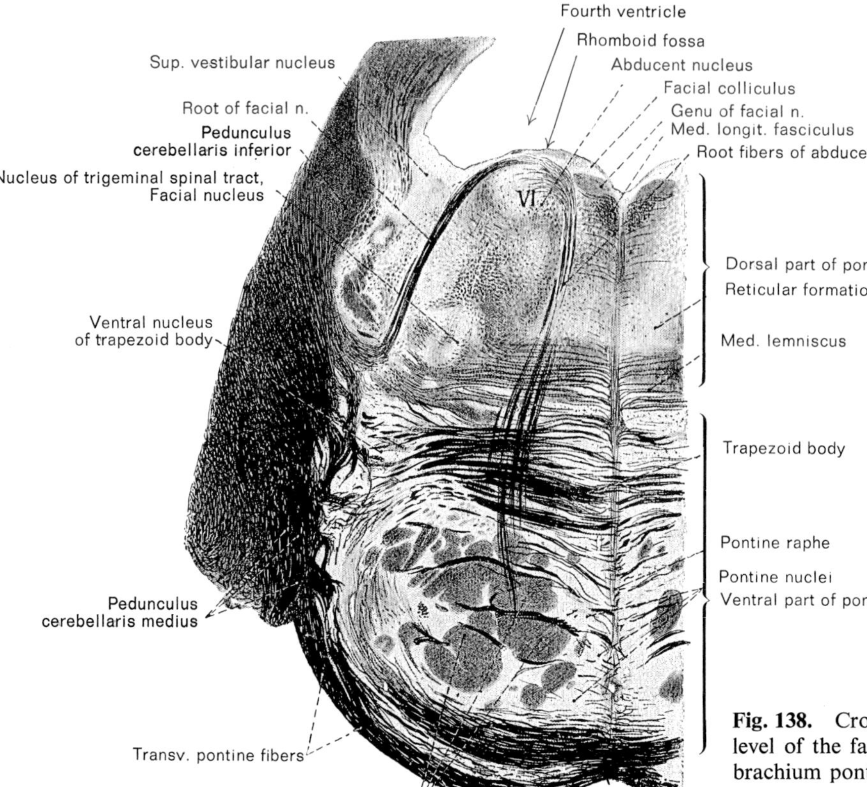
Fourth ventricle
Rhomboid fossa
Abducent nucleus
Facial colliculus
Genu of facial n.
Med. longit. fasciculus
Root fibers of abducent n.
Sup. vestibular nucleus
Root of facial n.
Pedunculus cerebellaris inferior
Nucleus of trigeminal spinal tract, Facial nucleus
VI
Dorsal part of pons
Reticular formation
Ventral nucleus of trapezoid body
Med. lemniscus
Trapezoid body
Pontine raphe
Pontine nuclei
Ventral part of pons
Pedunculus cerebellaris medius
Transv. pontine fibers
Longitudinal fascicles of pons (pyramidal tract)
Basilar sulcus of pons

Fig. 138. Cross section through the pons at the level of the facial colliculus. On the left side the brachium pontis is severed from the cerebellum. VI = abducent nucleus.

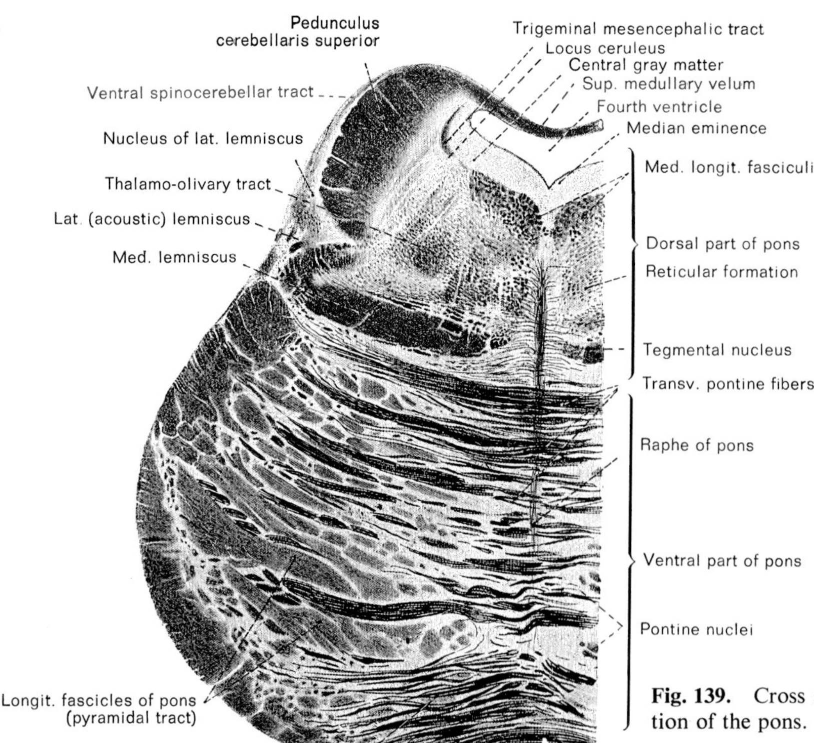
Pedunculus cerebellaris superior
Trigeminal mesencephalic tract
Locus ceruleus
Central gray matter
Sup. medullary velum
Ventral spinocerebellar tract
Fourth ventricle
Median eminence
Nucleus of lat. lemniscus
Med. longit. fasciculi
Thalamo-olivary tract
Lat. (acoustic) lemniscus
Dorsal part of pons
Med. lemniscus
Reticular formation
Tegmental nucleus
Transv. pontine fibers
Raphe of pons
Ventral part of pons
Pontine nuclei
Longit. fascicles of pons (pyramidal tract)
Transv. pontine fibers

Fig. 139. Cross section through the middle portion of the pons.

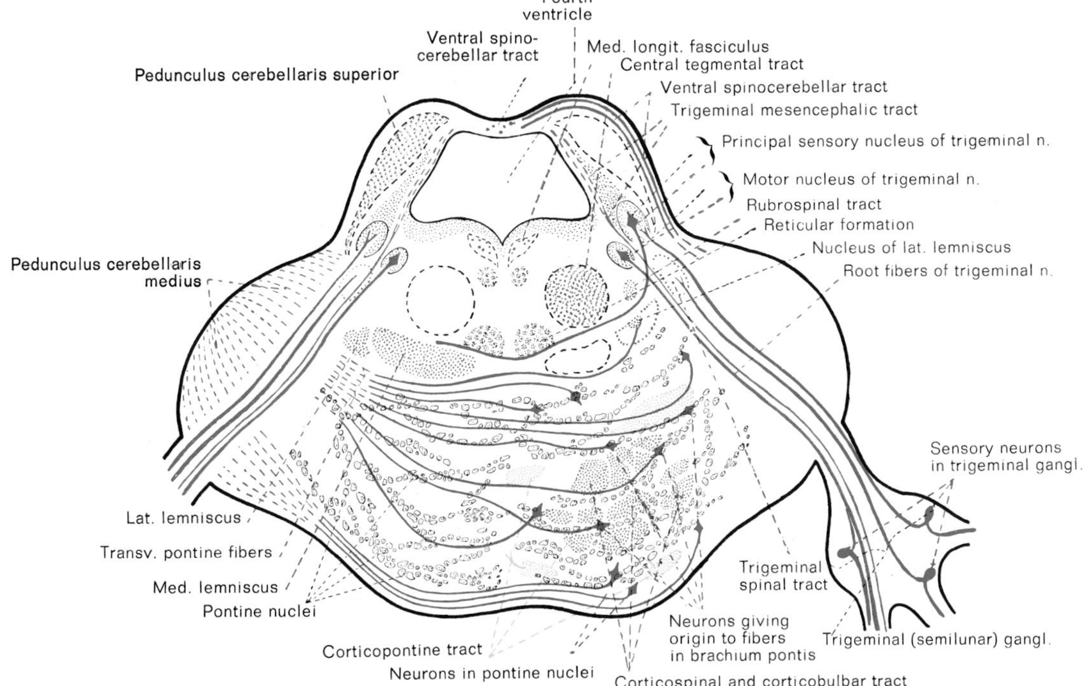
Fourth
ventricle
Ventral spino-
cerebellar tract
Med. longit. fasciculus
Central tegmental tract
Pedunculus cerebellaris superior
Ventral spinocerebellar tract
Trigeminal mesencephalic tract
Principal sensory nucleus of trigeminal n.
Motor nucleus of trigeminal n.
Rubrospinal tract
Reticular formation
Nucleus of lat. lemniscus
Root fibers of trigeminal n.
Pedunculus cerebellaris
medius
Sensory neurons
in trigeminal gangl.
Lat. lemniscus
Transv. pontine fibers
Med. lemniscus
Pontine nuclei
Trigeminal
spinal tract
Neurons giving
origin to fibers
in brachium pontis
Trigeminal (semilunar) gangl.
Corticopontine tract
Neurons in pontine nuclei
Corticospinal and corticobulbar tract

Fig. 140. Architecture of the pons at the level of the trigeminal nuclei. Schematic cross section.*

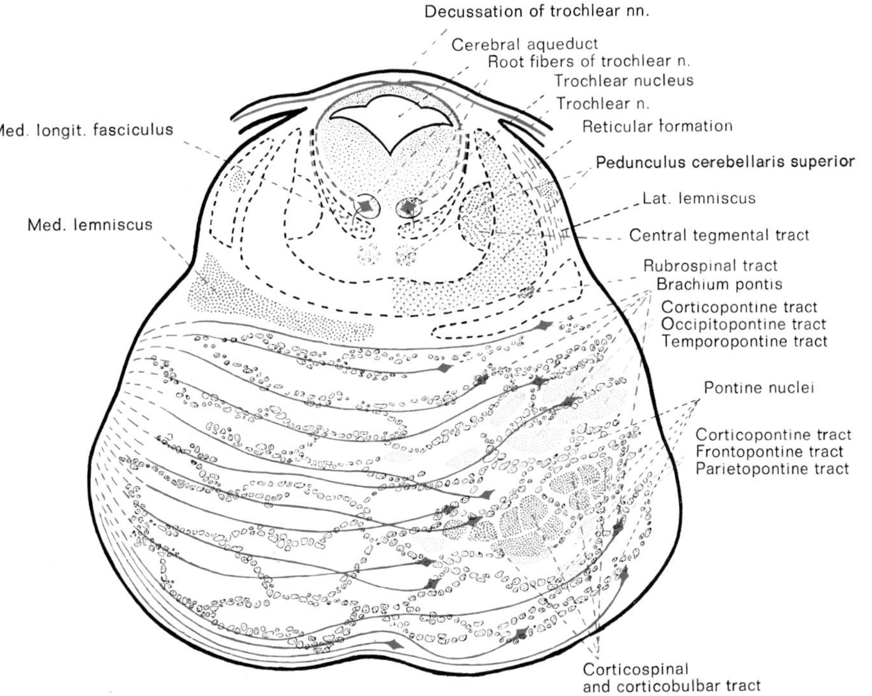
Decussation of trochlear nn.
Cerebral aqueduct
Root fibers of trochlear n.
Trochlear nucleus
Trochlear n.
Med. longit. fasciculus
Reticular formation
Pedunculus cerebellaris superior
Lat. lemniscus
Med. lemniscus
Central tegmental tract
Rubrospinal tract
Brachium pontis
Corticopontine tract
Occipitopontine tract
Temporopontine tract
Pontine nuclei
Corticopontine tract
Frontopontine tract
Parietopontine tract
Corticospinal
and corticobulbar tract

Fig. 141. Architecture of the pons at the level of the trochlear nuclei. Schematic cross section.*

* Red and yellow: descending pathways; blue: ascending pathways.

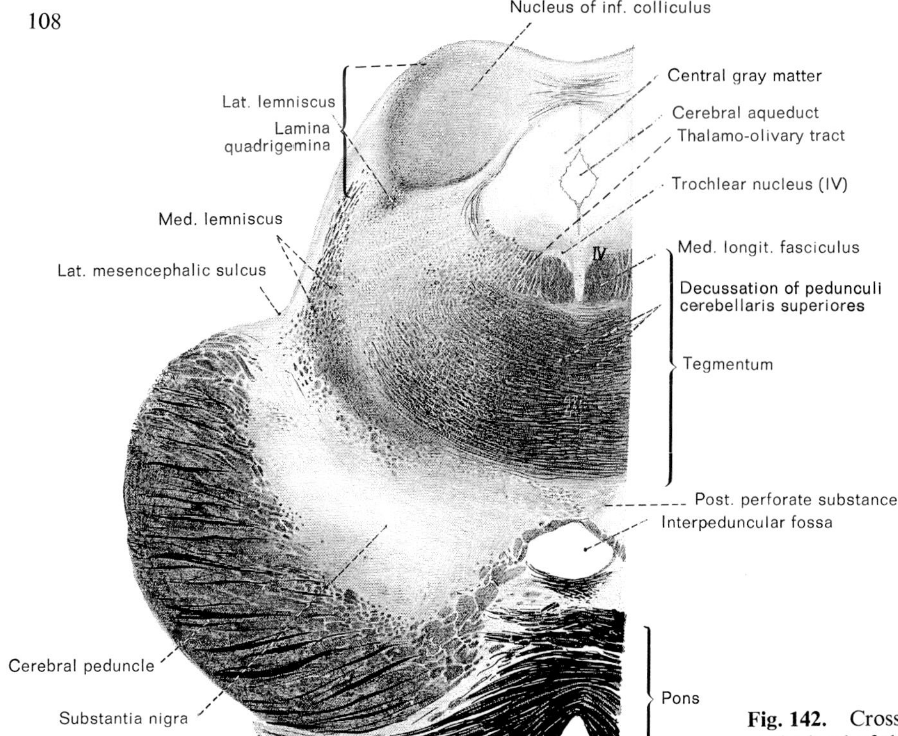
Nucleus of inf. colliculus
Central gray matter
Cerebral aqueduct
Thalamo-olivary tract
Trochlear nucleus (IV)
Lat. lemniscus
Lamina quadrigemina
Med. lemniscus
Lat. mesencephalic sulcus
IV
Med. longit. fasciculus
Decussation of pedunculi cerebellaris superiores
Tegmentum
Post. perforate substance
Interpeduncular fossa
Cerebral peduncle
Substantia nigra
Pons
Transv. pontine fibers

Fig. 142. Cross section through the midbrain at the level of the inferior colliculi.

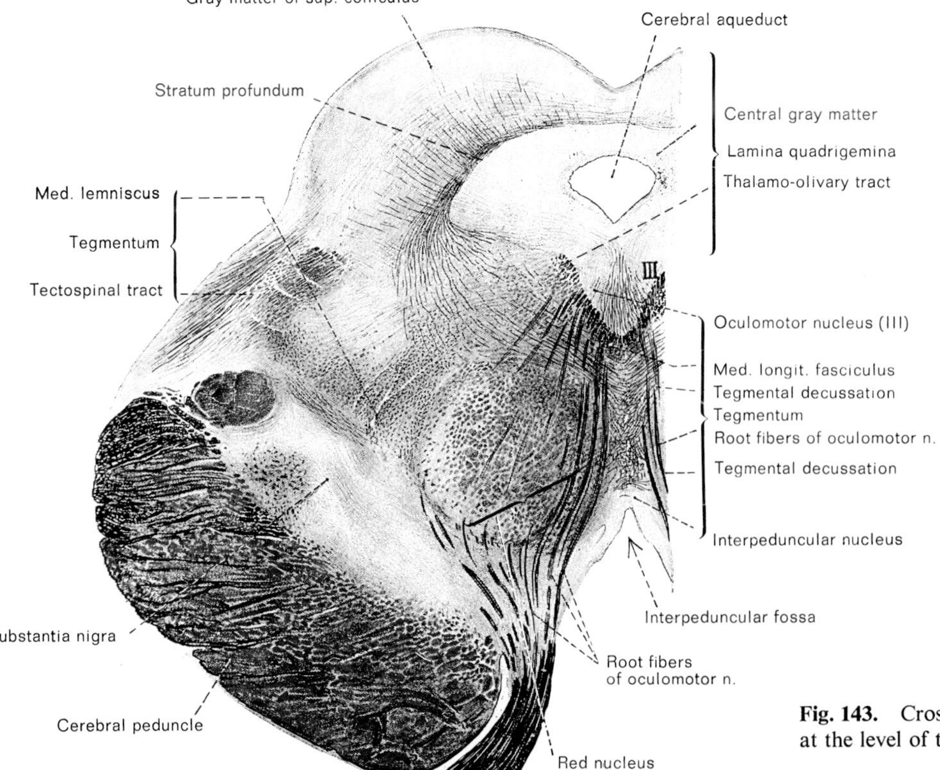
Gray matter of sup. colliculus
Cerebral aqueduct
Stratum profundum
Central gray matter
Lamina quadrigemina
Thalamo-olivary tract
Med. lemniscus
Tegmentum
Tectospinal tract
III
Oculomotor nucleus (III)
Med. longit. fasciculus
Tegmental decussation
Tegmentum
Root fibers of oculomotor n.
Tegmental decussation
Interpeduncular nucleus
Interpeduncular fossa
Substantia nigra
Root fibers of oculomotor n.
Cerebral peduncle
Red nucleus
Oculomotor n.

Fig. 143. Cross section through the midbrain at the level of the superior colliculi.

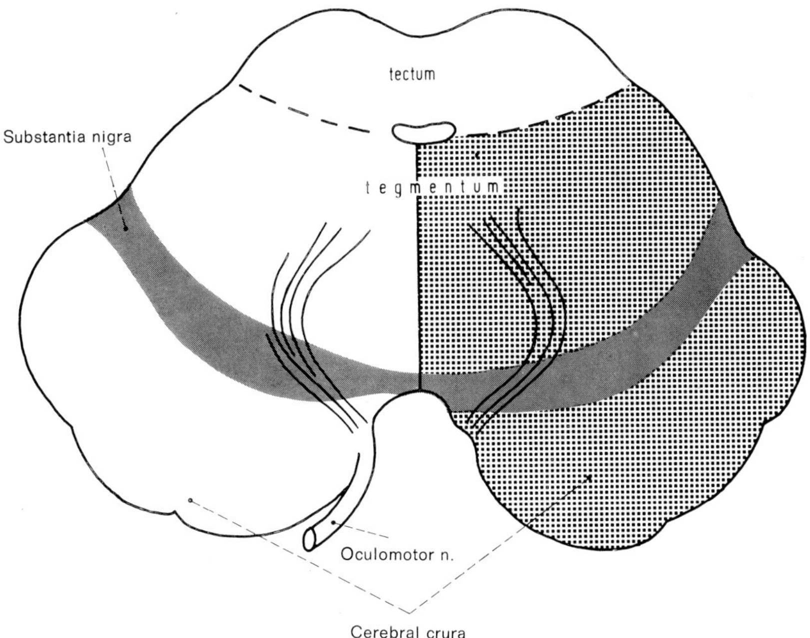
tectum
Substantia nigra
tegmentum
Oculomotor n.
Cerebral crura

Fig. 144. Subdivisions of the midbrain. Dotted area: cerebral peduncle (crus cerebri plus one half of the tegmentum).

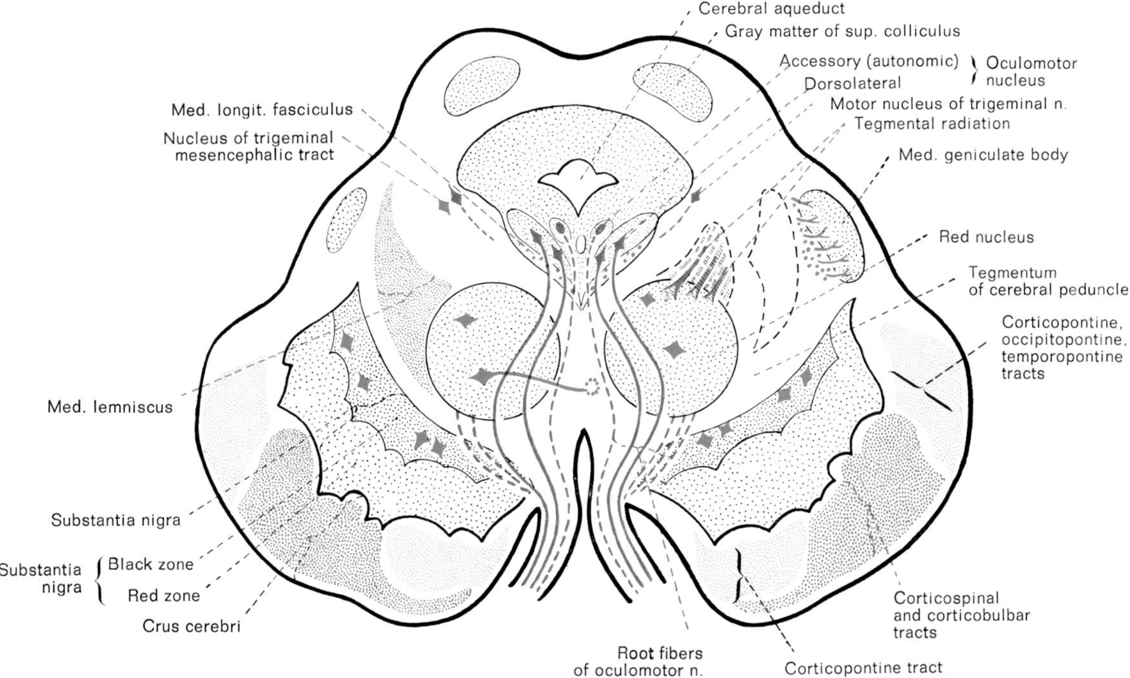
Cerebral aqueduct
Gray matter of sup. colliculus
Accessory (autonomic)
Dorsolateral
Oculomotor nucleus
Motor nucleus of trigeminal n.
Tegmental radiation
Med. geniculate body
Med. longit. fasciculus
Nucleus of trigeminal mesencephalic tract
Red nucleus
Tegmentum of cerebral peduncle
Corticopontine, occipitopontine, temporopontine tracts
Med. lemniscus
Substantia nigra
Substantia nigra
Black zone
Red zone
Crus cerebri
Corticospinal and corticobulbar tracts
Root fibers of oculomotor n.
Corticopontine tract

Fig. 145. Architecture of the midbrain at the level of the superior colliculi. Schematic cross section. Red and yellow: descending pathways, blue: ascending pathways.

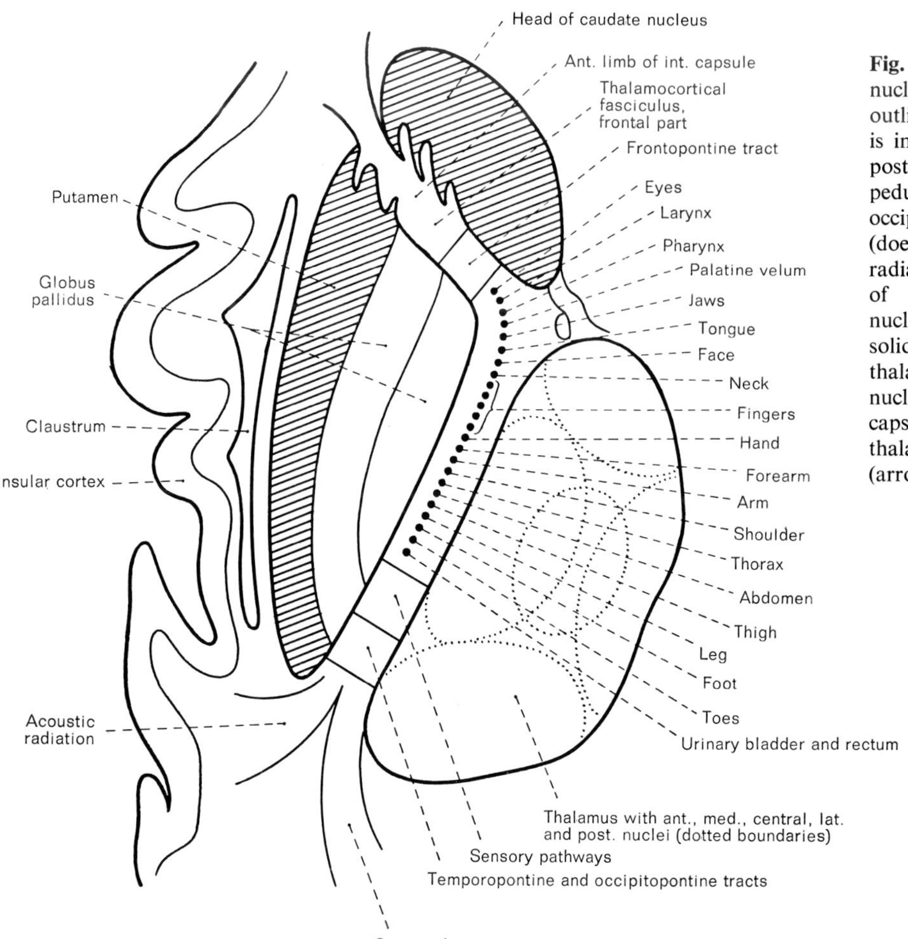
Head of caudate nucleus
Ant. limb of int. capsule
Thalamocortical fasciculus, frontal part
Frontopontine tract
Eyes
Larynx
Pharynx
Palatine velum
Jaws
Tongue
Face
Neck
Fingers
Hand
Forearm
Arm
Shoulder
Thorax
Abdomen
Thigh
Leg
Foot
Toes
Urinary bladder and rectum
Putamen
Globus pallidus
Claustrum
Insular cortex
Acoustic radiation
Thalamus with ant., med., central, lat. and post. nuclei (dotted boundaries)
Sensory pathways
Temporopontine and occipitopontine tracts
Optic radiation

Fig. 147. Thalamic radiation, caudate nucleus and putamen in lateral view. The outline of the medially located thalamus is indicated anteriorly by a dotted line, posteriorly by a solid line. 1: frontal peduncle; 2ab: parietal peduncle; 3: occipital peduncle; 4: inferior peduncle (does not actually belong to the thalamic radiation); 5: optic radiation. * Bridges of gray substance between caudate nucleus and putamen. ** This dotted and solid line indicates the position of the thalamus located medial to the lentiform nucleus. Between the two is the internal capsule through which the fibers of the thalamic radiation take their course (arrows).

Fig. 146. Disposition of the fiber systems within the internal capsule of the lentiform nucleus with special emphasis on the somatotopic arrangement of the motor pathways (pyramidal tract).

Note: Most of the long pathways between cerebral cortex and lower centers of brain stem and spinal cord (ascending and descending pathways) take their course through an L-shaped area located between the lentiform nucleus on the lateral side and the thalamus and caudate nucleus on the medial side. The entirety of these fibers forms the internal capsule in which can be distinguished an anterior limb, a genu, and a posterior limb. These designations are based upon the appearance of the internal capsule in a horizontally sectioned cerebral hemisphere. In three dimensional view, additionally, a sublentiform and a retrolentiform portion of the internal capsule may be distinguished. The anterior limb of the internal capsule contains the thalamocortical and frontopontine pathways, the genu contains the corticobulbar pathways, and in the posterior limb – arranged from rostral to caudal – are located the corticospinal tract, thalamocortical tract, temporo-occipital pontine pathways as well as the acoustic and optic radiations.

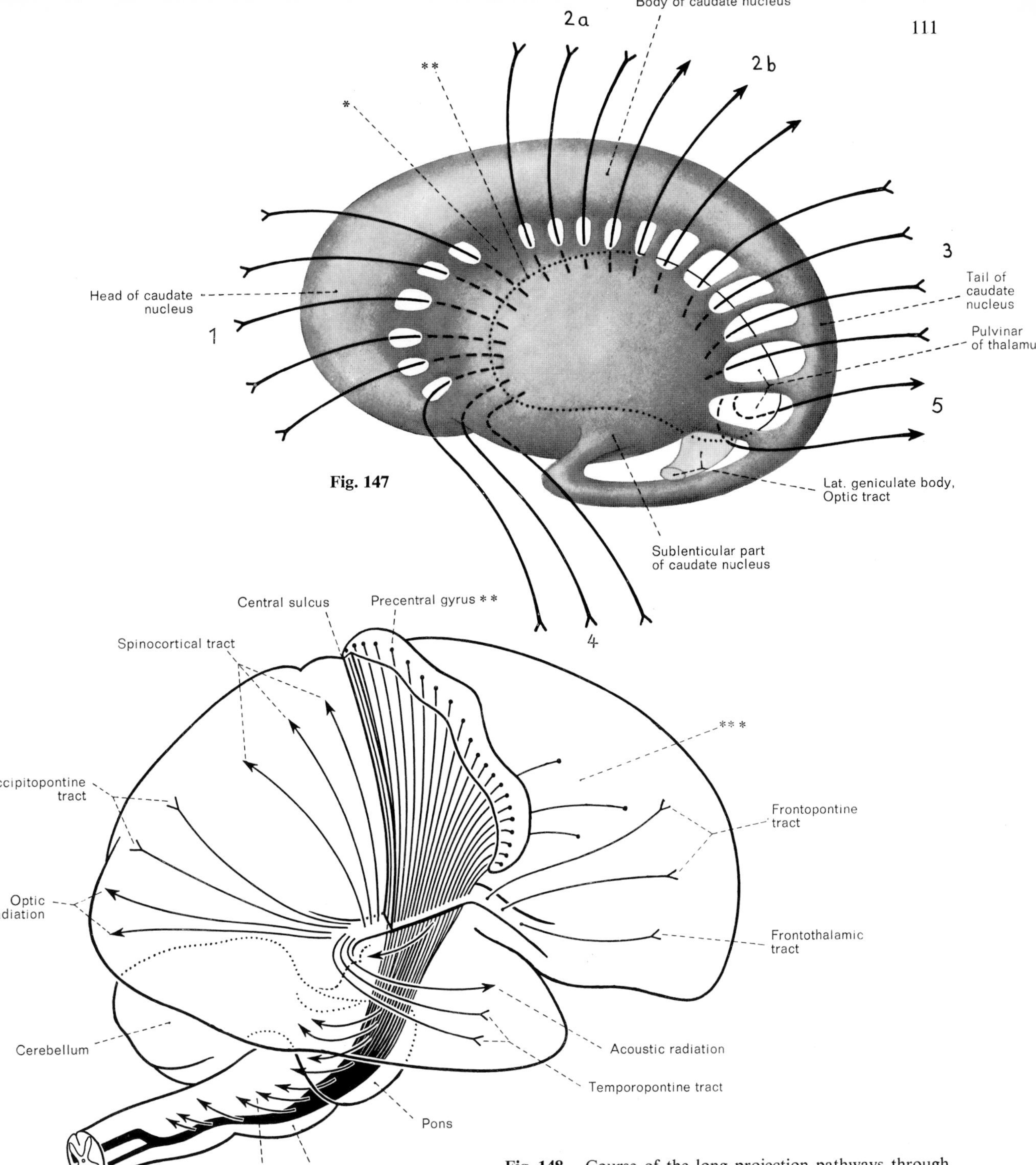

Body of caudate nucleus
2a
**
*
2b
Head of caudate nucleus
1
3
Tail of caudate nucleus
Pulvinar of thalamus
5
Lat. geniculate body, Optic tract
Sublenticular part of caudate nucleus
4
Central sulcus
Precentral gyrus **
Spinocortical tract
***
Occipitopontine tract
Frontopontine tract
Optic radiation
Frontothalamic tract
Cerebellum
Acoustic radiation
Temporopontine tract
Pons
Medulla oblongata
*

Fig. 147

Fig. 148. Course of the long projection pathways through internal capsule and brain stem. * Arrows = fibers leaving the pyramidal tract toward the lamina quadrigemina (corticotectal tract), toward the pontine nuclei (corticopontine tract), toward the cerebellum (corticocerebellar tract) and toward the nuclei of the medulla oblongata (corticobulbar tract). The pyramidal tract continues as crossed lateral corticospinal tract and as uncrossed ventral corticospinal tract. ** First neurons of the pyramidal tract; their fibers converge and occupy the anterior two thirds of the posterior limb of the internal capsule (compare Fig. 146). *** Motor pathways from medial the frontal gyrus.

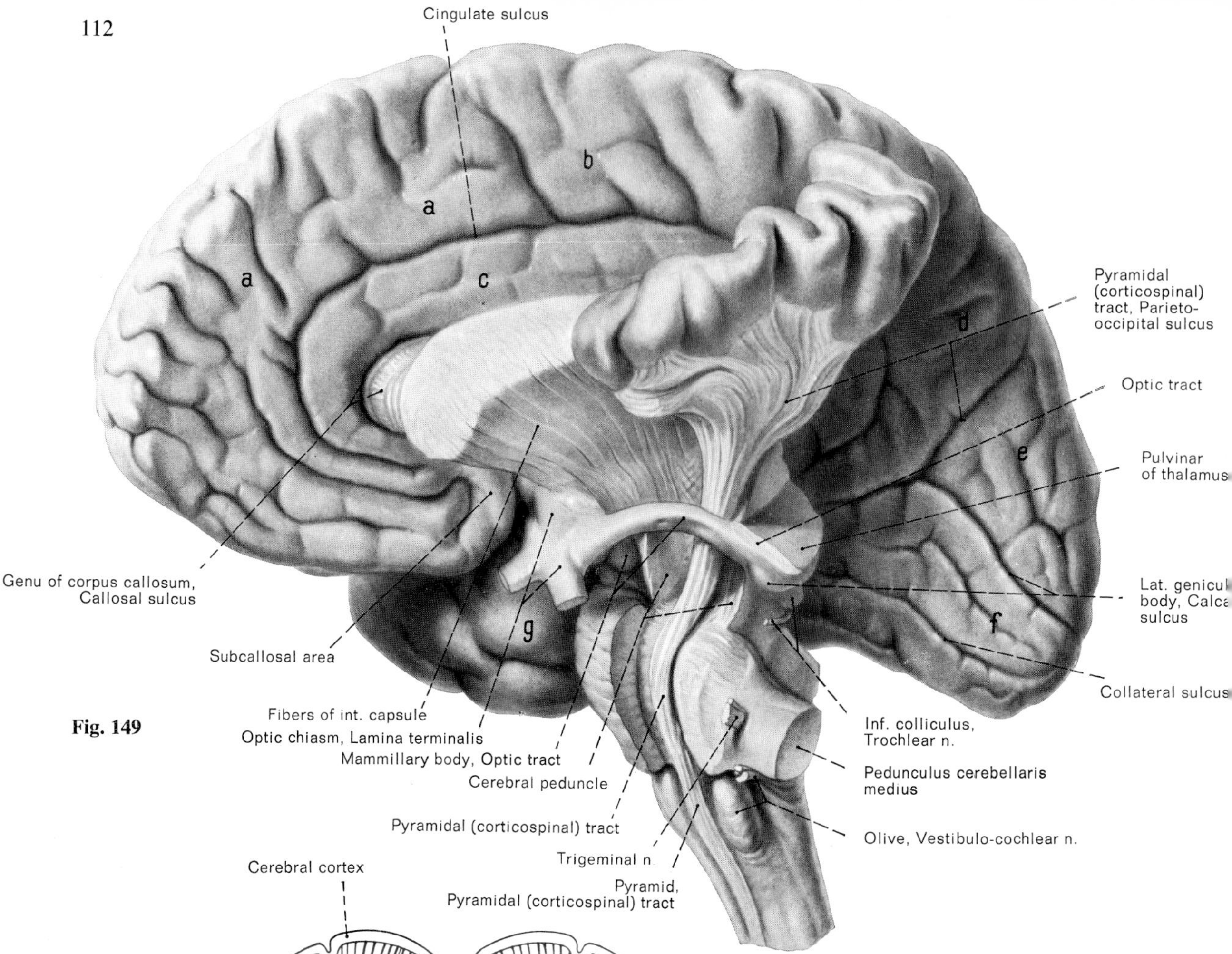

Cingulate sulcus

a

b

a

c

d

e

f

g

Pyramidal (corticospinal) tract, Parieto-occipital sulcus

Optic tract

Pulvinar of thalamus

Lat. genicul body, Calca sulcus

Collateral sulcus

Genu of corpus callosum, Callosal sulcus

Subcallosal area

Fibers of int. capsule

Optic chiasm, Lamina terminalis

Mammillary body, Optic tract

Cerebral peduncle

Pyramidal (corticospinal) tract

Trigeminal n.

Pyramid, Pyramidal (corticospinal) tract

Inf. colliculus, Trochlear n.

Pedunculus cerebellaris medius

Olive, Vestibulo-cochlear n.

Fig. 149

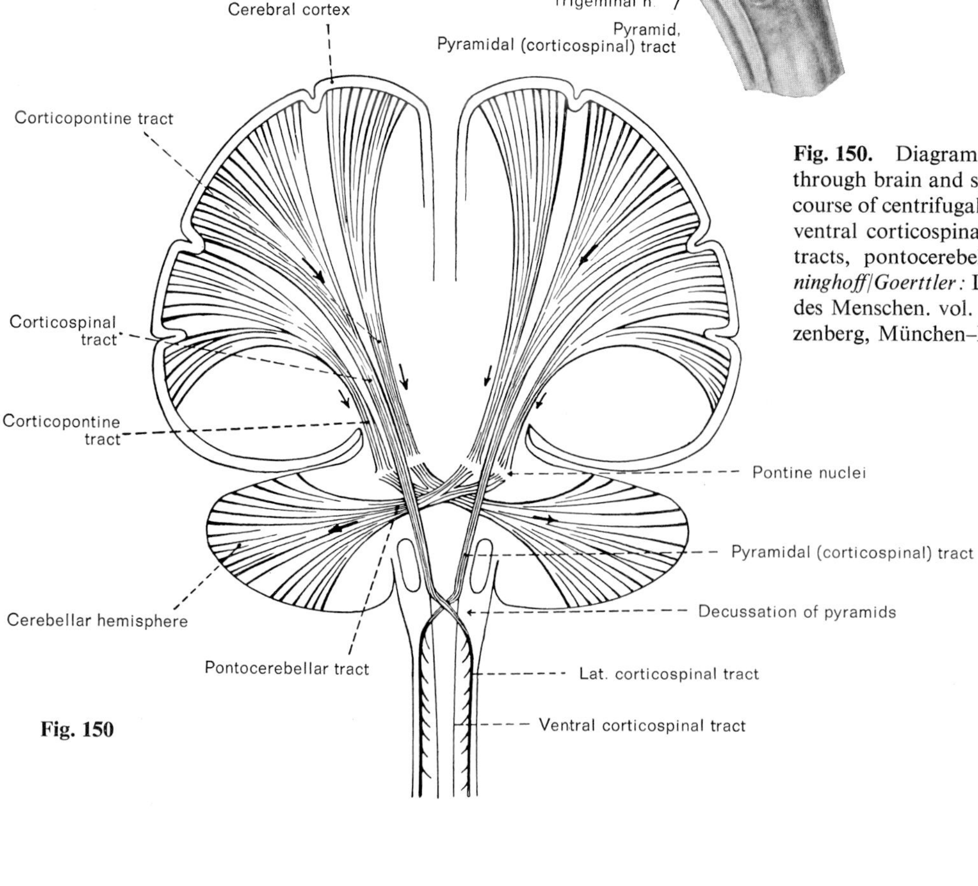

Cerebral cortex

Corticopontine tract

Corticospinal tract

Corticopontine tract

Pontine nuclei

Pyramidal (corticospinal) tract

Decussation of pyramids

Cerebellar hemisphere

Pontocerebellar tract

Lat. corticospinal tract

Ventral corticospinal tract

Fig. 150

Fig. 150. Diagram of a frontal section through brain and spinal cord showing the course of centrifugal pathways. Lateral and ventral corticospinal tracts, corticopontine tracts, pontocerebellar tracts (from *Benninghoff/Goerttler:* Lehrbuch der Anatomie des Menschen. vol. 3. Urban und Schwarzenberg, München–Berlin–Wien 1967).

Fig. 149. A fiber preparation demonstrating the left corticospinal (pyramidal) tract. Pons and cerebral peduncle have been resected as far as necessary, the lentiform nucleus has been removed so that the fibers within the internal capsule are exposed. Since only the precentral gyrus, the chief area of origin of the pyramidal tract, has been maintained all other fiber systems of the internal capsule are shown only in their intracapsular extent (from *Pernkopf / Ferner:* Atlas der angewandten und topographischen Anatomie des Menschen. vol. 1. Urban und Schwarzenberg, München–Berlin 1963).

a = superior frontal gyrus
b = paracentral lobulus
c = cingulate gyrus
d = precuneus
e = cuneus
f = medial occipitotemporal gyrus
g = uncus of parahippocampal gyrus

The psychomotor pathways: corticospinal and corticobulbar tracts

The pyramidal (corticospinal) tract is an exclusive possession of mammals and man, and has developed in connection with the development of the telencephalon. It originates in the precentral gyrus and in the paracentral lobule of the frontal lobe. Giant pyramidal cells *(Betz)* of the fifth cortical layer as well as numerous smaller neurons of cortical areas and deeper nuclei give rise to the tract which contains approximately one million fibers.

The pyramidal tract is concentrated in the posterior limb of the internal capsule (Fig. 146). From here it courses to the midbrain where it occupies the middle region of the cerebral crura (Fig. 145). In the base of the pons, it forms coarse bundles that are easily recognized in cross sections (Fig. 138). On the anterior aspect of the medulla oblongata, the fibers of the pyramidal tract are tightly bundled and cause surface elevations medial to the olives on both sides of the midline (Fig. 32) which are called pyramids, thus giving the pathway its name.

At the caudal tip of the pyramids about three quarters of the fibers cross to the contralateral side in the decussation of the pyramids (Figs. 127–130) and course downward in the lateral funiculus of the spinal cord (lateral corticospinal tract). The remainder of the fibers continues downward as the uncrossed ventral corticospinal tract in order to decussate at various segmental levels. The first neuron of the pyramidal tract synapses with ventral horn motor neurons either directly or via interneurons. The pyramidal tract transmits impulses to the ventral horn motor neurons whose myelinated axons leave the spinal cord through the ventral roots. They supply skeletal muscles either directly through spinal nerves or after having formed plexuses from which peripheral nerves reach skeletal musculature.

The corticobulbar tract is that shorter portion of the psycho-motor system that synapses on motor cranial nerve nuclei located in the midbrain tegmentum (III, IV), the pontine tegmentum (VI, V, VII), and in the medulla oblongata (nucleus ambiguus = IX, X, XI) (compare Fig. 37). In this tract, also, most fibers decussate to the nuclei of the contralateral side.

The corticobulbar tract originates in the lower part of the precentral gyrus and in the triangular portion (motor speech center) of the inferior frontal gyrus, where the neurons for the musculature of head and neck are located. The pathway courses through the genu of the internal capsule (Fig. 146) as well as through the crura of the midbrain and terminates upon the motor nuclei of the cranial nerves mentioned above. The axons of the peripheral neurons supply, via the motor cranial nerves (III–VII, IX, X), the extrinsic ocular muscles, speech musculature, mimic musculature, masticatory muscles as well as the muscles of pharynx and larynx.

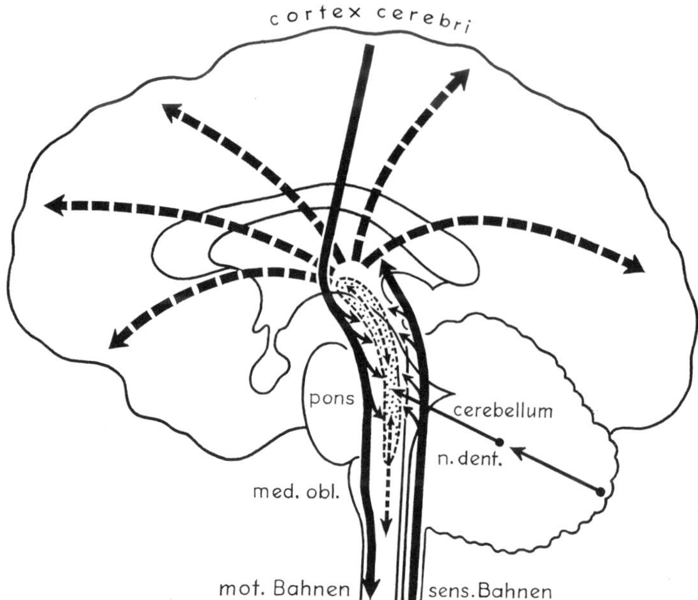
cortex cerebri
pons
cerebellum
n. dent.
med. obl.
mot. Bahnen
sens. Bahnen

Fig. 151. The reticular formation of the brain stem, stippled area. It extends from the diencephalon through the entire brain stem and is continuous with the reticular formation of the spinal cord. Black arrows indicate its connections with descending (motor) pathways and ascending (sensory) pathways including optic, acoustic and olfactory tracts. Dashed arrows indicate its connections to the cerebral cortex and to the pyramidal and extrapyramidal system of the spinal cord (after *H. W. Magoun,* 1950). (Cortex cerebri = cerebral cortex; sens. Bahnen = sensory pathways; mot. Bahnen = motor pathways; med. obl. = medulla oblongata.)

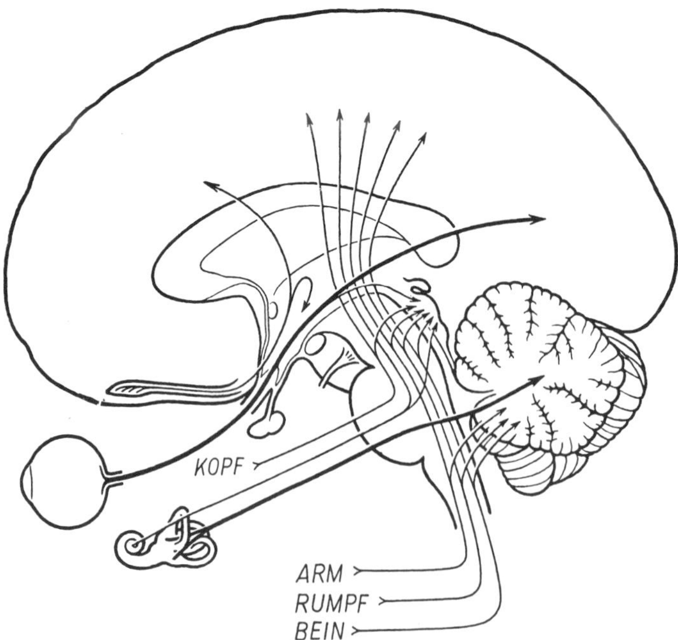
KOPF
ARM
RUMPF
BEIN

Fig. 152. The three integration areas of the human brain: telencephalon, anterior colliculi (optic tectum), and cerebellum. Incoming information from the entire body is collected here and new impulses are relayed to the motor neurons of the ventral horns. (Diagram after *Braus/Elze:* Anatomie des Menschen. vol. 3, 2nd ed. Springer, Berlin–Göttingen–Heidelberg 1960). (Kopf = head; Arm. = upper extremity; Rumpf = trunk; Bein = lower extremity.)

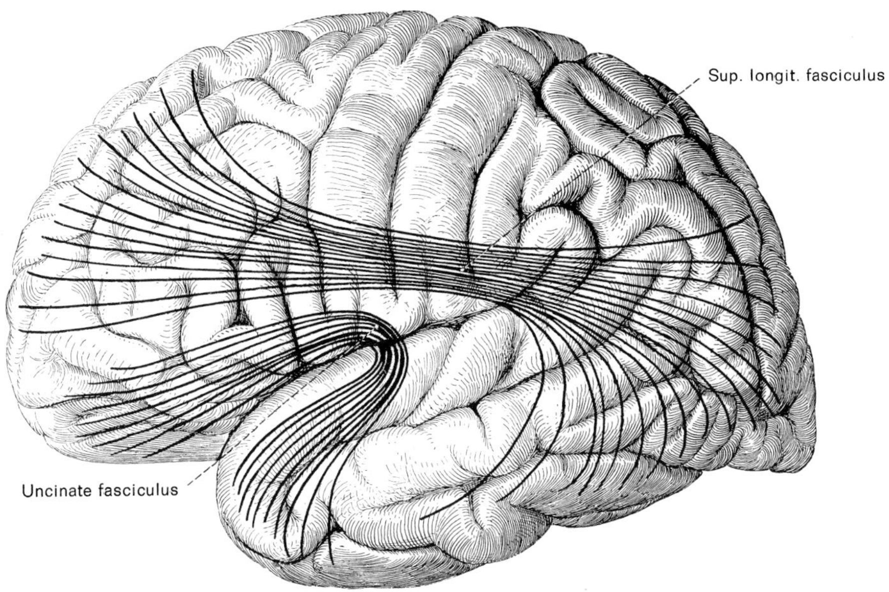
Sup. longit. fasciculus
Uncinate fasciculus

Fig. 153. Superior longitudinal fasciculus (fronto-occipital direction) and uncinate fasciculus (fronto-temporal direction) projected onto the lateral aspect of the left hemisphere (schematic).

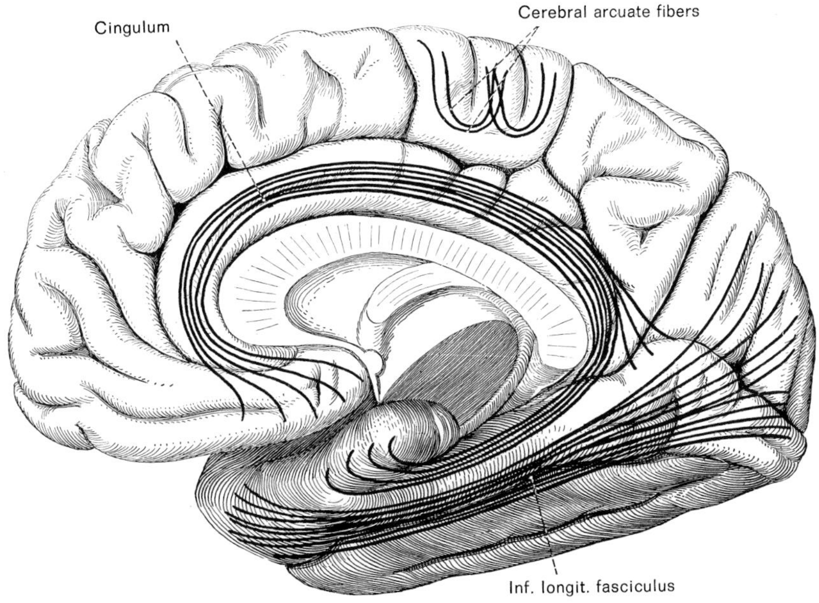
Cingulum
Cerebral arcuate fibers
Inf. longit. fasciculus

Fig. 154. Association pathways of the cerebral hemisphere projected onto the medial aspect of the right hemisphere (schematic).

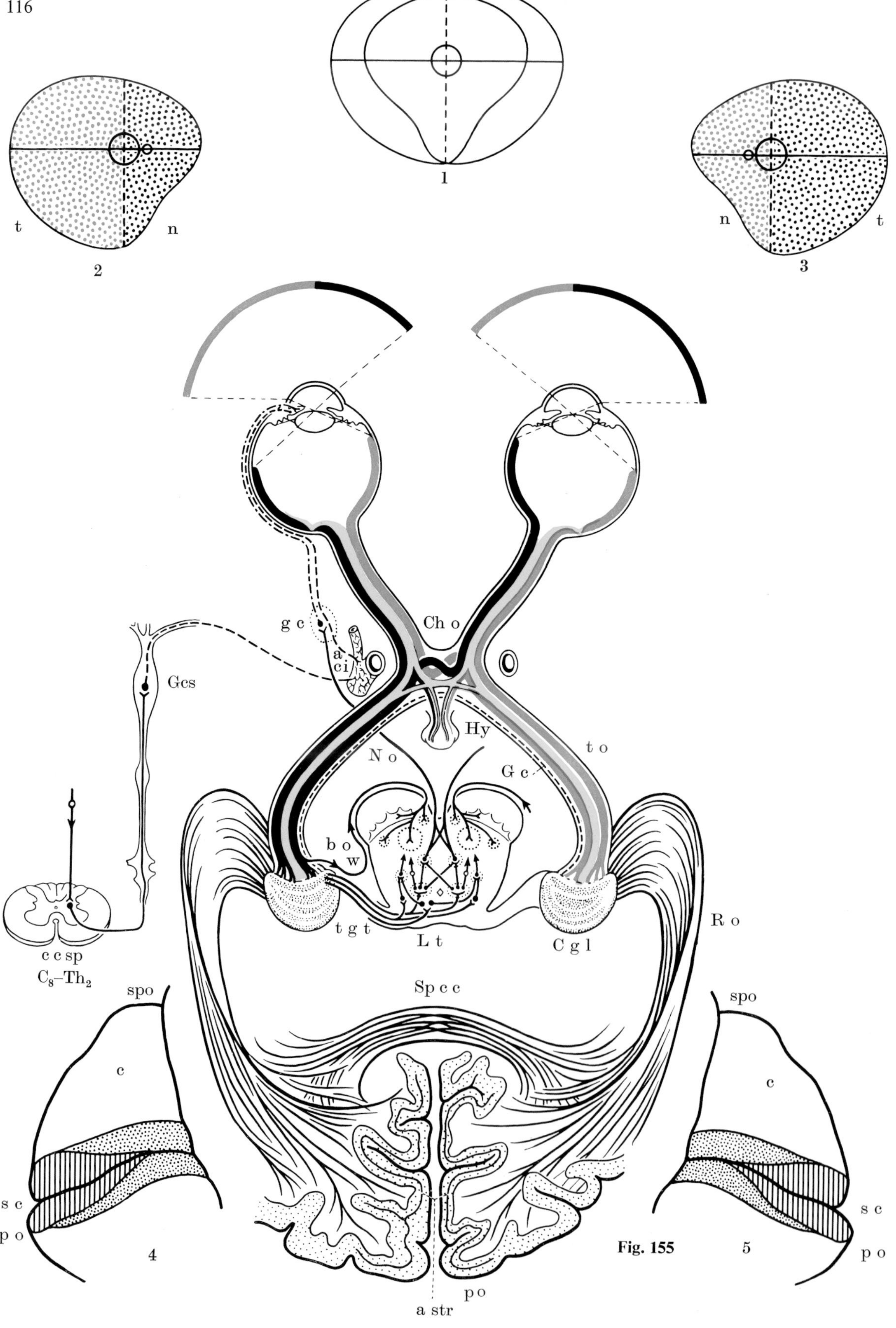
1
t
n
2
n
t
3
g c
a
ci
Gcs
Ch o
Hy
N o
t o
G c
b o
w
t g t
L t
C g l
R o
c c sp
C_8–Th_2
spo
Sp c c
spo
c
c
s c
p o
4
s c
p o
5
p o
a str

Fig. 155

The visual pathway

light

↓

pars optica of retina

1. Light sensitive cells (rod cells and cone cells) = photoreceptor cells.

2. *Retinal ganglion;* relay and integration system of predominantly bipolar neurons.

3. *Ganglion of optic nerve;* multipolar neurons whose axons pass through the optic disc into the optic nerve. The disc corresponds to the blind spot. The area of the most acute vision is the central fovea with its immediate vicinity, the macula lutea. Light rays from an object in the visual axis reach the fovea centralis which contains only cone cells.

↓

optic nerves

↓

optic chiasm

Partial decussation of fibers. About 60% do cross, 40% remain uncrossed. Nasal fibers decussate, temporal fibers remain uncrossed; fibers from the central fovea are crossed or uncrossed.

↓

optic trcat

↓

↓

secondary visual centers

1. *Lateral geniculate body.* Connection of both lateral geniculate bodies via Gudden's commissure.
2. *Pulvinar of thalamus*
3. *Nucleus of superior colliculus*

↓

Connections to extrinsic ocular muscle nuclei, muscle of accommodation, sphincter pupillae muscle and ciliospinal center (pupillary reflex).

Optic radiation. This large fiber system, fan-shaped and spiraled, courses through the posterior limb of the internal capsule, above the amygdala, lateral to the posterior horn of the lateral ventricle to the *visual cortex* in the occipital lobe, the *striate cortex* around the *calcarine sulcus.* The retina is represented in the striate area of the cortex with exact point-to-point projection (17 and 18 after Brodman). The representation of the central fovea occupies the largest part of the striate area. Furthermore, the optic region expands into the area of the cuneus and the medial occipitotemporal gyrus as well as the lateral surface of the occipital lobe. The optic radiations and the striate areas of both hemispheres may be interconnected through the splenium of the corpus callosum.

Fig. 155. Diagram of the visual pathway and its stations.

1	binocular visual field
2	visual field of the left eye
3	visual field of the right eye
n	nasal
t	temporal
4, 5	medial aspect of the occipital lobe of the telencephalon
Ch o	optic chiasm
a c i	internal carotid artery with sympathetic carotid plexus
g c	ciliary ganglion
Hy	hypophysis
t o	optic tract
G c	Gudden's commissure = connection of the lateral geniculate bodies
b o w	basal optic root = reflex pathway to the nuclear areas of the midbrain
L t	lamina tecti (quadrigemina)
t g t	geniculo-tectal tract
N o	oculomotor nerve
C g l	lateral geniculate body
R o	optic radiation
Sp c c	splenium of corpus callosum with possible connections of the optic radiations of both hemispheres
a str	striate cortex
p o	occipital pole
s c	calcarine sulcus; vertical hatching: projection area of the central fovea, the papillomacular bundle of the upper and lower half of the contralateral optic radiation; stippled area: projection area of the retinal periphery of the upper and lower quadrant
c	cuneus
Spo	parieto-occipital sulcus
G c s	superior cervical ganglion
cc sp	ciliospinal center C8–Th2 (dilatation of pupil)

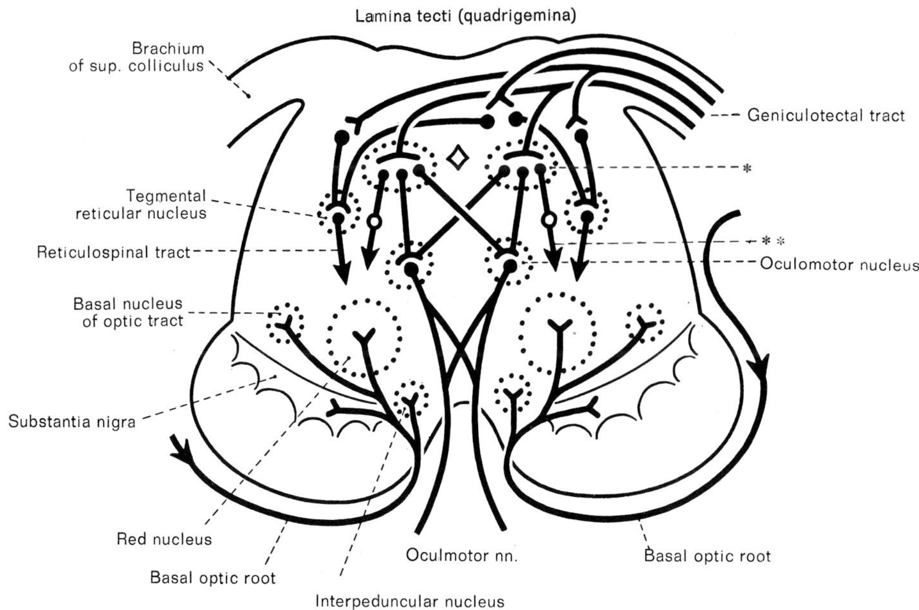
Lamina tecti (quadrigemina)
Brachium of sup. colliculus
Geniculotectal tract
*
Tegmental reticular nucleus
Reticulospinal tract
**
Oculomotor nucleus
Basal nucleus of optic tract
Substantia nigra
Red nucleus
Basal optic root
Oculmotor nn.
Basal optic root
Interpeduncular nucleus

Fig. 156. Diagrammatic cross section through the midbrain showing nuclei and connections subserving eye movements (enlarged portion from Fig. 155). * pupillary center, ** fibers to the ciliospinal center.

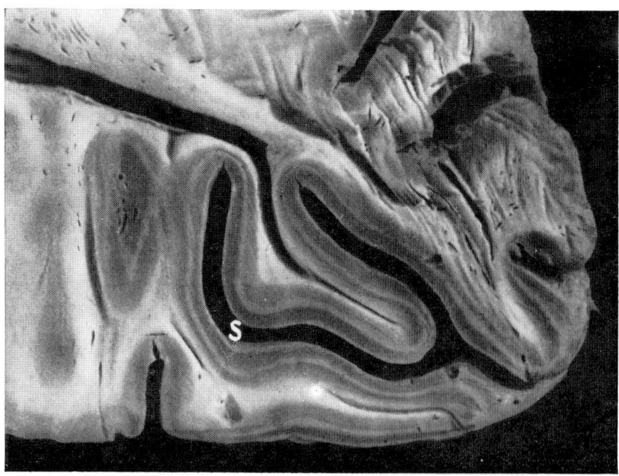
S

Fig. 157. Cortex of the occipital pole with the line of *Gennari* (or *Vicq d'Azyr*). S = calcarine sulcus, striate cortex, visual cortex.

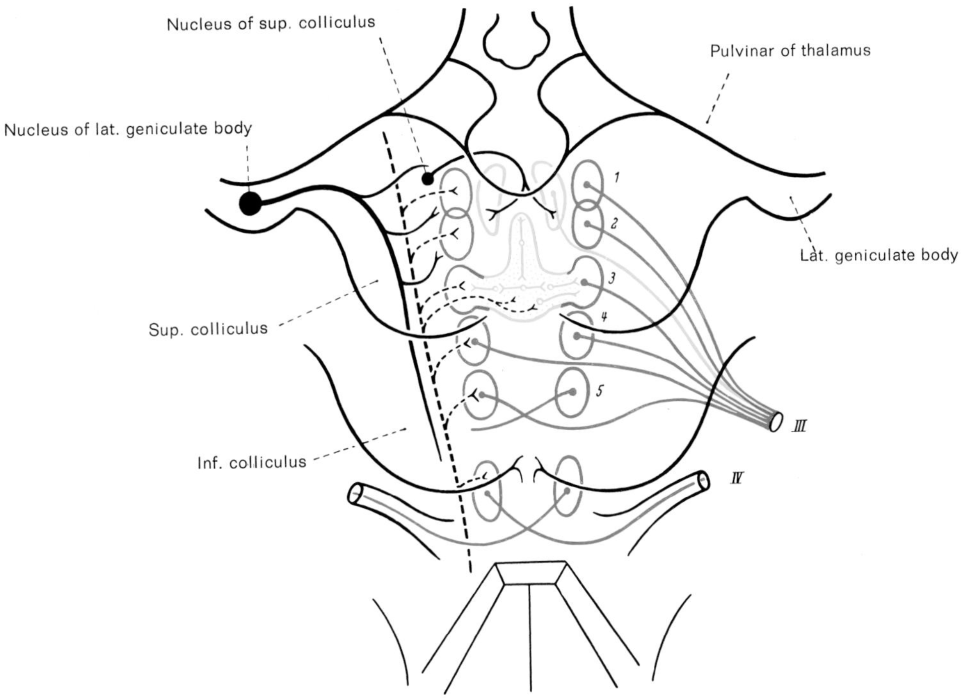

Nucleus of sup. colliculus
Pulvinar of thalamus
Nucleus of lat. geniculate body
1
2
Lat. geniculate body
3
4
Sup. colliculus
5
III
Inf. colliculus
IV

Fig. 158. Subdivisions of the oculomotor (III) and trochlear (IV) nuclei for the innervation of the extrinsic ocular muscles (nuclei proportionally larger than the outlines of the midbrain).

1 nucleus for inf. rectus m. ⎫
2 nucleus for inf. oblique m. ⎬ oculomotor n. (III)
3 nucleus for med. rectus m. ⎪
4 nucleus for sup. rectus m. ⎭
5 nucleus for sup. oblique m. = trochlear n. (IV)

yellow: parvocellular median nucleus *(Perlja)* for convergence
yellow paired: *Edinger-Westphal's* nucleus for intrinsic ocular muscles
black dashed: medial longitudinal fasciculus

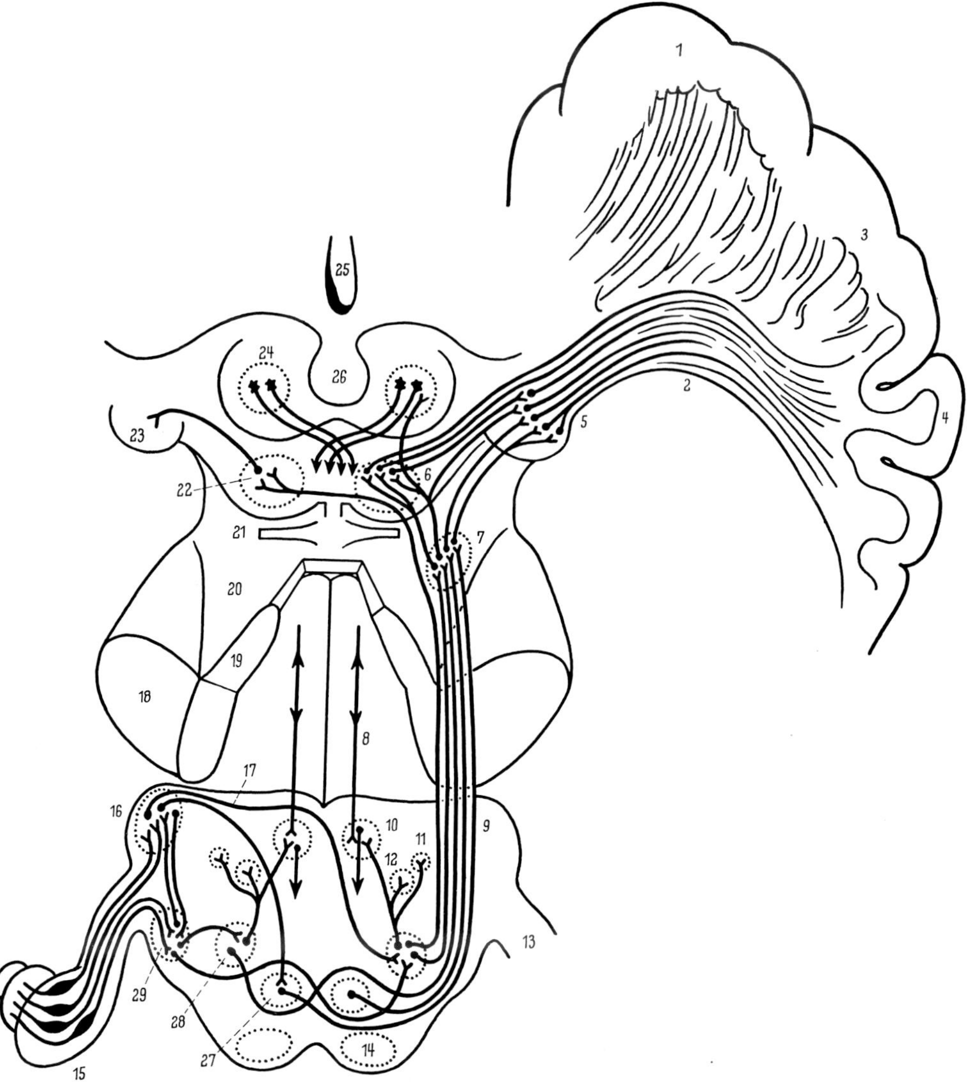
1
2
3
4
5
6
7
8
9
10
11
12
13
14
15
16
17
18
19
20
21
22
23
24
25
26
27
28
29

Fig. 159. Diagram of the auditory pathway and its stations. (The position of the nuclear areas is not exactly true; therefore, compare Fig. 134–145.)

1 temporal pole
2 acoustic radiation
3 superior temporal gyrus
4 transverse temporal gyrus
5 medial geniculate body, sixth neuron
6 nucleus of inferior colliculus, fifth neuron
7 nucleus of lateral lemniscus, fourth neuron
8 medial longitudinal fasciculus (ascending and descending fibers)
9 lateral lemniscus
10 abducent nucleus
11 trigeminal motor nucleus
12 facial nucleus
13 cochlear nerve
14 corticospinal tract
15 cochlea, first neuron
16 dorsal cochlear nerve, second neuron
17 medullary (acoustic) striae of fourth ventricle
18 pedunculus cerebellouis medius
19 pedunculus cerebellouis superior
20 trigone of lemniscus
21 trochlear nerve
22 nucleus of inferior colliculus
23 medial geniculate body
24 nucleus of superior colliculus
25 third ventricle
26 pineal body
27 trapezoid body
28 metencephalic olivary nucleus, third neuron
29 ventral cochlear nucleus, second neuron

The acoustic pathway

Auditory receptor cells (hair cells), surrounded by supporting cells, are located on the *basilar lamina* of the *spiral organ of Corti.* Their sensitivity encompasses a range from about 16 to 21 000 Hertz. There are 3–4 rows of outer hair cells and one row of inner hair cells running parallel to the inner tunnel.

Neuronal connections:

1. The hair cells are contacted by the peripheral extensions of neurons of the *spiral ganglion of the cochlea.* Their central extensions form the *cochlear portion of the vestibulocochlear nerve* which runs to

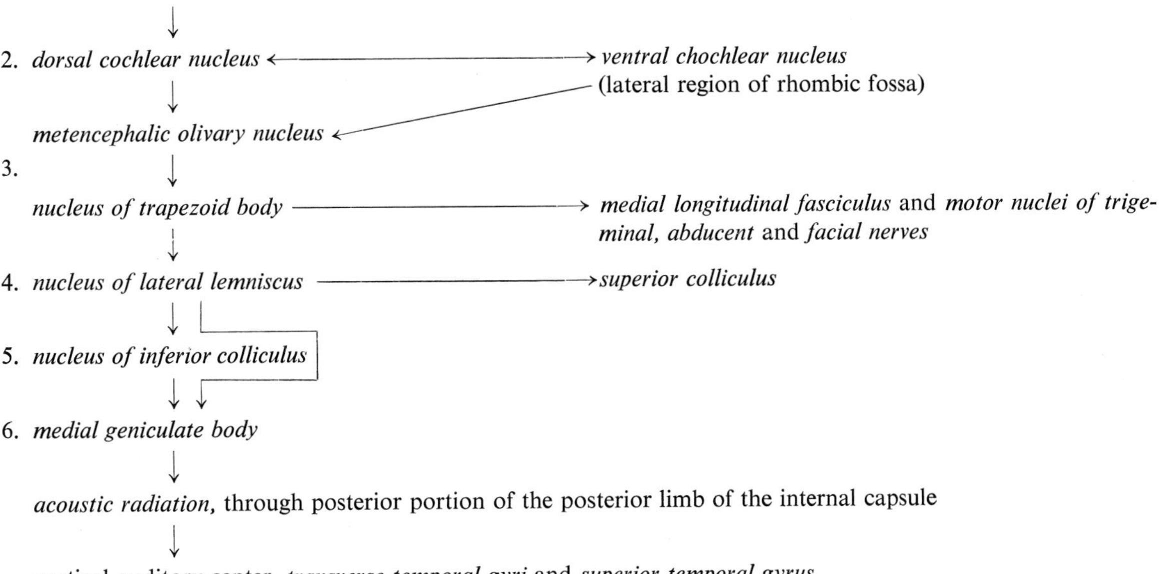
2. dorsal cochlear nucleus
ventral chochlear nucleus
(lateral region of rhombic fossa)
metencephalic olivary nucleus
3.
nucleus of trapezoid body
medial longitudinal fasciculus and motor nuclei of trigeminal, abducent and facial nerves
4. nucleus of lateral lemniscus
superior colliculus
5. nucleus of inferior colliculus
6. medial geniculate body
acoustic radiation, through posterior portion of the posterior limb of the internal capsule
cortical auditory center, transverse temporal gyri and superior temporal gyrus.

Autonomic Nervous System

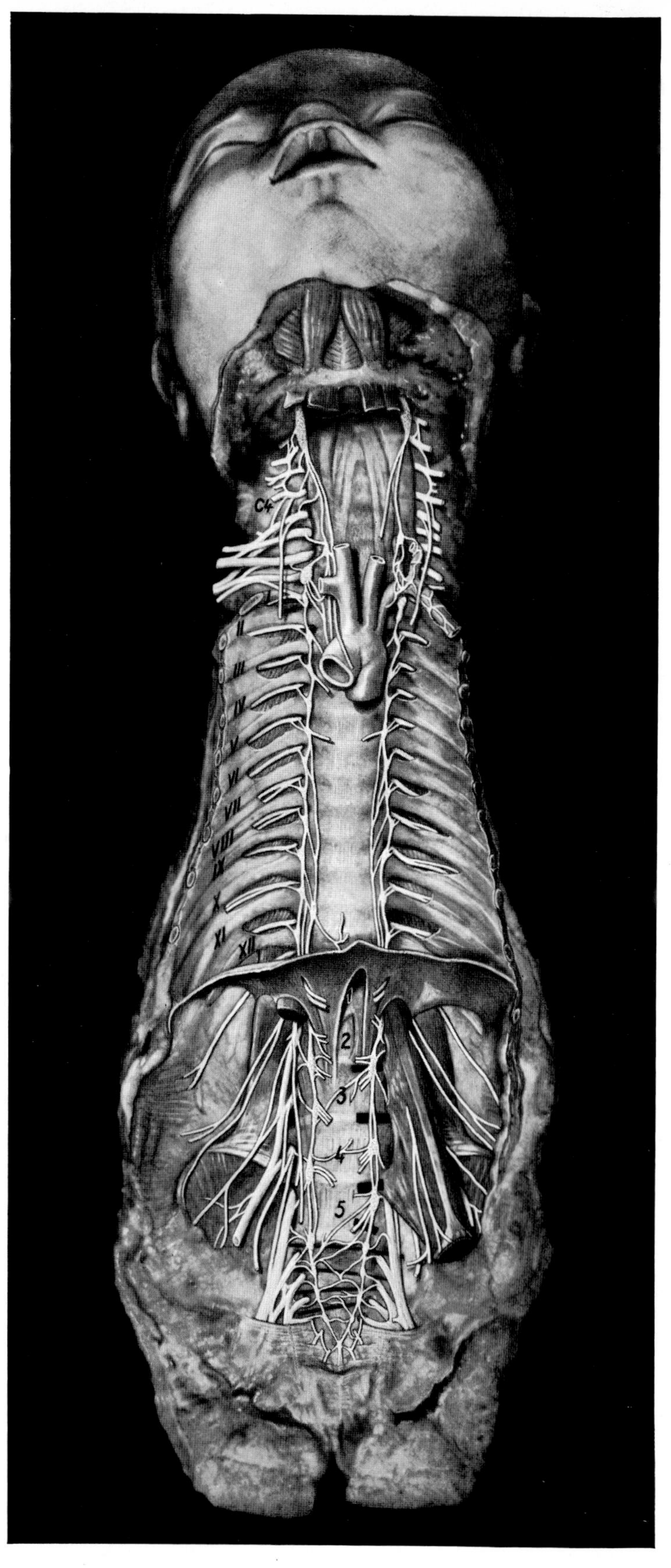
C4
II
III
IV
V
VI
VII
VIII
IX
X
XI
XII
2
3
4
5

Fig. 160

Fig. 160. The sympathetic trunk of the newborn. The brachial plexus and the lumbosacral plexus are depicted on the right side of the preparation. The sympathetic trunk and its ganglia in lumbar and sacral levels are emphasized by underlying markers (preparation in the Anatomical Institute Münster).

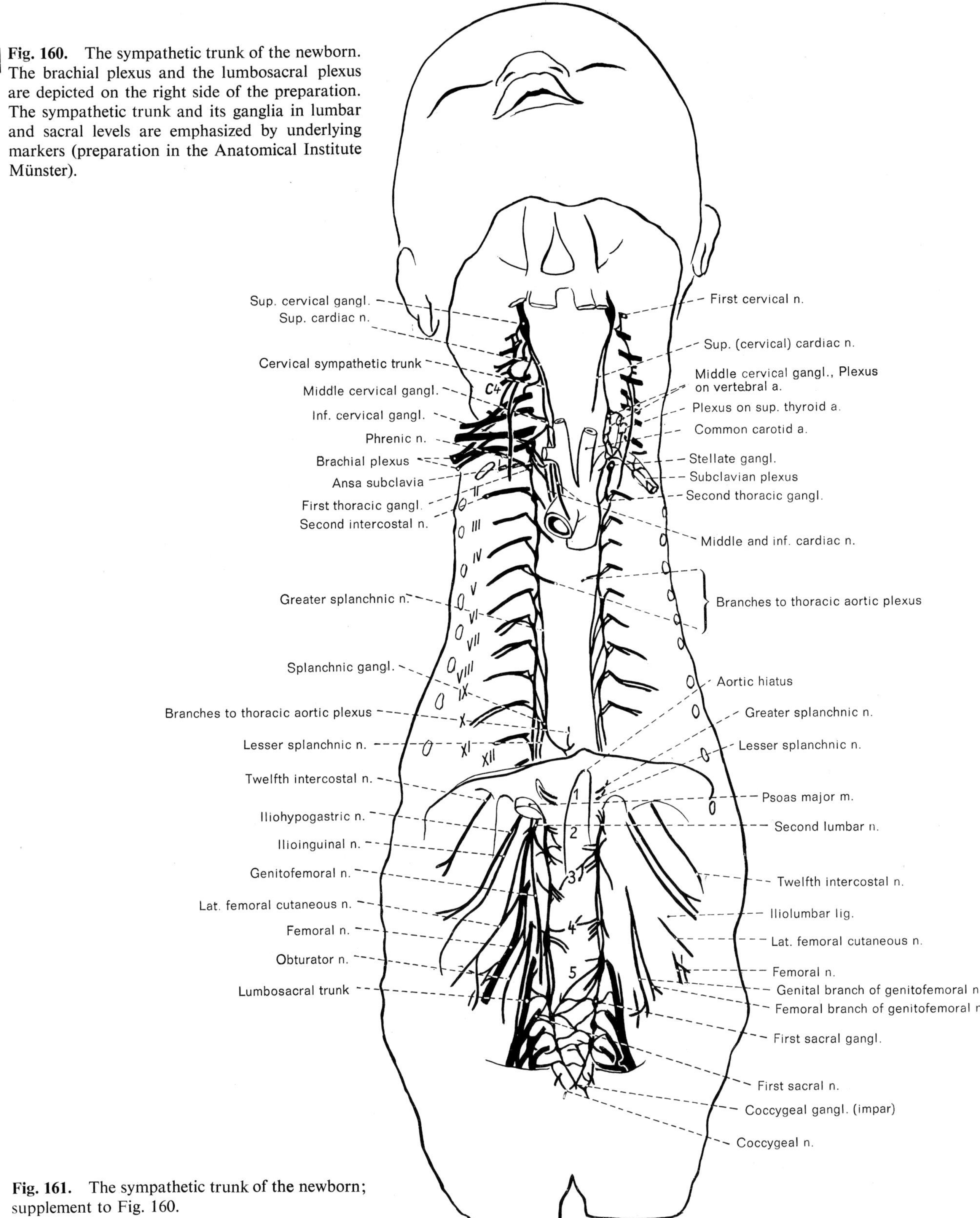

Sup. cervical gangl.
Sup. cardiac n.
Cervical sympathetic trunk
Middle cervical gangl.
Inf. cervical gangl.
Phrenic n.
Brachial plexus
Ansa subclavia
First thoracic gangl.
Second intercostal n.
Greater splanchnic n.
Splanchnic gangl.
Branches to thoracic aortic plexus
Lesser splanchnic n.
Twelfth intercostal n.
Iliohypogastric n.
Ilioinguinal n.
Genitofemoral n.
Lat. femoral cutaneous n.
Femoral n.
Obturator n.
Lumbosacral trunk
First cervical n.
Sup. (cervical) cardiac n.
Middle cervical gangl., Plexus on vertebral a.
Plexus on sup. thyroid a.
Common carotid a.
Stellate gangl.
Subclavian plexus
Second thoracic gangl.
Middle and inf. cardiac n.
Branches to thoracic aortic plexus
Aortic hiatus
Greater splanchnic n.
Lesser splanchnic n.
Psoas major m.
Second lumbar n.
Twelfth intercostal n.
Iliolumbar lig.
Lat. femoral cutaneous n.
Femoral n.
Genital branch of genitofemoral n.
Femoral branch of genitofemoral n.
First sacral gangl.
First sacral n.
Coccygeal gangl. (impar)
Coccygeal n.
C4
II
III
IV
V
VI
VII
VIII
IX
X
XI
XII
1
2
3
4
5

Fig. 161. The sympathetic trunk of the newborn; supplement to Fig. 160.

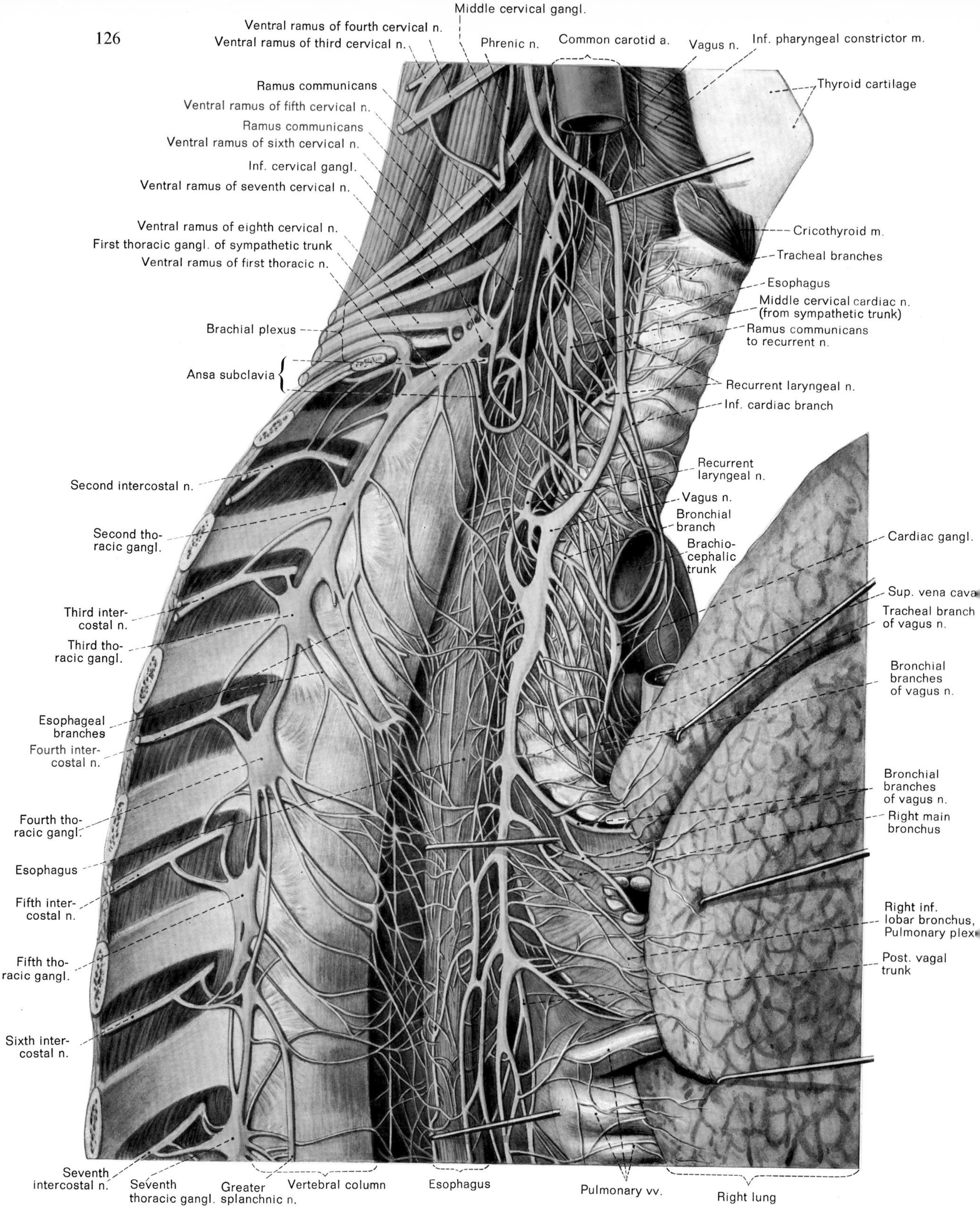

Middle cervical gangl.
Ventral ramus of fourth cervical n.
Ventral ramus of third cervical n.
Phrenic n.
Common carotid a.
Vagus n.
Inf. pharyngeal constrictor m.
Ramus communicans
Ventral ramus of fifth cervical n.
Ramus communicans
Ventral ramus of sixth cervical n.
Inf. cervical gangl.
Ventral ramus of seventh cervical n.
Ventral ramus of eighth cervical n.
First thoracic gangl. of sympathetic trunk
Ventral ramus of first thoracic n.
Brachial plexus
Ansa subclavia
Thyroid cartilage
Cricothyroid m.
Tracheal branches
Esophagus
Middle cervical cardiac n. (from sympathetic trunk)
Ramus communicans to recurrent n.
Recurrent laryngeal n.
Inf. cardiac branch
Second intercostal n.
Second thoracic gangl.
Recurrent laryngeal n.
Vagus n.
Bronchial branch
Brachiocephalic trunk
Cardiac gangl.
Sup. vena cava
Tracheal branch of vagus n.
Third intercostal n.
Third thoracic gangl.
Bronchial branches of vagus n.
Esophageal branches
Fourth intercostal n.
Fourth thoracic gangl.
Bronchial branches of vagus n.
Right main bronchus
Esophagus
Fifth intercostal n.
Fifth thoracic gangl.
Right inf. lobar bronchus, Pulmonary plexus
Post. vagal trunk
Sixth intercostal n.
Seventh intercostal n.
Seventh thoracic gangl.
Greater splanchnic n.
Vertebral column
Esophagus
Pulmonary vv.
Right lung

Fig. 162. Lower cervical and upper thoracic portion of autonomic nervous system; lateral view.
Fig. 163. Lower thoracic portion of the autonomic nervous system; lateral view.

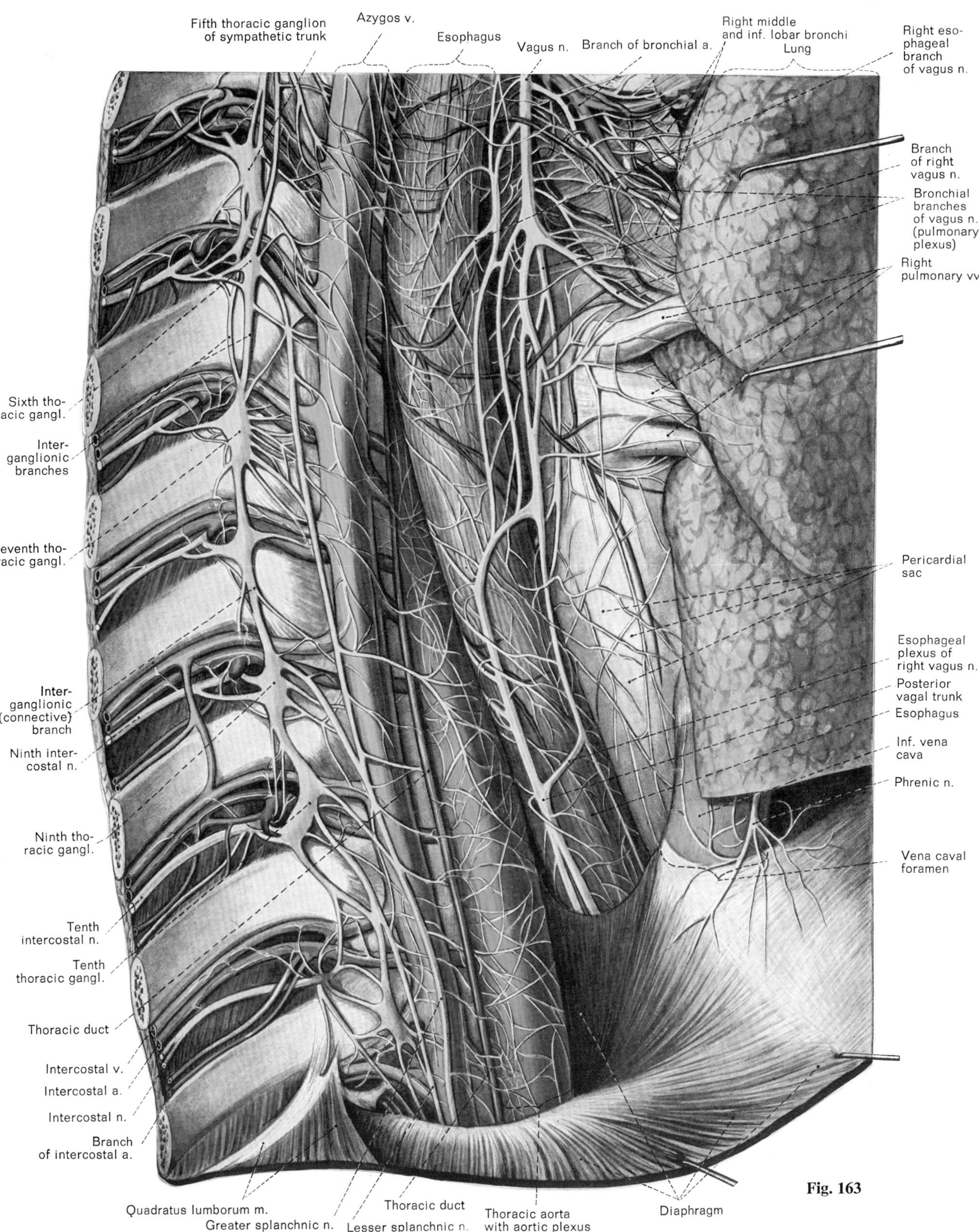

Fifth thoracic ganglion of sympathetic trunk
Azygos v.
Esophagus
Vagus n.
Branch of bronchial a.
Right middle and inf. lobar bronchi
Lung
Right esophageal branch of vagus n.
Branch of right vagus n.
Bronchial branches of vagus n. (pulmonary plexus)
Right pulmonary vv.
Sixth thoracic gangl.
Interganglionic branches
Seventh thoracic gangl.
Pericardial sac
Interganglionic (connective) branch
Esophageal plexus of right vagus n.
Posterior vagal trunk
Esophagus
Ninth intercostal n.
Inf. vena cava
Phrenic n.
Ninth thoracic gangl.
Vena caval foramen
Tenth intercostal n.
Tenth thoracic gangl.
Thoracic duct
Intercostal v.
Intercostal a.
Intercostal n.
Branch of intercostal a.
Quadratus lumborum m.
Greater splanchnic n.
Thoracic duct
Lesser splanchnic n.
Thoracic aorta with aortic plexus
Diaphragm

Fig. 163

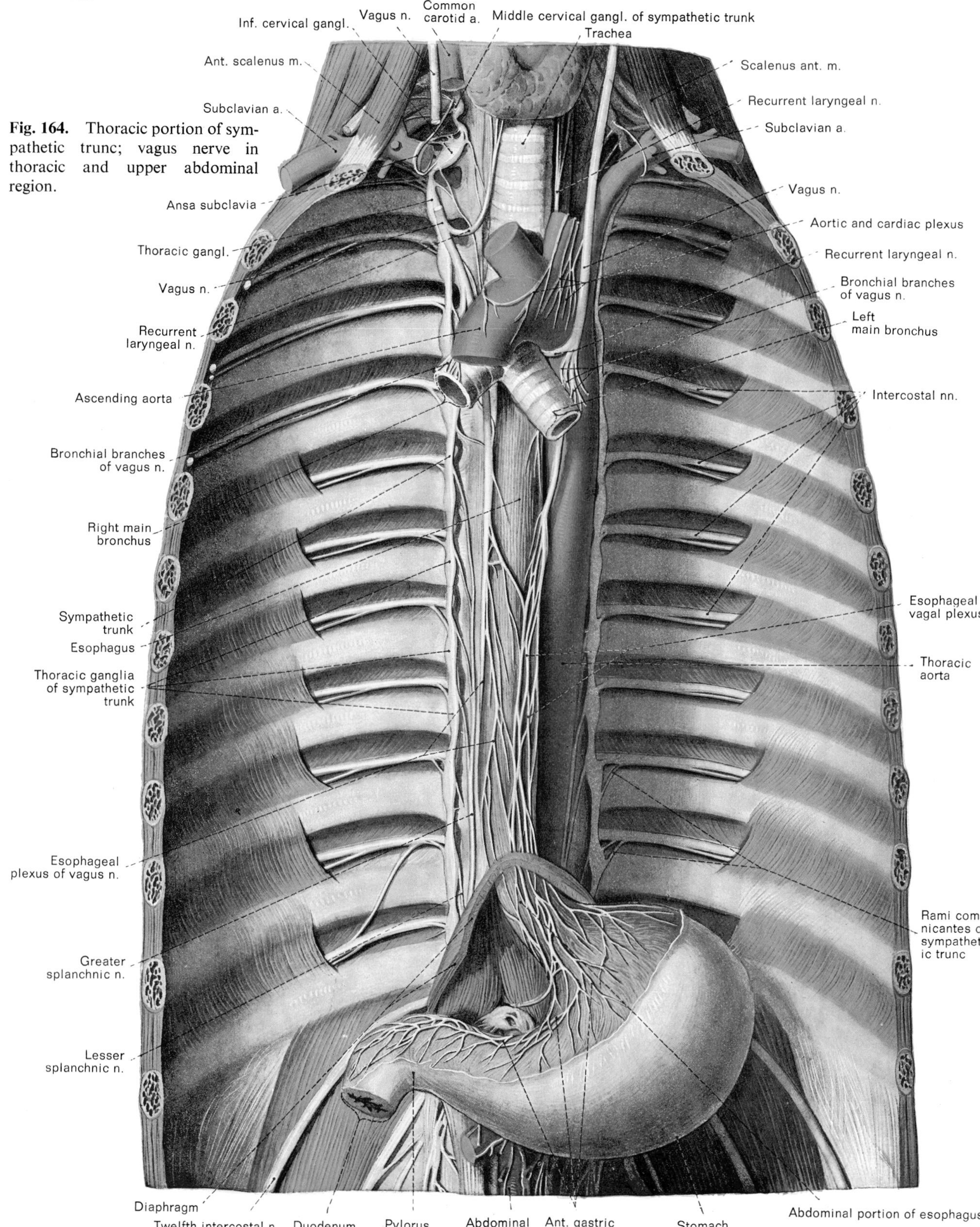
Inf. cervical gangl.
Vagus n.
Common carotid a.
Middle cervical gangl. of sympathetic trunk
Trachea
Ant. scalenus m.
Subclavian a.
Ansa subclavia
Thoracic gangl.
Vagus n.
Recurrent laryngeal n.
Ascending aorta
Bronchial branches of vagus n.
Right main bronchus
Sympathetic trunk
Esophagus
Thoracic ganglia of sympathetic trunk
Esophageal plexus of vagus n.
Greater splanchnic n.
Lesser splanchnic n.
Diaphragm
Twelfth intercostal n.
Duodenum
Pylorus
Abdominal aorta
Ant. gastric branches
Stomach
Abdominal portion of esophagus
Scalenus ant. m.
Recurrent laryngeal n.
Subclavian a.
Vagus n.
Aortic and cardiac plexus
Recurrent laryngeal n.
Bronchial branches of vagus n.
Left main bronchus
Intercostal nn.
Esophageal vagal plexus
Thoracic aorta
Rami communicantes of sympathetic trunc

Fig. 164. Thoracic portion of sympathetic trunc; vagus nerve in thoracic and upper abdominal region.

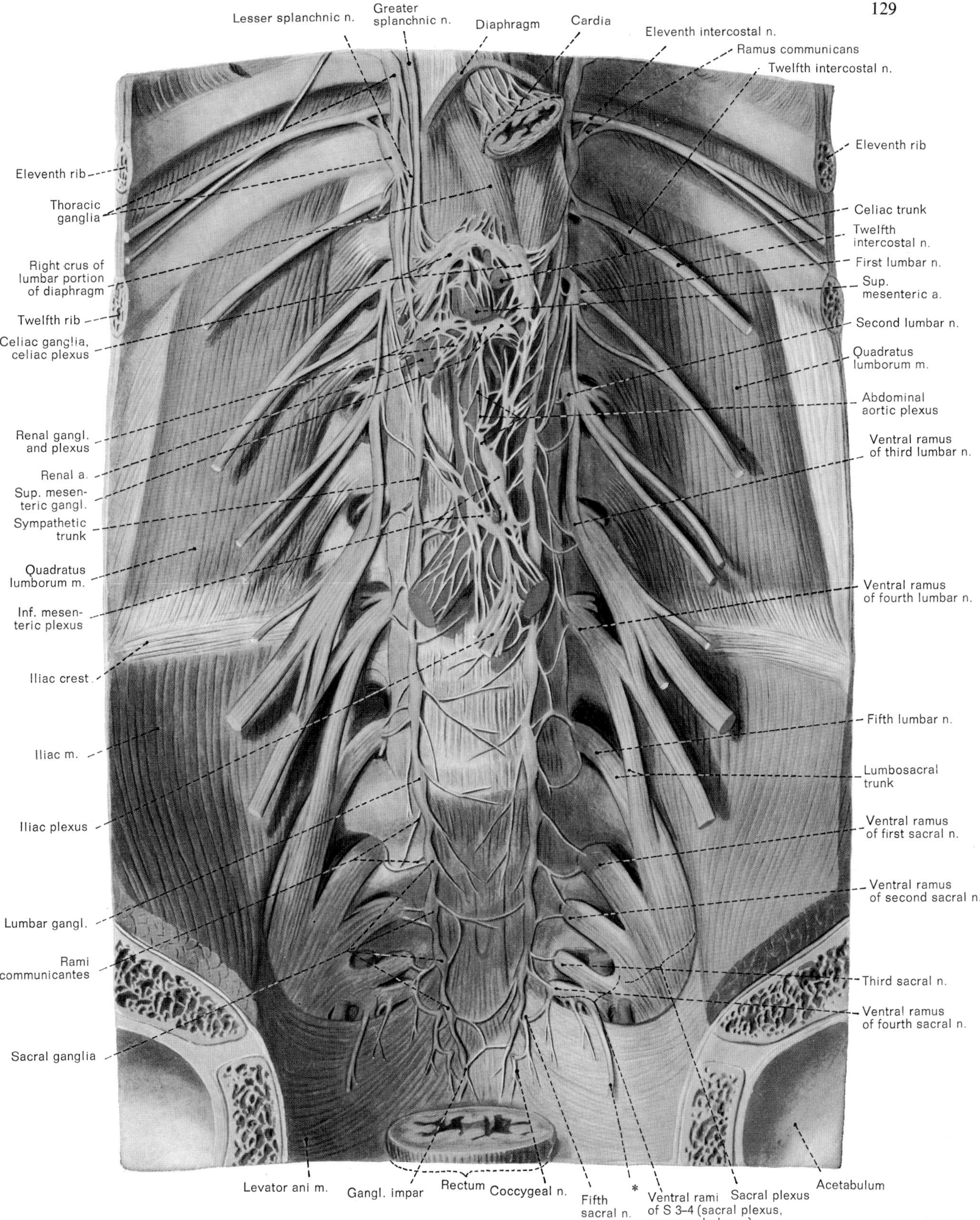
Lesser splanchnic n.
Greater splanchnic n.
Diaphragm
Cardia
Eleventh intercostal n.
Ramus communicans
Twelfth intercostal n.
Eleventh rib
Eleventh rib
Thoracic ganglia
Celiac trunk
Twelfth intercostal n.
Right crus of lumbar portion of diaphragm
First lumbar n.
Sup. mesenteric a.
Twelfth rib
Second lumbar n.
Celiac ganglia, celiac plexus
Quadratus lumborum m.
Abdominal aortic plexus
Renal gangl. and plexus
Ventral ramus of third lumbar n.
Renal a.
Sup. mesenteric gangl.
Sympathetic trunk
Quadratus lumborum m.
Ventral ramus of fourth lumbar n.
Inf. mesenteric plexus
Iliac crest
Fifth lumbar n.
Iliac m.
Lumbosacral trunk
Iliac plexus
Ventral ramus of first sacral n.
Ventral ramus of second sacral n.
Lumbar gangl.
Rami communicantes
Third sacral n.
Ventral ramus of fourth sacral n.
Sacral ganglia
Levator ani m.
Gangl. impar
Rectum
Coccygeal n.
Fifth sacral n.
*
Ventral rami of S 3–4 (sacral plexus, coccygeal plexus)
Sacral plexus
Acetabulum

Fig. 165. Abdominal and pelvic portions of the sympathetic trunk. The lumbar plexus is exposed by removal of the psoas muscle, the aortic bifurcation has been maintained. * Pudendal nerve.

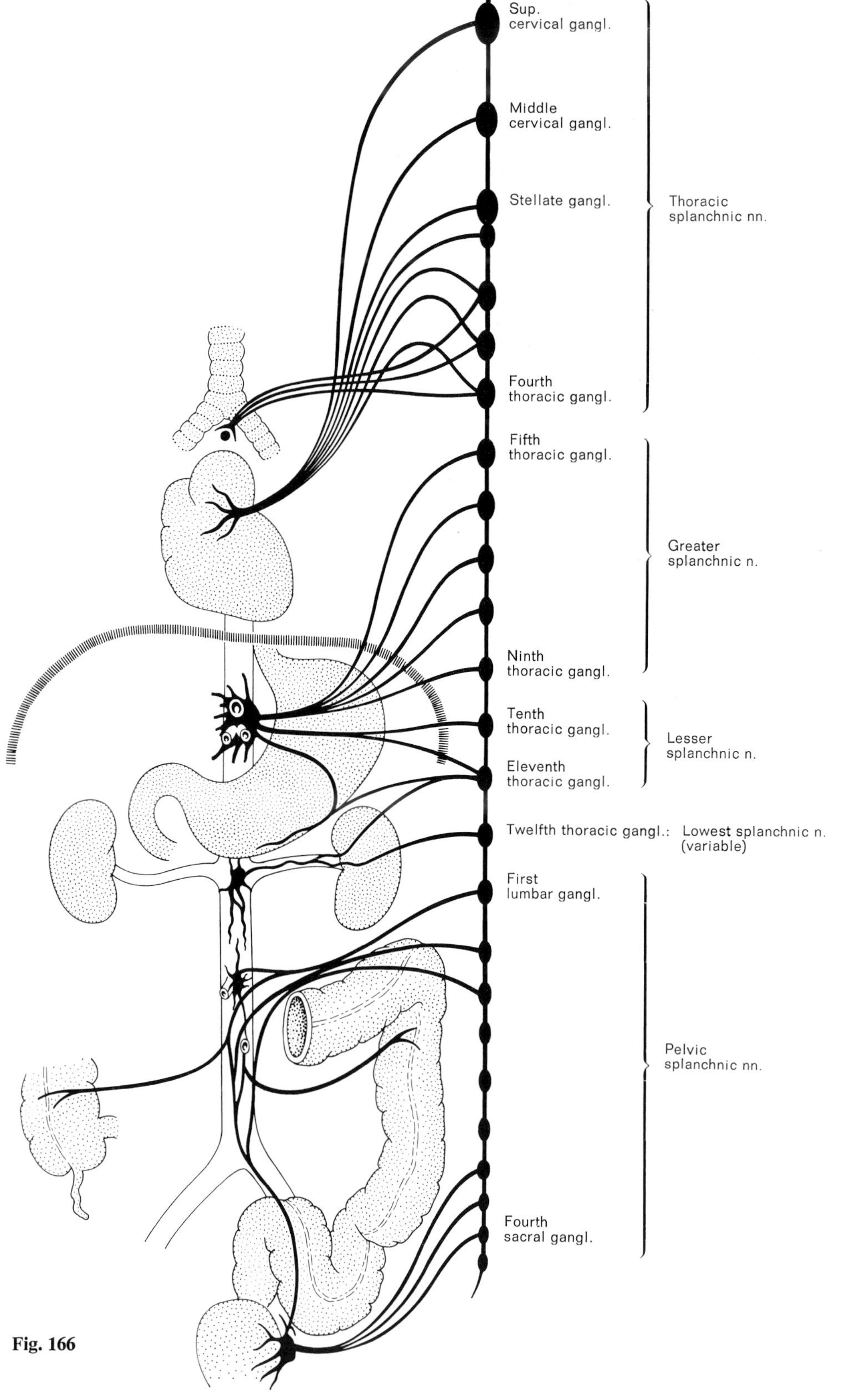
Sup.
cervical gangl.
Middle
cervical gangl.
Stellate gangl.
Thoracic
splanchnic nn.
Fourth
thoracic gangl.
Fifth
thoracic gangl.
Greater
splanchnic n.
Ninth
thoracic gangl.
Tenth
thoracic gangl.
Lesser
splanchnic n.
Eleventh
thoracic gangl.
Twelfth thoracic gangl.: Lowest splanchnic n.
(variable)
First
lumbar gangl.
Pelvic
splanchnic nn.
Fourth
sacral gangl.

Fig. 166

Fig. 166. Diagram of the three main groups of splanchnic nerves. The thoracic splanchnic nerves include the sympathetic cardiac nerves as well as the sympathetic fibers to the lungs, esophagus, aorta and azygos vein. The splanchnic nerves proper (greater and lesser splanchnic nerve) are the largest of these independent nerves and supply the abdominal viscera = abdominal splanchnic nerves. The fibers for the sympathetic innervation of the viscera of the lesser pelvis are called pelvic splanchnic nerves (after *M. Clara:* Das Nervensystem des Menschen. J. A. Barth, Leipzig 1942).

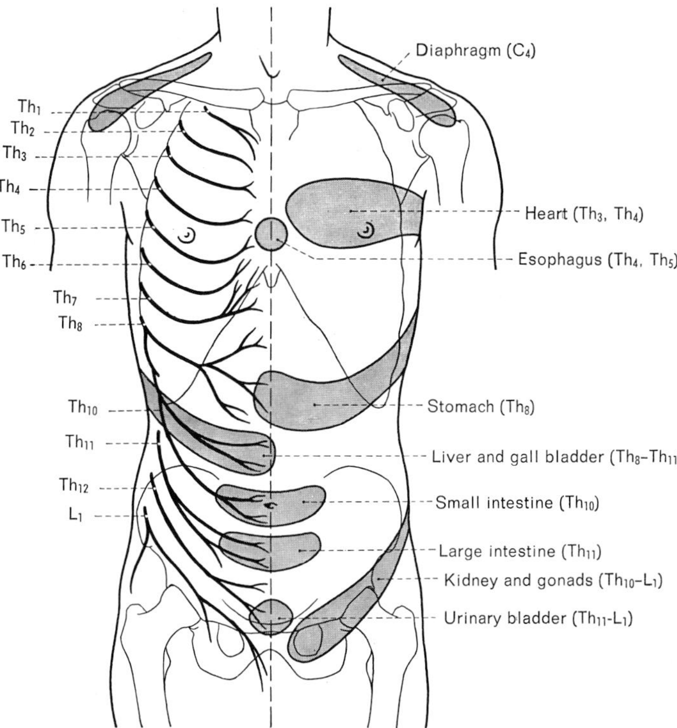
Diaphragm (C_4)
Th_1
Th_2
Th_3
Th_4
Th_5
Th_6
Th_7
Th_8
Th_{10}
Th_{11}
Th_{12}
L_1
Heart (Th_3, Th_4)
Esophagus (Th_4, Th_5)
Stomach (Th_8)
Liver and gall bladder (Th_8-Th_{11})
Small intestine (Th_{10})
Large intestine (Th_{11})
Kidney and gonads (Th_{10}-L_1)
Urinary bladder (Th_{11}-L_1)

Fig. 167. Segmental, sensory innervation of the viscera. Frequently, the pain associated with certain irritative visceral diseases is referred to the corresponding skin segment or dermatome (hyperesthesia and hyperalgesia). Explanation: The afferent dorsal roots of spinal nerves contain not only fibers from dermatomes but also afferent, vegetative fibers from corresponding viscera. The hyperesthetic and hyperalgesic skin areas are called *Head*'s zones (*Head,* English neurologist, 1861–1940). These are of practical importance for the diagnosis of visceral diseases. Reflex pain may be treated by anesthesia or transection of dorsal roots (after *Treves/Keith:* Chirurgische Anatomie. Springer, Berlin 1914).

Sense Organs and Skin

Eye and Accessory Organs

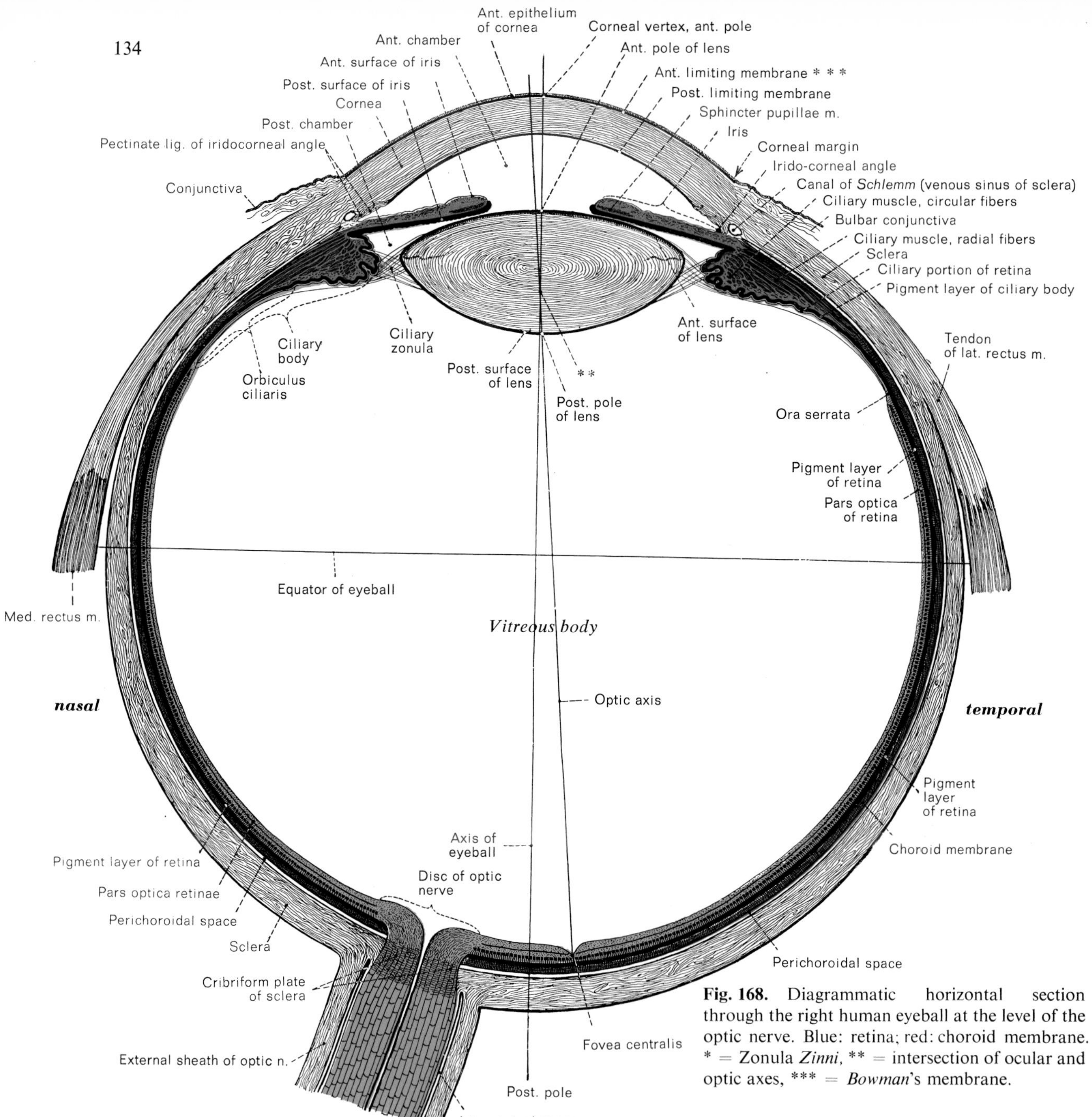
Ant. epithelium of cornea
Corneal vertex, ant. pole
Ant. chamber
Ant. pole of lens
Ant. surface of iris
Ant. limiting membrane * * *
Post. surface of iris
Post. limiting membrane
Cornea
Sphincter pupillae m.
Post. chamber
Iris
Pectinate lig. of iridocorneal angle
Corneal margin
Irido-corneal angle
Conjunctiva
Canal of Schlemm (venous sinus of sclera)
Ciliary muscle, circular fibers
Bulbar conjunctiva
Ciliary muscle, radial fibers
Sclera
Ciliary portion of retina
Pigment layer of ciliary body
Ciliary body
Ciliary zonula
Ant. surface of lens
Tendon of lat. rectus m.
Orbiculus ciliaris
Post. surface of lens
* *
Post. pole of lens
Ora serrata
Pigment layer of retina
Pars optica of retina
Equator of eyeball
Med. rectus m.
Vitreous body
Optic axis
nasal
temporal
Pigment layer of retina
Choroid membrane
Axis of eyeball
Pigment layer of retina
Disc of optic nerve
Pars optica retinae
Perichoroidal space
Sclera
Perichoroidal space
Cribriform plate of sclera
Fovea centralis
External sheath of optic n.
Post. pole
Intervaginal space

Fig. 168. Diagrammatic horizontal section through the right human eyeball at the level of the optic nerve. Blue: retina; red: choroid membrane. * = Zonula *Zinni*, ** = intersection of ocular and optic axes, *** = *Bowman*'s membrane.

Measurements of the human eyeball (average values from the anatomical and ophthalmological literature):

↕ outer diameter (axis) 24.27 mm,	sagittal axis of lens 3 mm,
↕ inner diameter (axis) 21.74 mm,	diameter of lens at equator 9–10 mm,
diameter at equator 24.32 mm,	distance from lens to retina 14.5 mm,
vertical diameter 23.60 mm,	interpupillary distance right ↔ left 56–61 mm,
radius of scleral curvature 12.70 mm,	horizontal diameter of cornea 11.9 mm,
radius of corneal curvature 7.75 mm,	vertical diameter of cornea 11.0 mm.
depth of anterior chamber 3 mm,	

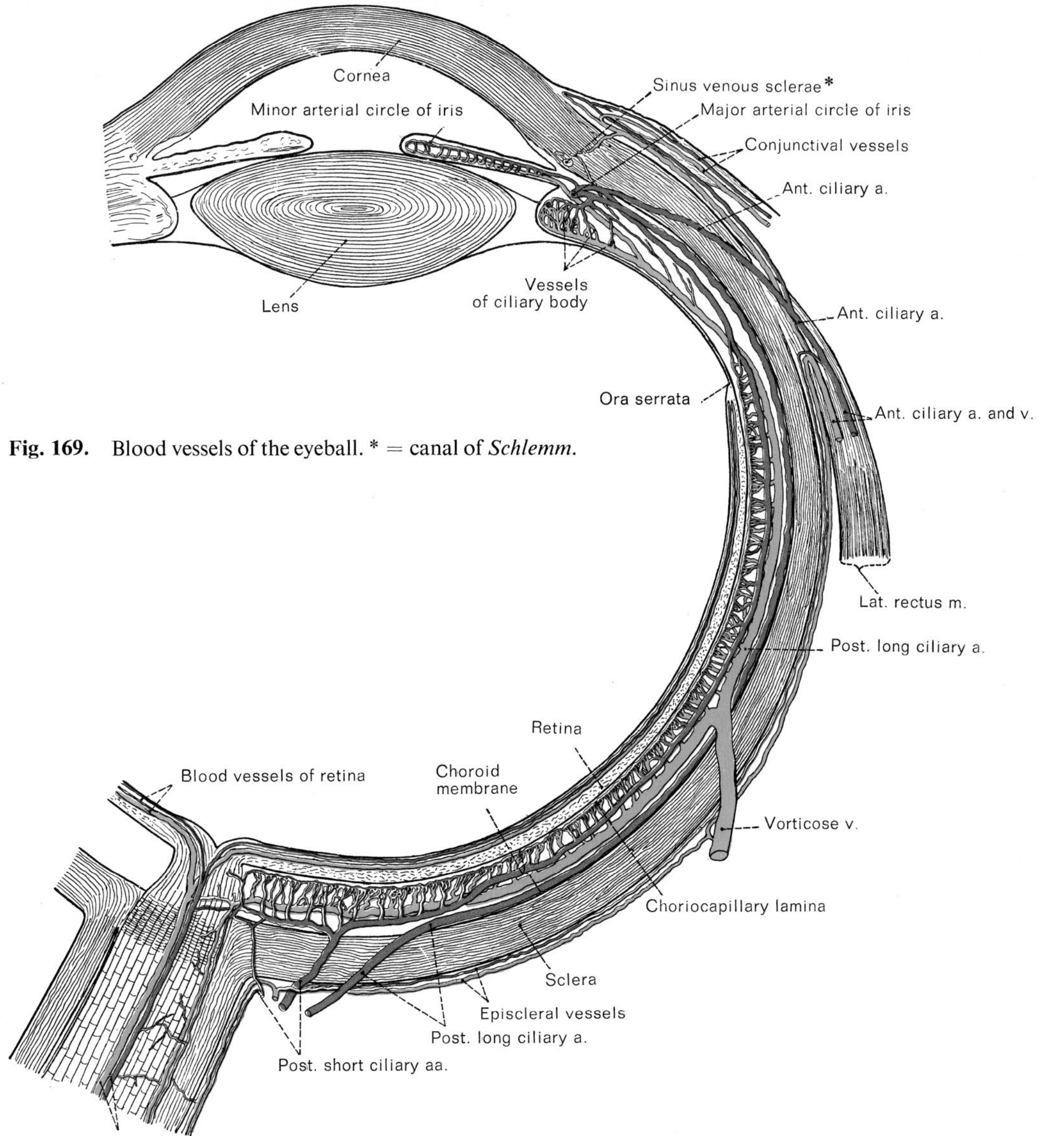
Cornea
Minor arterial circle of iris
Sinus venous sclerae*
Major arterial circle of iris
Conjunctival vessels
Ant. ciliary a.
Lens
Vessels
of ciliary body
Ant. ciliary a.
Ora serrata
Ant. ciliary a. and v.
Lat. rectus m.
Post. long ciliary a.
Retina
Blood vessels of retina
Choroid
membrane
Vorticose v.
Choriocapillary lamina
Sclera
Episcleral vessels
Post. long ciliary a.
Post. short ciliary aa.
Central vessels of retina

Fig. 169. Blood vessels of the eyeball. * = canal of *Schlemm.*

The Tunics of the Eyeball

I. Fibrous tunic *(corneo-scleral coat)*

a) Cornea, anterior smaller portion (1/5), pronounced curvature, transparent.
b) Sclera, white appearance, larger portion (4/5), less pronounced curvature, opaque, in infancy bluish-white, in senescence yellowish-white (in icteric conditions yellow).

II. Middle, vascular tunic *(uvea)*

a) iris with central, round opening = pupil
b) ciliary body with ciliary muscle, ciliary process, ciliary zonule
c) choroid membrane.

III. Innermost tunic, *retina proper* (inner layer of optic cup)

a) pars caeca, from pupillary margin of iris to ora serrata
   1. iridial portion of retina; simple, low, pigmented epithelium
   2. ciliary portion of retina; simple, non-pigmented epithelium
b) pars optica, stratified. Three-neuron-system. Ist neuron, outward location, bordering on pigment layer, neuroepithelium, rod cells, cone cells, avascular. 2nd and 3rd neuron, inward location, vascularized. Specialized areas in the posterior segment of eyeball: macula lutea with central fovea (area of most acute vision), papilla of optic nerve (blind spot, exit of optic nerve containing central vessels).

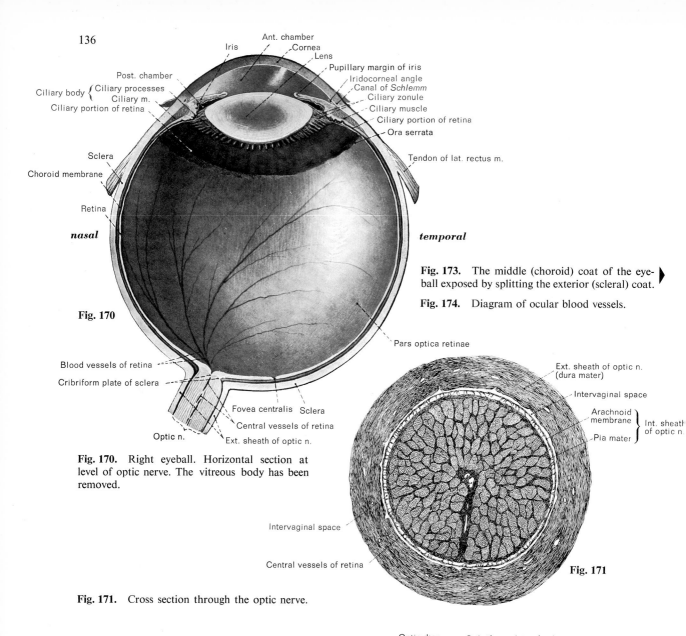

Ant. chamber
Iris
Cornea
Lens
Pupillary margin of iris
Post. chamber
Iridocorneal angle
Canal of *Schlemm*
Ciliary body { Ciliary processes, Ciliary m.
Ciliary zonule
Ciliary portion of retina
Ciliary muscle
Ciliary portion of retina
Ora serrata
Sclera
Tendon of lat. rectus m.
Choroid membrane
Retina
nasal
temporal

Fig. 173. The middle (choroid) coat of the eyeball exposed by splitting the exterior (scleral) coat.

Fig. 174. Diagram of ocular blood vessels.

Fig. 170

Pars optica retinae
Blood vessels of retina
Cribriform plate of sclera
Fovea centralis
Sclera
Central vessels of retina
Optic n.
Ext. sheath of optic n.

Fig. 170. Right eyeball. Horizontal section at level of optic nerve. The vitreous body has been removed.

Ext. sheath of optic n. (dura mater)
Intervaginal space
Arachnoid membrane } Int. sheath of optic n.
Pia mater
Intervaginal space
Central vessels of retina

Fig. 171

Fig. 171. Cross section through the optic nerve.

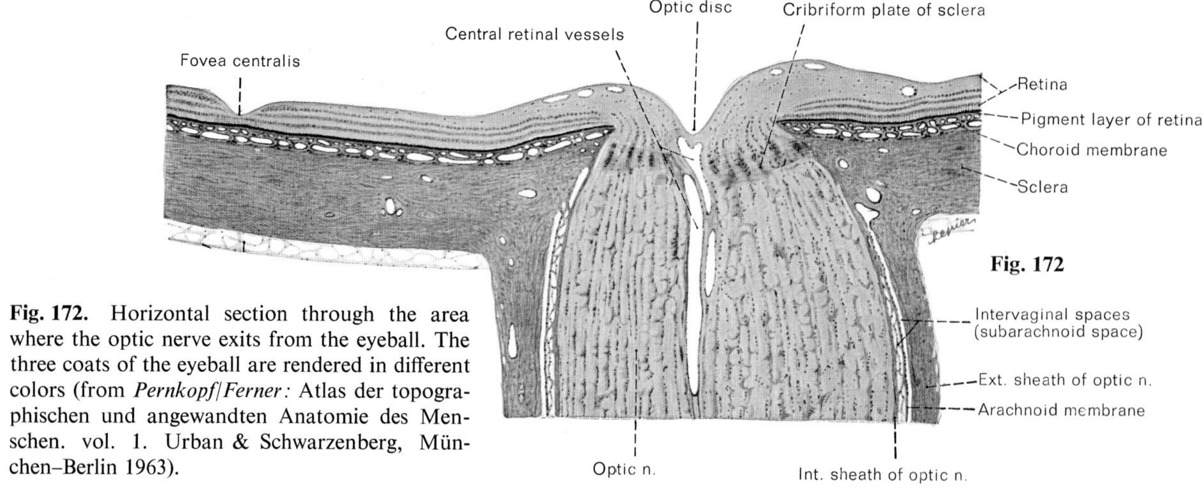
Optic disc
Cribriform plate of sclera
Central retinal vessels
Fovea centralis
Retina
Pigment layer of retina
Choroid membrane
Sclera
Fig. 172
Intervaginal spaces (subarachnoid space)
Ext. sheath of optic n.
Arachnoid membrane
Optic n.
Int. sheath of optic n.

Fig. 172. Horizontal section through the area where the optic nerve exits from the eyeball. The three coats of the eyeball are rendered in different colors (from *Pernkopf/Ferner:* Atlas der topographischen und angewandten Anatomie des Menschen. vol. 1. Urban & Schwarzenberg, München–Berlin 1963).

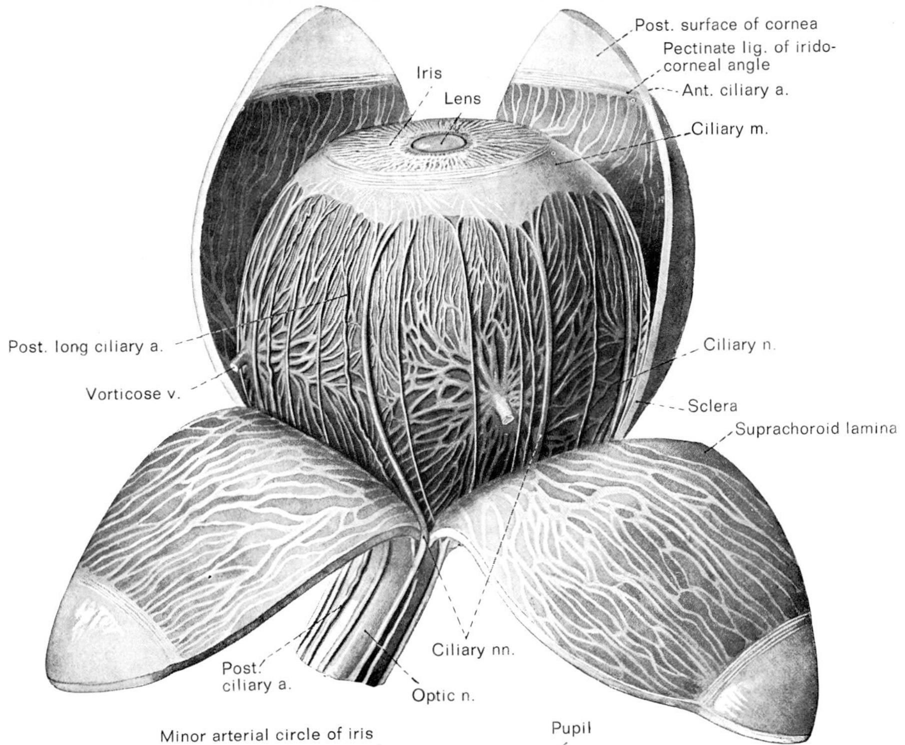

Post. surface of cornea
Pectinate lig. of irido-corneal angle
Iris
Lens
Ant. ciliary a.
Ciliary m.
Post. long ciliary a.
Ciliary n.
Vorticose v.
Sclera
Suprachoroid lamina
Post. ciliary a.
Ciliary nn.
Optic n.

Fig. 173

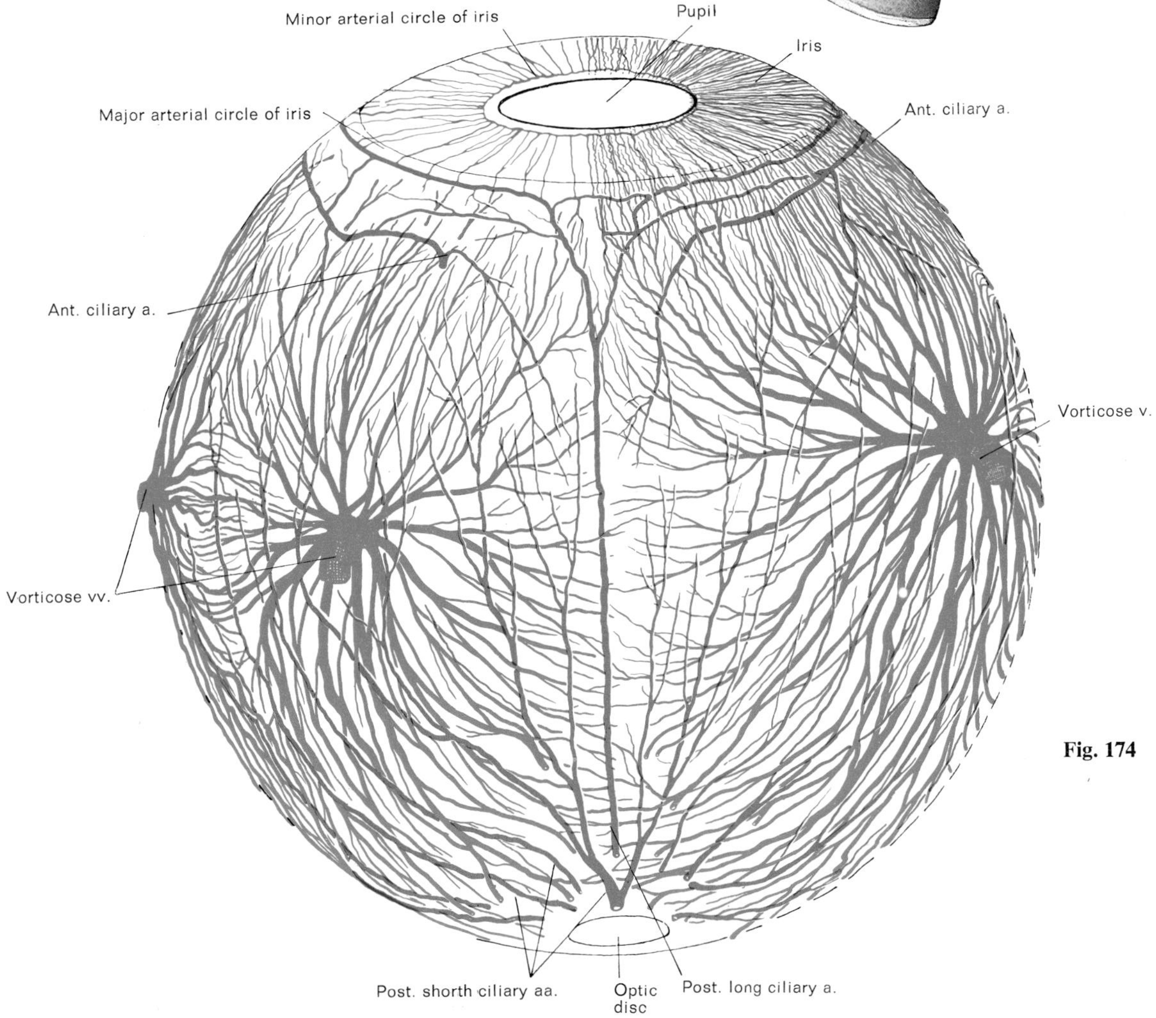

Minor arterial circle of iris
Pupil
Iris
Major arterial circle of iris
Ant. ciliary a.
Ant. ciliary a.
Vorticose v.
Vorticose vv.
Post. shorth ciliary aa.
Optic disc
Post. long ciliary a.

Fig. 174

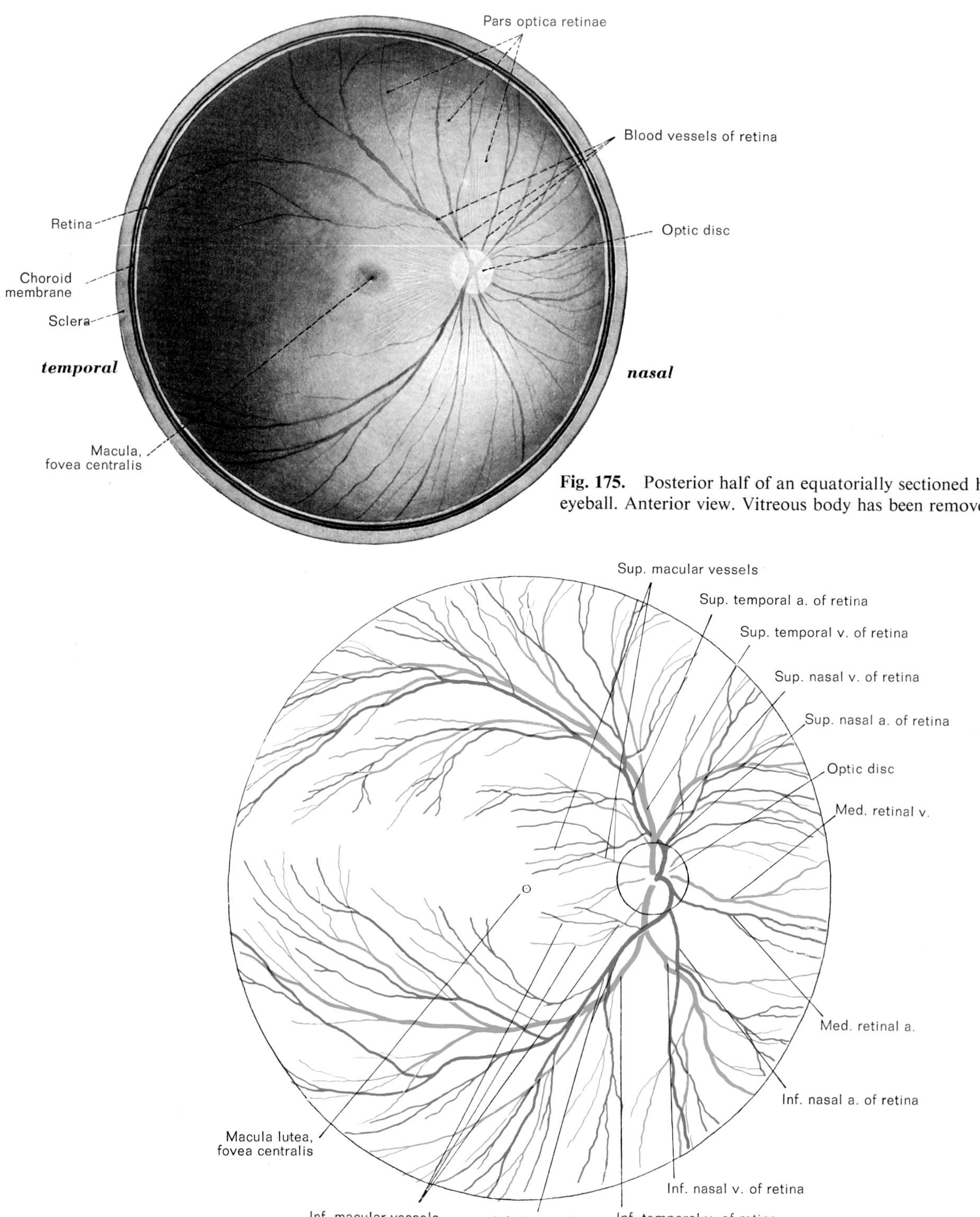
Pars optica retinae
Blood vessels of retina
Retina
Optic disc
Choroid membrane
Sclera
temporal
nasal
Macula, fovea centralis
Sup. macular vessels
Sup. temporal a. of retina
Sup. temporal v. of retina
Sup. nasal v. of retina
Sup. nasal a. of retina
Optic disc
Med. retinal v.
Med. retinal a.
Inf. nasal a. of retina
Macula lutea, fovea centralis
Inf. nasal v. of retina
Inf. macular vessels
Inf. temporal a. of retina
Inf. temporal v. of retina

Fig. 175. Posterior half of an equatorially sectioned human eyeball. Anterior view. Vitreous body has been removed.

Fig. 176. Diagram of the fundus of the right eye with retinal vessels as seen through an opthalmoscope.

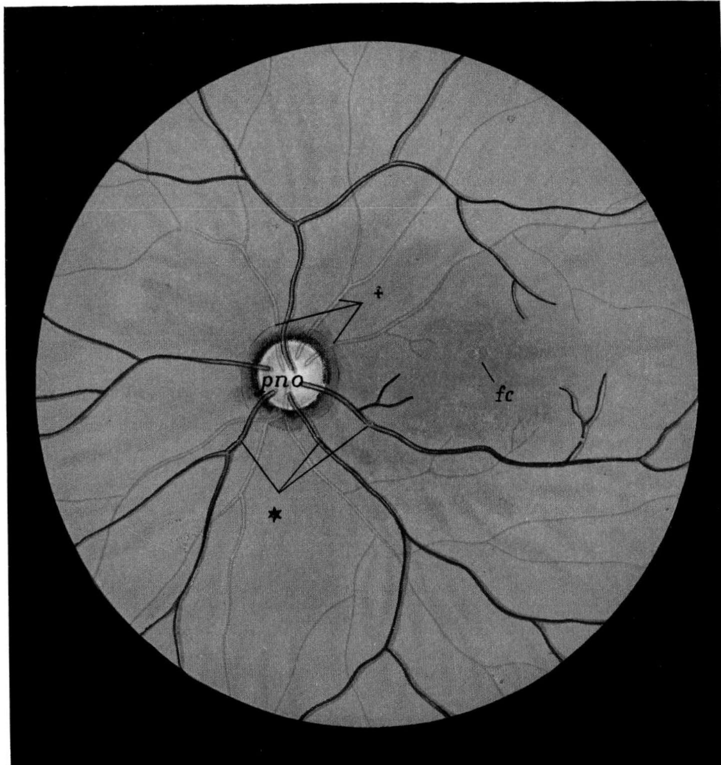
pno
fc

Fig. 177. Fundus of a normal eye as seen through an opthalmoscope. Arteries red, veins outlined in black. Medium pigmentation.

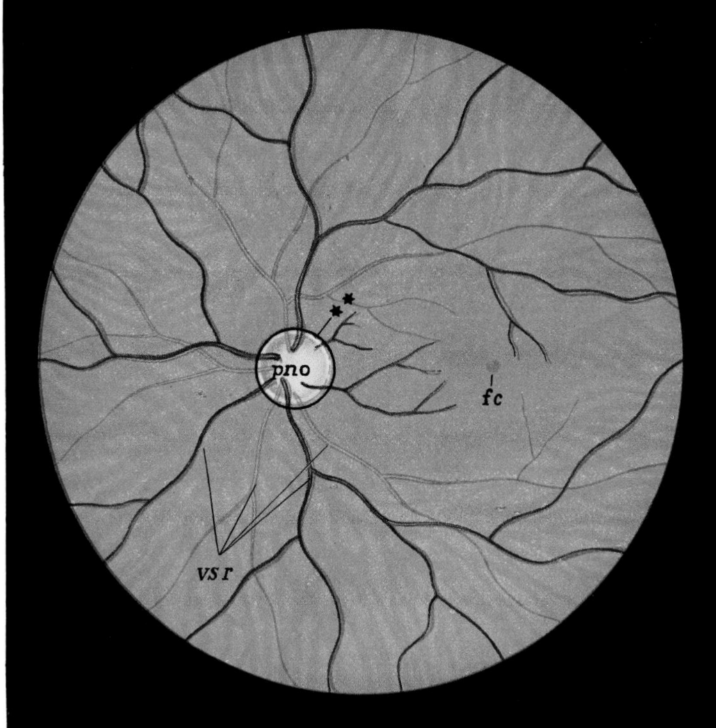
pno
fc
vsr

pno = Optic disc
fc = Fovea centralis
vsr = Blood vessels of retina
* = Retinal veins
* * = Choroidal ring
+ = Retinal arteries

Fig. 178. Fundus of a normal eye as seen through an ophthalmoscope. Slight pigmentation. The choroidal vessels can be recognized. At the optic disc choroidal ring and scleral ring can be distinctly seen.

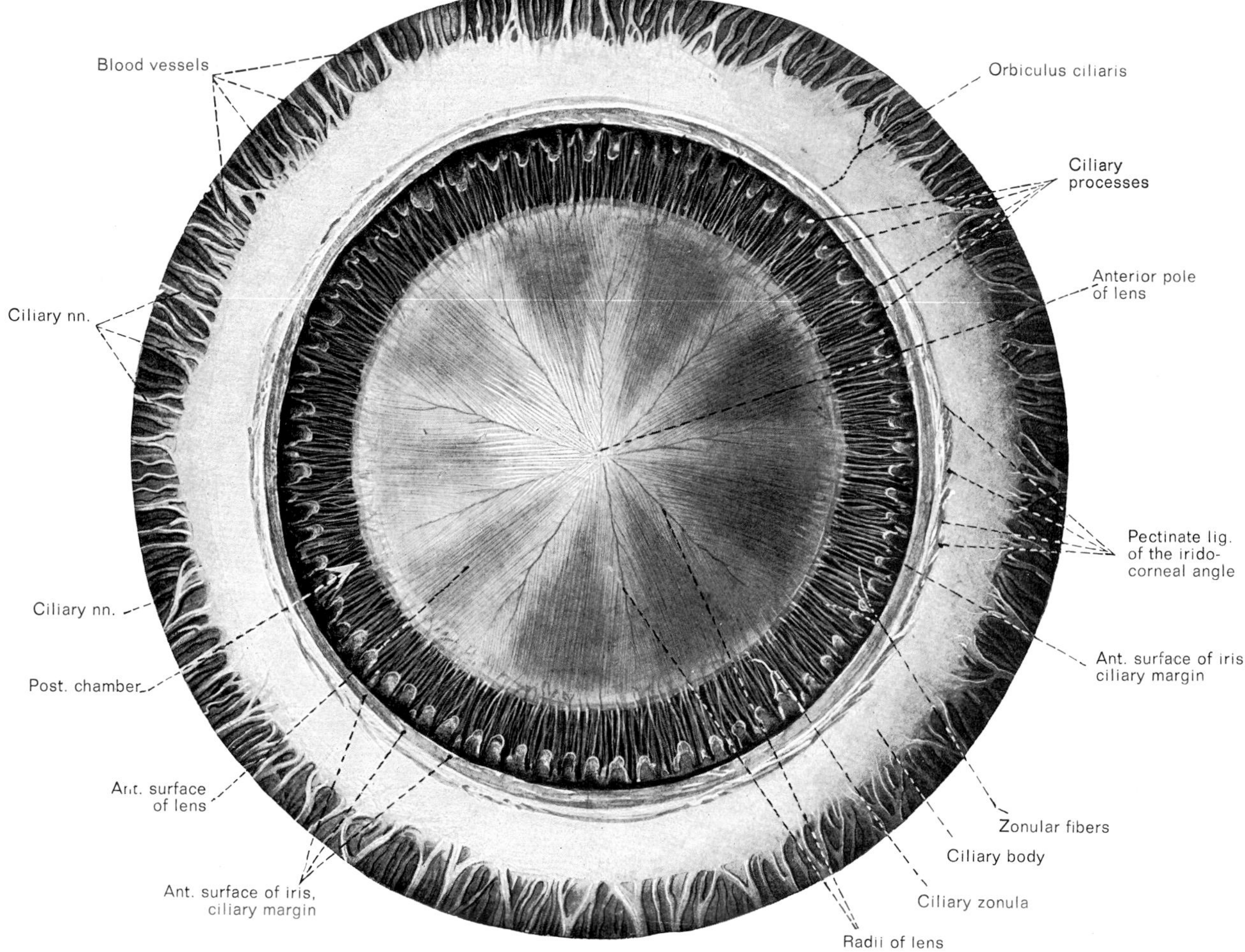
Blood vessels
Orbiculus ciliaris
Ciliary processes
Anterior pole of lens
Ciliary nn.
Pectinate lig. of the irido-corneal angle
Ciliary nn.
Ant. surface of iris, ciliary margin
Post. chamber
Ant. surface of lens
Zonular fibers
Ciliary body
Ant. surface of iris, ciliary margin
Ciliary zonula
Radii of lens

Fig. 183. Suspensory apparatus of the lens, anterior view. Cornea and iris have been removed. The anterior ends of the ciliary processes can be seen. Between them are the zonular fibers of the suspensory apparatus of the lens. They insert at the equator of the lens as well as at the anterior and posterior surface of the lens capsule. The lens star and lens fibers are also illustrated.

Note: The ring-shaped suspensory apparatus of the lens, the zonula, consists of meridionally arranged very fine, yet rigid fibrils, the zonular fibers. They originate from the ciliary orbiculus and the valleys between the ciliary processes. These fine fibers are grouped into dense bundles. They course in the valleys between the ciliary processes toward the lens where, the in area of the equator, they insert in the lens capsule thereby causing small, yet distinct notches on the equatorial surface. Fine interstices, spatia zonularia, exist between the main fiber bundles.

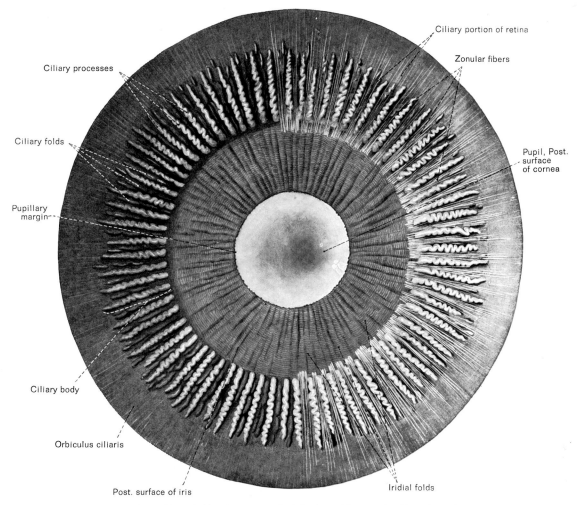

Ciliary portion of retina
Ciliary processes
Zonular fibers
Ciliary folds
Pupil, Post. surface of cornea
Pupillary margin
Ciliary body
Orbiculus ciliaris
Post. surface of iris
Iridial folds

Fig. 184. Posterior surface of the iris and the ciliary body after removal of the lens. The zonular fibers have been removed on the left side, on the right they are sectioned close to the ciliary body; through the pupil one looks onto the posterior surface of the cornea.

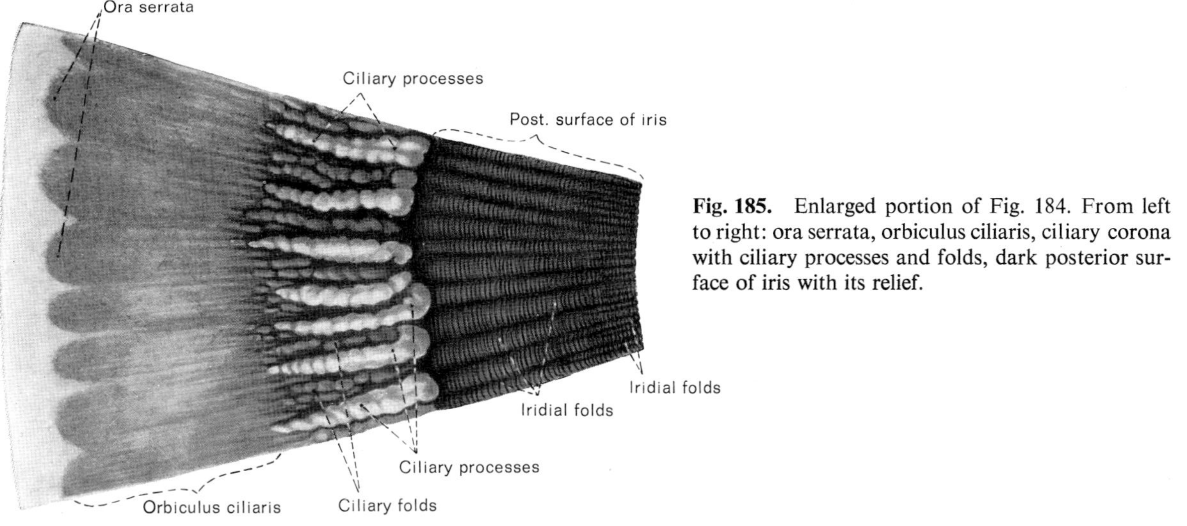
Ora serrata
Ciliary processes
Post. surface of iris
Iridial folds
Iridial folds
Ciliary processes
Orbiculus ciliaris
Ciliary folds

Fig. 185. Enlarged portion of Fig. 184. From left to right: ora serrata, orbiculus ciliaris, ciliary corona with ciliary processes and folds, dark posterior surface of iris with its relief.

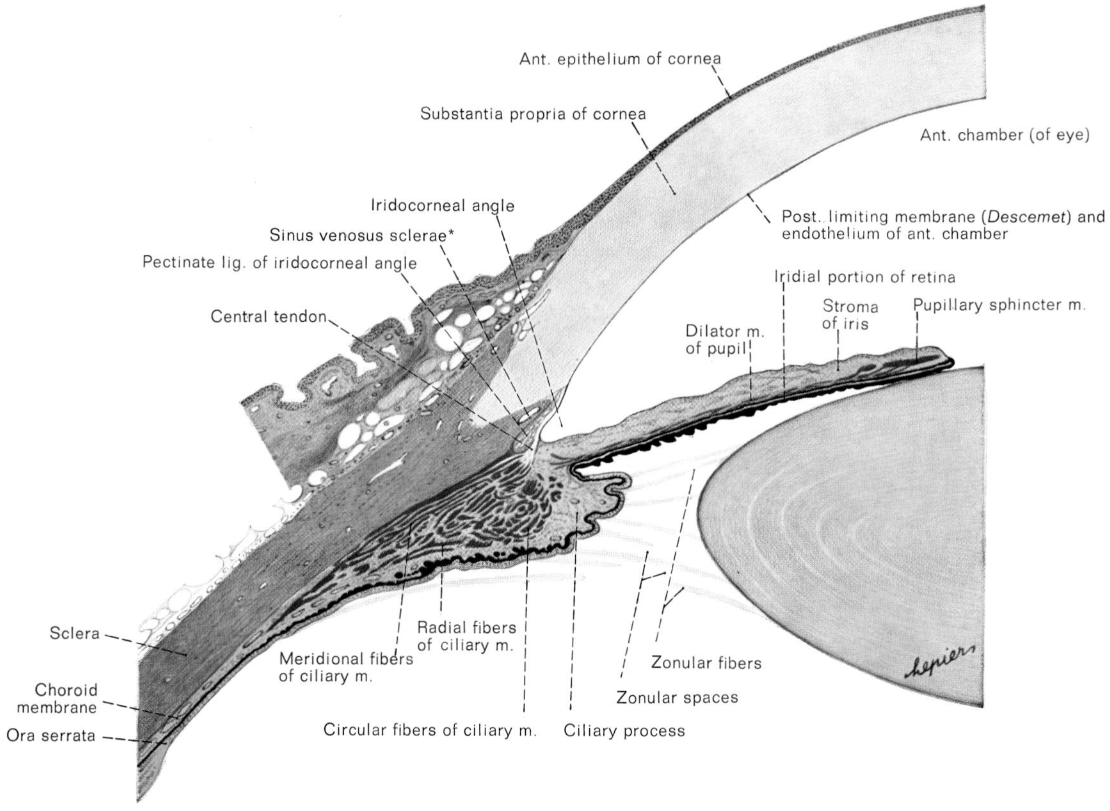
Ant. epithelium of cornea
Substantia propria of cornea
Ant. chamber (of eye)
Iridocorneal angle
Sinus venosus sclerae*
Pectinate lig. of iridocorneal angle
Post. limiting membrane (Descemet) and endothelium of ant. chamber
Iridial portion of retina
Central tendon
Stroma of iris
Pupillary sphincter m.
Dilator m. of pupil
Sclera
Radial fibers of ciliary m.
Meridional fibers of ciliary m.
Zonular fibers
Choroid membrane
Zonular spaces
Ora serrata
Circular fibers of ciliary m.
Ciliary process

Fig. 186. Horinzontal section through the anterior part of the eyeball (from *Pernkopf/Ferber:* Atlas der topographischen und angewandten Anatomie der Menschen. vol. 1. Urban & Schwarzenberg, München–Berlin 1963). * canal of *Schlemm.*

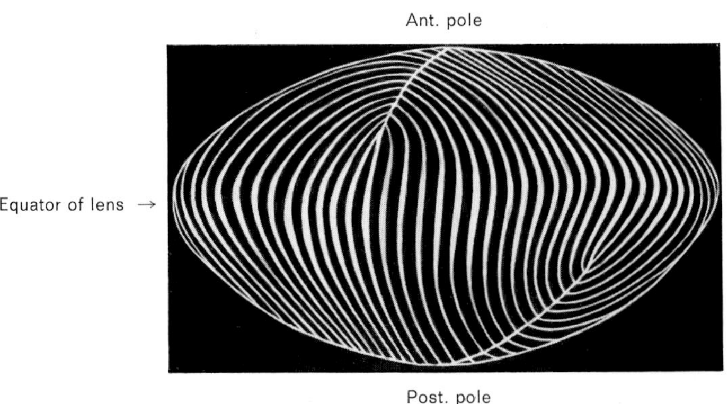
Ant. pole
Equator of lens →
Post. pole

Fig. 187. Diagram of the lens of a newborn; equatorial view. Course of the lens fibers. Note their beginning and ending at the anterior and posterior lens star, respectively.

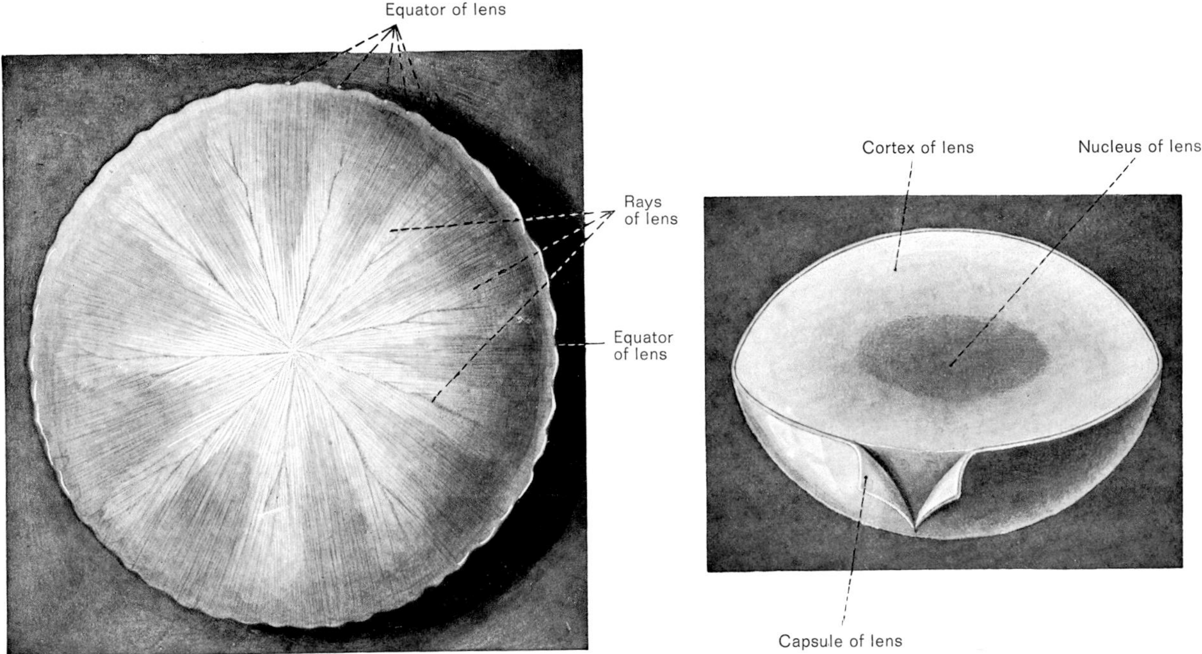
Equator of lens
Rays of lens
Equator of lens
Cortex of lens
Nucleus of lens
Capsule of lens

Fig. 188. Lens of an adult in frontal view; lens star with multiple rays.

Fig. 190. Lens halved through the equator, capsule partially elevated.

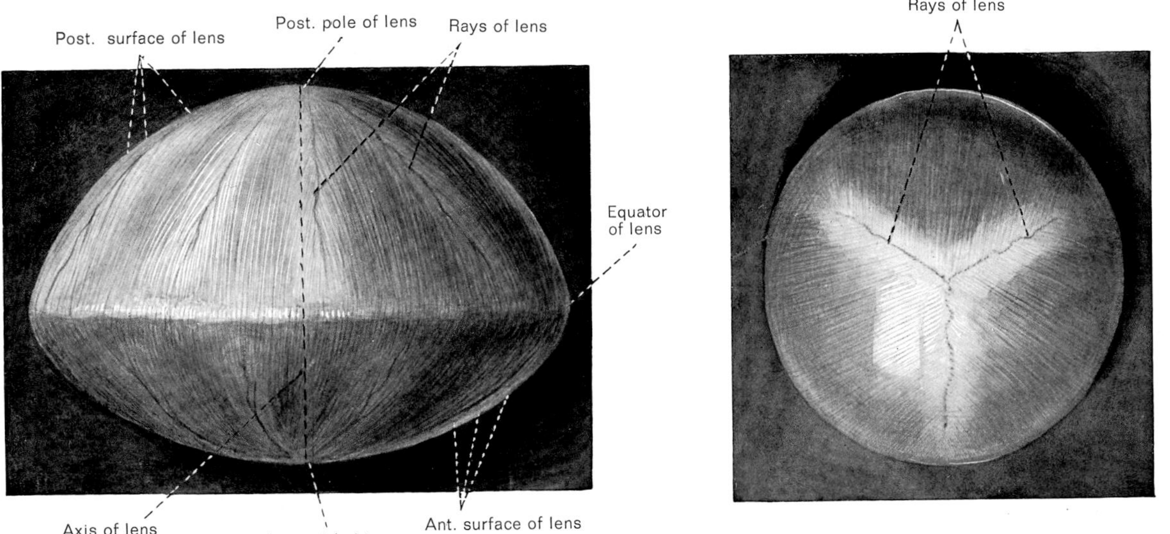
Post. surface of lens
Post. pole of lens
Rays of lens
Equator of lens
Axis of lens
Ant. pole of lens
Ant. surface of lens
Rays of lens

Fig. 189. Lens in equatorial view.

Fig. 191. Lens of a child in ventral view; lens star with three rays.

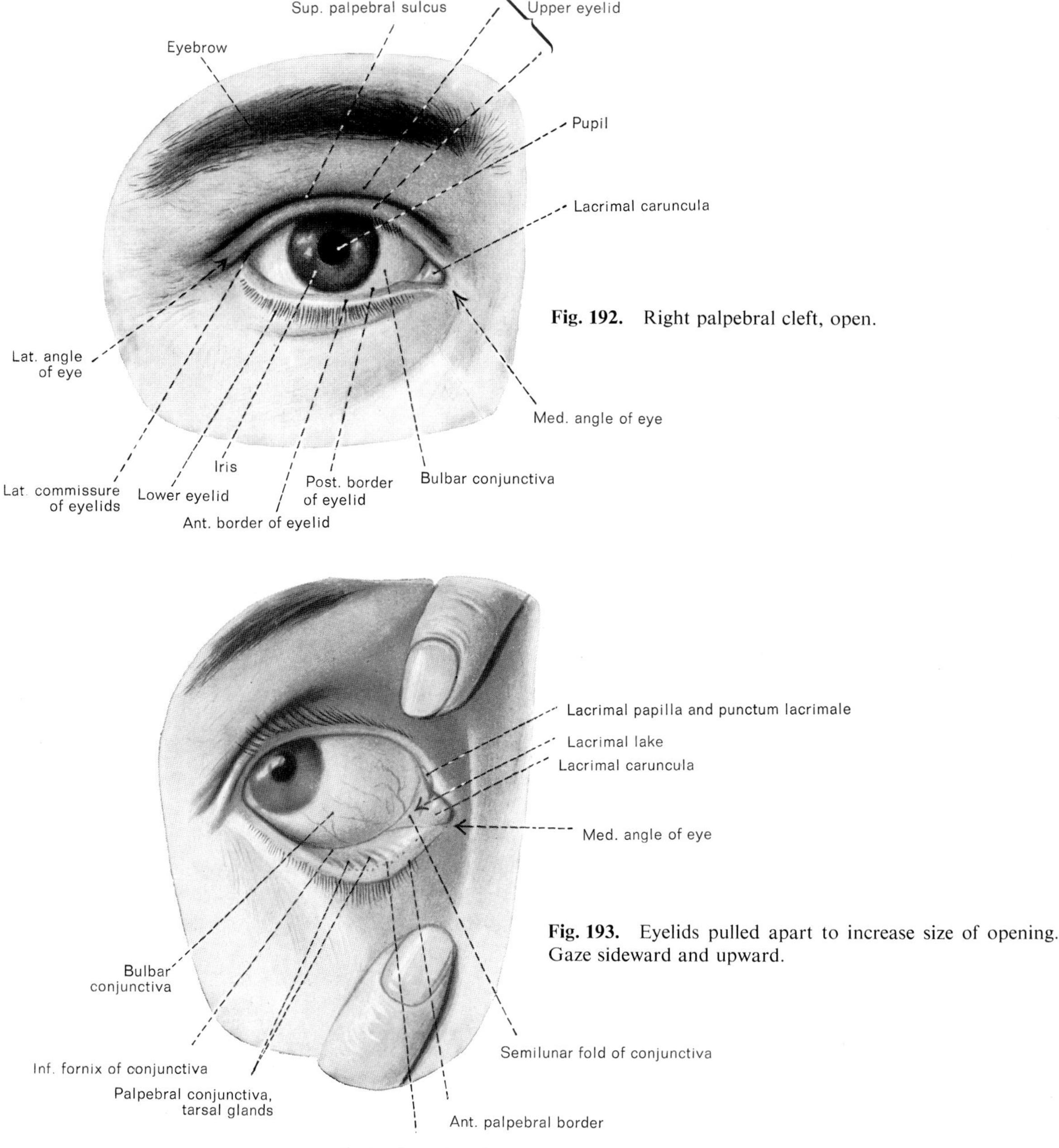
Sup. palpebral sulcus
Upper eyelid
Eyebrow
Pupil
Lacrimal caruncula
Lat. angle of eye
Med. angle of eye
Iris
Lat. commissure of eyelids
Lower eyelid
Post. border of eyelid
Bulbar conjunctiva
Ant. border of eyelid
Lacrimal papilla and punctum lacrimale
Lacrimal lake
Lacrimal caruncula
Med. angle of eye
Bulbar conjunctiva
Inf. fornix of conjunctiva
Palpebral conjunctiva, tarsal glands
Semilunar fold of conjunctiva
Ant. palpebral border
Post. palpebral border

Fig. 192. Right palpebral cleft, open.

Fig. 193. Eyelids pulled apart to increase size of opening. Gaze sideward and upward.

Fig. 194. The orbital septum of the right eye in anterior view. In the lateral part of the upper lid the orbital septum is sectioned and reflected to expose the orbital and palpebral portions of the lacrimal gland. Between these two portions one sees the tendon of the levator palpebrae superioris muscle. Compare with Fig. 216.

Fig. 195. The lacrimal apparatus. The eyelids have been pulled away from the eyeball to expose the conjunctival sac. At the medial palebral angle the lacrimal canaliculi and their entry into the lacrimal sac can be seen. Note the small muscle bundles from the orbicularis oculi muscle that surround the lacrimal canaliculi; their contraction causes tear fluid to enter the canaliculi. The lacrimal sac and the nasolacrimal duct have been opened and its orifice under the inferior nasal concha is shown. Part of the outer nose and of the inferior concha have been removed (preparation in the Anatomical Institute Münster). Compare with Fig. 199.

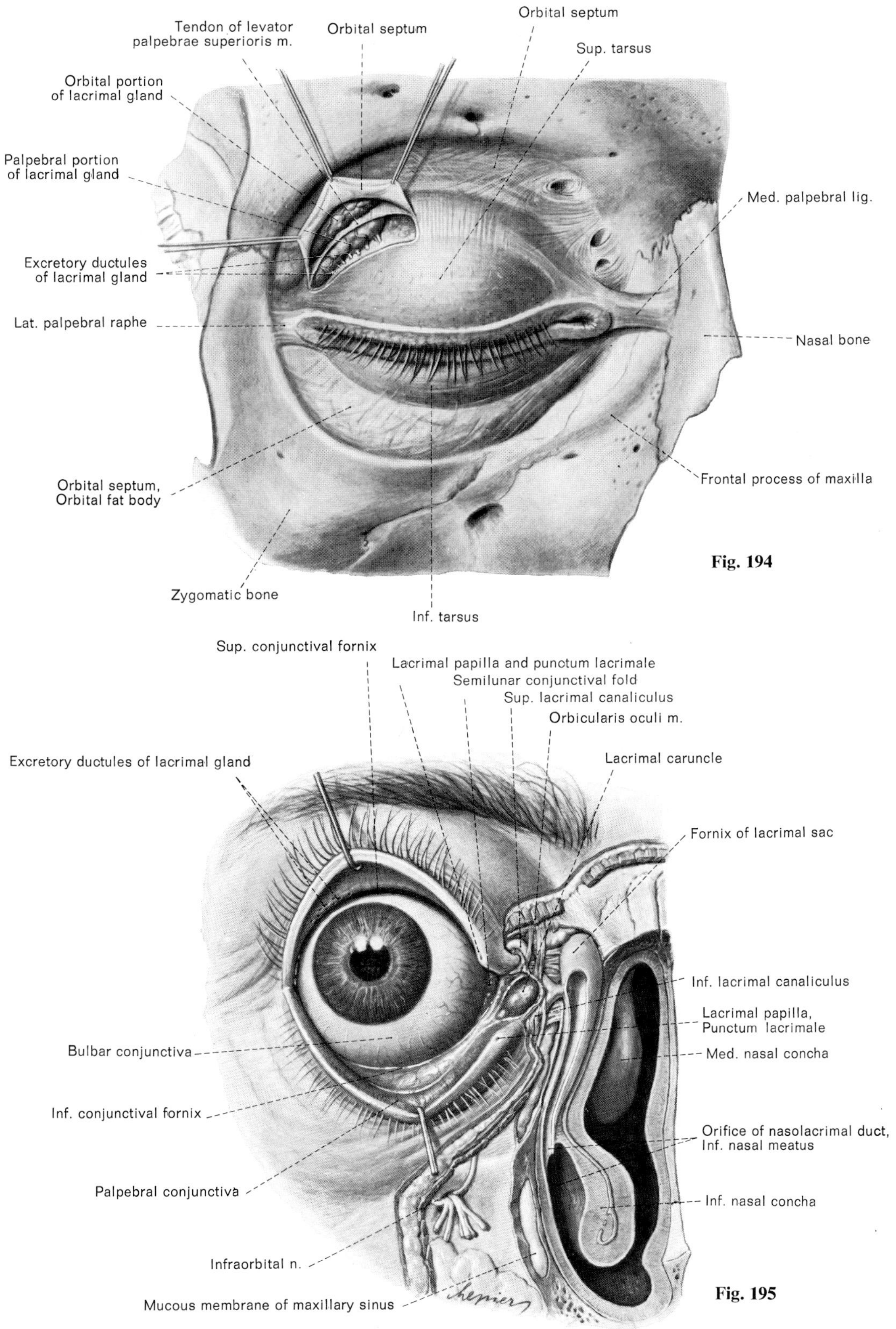
Tendon of levator palpebrae superioris m.
Orbital septum
Orbital septum
Sup. tarsus
Orbital portion of lacrimal gland
Palpebral portion of lacrimal gland
Med. palpebral lig.
Excretory ductules of lacrimal gland
Lat. palpebral raphe
Nasal bone
Orbital septum, Orbital fat body
Frontal process of maxilla
Zygomatic bone
Inf. tarsus
Sup. conjunctival fornix
Lacrimal papilla and punctum lacrimale
Semilunar conjunctival fold
Sup. lacrimal canaliculus
Orbicularis oculi m.
Excretory ductules of lacrimal gland
Lacrimal caruncle
Fornix of lacrimal sac
Inf. lacrimal canaliculus
Lacrimal papilla, Punctum lacrimale
Bulbar conjunctiva
Med. nasal concha
Inf. conjunctival fornix
Orifice of nasolacrimal duct, Inf. nasal meatus
Palpebral conjunctiva
Inf. nasal concha
Infraorbital n.
Mucous membrane of maxillary sinus

Fig. 194

Fig. 195

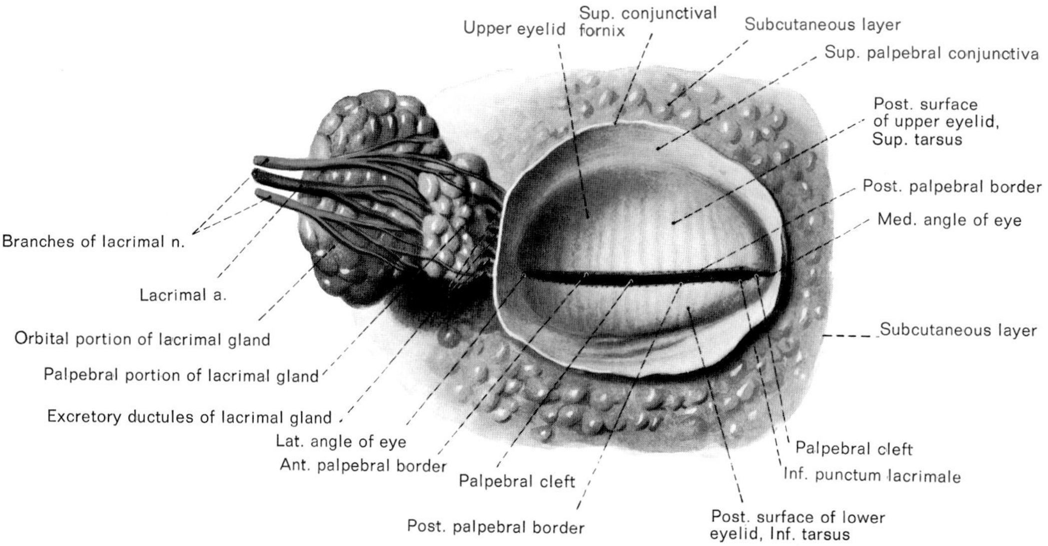
Upper eyelid
Sup. conjunctival fornix
Subcutaneous layer
Sup. palpebral conjunctiva
Post. surface of upper eyelid, Sup. tarsus
Post. palpebral border
Med. angle of eye
Subcutaneous layer
Palpebral cleft
Inf. punctum lacrimale
Post. surface of lower eyelid, Inf. tarsus
Post. palpebral border
Palpebral cleft
Ant. palpebral border
Lat. angle of eye
Excretory ductules of lacrimal gland
Palpebral portion of lacrimal gland
Orbital portion of lacrimal gland
Lacrimal a.
Branches of lacrimal n.

Fig. 196. Eyelids and lacrimal gland; dorsal aspect, left side.

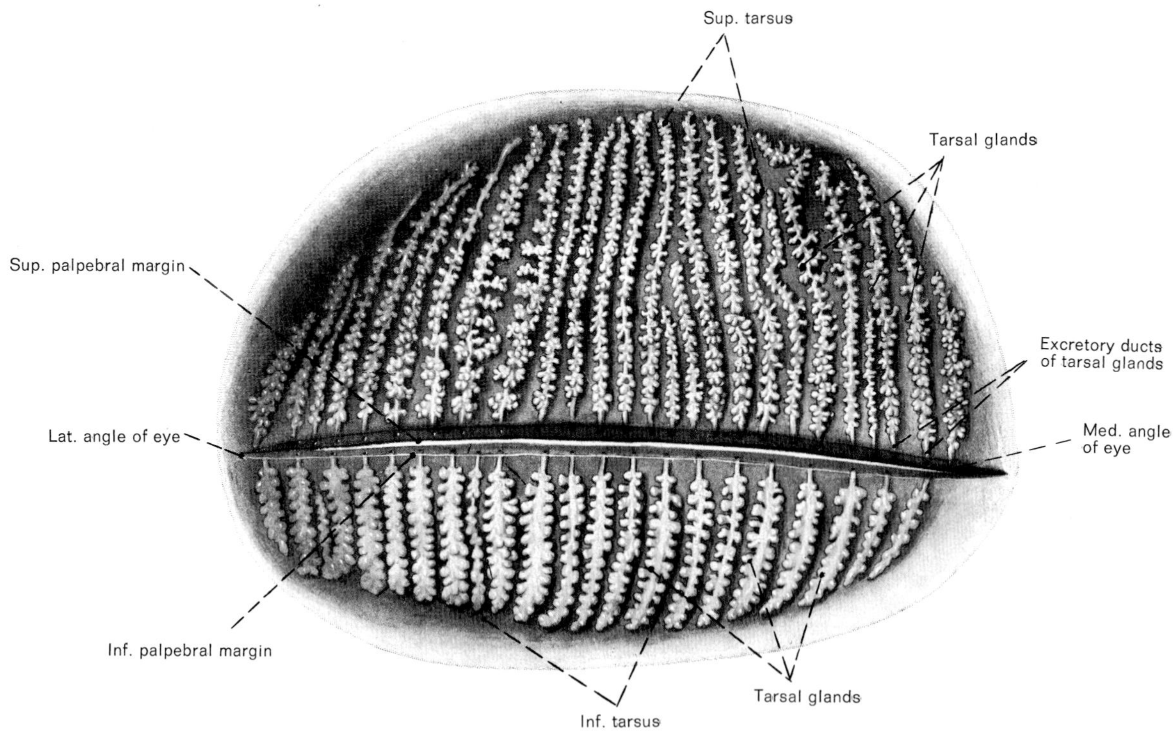
Sup. tarsus
Tarsal glands
Sup. palpebral margin
Excretory ducts of tarsal glands
Lat. angle of eye
Med. angle of eye
Inf. palpebral margin
Tarsal glands
Inf. tarsus

Fig. 197. Dorsal view of the eyelids made transparent by treatment with sodium hydroxide-glycerin to demonstrate the tarsal glands *(Meibom)*.

Fig. 199. Lacrimal canaliculi, lacrimal sac and nasolacrimal duct opened and viewed from ventral and lateral. Preparation similar to the one in Fig. 198 except for partial opening of the maxillary bone in order to expose a portion of the nasolacrimal duct. Compare with Fig. 195.

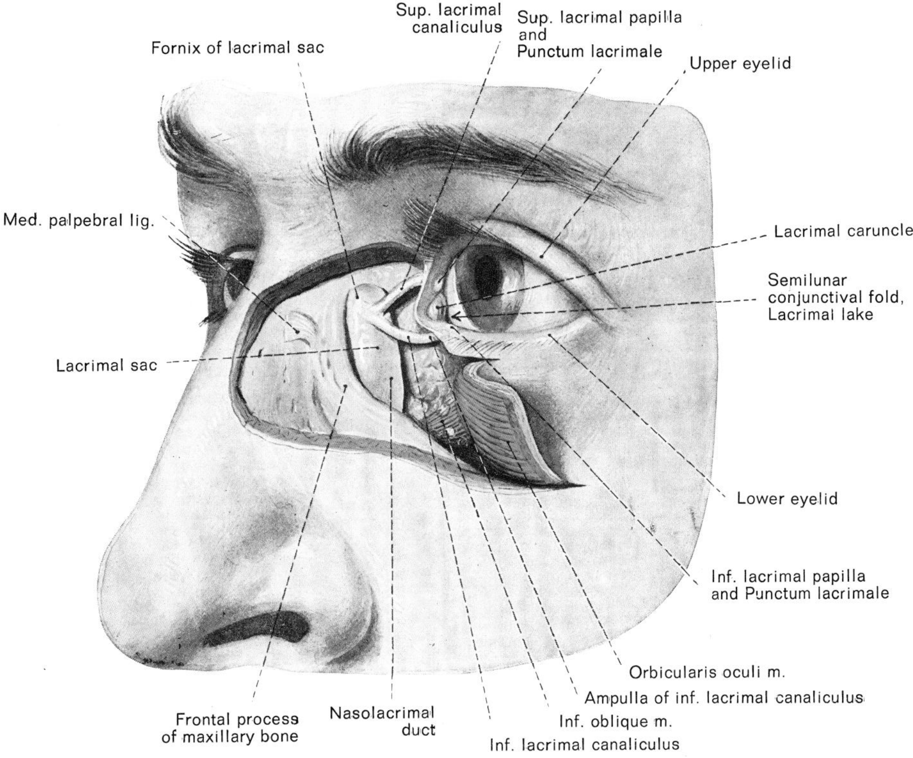
Sup. lacrimal canaliculus
Sup. lacrimal papilla and Punctum lacrimale
Fornix of lacrimal sac
Upper eyelid
Med. palpebral lig.
Lacrimal caruncle
Semilunar conjunctival fold, Lacrimal lake
Lacrimal sac
Lower eyelid
Inf. lacrimal papilla and Punctum lacrimale
Orbicularis oculi m.
Ampulla of inf. lacrimal canaliculus
Frontal process of maxillary bone
Nasolacrimal duct
Inf. oblique m.
Inf. lacrimal canaliculus

Fig. 198. Lacrimal sac and lacrimal canaliculi seen from ventral and lateral. Skin and musculature are partially removed and the medial palpebral ligament has been transected.

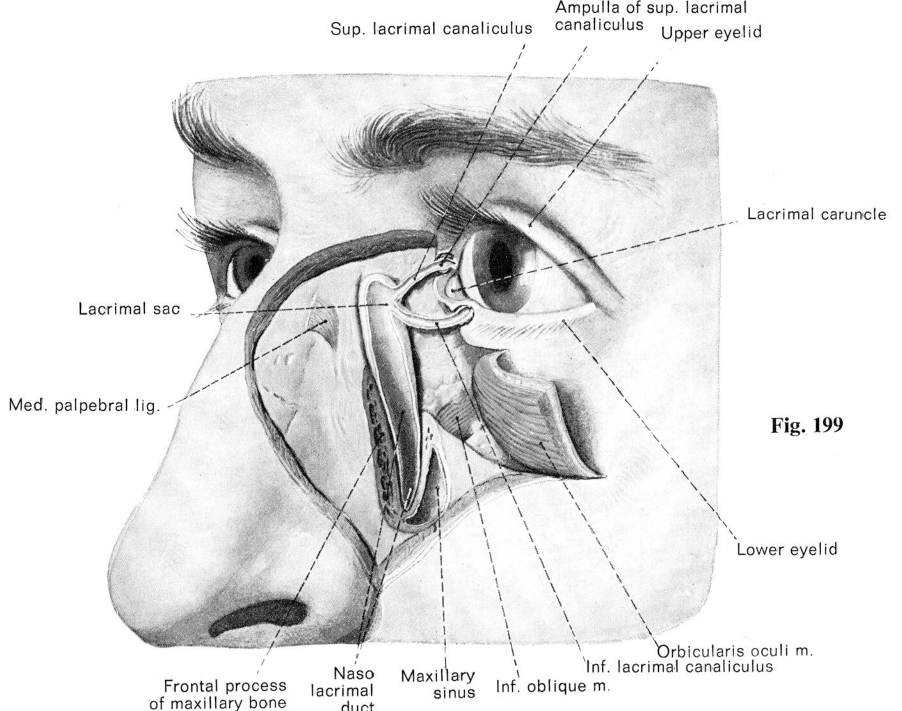
Ampulla of sup. lacrimal canaliculus
Sup. lacrimal canaliculus
Upper eyelid
Lacrimal caruncle
Lacrimal sac
Med. palpebral lig.
Lower eyelid
Orbicularis oculi m.
Inf. lacrimal canaliculus
Frontal process of maxillary bone
Naso lacrimal duct
Maxillary sinus
Inf. oblique m.

Fig. 199

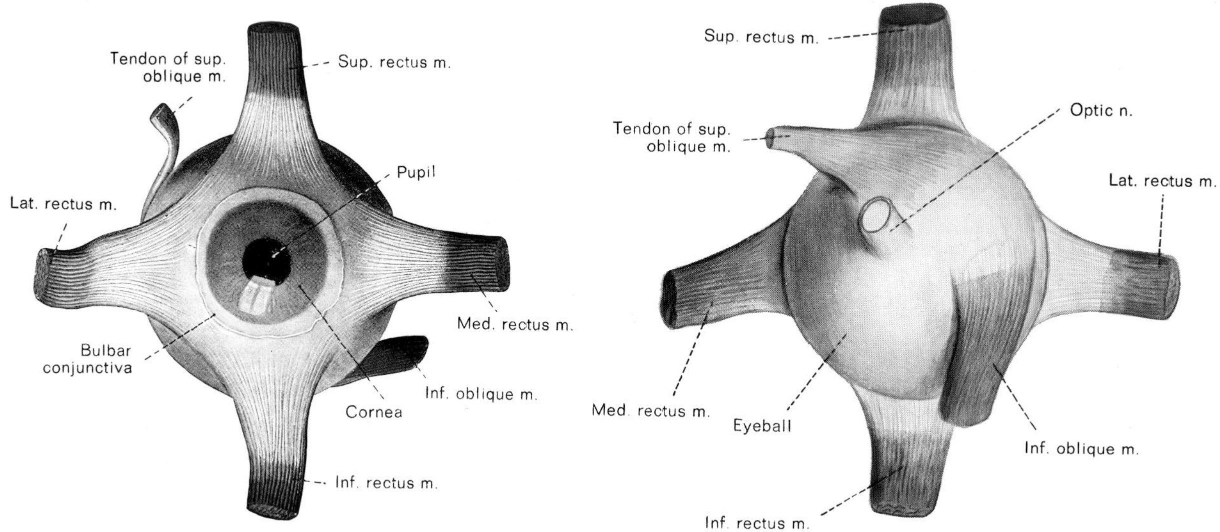
Tendon of sup. oblique m.
Sup. rectus m.
Pupil
Lat. rectus m.
Med. rectus m.
Bulbar conjunctiva
Inf. oblique m.
Cornea
Inf. rectus m.
Sup. rectus m.
Optic n.
Tendon of sup. oblique m.
Lat. rectus m.
Med. rectus m.
Eyeball
Inf. oblique m.
Inf. rectus m.

Fig. 200. Right eyeball with insertions of extrinsic eye muscles; ventral view; the tendon of the superior oblique muscle has been pulled sideward.

Fig. 201. Right eyeball with insertions of extrinsic eye muscles; viewed from dorsal and below.

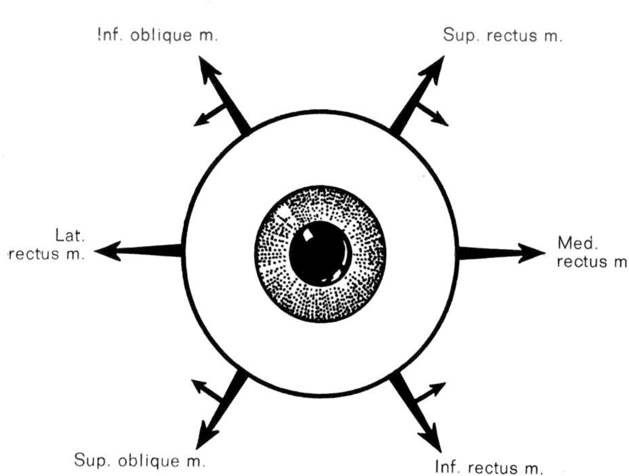
Inf. oblique m.
Sup. rectus m.
Lat. rectus m.
Med. rectus m.
Sup. oblique m.
Inf. rectus m.

Fig. 203. Diagram to illustrate the direction of traction of the extrinsic eye muscles; right eye.

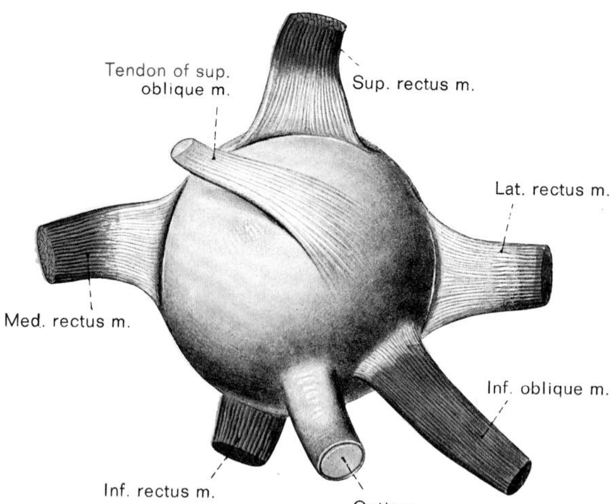
Tendon of sup. oblique m.
Sup. rectus m.
Lat. rectus m.
Med. rectus m.
Inf. oblique m.
Inf. rectus m.
Optic n.

Fig. 202. Right eyeball with insertions of extrinsic eye muscles; viewed from behind and above. The inferior oblique muscle has been deflected from the eyeball.

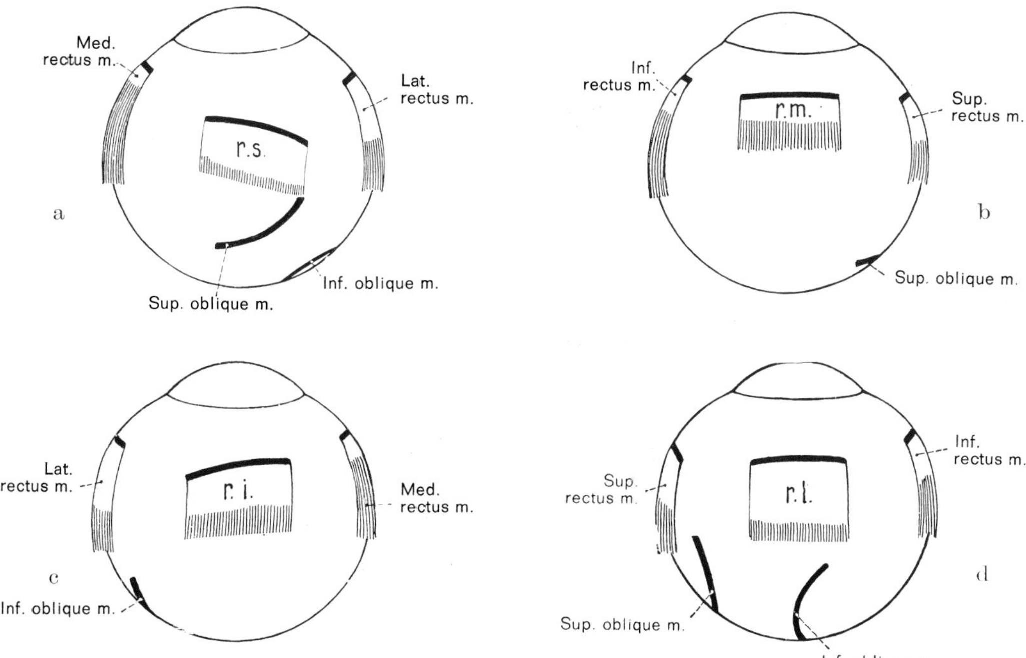
Med.
rectus m.
Lat.
rectus m.
r.s.
a
Inf. oblique m.
Sup. oblique m.
Inf.
rectus m.
r.m.
Sup.
rectus m.
b
Sup. oblique m.
Lat.
rectus m.
r.i.
Med.
rectus m.
c
Inf. oblique m.
Inf.
rectus m.
Sup.
rectus m.
r.l.
d
Sup. oblique m.
Inf. oblique m.

Fig. 204. Diagram to illustrate the insertions of the six extrinsic eye muscles on the right eye. a = seen from above, b = from medial, c = from below, d = from lateral. r.c. = inferior rectus muscle, r.l. = lateral rectus muscle, r.m. = medial rectus muscle, r.s. = superior rectus mucsle.

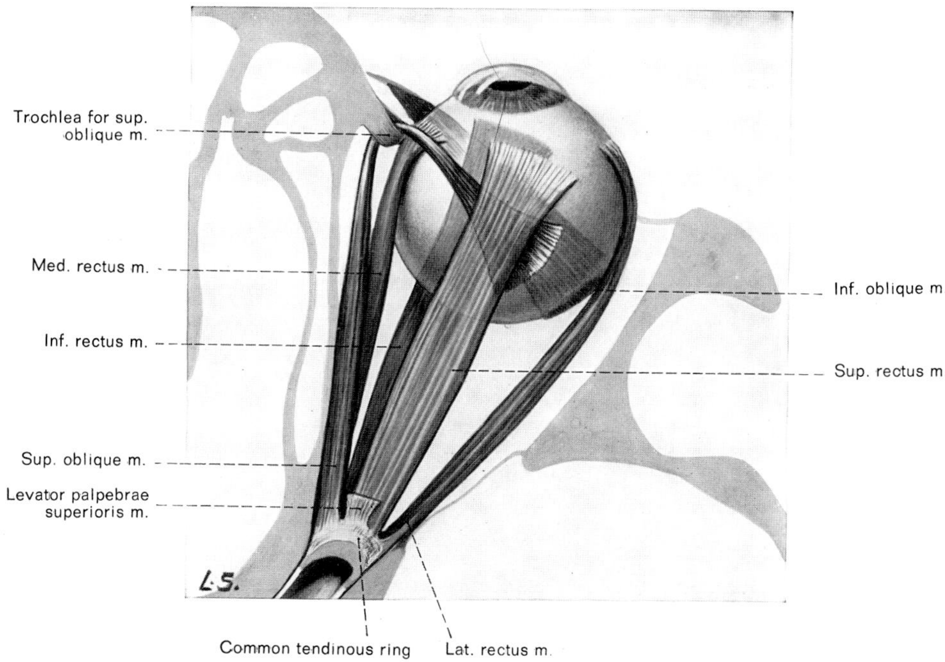
Trochlea for sup.
oblique m.
Med. rectus m.
Inf. rectus m.
Sup. oblique m.
Levator palpebrae
superioris m.
Inf. oblique m.
Sup. rectus m.
Common tendinous ring
Lat. rectus m.

Fig. 205. Diagram of the extrinsic muscles of the right eyeball seen from above; muscles partially transparent (from *Pernkopf/Ferner:* Atlas der topographischen und angewandten Anatomie des Menschen. vol. 1. Urban & Schwarzenberg, München–Berlin 1963).

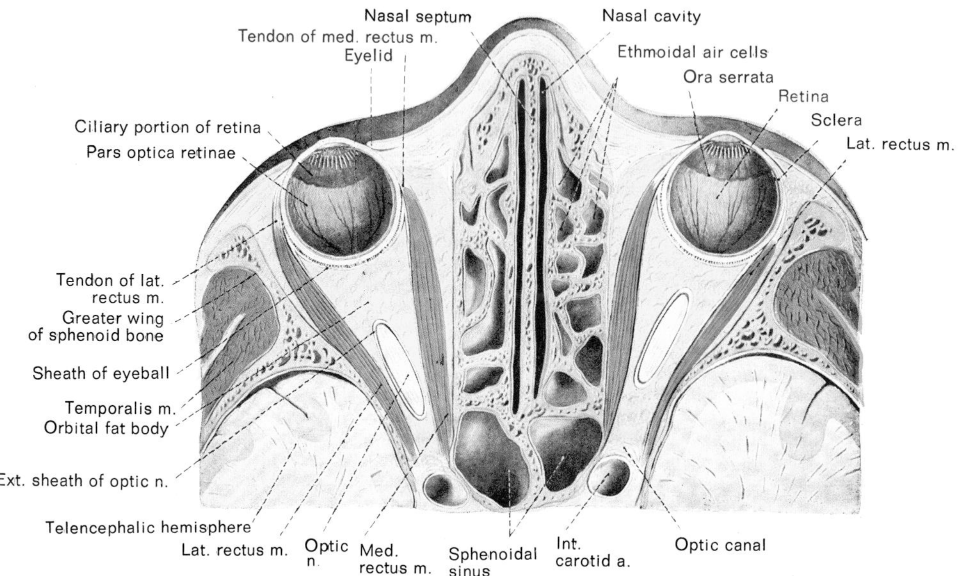
Nasal septum
Tendon of med. rectus m.
Eyelid
Nasal cavity
Ethmoidal air cells
Ora serrata
Retina
Sclera
Lat. rectus m.
Ciliary portion of retina
Pars optica retinae
Tendon of lat. rectus m.
Greater wing of sphenoid bone
Sheath of eyeball
Temporalis m.
Orbital fat body
Ext. sheath of optic n.
Telencephalic hemisphere
Lat. rectus m.
Optic n.
Med. rectus m.
Sphenoidal sinus
Int. carotid a.
Optic canal

Fig. 206. Horinzontal section through both orbits.

Tendon of sup. oblique m.
Orbital fat body
Sup. oblique m.
Crista galli
Levator palpebrae superioris m.
Tendon of sup. oblique m.
Eyeball
Trochlea for sup. oblique m.
Levator palpebrae superioris m.
Orbital portion of lacrimal gland
Med. rectus m.
Lat. rectus m.
Greater wing of sphenoid bone
Sup. rectus m.
Lat. rectus m.
Common tendinous ring
Sup. rectus m.
Dura mater of ant. cranial fossa
Optic chiasm
Optic n.
Sup. oblique m.
Levator palpebrae superioris m.

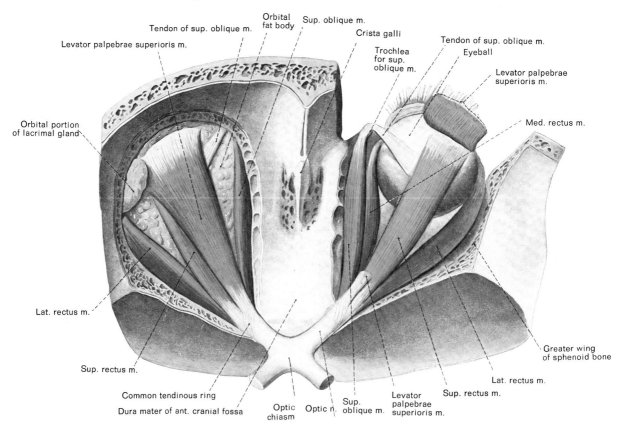

Fig. 207. The muscles of the orbit seen from above. Left side: the roof of the orbit and the periorbit have been removed to expose the superficial layer; right side: the levator palpebrae superioris muscle and the orbital fat body have been removed to expose the deep layer.

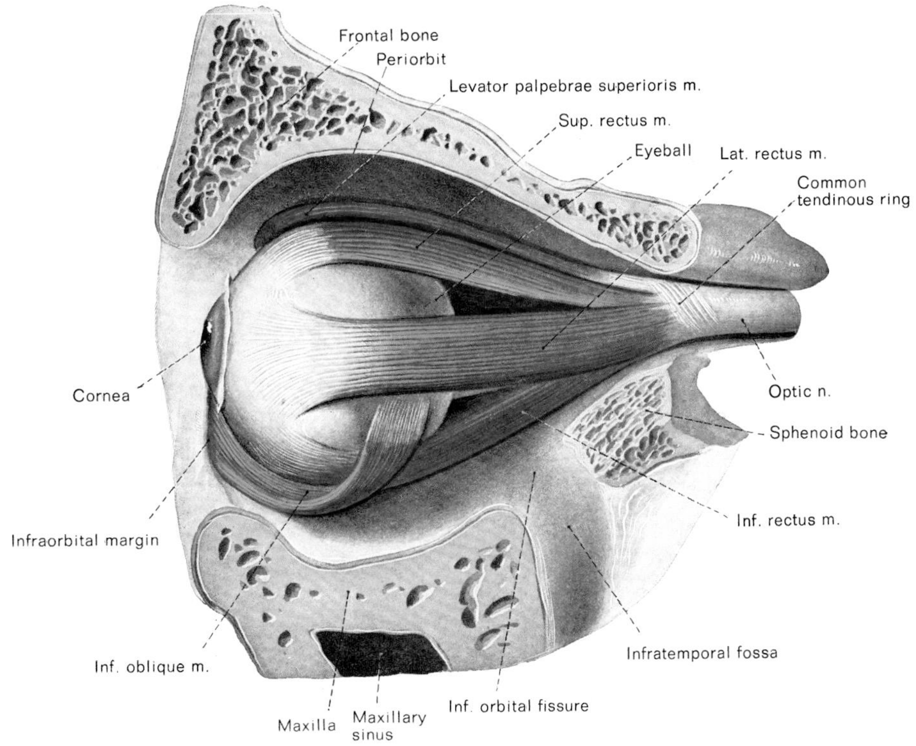
Frontal bone
Periorbit
Levator palpebrae superioris m.
Sup. rectus m.
Eyeball
Lat. rectus m.
Common tendinous ring
Cornea
Optic n.
Sphenoid bone
Inf. rectus m.
Infraorbital margin
Infratemporal fossa
Inf. oblique m.
Inf. orbital fissure
Maxilla
Maxillary sinus

Fig. 208. The extrinsic muscles of the left eye in lateral view. The lateral wall of the left orbit and most of the contents of the orbit including the fascia, the eyelids and the anterior end of the levator palpabrae superioris muscle have been removed.

Fig. 209. The extrinsic muscles of the left eyeball in lateral view. The lateral rectus muscle and the optic nerve have been divided. The eyeball has been rotated to expose the dorsal pole with the stump of the optic nerve. Most of the levator palpebrae superioris muscle has been removed.

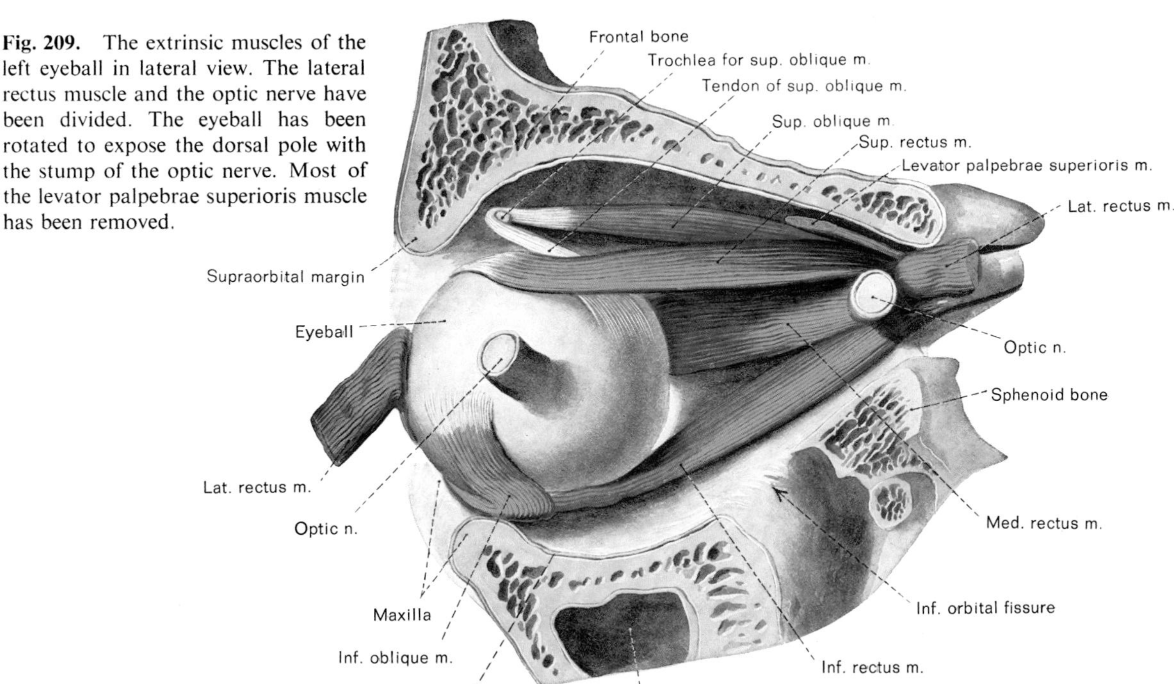
Frontal bone
Trochlea for sup. oblique m.
Tendon of sup. oblique m.
Sup. oblique m.
Sup. rectus m.
Levator palpebrae superioris m.
Lat. rectus m.
Supraorbital margin
Eyeball
Optic n.
Sphenoid bone
Lat. rectus m.
Optic n.
Med. rectus m.
Maxilla
Inf. orbital fissure
Inf. oblique m.
Inf. rectus m.
Periorbit
Maxillary sinus

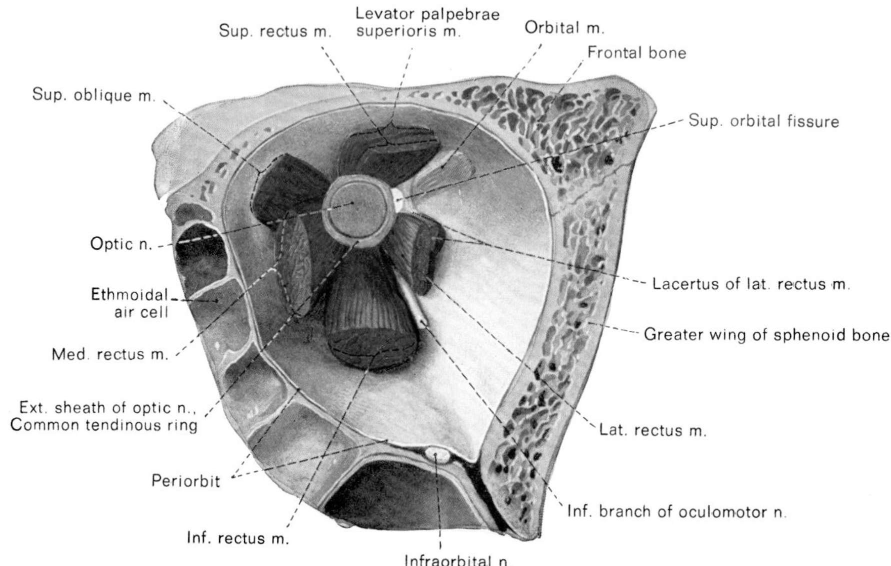
Sup. rectus m.
Levator palpebrae superioris m.
Orbital m.
Frontal bone
Sup. oblique m.
Sup. orbital fissure
Optic n.
Ethmoidal air cell
Med. rectus m.
Ext. sheath of optic n., Common tendinous ring
Periorbit
Inf. rectus m.
Infraorbital n.
Lacertus of lat. rectus m.
Greater wing of sphenoid bone
Lat. rectus m.
Inf. branch of oculomotor n.

Fig. 210. The origins of the extrinsic ocular muscles from the common tendinous ring; frontal section through the orbit viewed from ventral. The optic nerve has been cut off close to the optic canal. The stumps of the muscles as well as the lower branch of the oculomotor nerve have been retained.

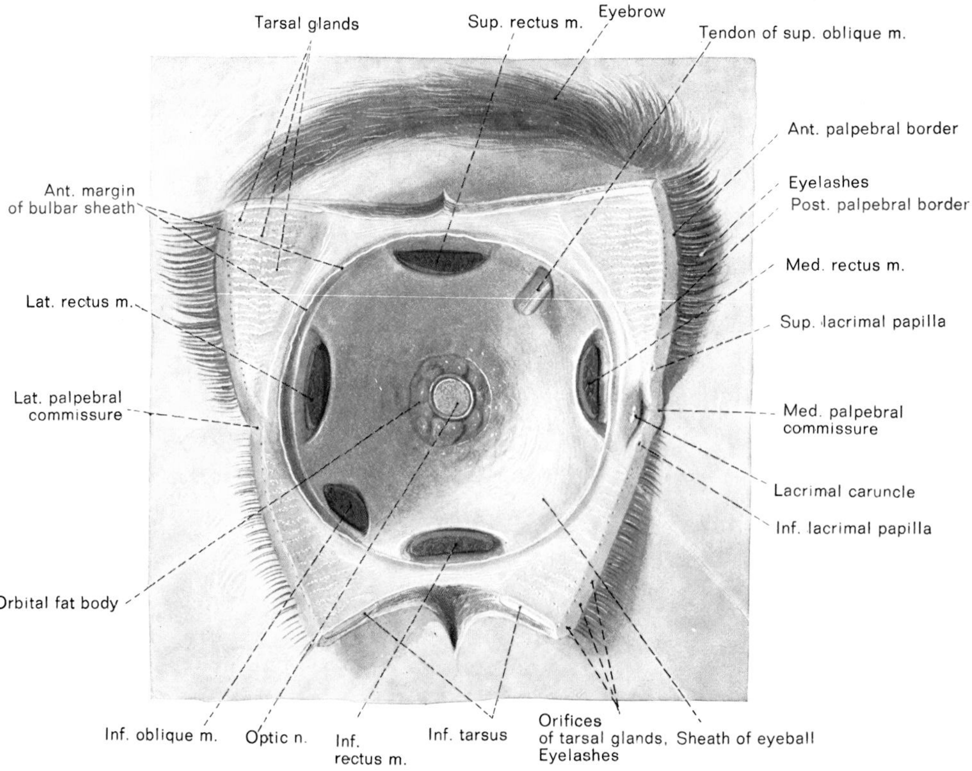
Tarsal glands
Sup. rectus m.
Eyebrow
Tendon of sup. oblique m.
Ant. palpebral border
Eyelashes
Post. palpebral border
Ant. margin of bulbar sheath
Med. rectus m.
Lat. rectus m.
Sup. lacrimal papilla
Lat. palpebral commissure
Med. palpebral commissure
Lacrimal caruncle
Inf. lacrimal papilla
Orbital fat body
Inf. oblique m.
Optic n.
Inf. rectus m.
Inf. tarsus
Orifices of tarsal glands, Sheath of eyeball
Eyelashes

Fig. 211. Bulbar fascia (*Tenon's* capsule) of the right eyeball with its openings. The eyeball has been removed. Both eyelids have been divided and reflected.

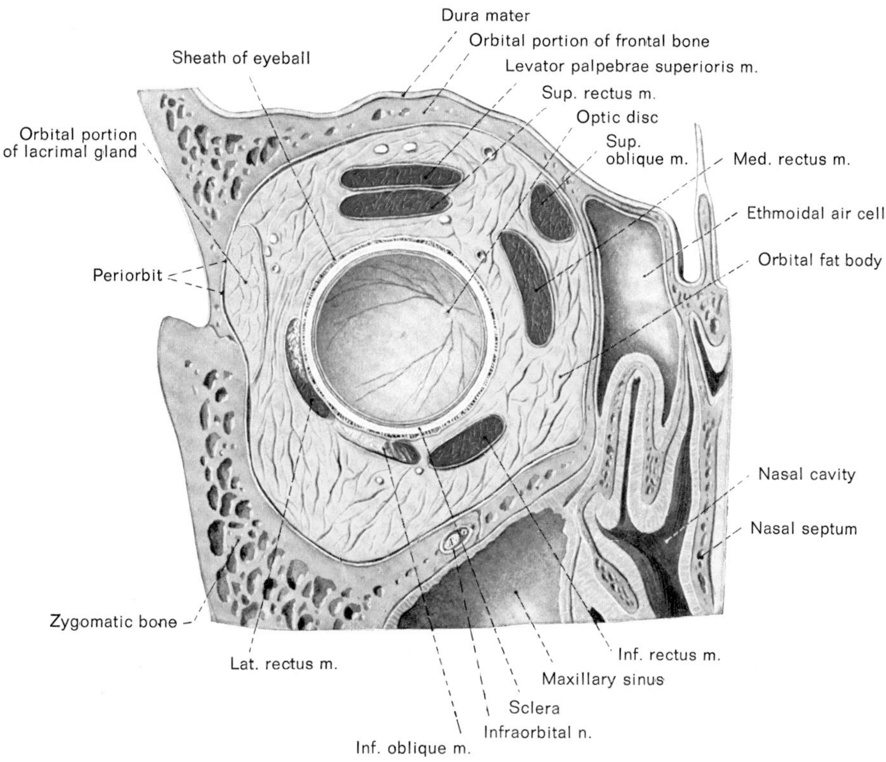
Dura mater
Orbital portion of frontal bone
Sheath of eyeball
Levator palpebrae superioris m.
Sup. rectus m.
Optic disc
Orbital portion of lacrimal gland
Sup. oblique m.
Med. rectus m.
Ethmoidal air cell
Orbital fat body
Periorbit
Nasal cavity
Nasal septum
Zygomatic bone
Inf. rectus m.
Lat. rectus m.
Maxillary sinus
Sclera
Infraorbital n.
Inf. oblique m.

Fig. 212. Frontal section of the right orbit through the dorsal third of the eyeball. Anterior view.

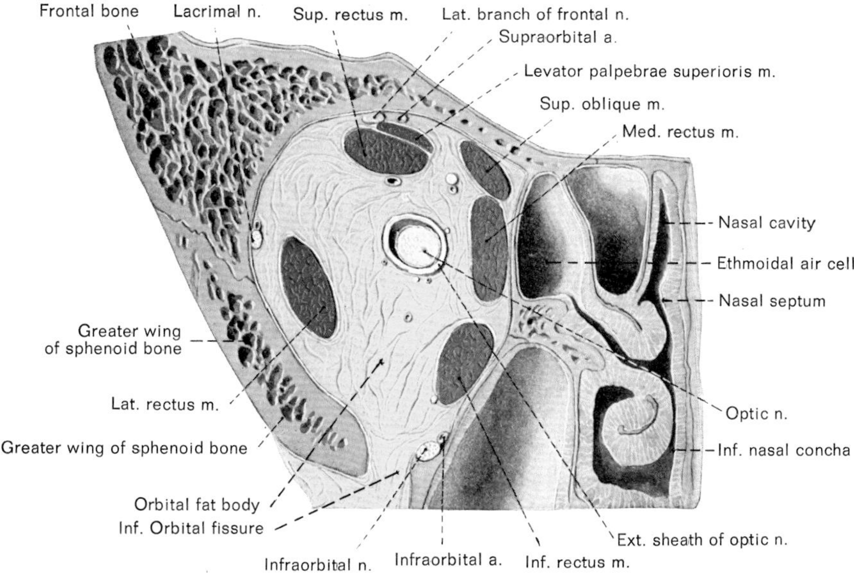
Frontal bone
Lacrimal n.
Sup. rectus m.
Lat. branch of frontal n.
Supraorbital a.
Levator palpebrae superioris m.
Sup. oblique m.
Med. rectus m.
Nasal cavity
Ethmoidal air cell
Nasal septum
Greater wing of sphenoid bone
Lat. rectus m.
Optic n.
Greater wing of sphenoid bone
Inf. nasal concha
Orbital fat body
Inf. Orbital fissure
Ext. sheath of optic n.
Infraorbital n.
Infraorbital a.
Inf. rectus m.

Fig. 213. Frontal section through the right orbit behind the eyeball. Ventral view.

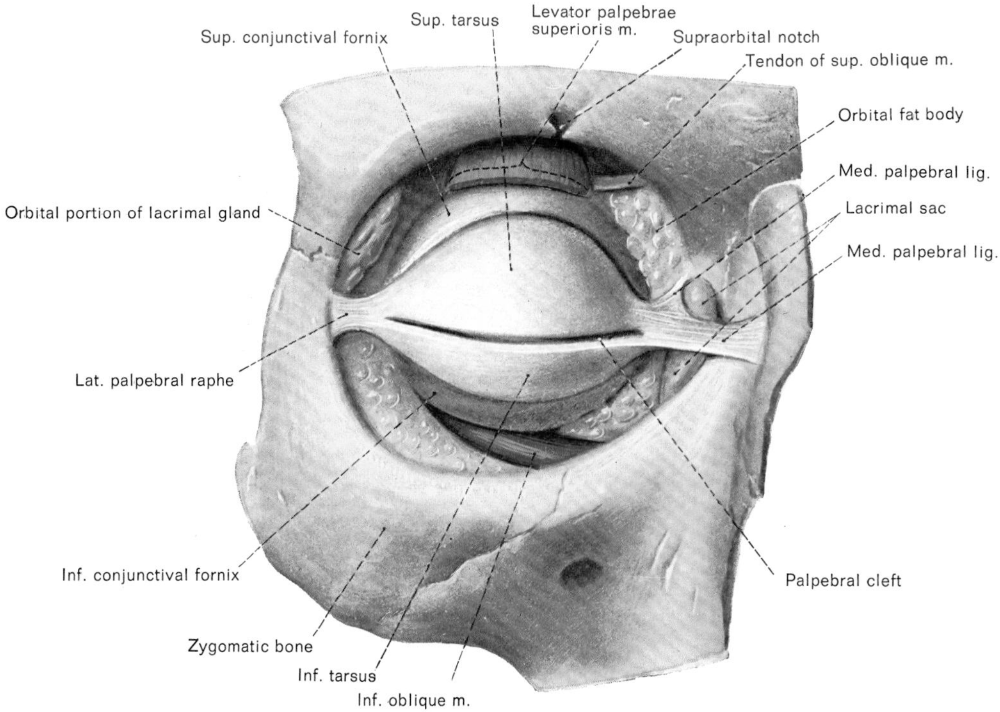
Sup. tarsus
Levator palpebrae superioris m.
Sup. conjunctival fornix
Supraorbital notch
Tendon of sup. oblique m.
Orbital fat body
Med. palpebral lig.
Lacrimal sac
Med. palpebral lig.
Orbital portion of lacrimal gland
Lat. palpebral raphe
Inf. conjunctival fornix
Palpebral cleft
Zygomatic bone
Inf. tarsus
Inf. oblique m.

Fig. 214. Tarsal plates, medial palpebral ligament, lateral palpebral raphe and lacrimal sac of the right eye. Most parts of the lids have been removed and the tendon of the levator palpebrae superioris muscle has been cut off.

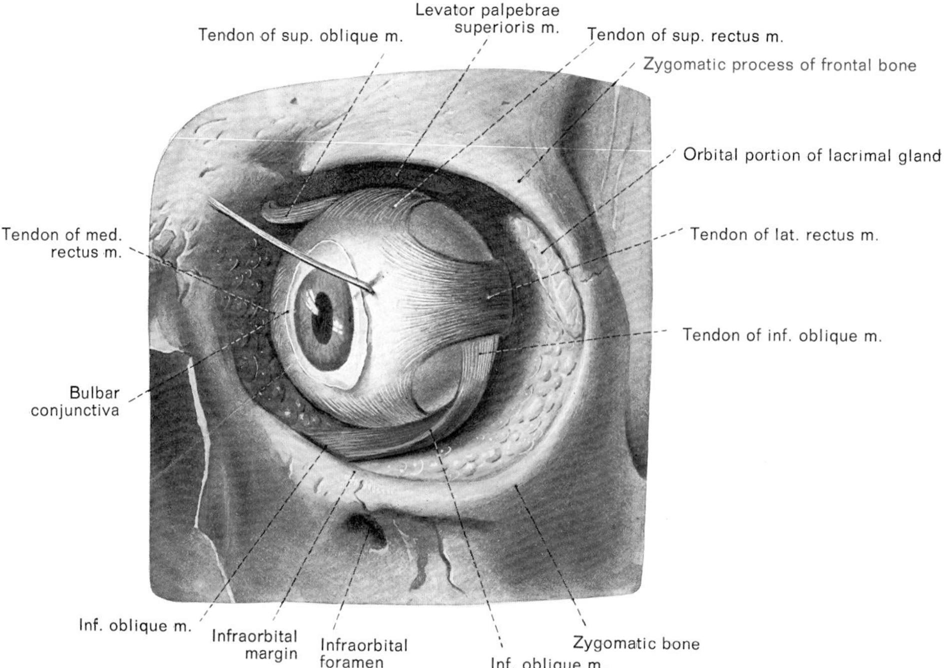
Levator palpebrae superioris m.
Tendon of sup. oblique m.
Tendon of sup. rectus m.
Zygomatic process of frontal bone
Orbital portion of lacrimal gland
Tendon of med. rectus m.
Tendon of lat. rectus m.
Tendon of inf. oblique m.
Bulbar conjunctiva
Inf. oblique m.
Infraorbital margin
Infraorbital foramen
Zygomatic bone
Inf. oblique m.

Fig. 215. Extrinsic muscles of left eyeball, ventrolateral view. Skin, eyelids and fascia have been removed.

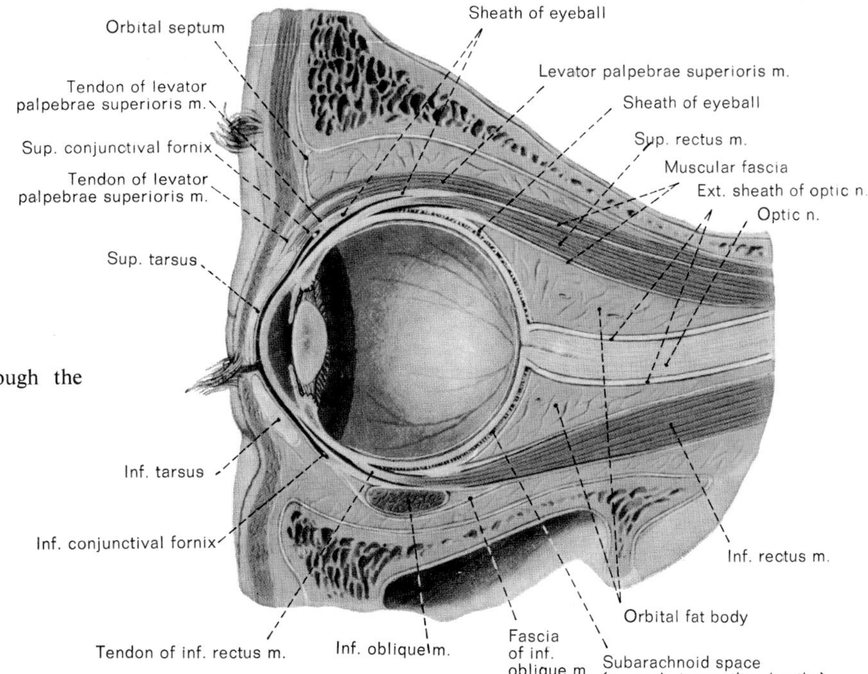
Orbital septum
Sheath of eyeball
Tendon of levator palpebrae superioris m.
Levator palpebrae superioris m.
Sheath of eyeball
Sup. conjunctival fornix
Sup. rectus m.
Tendon of levator palpebrae superioris m.
Muscular fascia
Ext. sheath of optic n.
Optic n.
Sup. tarsus
Inf. tarsus
Inf. conjunctival fornix
Inf. rectus m.
Orbital fat body
Tendon of inf. rectus m.
Inf. oblique m.
Fascia of inf. oblique m.
Subarachnoid space (space between the sheaths)

Fig. 216. Sagittal section through the orbit and its contents.

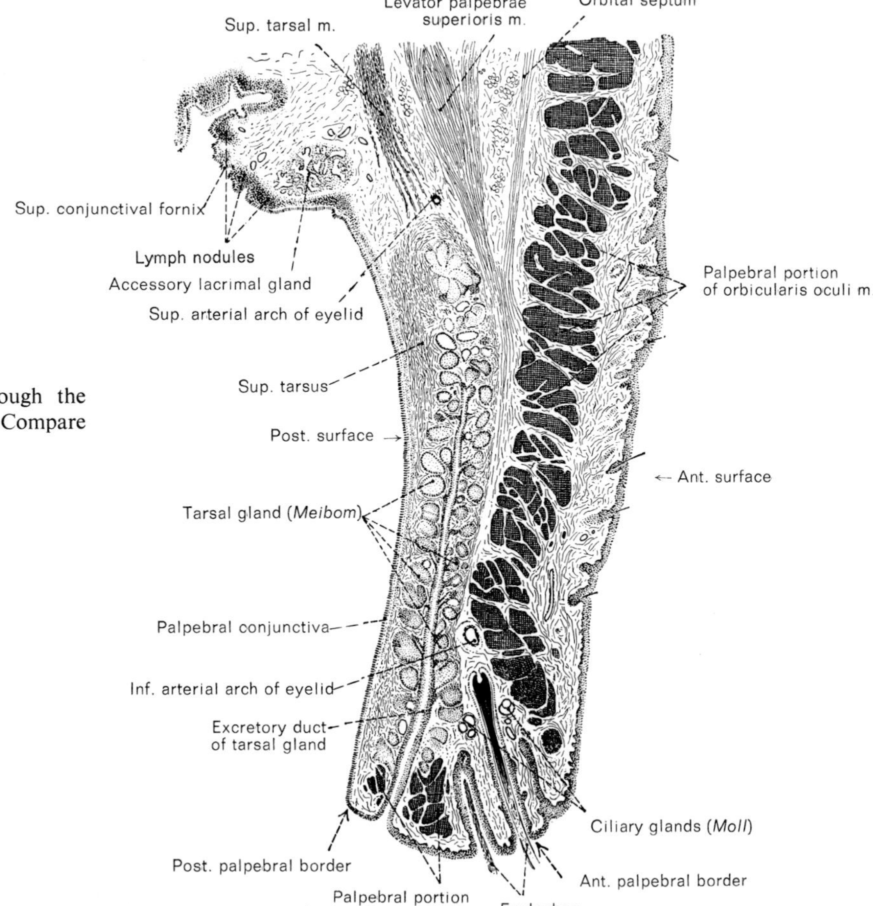
Levator palpebrae superioris m.
Orbital septum
Sup. tarsal m.
Sup. conjunctival fornix
Lymph nodules
Accessory lacrimal gland
Sup. arterial arch of eyelid
Palpebral portion of orbicularis oculi m.
Sup. tarsus
Post. surface
Ant. surface
Tarsal gland (Meibom)
Palpebral conjunctiva
Inf. arterial arch of eyelid
Excretory duct of tarsal gland
Ciliary glands (Moll)
Post. palpebral border
Ant. palpebral border
Palpebral portion of orbicularis oculi m.
Eyelashes

Fig. 217. Sagittal section through the upper eyelid; low magnification. Compare with Fig. 197.

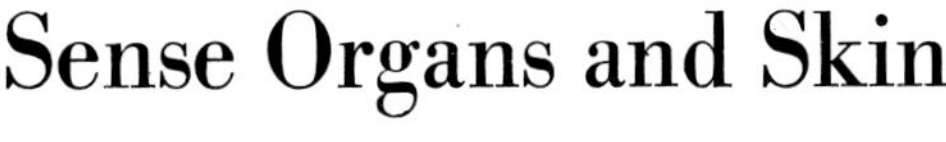

Sense Organs and Skin

Ear and Vestibular Apparatus

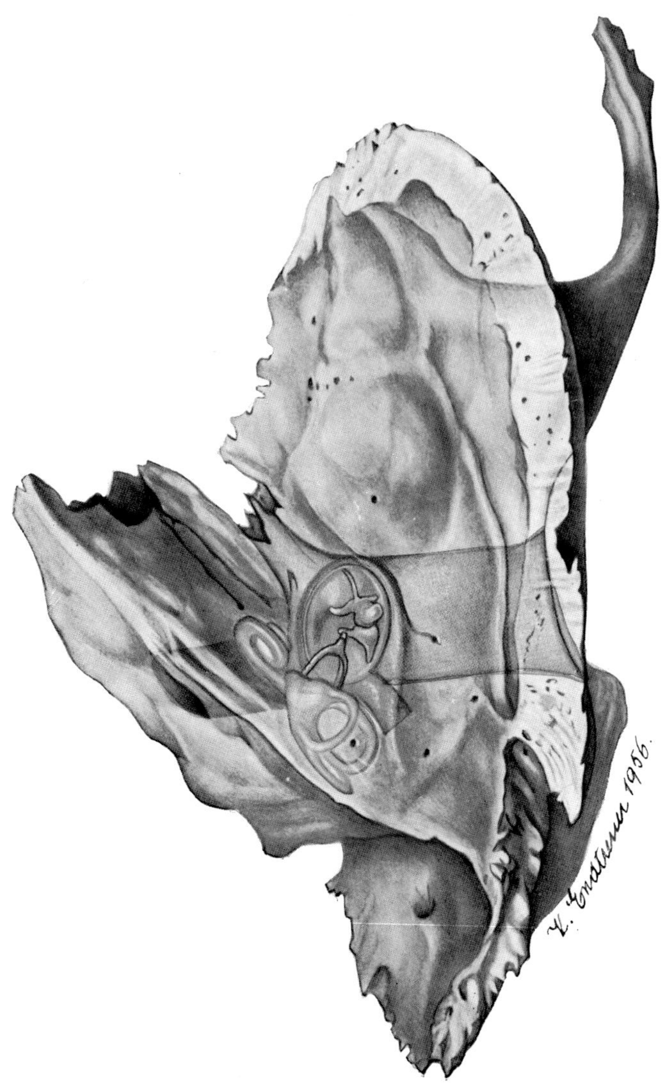
K. Endtresser 1956.

Fig. 218. Topographical overview of the vestibulo-cochlear apparatus located within the right temporal bone. Red: external auditory meatus; green: tympanic cavity with middle ear ossicles; blue: inner ear (membranous labyrinth and cochlear duct). (From *Pernkopf/Ferner:* Atlas der topographischen und angewandten Anatomie des Menschen. vol. 1. Urban & Schwarzenberg, München–Berlin 1963.)

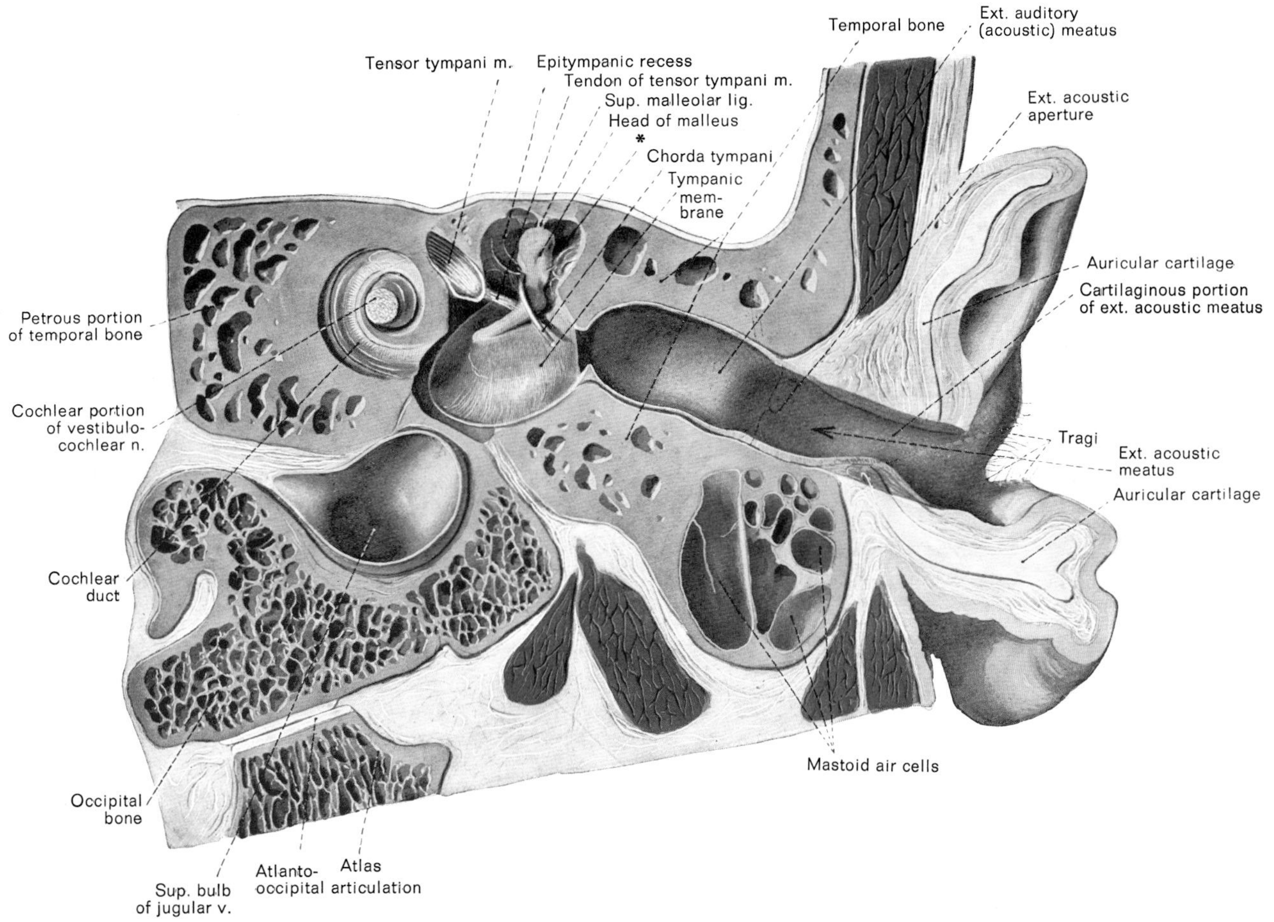
Temporal bone
Ext. auditory (acoustic) meatus
Tensor tympani m.
Epitympanic recess
Tendon of tensor tympani m.
Sup. malleolar lig.
Head of malleus
*
Chorda tympani
Tympanic mem-brane
Ext. acoustic aperture
Auricular cartilage
Cartilaginous portion of ext. acoustic meatus
Petrous portion of temporal bone
Cochlear portion of vestibulo-cochlear n.
Tragi
Ext. acoustic meatus
Auricular cartilage
Cochlear duct
Mastoid air cells
Occipital bone
Atlanto- occipital articulation
Atlas
Sup. bulb of jugular v.

Fig. 219. Frontal section through external auditory meatus, tympanic cavity, and cochlea. * Epitympanic recess, apical part.

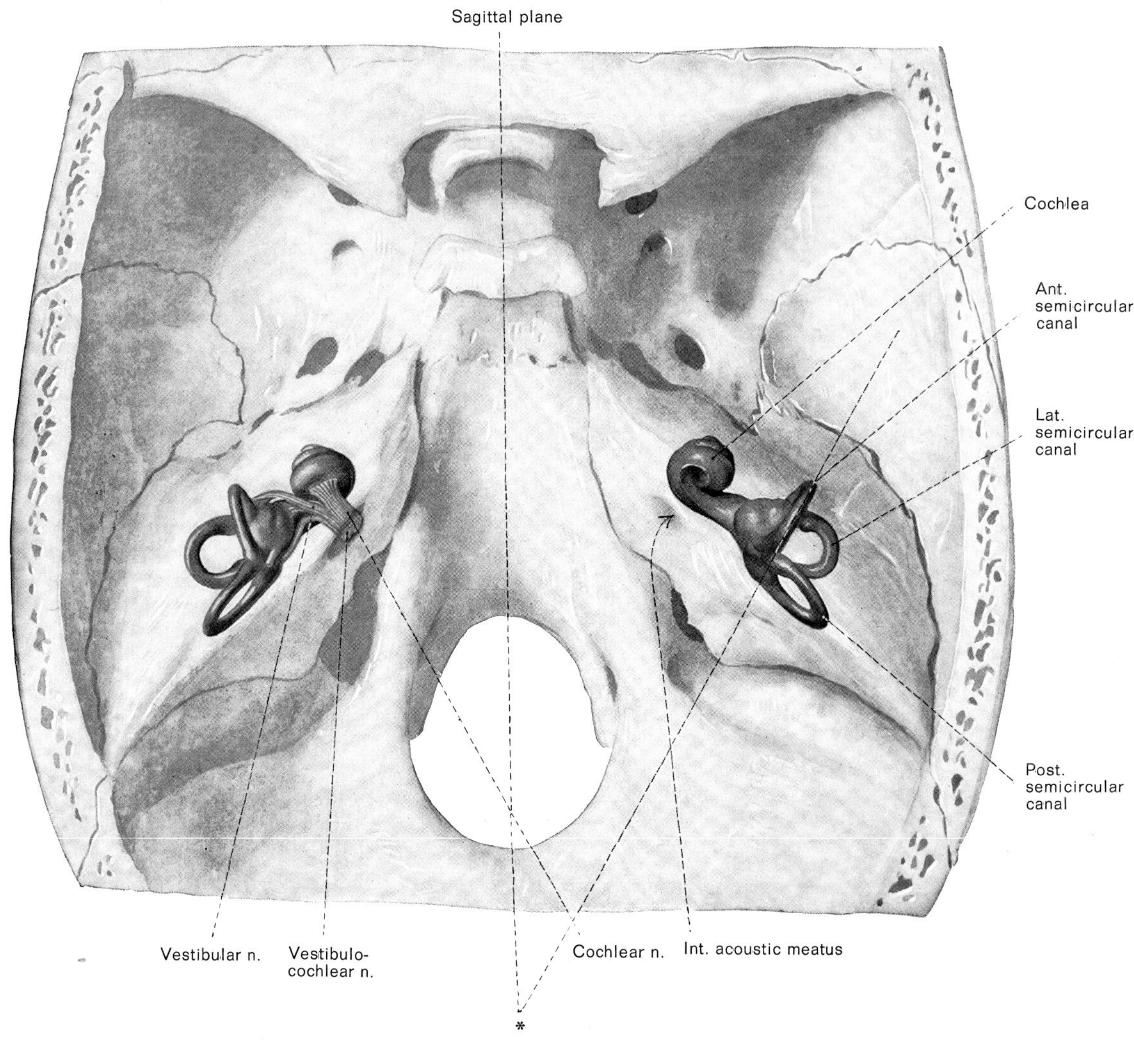

Sagittal plane
Cochlea
Ant. semicircular canal
Lat. semicircular canal
Post. semicircular canal
Vestibular n.
Vestibulo-cochlear n.
Cochlear n.
Int. acoustic meatus
*

Fig. 220. Phantom view of osseous labyrinths in natural position projected onto the inside of the cranial base with nerve supply on the left. Note the oblique orientation of the cochlear axis. The cochlea points in the lateral anterior caudal direction. * indicates the plane of the anterior semicircular canal and its intersection with the sagittal plane.

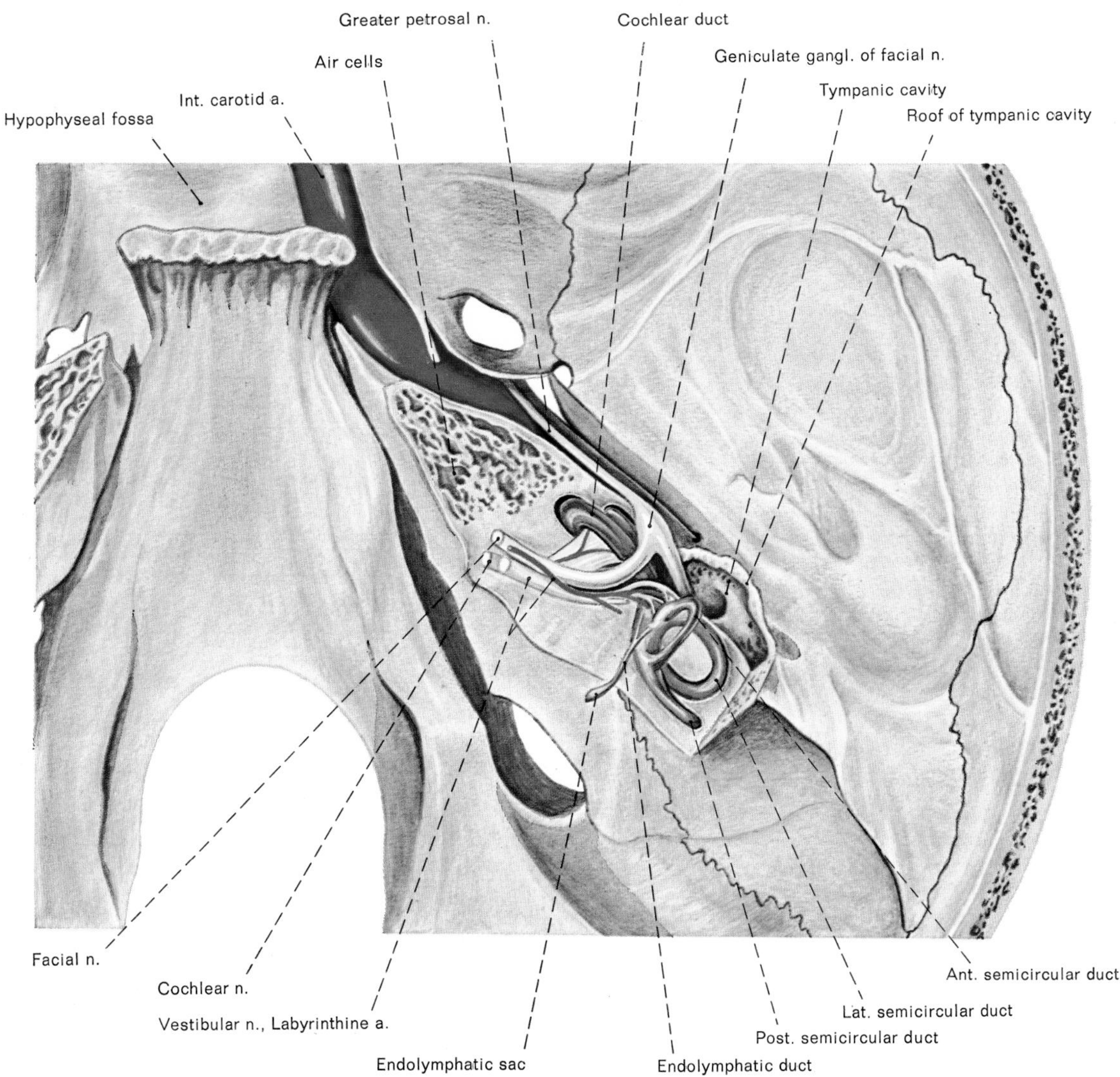
Greater petrosal n.
Cochlear duct
Air cells
Geniculate gangl. of facial n.
Int. carotid a.
Tympanic cavity
Hypophyseal fossa
Roof of tympanic cavity
Facial n.
Cochlear n.
Vestibular n., Labyrinthine a.
Endolymphatic sac
Endolymphatic duct
Post. semicircular duct
Lat. semicircular duct
Ant. semicircular duct

Fig. 221. Right internal ear with membranous labyrinth, cochlear duct, vestibulo-cochlear nerve and facial nerve within the petrous part of temporal bone. The upper portion of the petrous bone has been removed (from *Pernkopf/Ferner:* Atlas der topographischen und angewandten Anatomie des Menschen. vol. 1. Urban & Schwarzenberg, München–Berlin 1963).

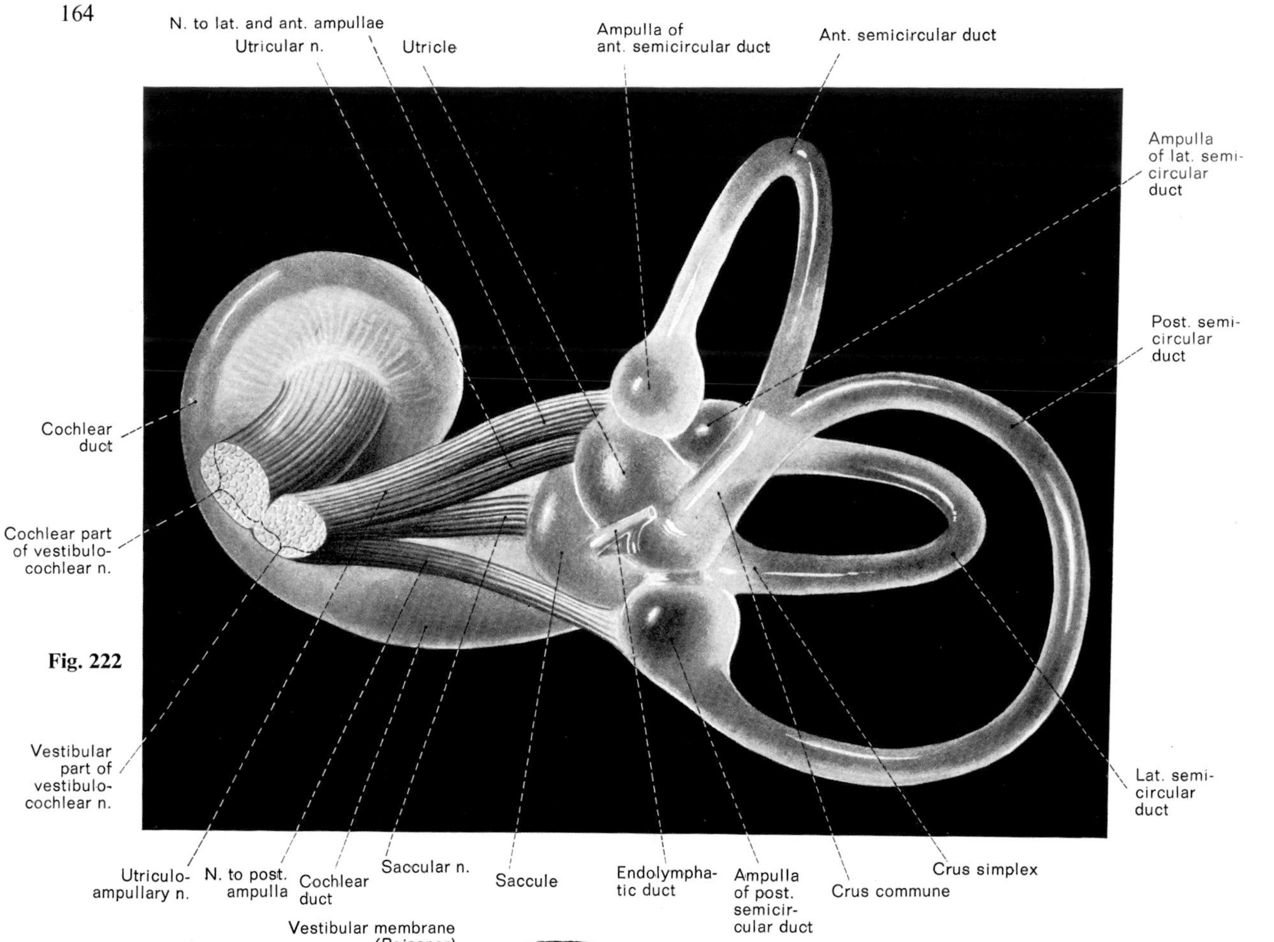

N. to lat. and ant. ampullae
Utricular n.
Utricle
Ampulla of ant. semicircular duct
Ant. semicircular duct
Ampulla of lat. semicircular duct
Post. semicircular duct
Cochlear duct
Cochlear part of vestibulocochlear n.
Vestibular part of vestibulocochlear n.
Lat. semicircular duct
Utriculoampullary n.
N. to post. ampulla
Cochlear duct
Saccular n.
Saccule
Endolymphatic duct
Ampulla of post. semicircular duct
Crus commune
Crus simplex

Fig. 222

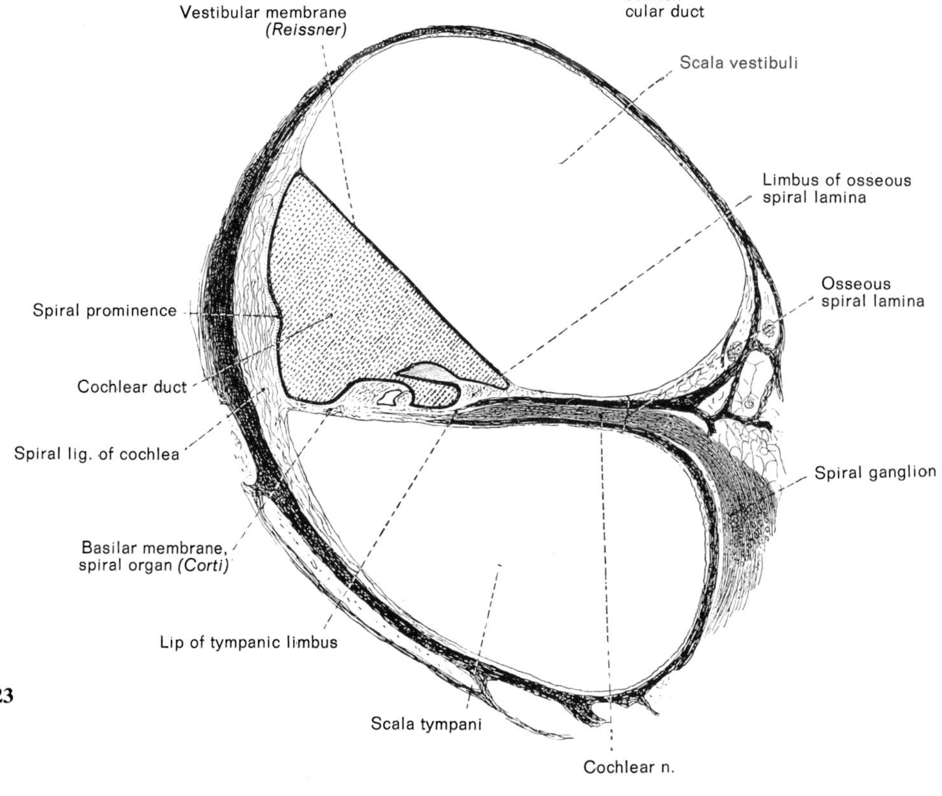

Vestibular membrane *(Reissner)*
Scala vestibuli
Limbus of osseous spiral lamina
Osseous spiral lamina
Spiral prominence
Cochlear duct
Spiral lig. of cochlea
Spiral ganglion
Basilar membrane, spiral organ *(Corti)*
Lip of tympanic limbus
Scala tympani
Cochlear n.

Fig. 223

◀ **Fig. 222.** Right membranous labyrinth and branches of vestibulocochlear nerve.

Fig. 223. Diagrammatic cross section of cochlear coil. Endolymphatic space marked by stippling.

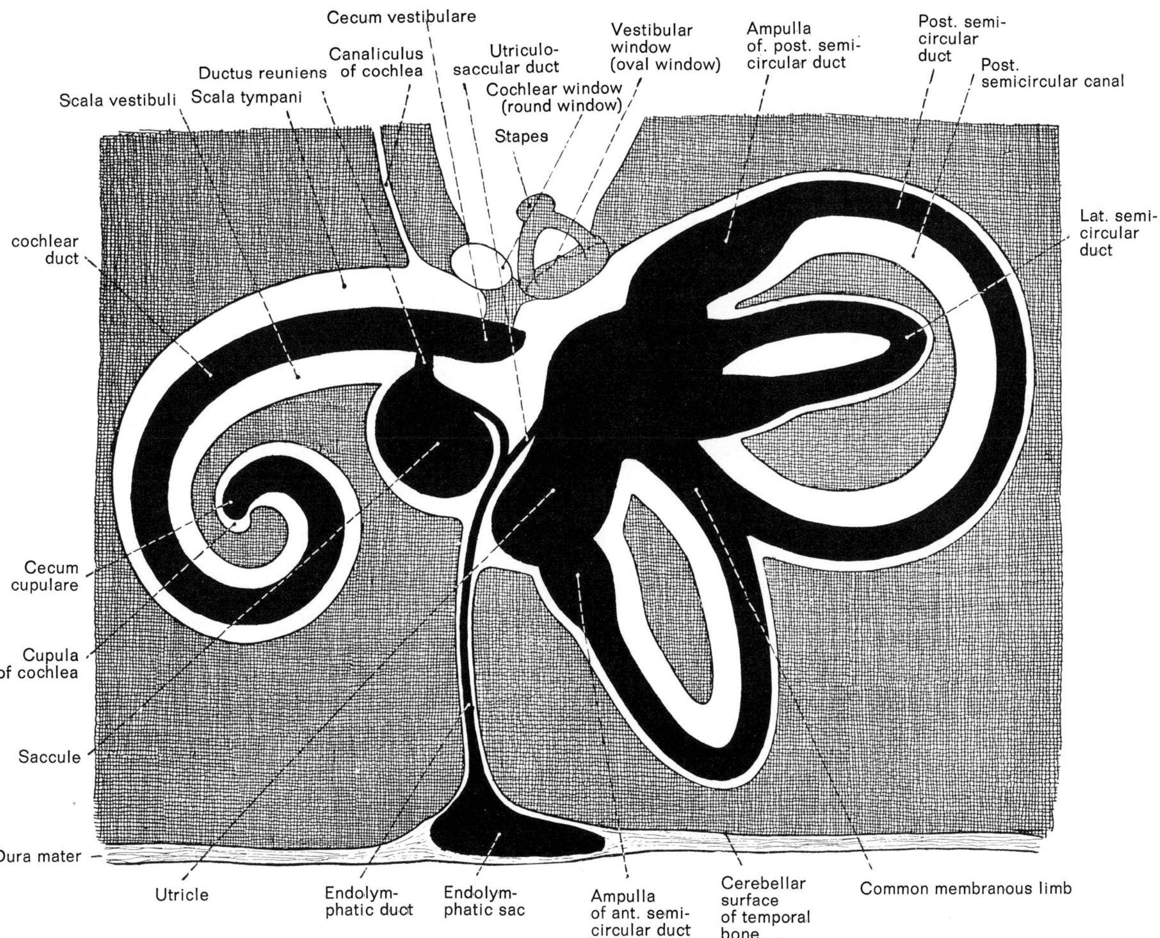
Cecum vestibulare
Canaliculus of cochlea
Ductus reuniens
Scala vestibuli
Scala tympani
Utriculo-saccular duct
Vestibular window (oval window)
Cochlear window (round window)
Stapes
Ampulla of post. semi-circular duct
Post. semi-circular duct
Post. semicircular canal
cochlear duct
Lat. semi-circular duct
Cecum cupulare
Cupula of cochlea
Saccule
Dura mater
Utricle
Endolym-phatic duct
Endolym-phatic sac
Ampulla of ant. semi-circular duct
Cerebellar surface of temporal bone
Common membranous limb

Fig. 224. Diagram of the right membranous labyrinth. Black: endolymphatic spaces; cross-hatched: bone; white: perilymphatic spaces.

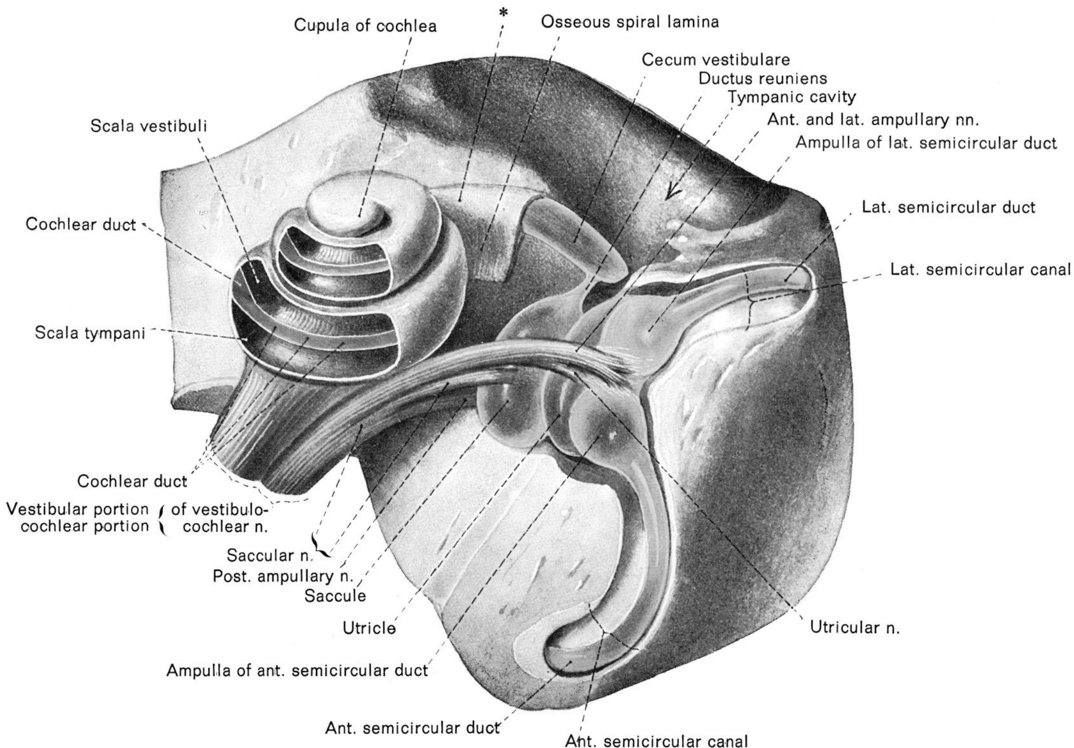
Cupula of cochlea
*
Osseous spiral lamina
Cecum vestibulare
Ductus reuniens
Tympanic cavity
Ant. and lat. ampullary nn.
Ampulla of lat. semicircular duct
Scala vestibuli
Cochlear duct
Lat. semicircular duct
Lat. semicircular canal
Scala tympani
Cochlear duct
Vestibular portion of vestibulo-
cochlear portion cochlear n.
Saccular n.
Post. ampullary n.
Saccule
Utricle
Utricular n.
Ampulla of ant. semicircular duct
Ant. semicircular duct
Ant. semicircular canal

Fig. 225. Right membranous labyrinth with nerve supply partly exposed by chiseling away wall of bony labyrinth (somewhat diagrammatic). Blue: membranous labyrinth containing endolymph; * = basal coil of chochlea.

Fig. 226. Right internal acoustic meatus after partial removal of its wall; medial view.

Fig. 227. Internal acoustic meatus. Same preparation as in Fig. 226, but more of the dorsomedial wall has been removed.

Fig. 228. Left bony cochlea sectioned along the axis of the modiolus.

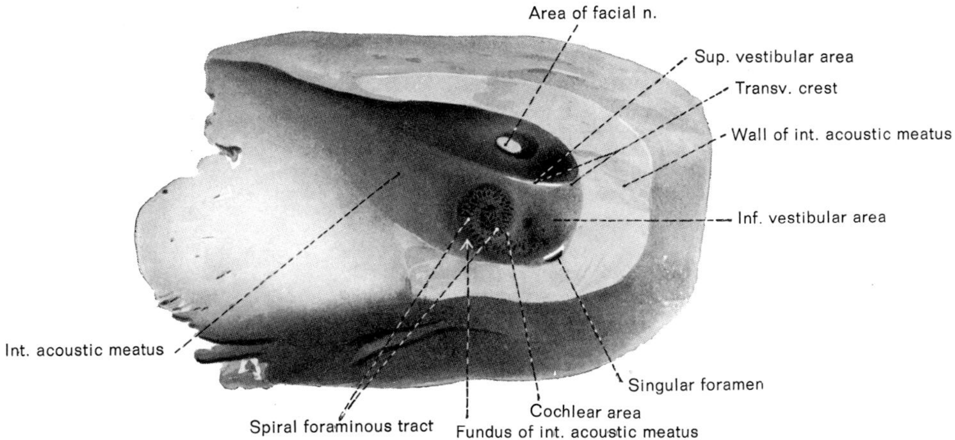
Area of facial n.
Sup. vestibular area
Transv. crest
Wall of int. acoustic meatus
Inf. vestibular area
Int. acoustic meatus
Singular foramen
Cochlear area
Spiral foraminous tract
Fundus of int. acoustic meatus

Fig. 226

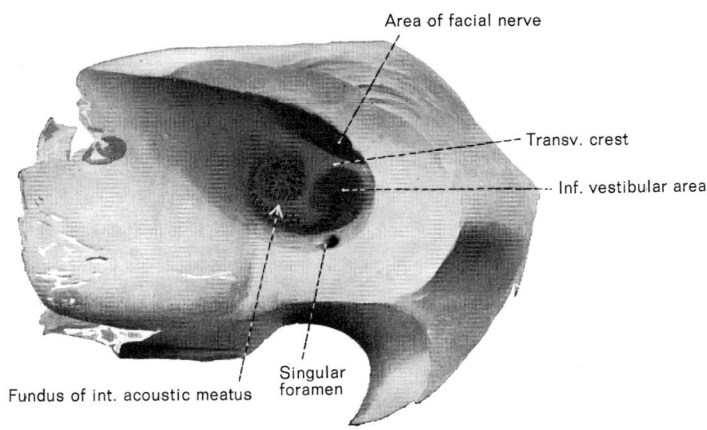
Area of facial nerve
Transv. crest
Inf. vestibular area
Fundus of int. acoustic meatus
Singular foramen

Fig. 227

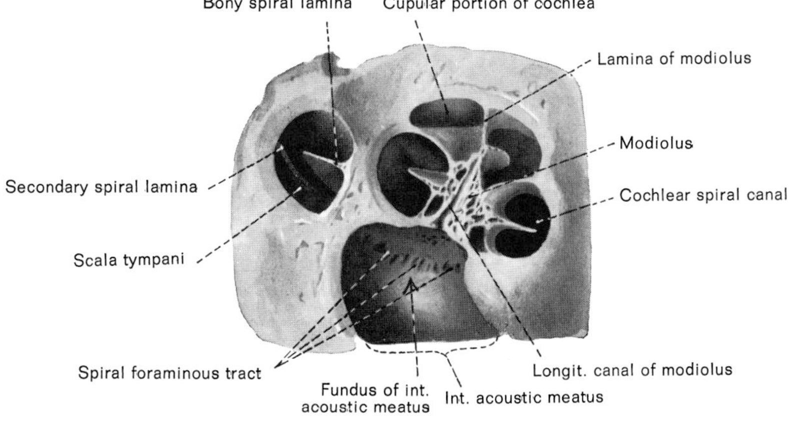
Bony spiral lamina
Cupular portion of cochlea
Lamina of modiolus
Modiolus
Secondary spiral lamina
Cochlear spiral canal
Scala tympani
Spiral foraminous tract
Longit. canal of modiolus
Fundus of int. acoustic meatus
Int. acoustic meatus

Fig. 228

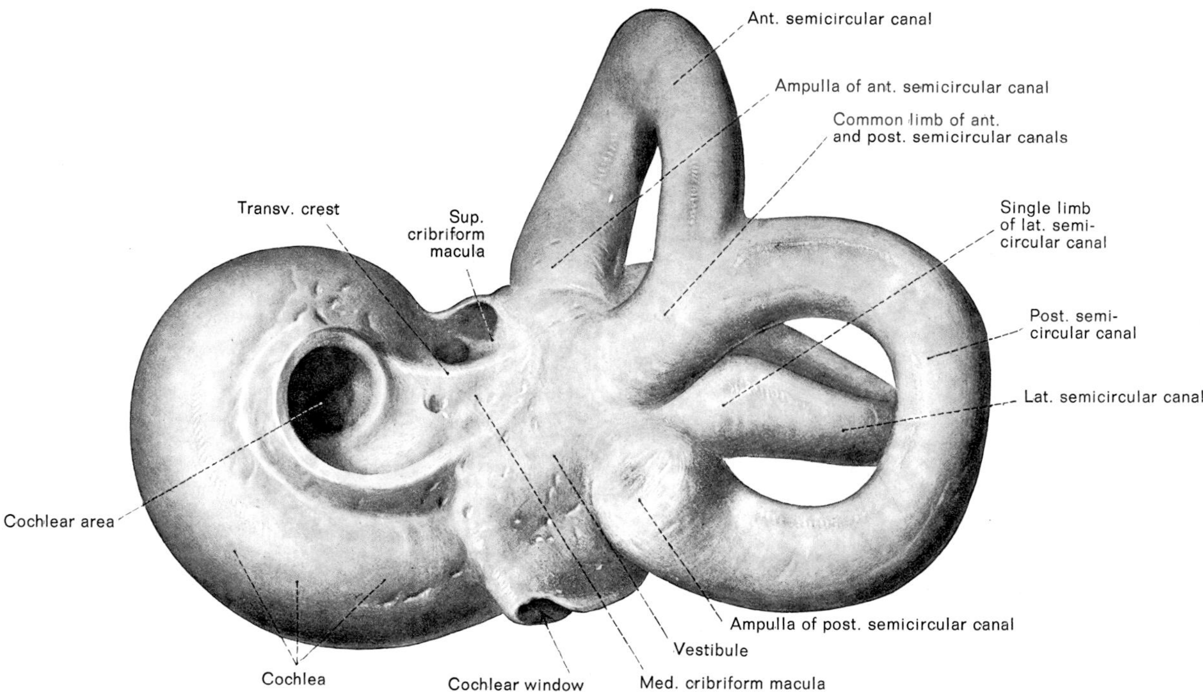
Ant. semicircular canal
Ampulla of ant. semicircular canal
Common limb of ant. and post. semicircular canals
Transv. crest
Sup. cribriform macula
Single limb of lat. semicircular canal
Post. semicircular canal
Lat. semicircular canal
Cochlear area
Ampulla of post. semicircular canal
Vestibule
Cochlea
Cochlear window
Med. cribriform macula

Fig. 229. Right bony labyrinth, carved out of the petrous bone; seen from medial and behind.

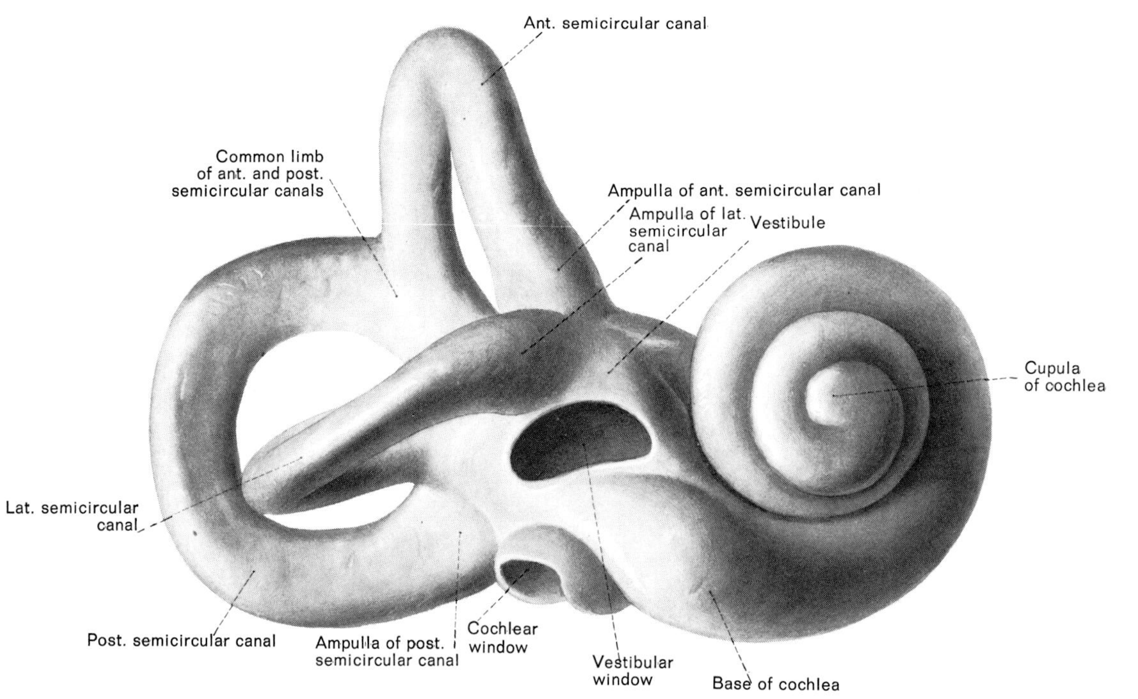
Ant. semicircular canal
Common limb of ant. and post. semicircular canals
Ampulla of ant. semicircular canal
Ampulla of lat. semicircular canal
Vestibule
Cupula of cochlea
Lat. semicircular canal
Post. semicircular canal
Ampulla of post. semicircular canal
Cochlear window
Vestibular window
Base of cochlea

Fig. 230. Right bony labyrinth, carved out of the petrous bone; antero-lateral view.

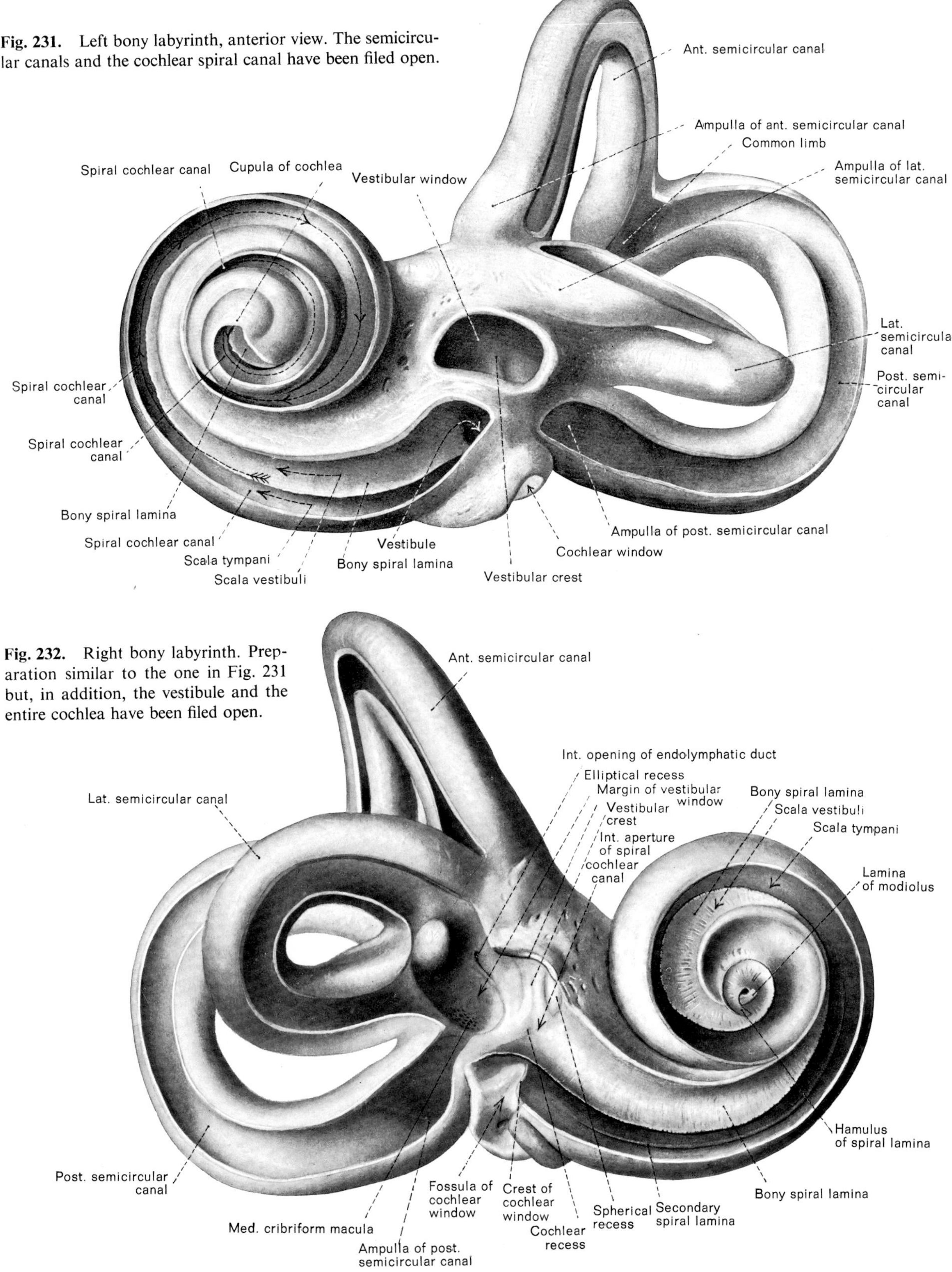

Ant. semicircular canal
Ampulla of ant. semicircular canal
Common limb
Ampulla of lat. semicircular canal
Spiral cochlear canal
Cupula of cochlea
Vestibular window
Lat. semicircular canal
Post. semicircular canal
Spiral cochlear canal
Spiral cochlear canal
Bony spiral lamina
Spiral cochlear canal
Scala tympani
Scala vestibuli
Vestibule
Bony spiral lamina
Vestibular crest
Cochlear window
Ampulla of post. semicircular canal
Ant. semicircular canal
Int. opening of endolymphatic duct
Elliptical recess
Margin of vestibular window
Vestibular crest
Int. aperture of spiral cochlear canal
Bony spiral lamina
Scala vestibuli
Scala tympani
Lamina of modiolus
Lat. semicircular canal
Hamulus of spiral lamina
Bony spiral lamina
Post. semicircular canal
Med. cribriform macula
Ampulla of post. semicircular canal
Fossula of cochlear window
Crest of cochlear window
Cochlear recess
Spherical recess
Secondary spiral lamina

Fig. 231. Left bony labyrinth, anterior view. The semicircular canals and the cochlear spiral canal have been filed open.

Fig. 232. Right bony labyrinth. Preparation similar to the one in Fig. 231 but, in addition, the vestibule and the entire cochlea have been filed open.

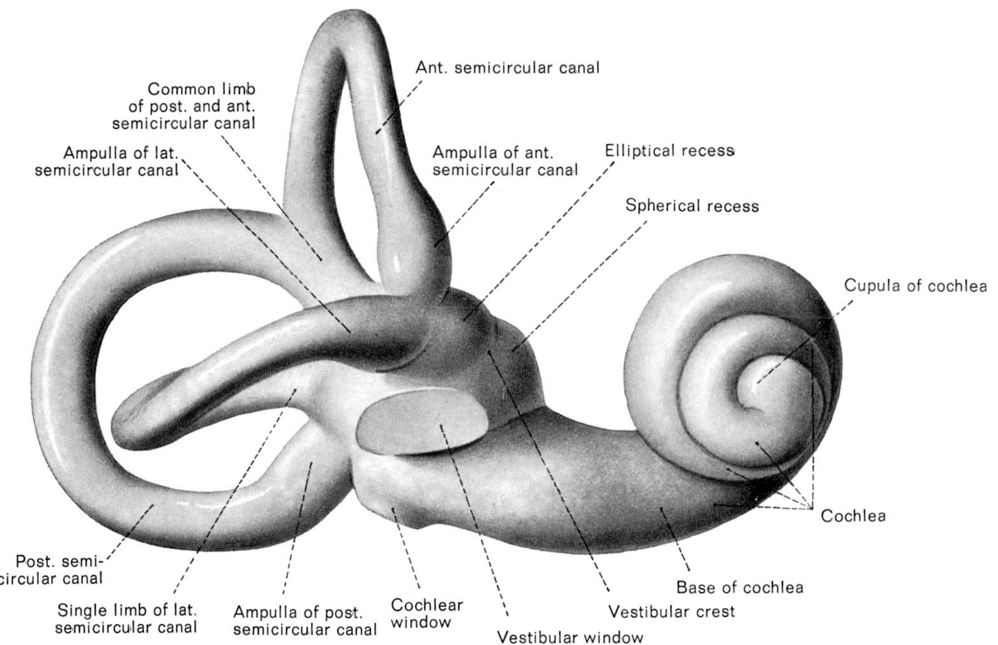

Ant. semicircular canal
Common limb of post. and ant. semicircular canal
Ampulla of lat. semicircular canal
Ampulla of ant. semicircular canal
Elliptical recess
Spherical recess
Cupula of cochlea
Cochlea
Post. semicircular canal
Single limb of lat. semicircular canal
Ampulla of post. semicircular canal
Cochlear window
Vestibular window
Vestibular crest
Base of cochlea

Fig. 233. Cast of spaces in the right bony labyrinth, lateral view.

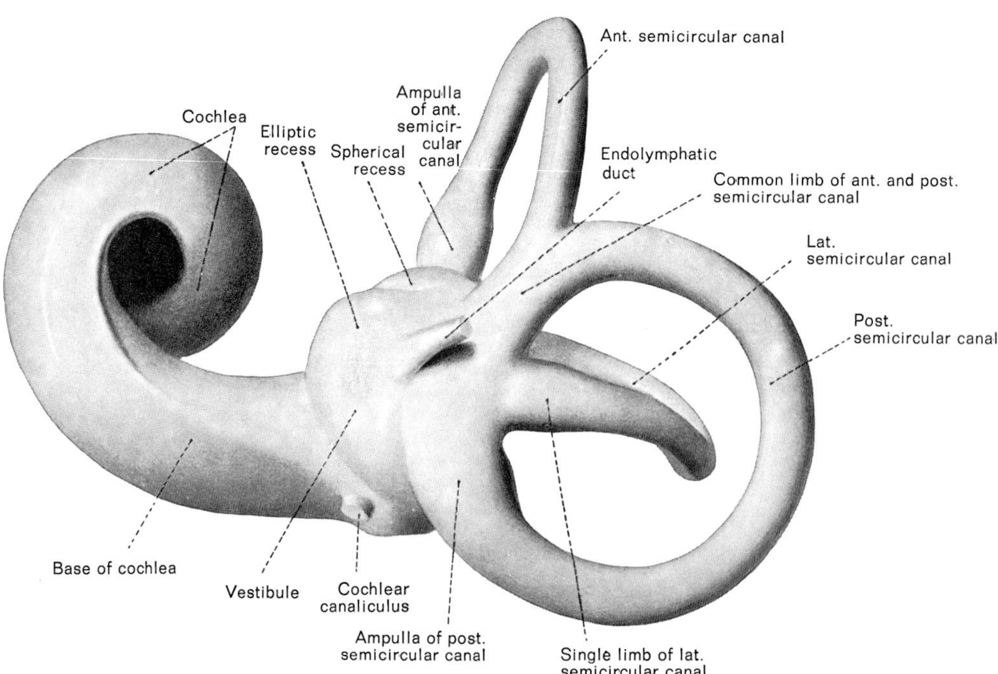

Ant. semicircular canal
Cochlea
Elliptic recess
Spherical recess
Ampulla of ant. semicircular canal
Endolymphatic duct
Common limb of ant. and post. semicircular canal
Lat. semicircular canal
Post. semicircular canal
Base of cochlea
Vestibule
Cochlear canaliculus
Ampulla of post. semicircular canal
Single limb of lat. semicircular canal

Fig. 234. Cast of the spaces of the right bony labyrinth, medial view.

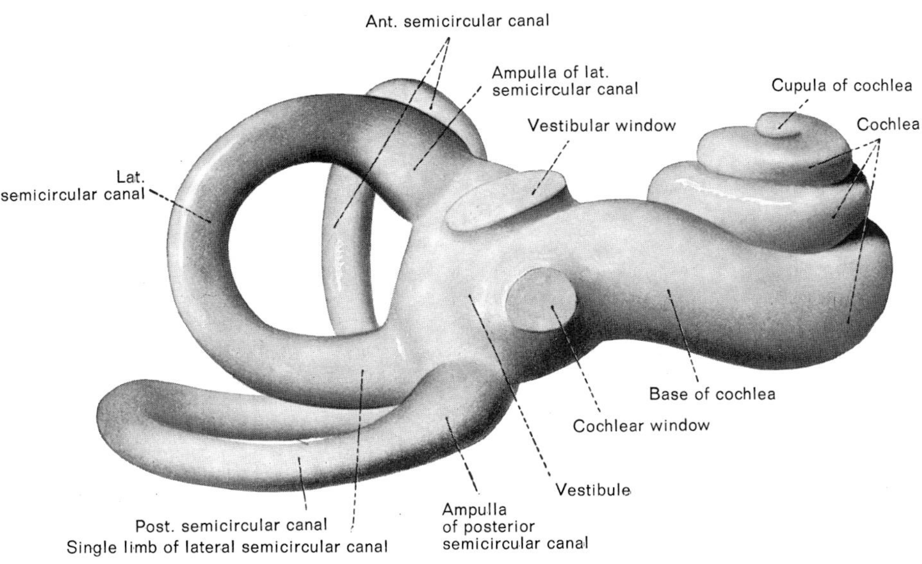
Ant. semicircular canal
Ampulla of lat. semicircular canal
Cupula of cochlea
Vestibular window
Cochlea
Lat. semicircular canal
Base of cochlea
Cochlear window
Vestibule
Post. semicircular canal
Single limb of lateral semicircular canal
Ampulla of posterior semicircular canal

Fig. 235. Cast of the spaces in the right bony labyrinth, viewed from below.

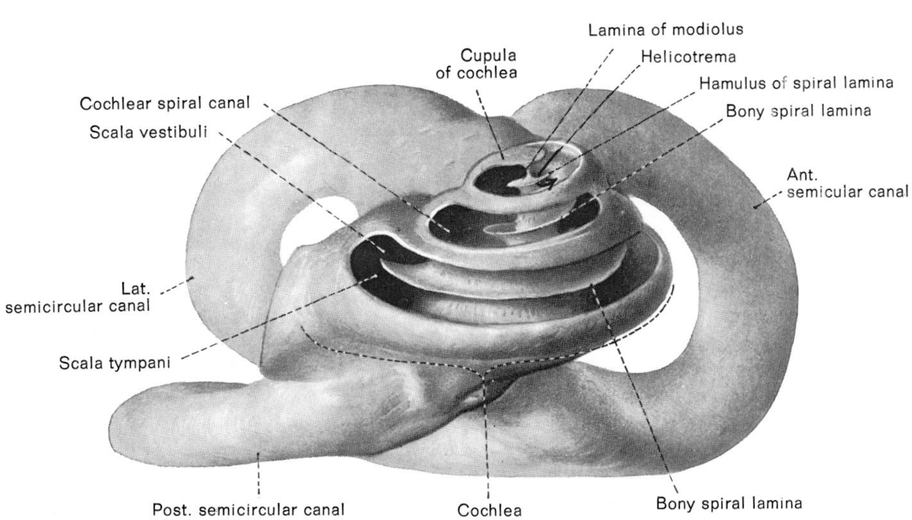
Lamina of modiolus
Helicotrema
Cupula of cochlea
Hamulus of spiral lamina
Cochlear spiral canal
Bony spiral lamina
Scala vestibuli
Ant. semicular canal
Lat. semicircular canal
Scala tympani
Post. semicircular canal
Cochlea
Bony spiral lamina

Fig. 236. Right bony labyrinth; frontal view. The cochlear canal has been filed open on one side.

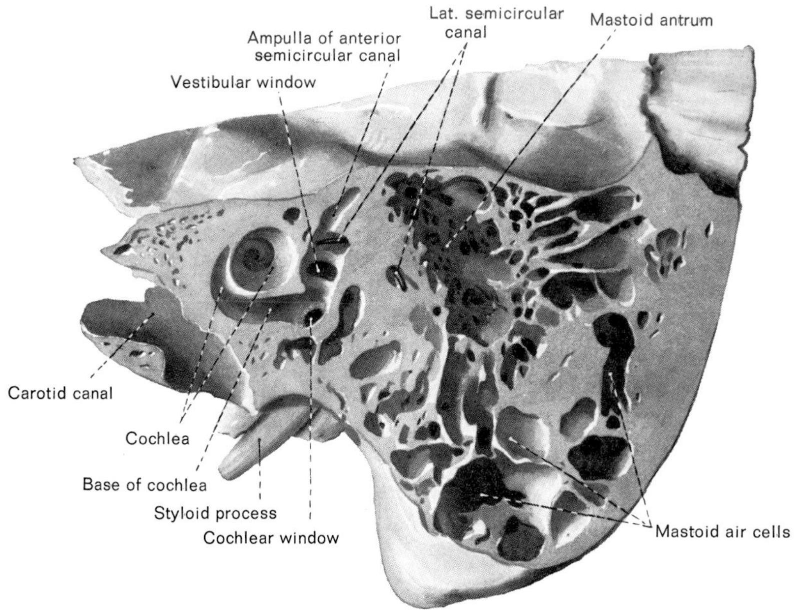
Lat. semicircular canal
Mastoid antrum
Ampulla of anterior semicircular canal
Vestibular window
Carotid canal
Cochlea
Base of cochlea
Styloid process
Cochlear window
Mastoid air cells

Fig. 237. Lateral wall of the right vestibule. The temporal bone has been sectioned along the axis of the petrous portion.

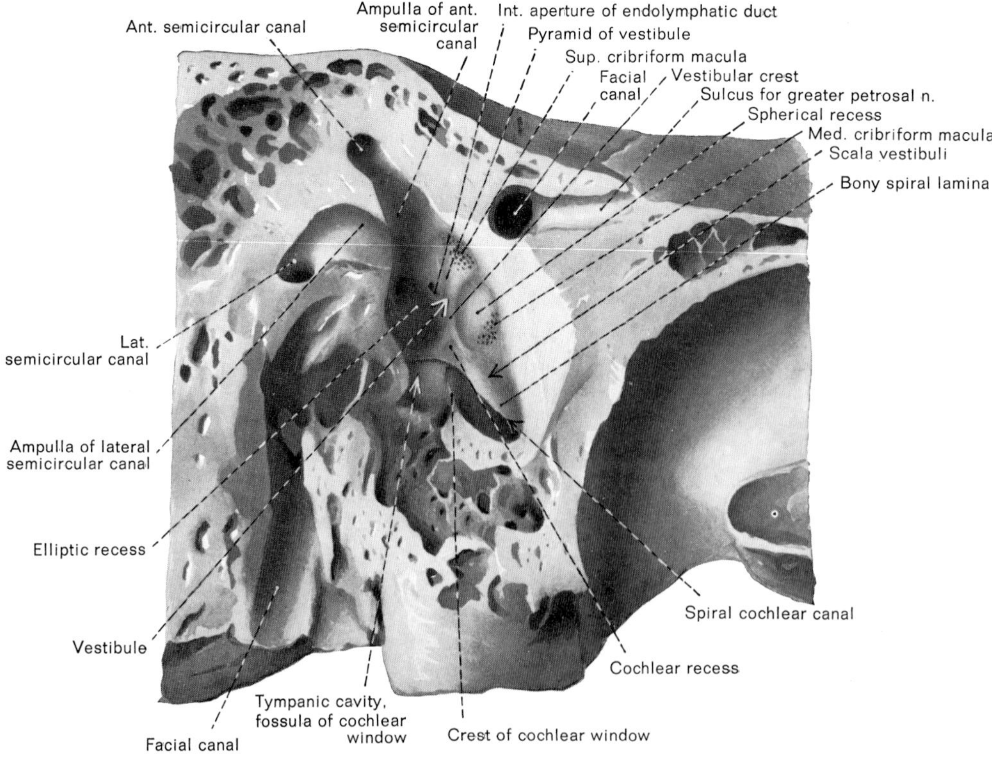
Ampulla of ant. semicircular canal
Int. aperture of endolymphatic duct
Ant. semicircular canal
Pyramid of vestibule
Sup. cribriform macula
Facial canal
Vestibular crest
Sulcus for greater petrosal n.
Spherical recess
Med. cribriform macula
Scala vestibuli
Bony spiral lamina
Lat. semicircular canal
Ampulla of lateral semicircular canal
Elliptic recess
Vestibule
Spiral cochlear canal
Cochlear recess
Tympanic cavity, fossula of cochlear window
Crest of cochlear window
Facial canal

Fig. 238. Medial wall of right vestibule, exposed by removal of the lateral wall.

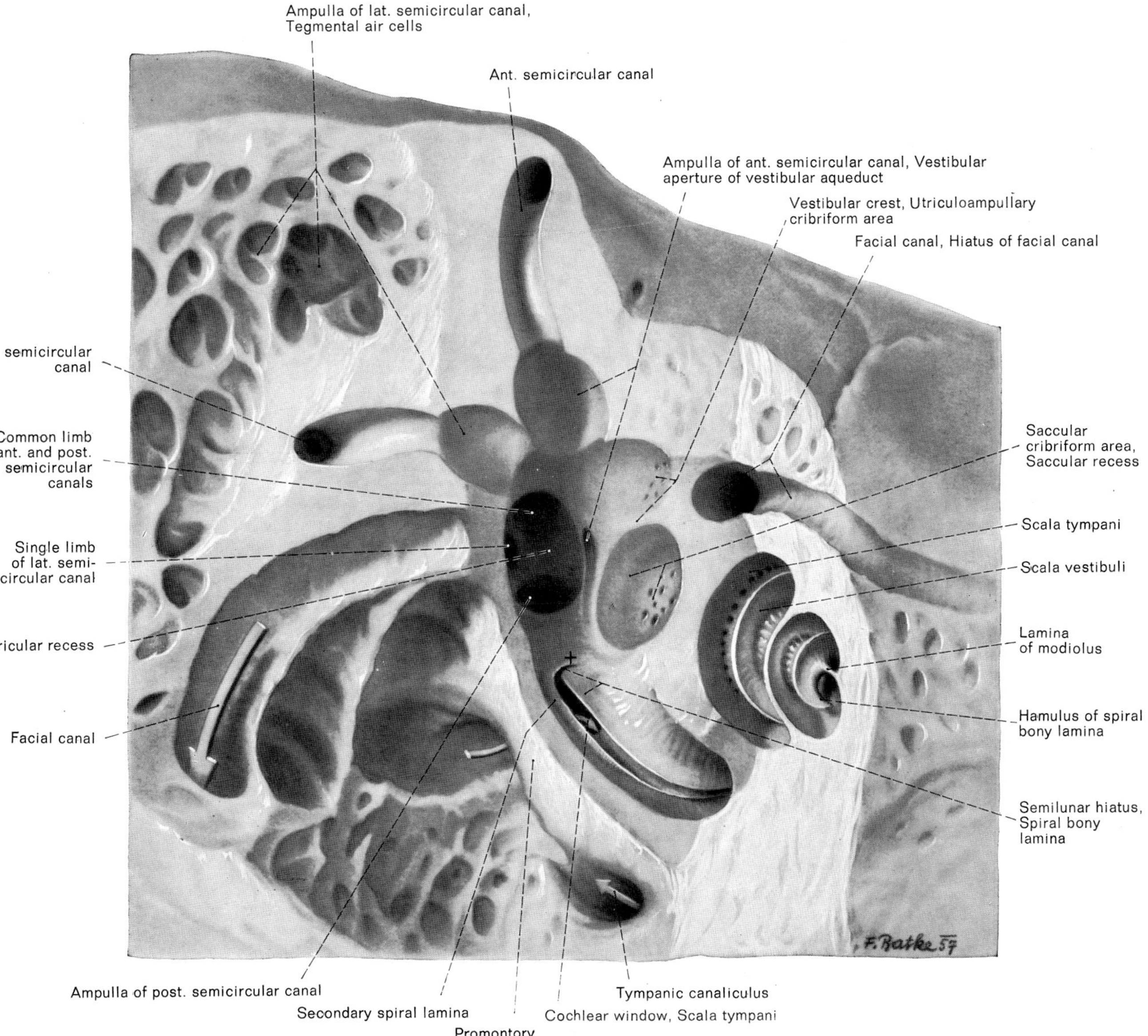
Ampulla of lat. semicircular canal, Tegmental air cells
Ant. semicircular canal
Ampulla of ant. semicircular canal, Vestibular aperture of vestibular aqueduct
Vestibular crest, Utriculoampullary cribriform area
Facial canal, Hiatus of facial canal
semicircular canal
Common limb ant. and post. semicircular canals
Single limb of lat. semicircular canal
ricular recess
Facial canal
Saccular cribriform area, Saccular recess
Scala tympani
Scala vestibuli
Lamina of modiolus
Hamulus of spiral bony lamina
Semilunar hiatus, Spiral bony lamina
F. Batke 57
Ampulla of post. semicircular canal
Secondary spiral lamina
Promontory
Cochlear window, Scala tympani
Tympanic canaliculus

Fig. 239. Stepwise frontal section through the petrous portion of the right temporal bone to illustrate the medial wall of the vestibule. The basal cochlear coil has been opened so that the scala vestibuli faces the viewer (from *Pernkopf/Ferner:* Atlas der topographischen und angewandten Anatomie des Menschen. vol. 1. Urban & Schwarzenberg, München–Berlin 1963).

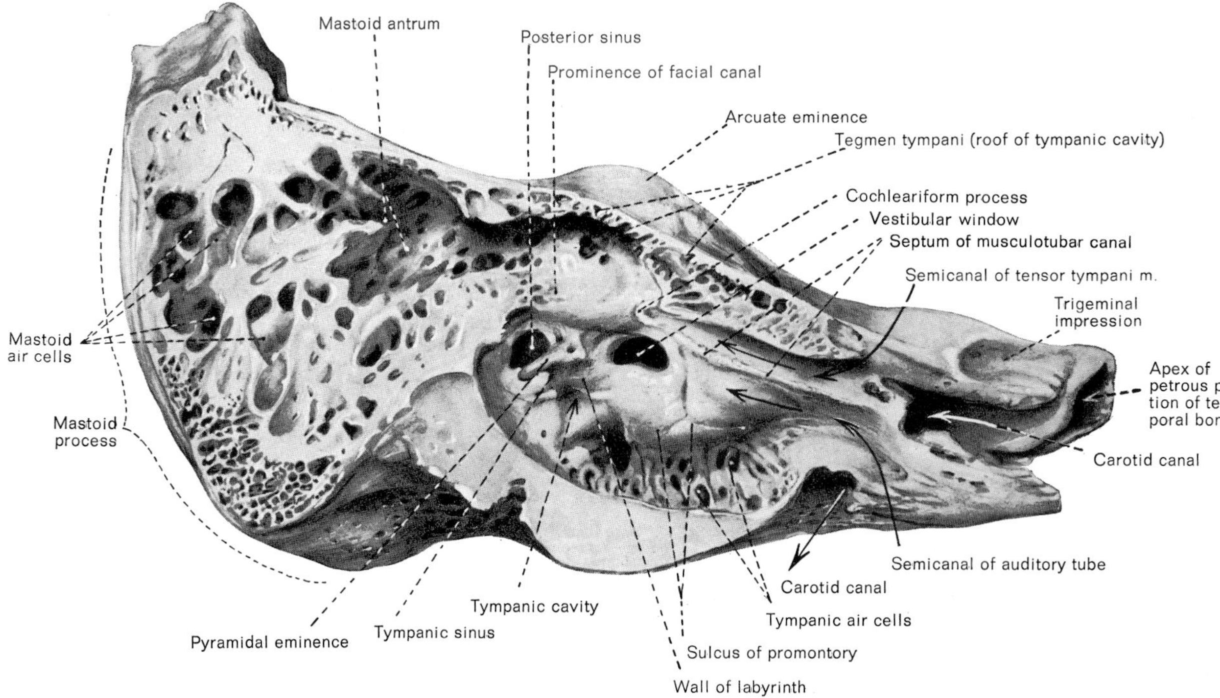
Mastoid antrum
Posterior sinus
Prominence of facial canal
Arcuate eminence
Tegmen tympani (roof of tympanic cavity)
Cochleariform process
Vestibular window
Septum of musculotubar canal
Semicanal of tensor tympani m.
Trigeminal impression
Apex of petrous portion of temporal bone
Carotid canal
Mastoid air cells
Mastoid process
Semicanal of auditory tube
Carotid canal
Tympanic cavity
Tympanic air cells
Pyramidal eminence
Tympanic sinus
Sulcus of promontory
Wall of labyrinth

Fig. 240. Section through the right tympanic cavity and mastoid antrum parallel to the long axis of the petrous portion of the temporal bone.

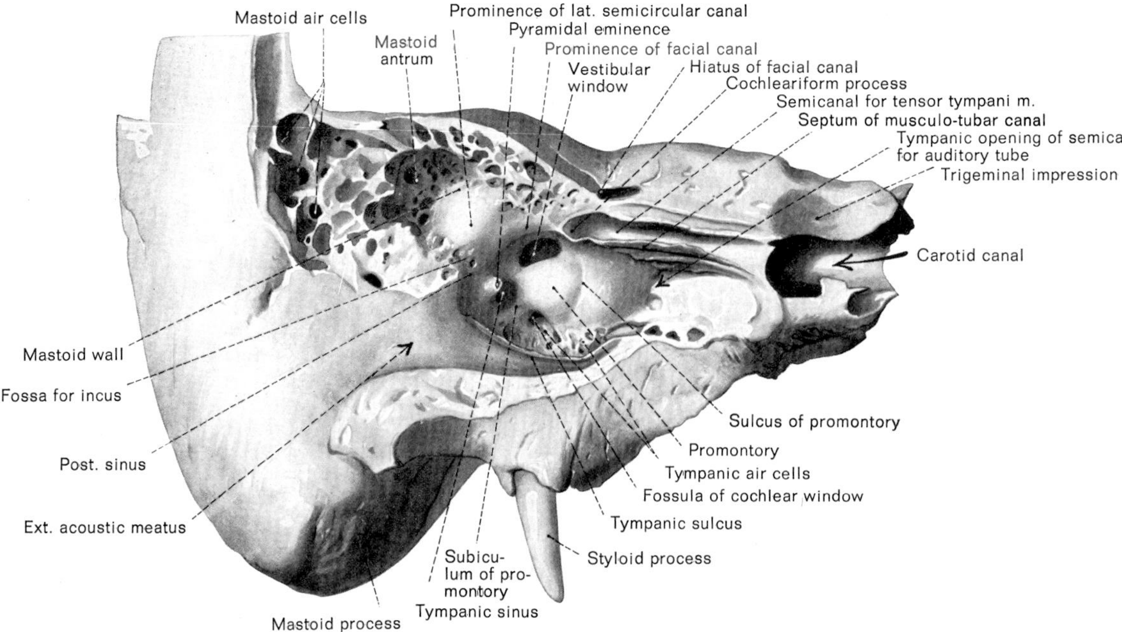
Mastoid air cells
Mastoid antrum
Prominence of lat. semicircular canal
Pyramidal eminence
Prominence of facial canal
Vestibular window
Hiatus of facial canal
Cochleariform process
Semicanal for tensor tympani m.
Septum of musculo-tubar canal
Tympanic opening of semicanal for auditory tube
Trigeminal impression
Carotid canal
Mastoid wall
Fossa for incus
Sulcus of promontory
Promontory
Post. sinus
Tympanic air cells
Fossula of cochlear window
Ext. acoustic meatus
Tympanic sulcus
Subiculum of promontory
Styloid process
Tympanic sinus
Mastoid process

Fig. 241. Right tympanic cavity. Some parts of the lateral, anterior and superior wall have been removed. Fronto-lateral view.

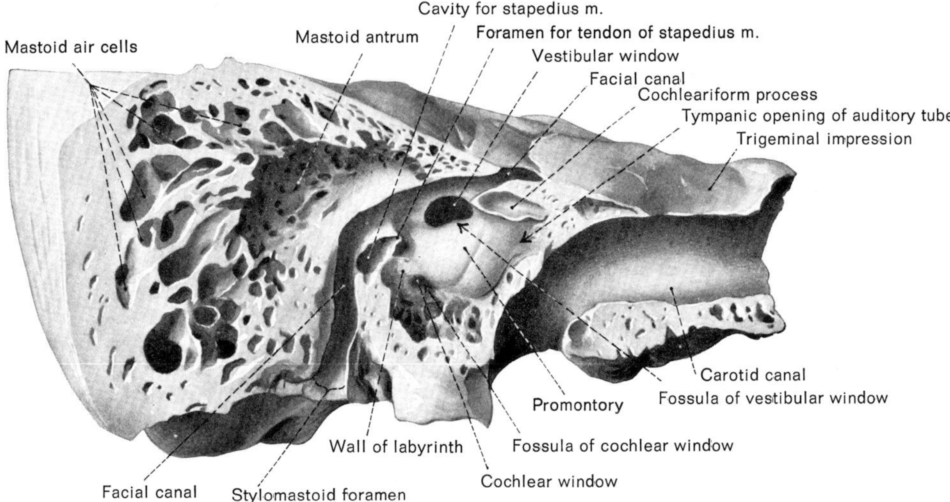
Cavity for stapedius m.
Mastoid antrum
Foramen for tendon of stapedius m.
Mastoid air cells
Vestibular window
Facial canal
Cochleariform process
Tympanic opening of auditory tube
Trigeminal impression
Carotid canal
Promontory
Fossula of vestibular window
Wall of labyrinth
Fossula of cochlear window
Cochlear window
Facial canal
Stylomastoid foramen

Fig. 242. Right tympanic cavity, sectioned more medial than in Fig. 241. The carotid, facial and musculotubar canals as well as the mastoid air cells have been opened, the external acoustic meatus has been completely removed.

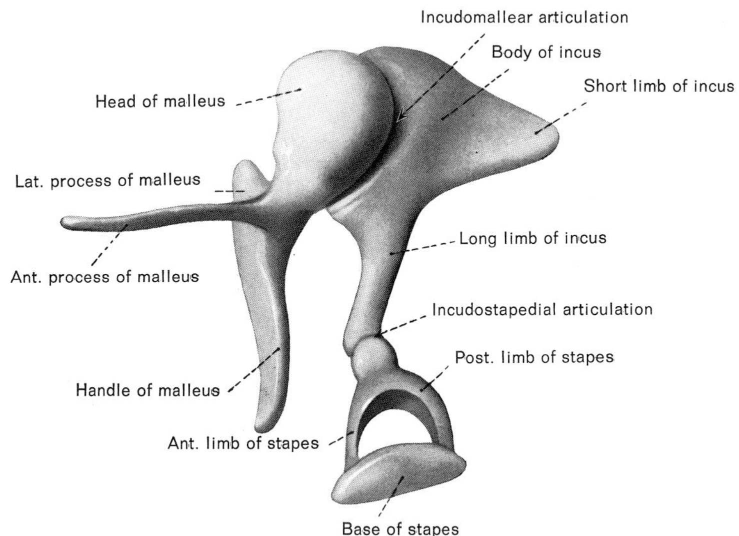
Incudomallear articulation
Body of incus
Head of malleus
Short limb of incus
Lat. process of malleus
Long limb of incus
Ant. process of malleus
Incudostapedial articulation
Post. limb of stapes
Handle of malleus
Ant. limb of stapes
Base of stapes

Fig. 243. The auditory ossicles of the right ear, shown in their natural relationship.

Note: Curtailment of the motility of the middle ear ossicles leads to hearing impairment (hypacusis). In the condition, stapes ankylosis, the motility of the stapedial footplate within the oval window is impaired or completely blocked by newly formed bone (otosclerosis).

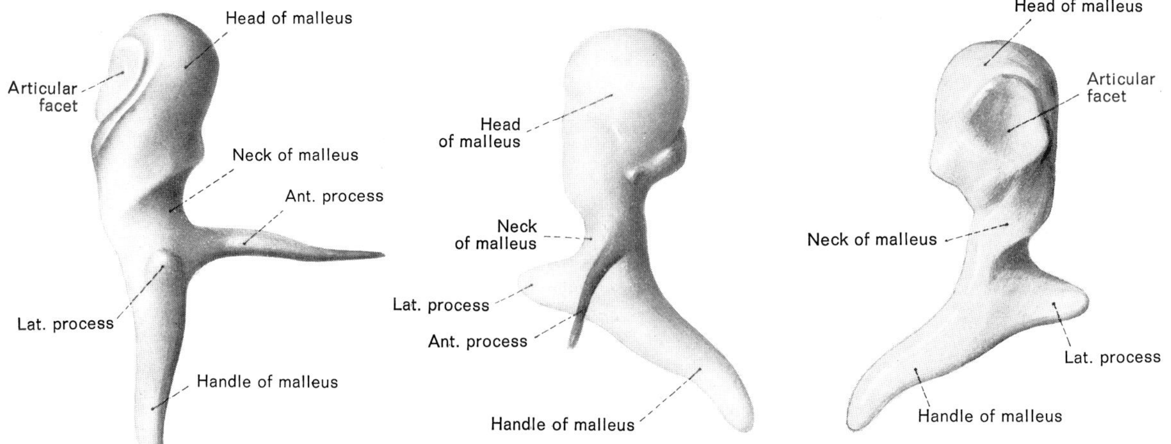
Head of malleus
Articular facet
Neck of malleus
Ant. process
Lat. process
Handle of malleus
Head of malleus
Neck of malleus
Lat. process
Ant. process
Handle of malleus
Head of malleus
Articular facet
Neck of malleus
Lat. process
Handle of malleus

Fig. 244. Right malleus, lateral view. **Fig. 245.** Right malleus, anterior view. **Fig. 246.** Right malleus, dorsal view.

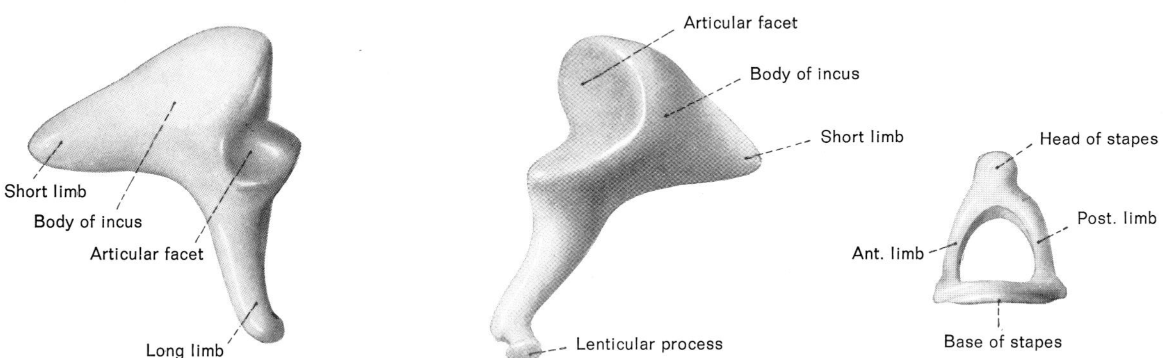
Short limb
Body of incus
Articular facet
Long limb
Articular facet
Body of incus
Short limb
Lenticular process
Head of stapes
Post. limb
Ant. limb
Base of stapes

Fig. 247. Right incus, lateral view. **Fig. 248.** Right incus, medial view. **Fig. 249.** Right stapes, seen from above.

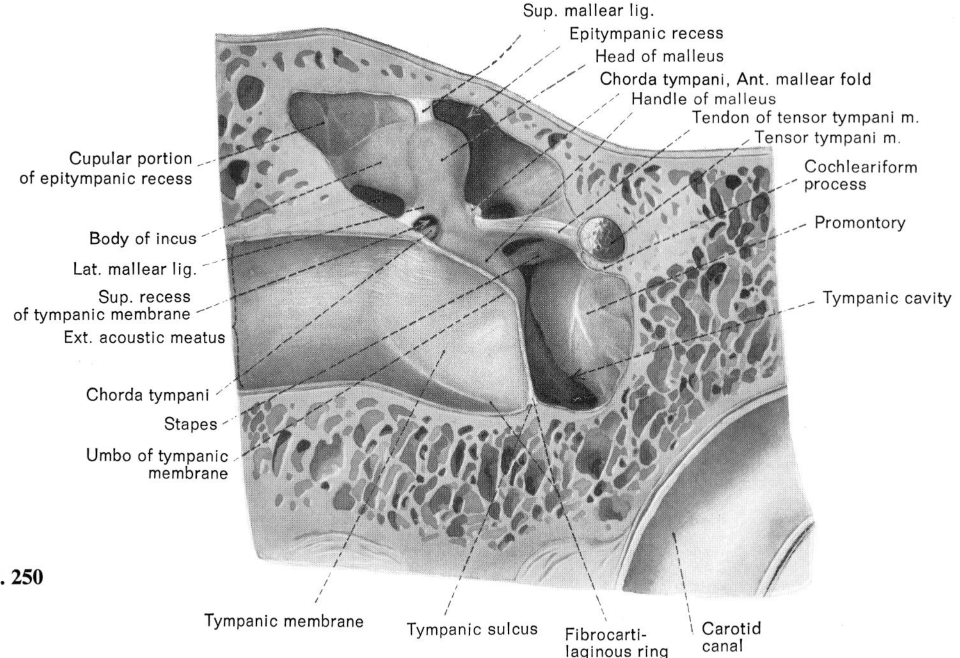
Sup. mallear lig.
Epitympanic recess
Head of malleus
Chorda tympani, Ant. mallear fold
Handle of malleus
Tendon of tensor tympani m.
Tensor tympani m.
Cochleariform process
Promontory
Tympanic cavity
Cupular portion of epitympanic recess
Body of incus
Lat. mallear lig.
Sup. recess of tympanic membrane
Ext. acoustic meatus
Chorda tympani
Stapes
Umbo of tympanic membrane
Tympanic membrane
Tympanic sulcus
Fibrocartilaginous ring
Carotid canal

Fig. 250

The boundaries of the tympanic cavity with reference to their clinical significance
(after O. Groner)

name	constituents	neighboring organs	peculiarities	clinical complications
roof	epitympanic recess, tegmen tympani of temporal bone, petrosquamous suture	middle cranial fossa, meninges, temporal lobe of telencephalon	vascular channels in the roof and suture: route for infections	meningitis, abscess of temporal lobe
floor	floor of tympanic cavity, jugular air cells, styloid prominence	jugular fossa, superior bulb of jugular vein	variable form and size of air cells, bony lamina may be partially absent	septic thrombosis of internal jugular vein → pyemia
medial (labyrinthine) wall	promontory, oval and round window, prominence of facial canal, tympanic nervous plexus	membranous labyrinth, facial nerve		infections of the labyrinth (deafness), facial paresis
lateral (membranous) wall	tympanic membrane, manubrium of malleus, (chorda tympani)	external acoustic meatus		perforation of tympanic membrane
posterior (mastoid) wall	mastoid antrum, mastoid air cells, prominence of lat. semicircular canal, facial canal	facial nerve, sigmoid sinus, posterior cranial fossa, cerebellum	variable pneumatization of the mastoid process	sinus thrombosis, meningitis, cerebellar abscess, facial paresis
anterior (carotid) wall	tympanic opening of auditory tube, musculo-tubular canal	carotid canal, cavernous sinus, abducent nerve, trigeminal ganglion	apical pneumatization of the pyramid	auditory tube as route for infections, infection of apical air cells, abducent paresis

Fig. 250. Frontal section through right external auditory meatus, tympanic membrane and tympanic cavity. Note the narrowest area of the tympanic cavity between the promontory and the umbo of the tympanic membrane. The epitympanic cupular recess is the highest point of the tympanic cavity. The surgical access to the upper tympanic cavity is through that portion of the temporal squama that reaches as "mur de la loguette" to the flaccid portion of the tympanic membrane.

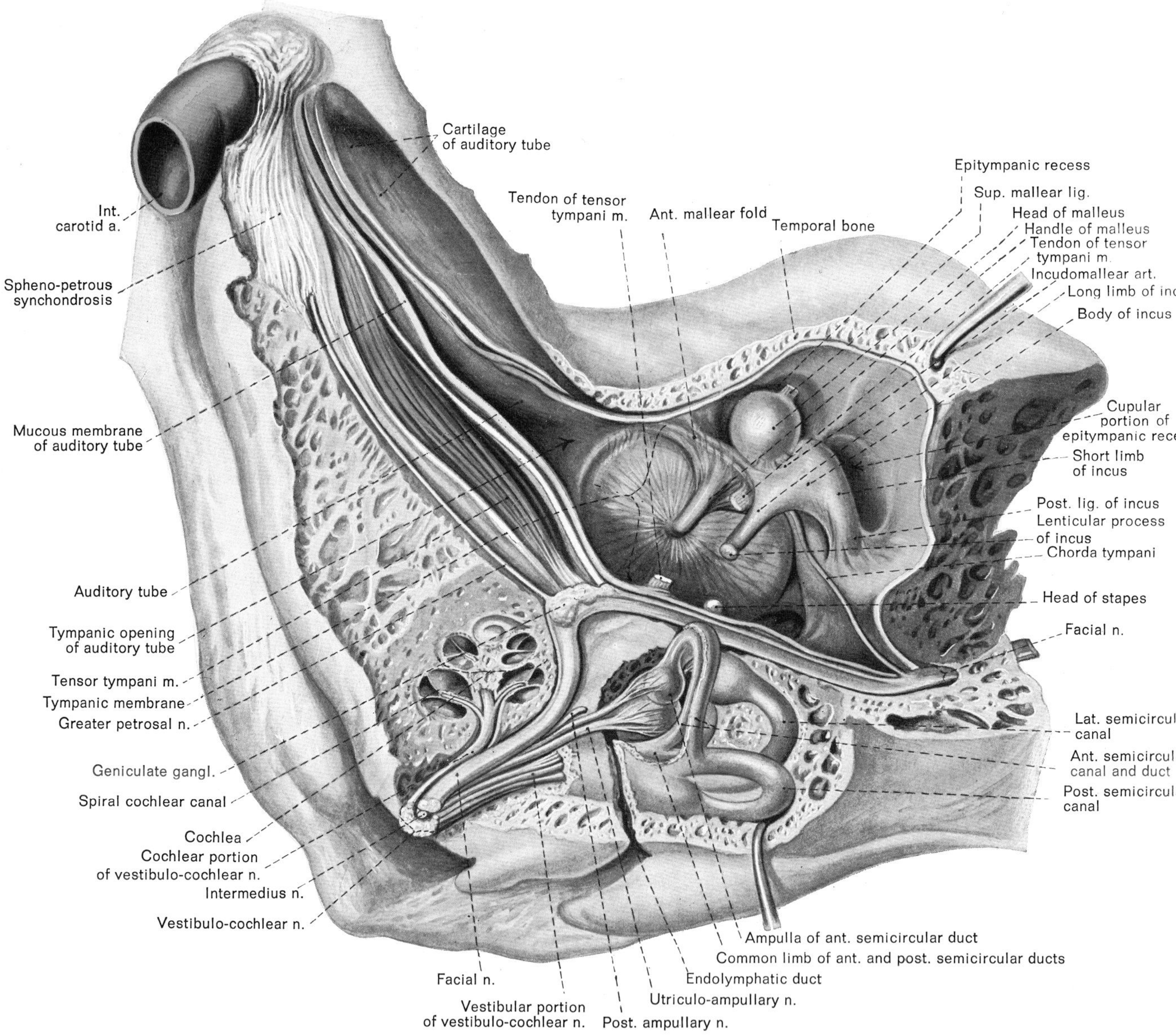
Cartilage
of auditory tube
Int.
carotid a.
Spheno-petrous
synchondrosis
Mucous membrane
of auditory tube
Tendon of tensor
tympani m.
Ant. mallear fold
Temporal bone
Epitympanic recess
Sup. mallear lig.
Head of malleus
Handle of malleus
Tendon of tensor
tympani m.
Incudomallear art.
Body of incus
Cupular
portion of
Short limb
of incus
Post. lig. of incus
Lenticular process
of incus
Chorda tympani
Head of stapes
Facial n.
Auditory tube
Tympanic opening
of auditory tube
Tensor tympani m.
Tympanic membrane
Greater petrosal n.
Geniculate gangl.
Spiral cochlear canal
Cochlea
Cochlear portion
of vestibulo-cochlear n.
Intermedius n.
Vestibulo-cochlear n.
Ampulla of ant. semicircular duct
Common limb of ant. and post. semicircular ducts
Endolymphatic duct
Utriculo-ampullary n.
Post. ampullary n.
Facial n.
Vestibular portion
of vestibulo-cochlear n.

Fig. 251. Right middle and inner ear, survey preparation of a decalcified temporal bone. The tendon of the tensor tympani muscle has been cut and the joint between stapes and incus has been divided. Both halves of the preparation have been bent and pulled up and down in the arc of the section through the tympanic cavity. Note the course of the facial and vestibulo-cochlear nerves as well as the relationship of the labyrinth to the tympanic cavity and its walls (compare with table on page 177).

Fig. 252. Lateral wall of right tympanic cavity, medial view. Sectional plane approximately parallel to the tympanic membrane. The medial wall of the tympanic cavity, the semicanal for the tensor tympani muscle, the muscle itself and its insertion on the malleus have been removed to demonstrate the relationships between malleus, incus, tympanic membrane, and auditory tube.

Fig. 253. Lateral wall of the right tympanic cavity, medial view. Dissection is similar to that illustrated in Fig. 252, but the bone has been sectioned so that the chorda tympani and the tympanic opening of the canaliculus for the chorda tympani as well as a portion of the facial nerve are exposed. The carotid canal has been opened. The tendon of the tensor tympani muscle has been divided, its insertion on the malleus has been retained. In both figures 252 and 253 the mucous membrane of the tympanic cavity is shown in pink, the bone in yellow.

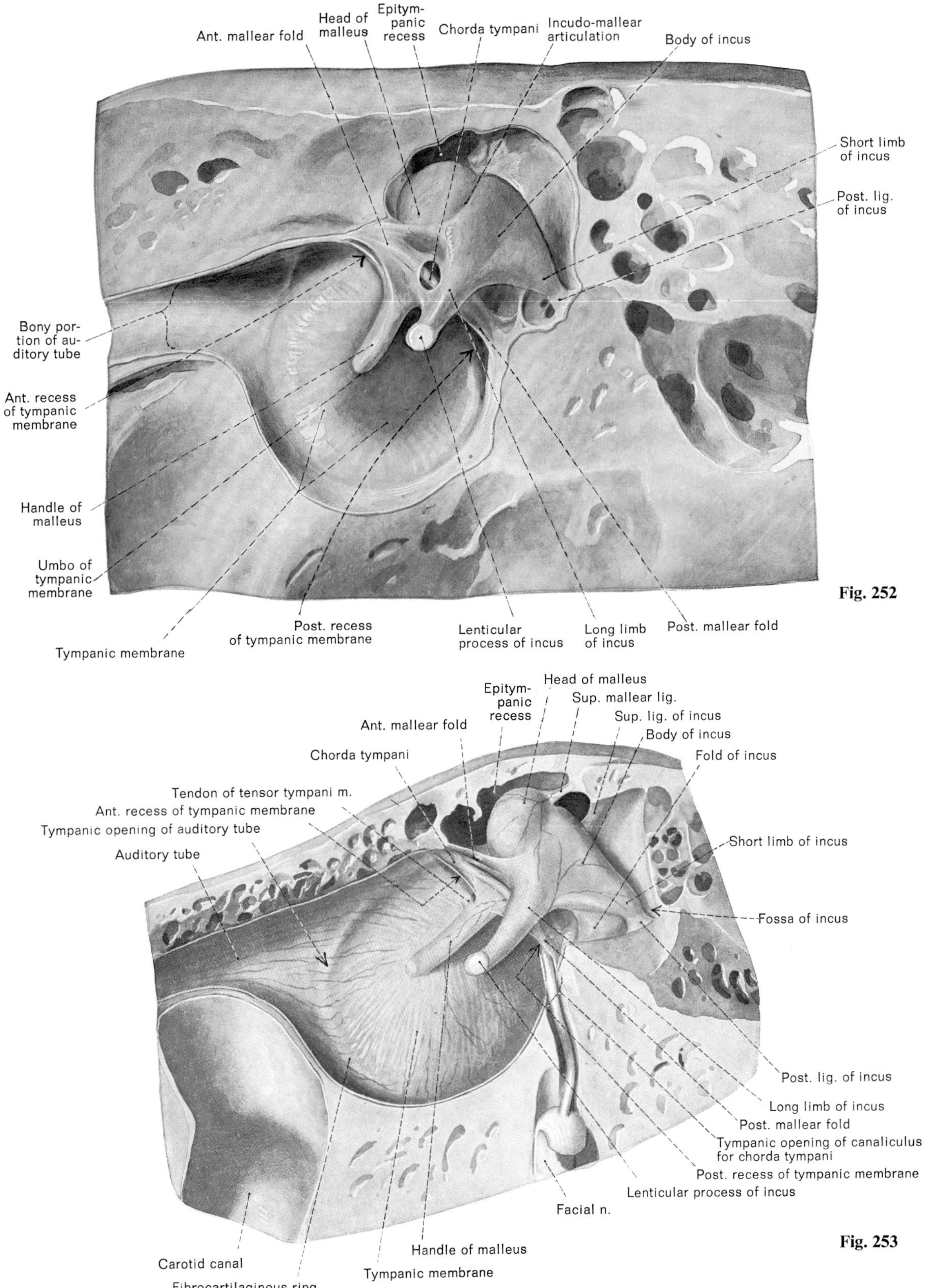

Ant. mallear fold
Head of malleus
Epitympanic recess
Chorda tympani
Incudo-mallear articulation
Body of incus
Short limb of incus
Post. lig. of incus
Bony portion of auditory tube
Ant. recess of tympanic membrane
Handle of malleus
Umbo of tympanic membrane
Tympanic membrane
Post. recess of tympanic membrane
Lenticular process of incus
Long limb of incus
Post. mallear fold
Head of malleus
Epitympanic recess
Sup. mallear lig.
Sup. lig. of incus
Ant. mallear fold
Body of incus
Chorda tympani
Fold of incus
Tendon of tensor tympani m.
Ant. recess of tympanic membrane
Tympanic opening of auditory tube
Auditory tube
Short limb of incus
Fossa of incus
Post. lig. of incus
Long limb of incus
Post. mallear fold
Tympanic opening of canaliculus for chorda tympani
Post. recess of tympanic membrane
Lenticular process of incus
Facial n.
Handle of malleus
Carotid canal
Tympanic membrane
Fibrocartilaginous ring

Fig. 252

Fig. 253

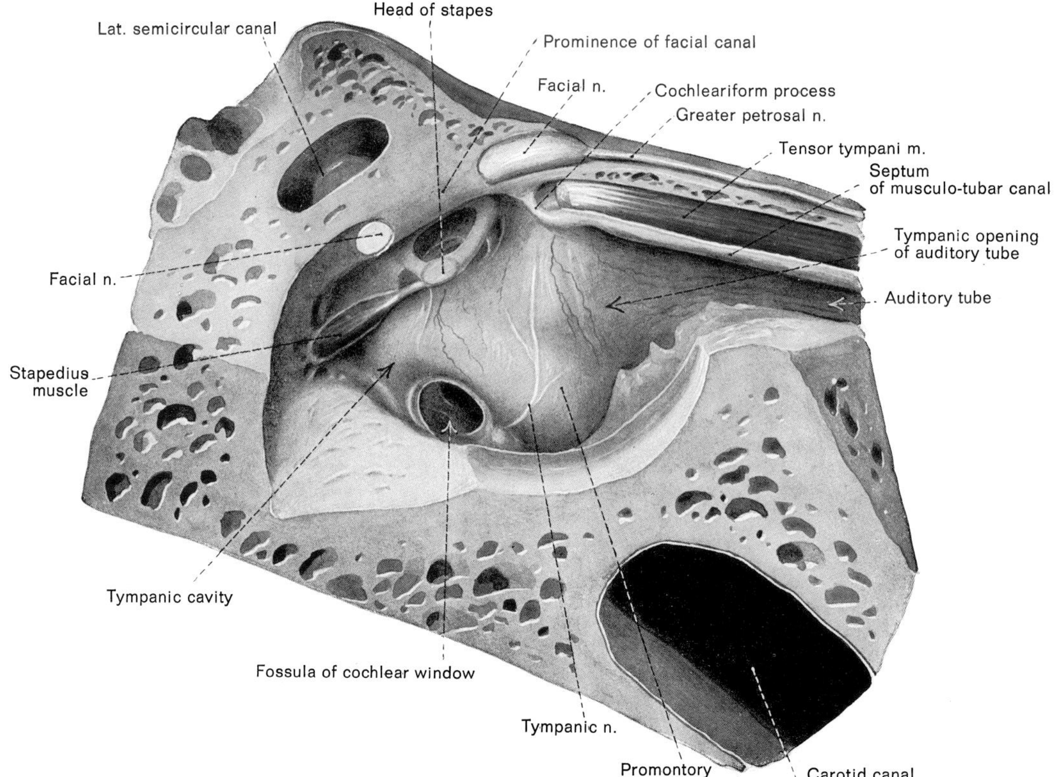
Head of stapes
Lat. semicircular canal
Prominence of facial canal
Facial n.
Cochleariform process
Greater petrosal n.
Tensor tympani m.
Septum of musculo-tubar canal
Tympanic opening of auditory tube
Auditory tube
Facial n.
Stapedius muscle
Tympanic cavity
Fossula of cochlear window
Tympanic n.
Promontory
Carotid canal

Fig. 254. Medial (labyrinthine) wall of the right tympanic cavity, lateral view. The posterior wall of the tympanic cavity has been partially removed, the stapedius muscle has been partially exposed by removal of the bony wall of the pyramidal eminence. The lower portion of the facial canal has been removed; the lateral semicircular canal and the carotid canal have been opened. Compare with Fig. 256.

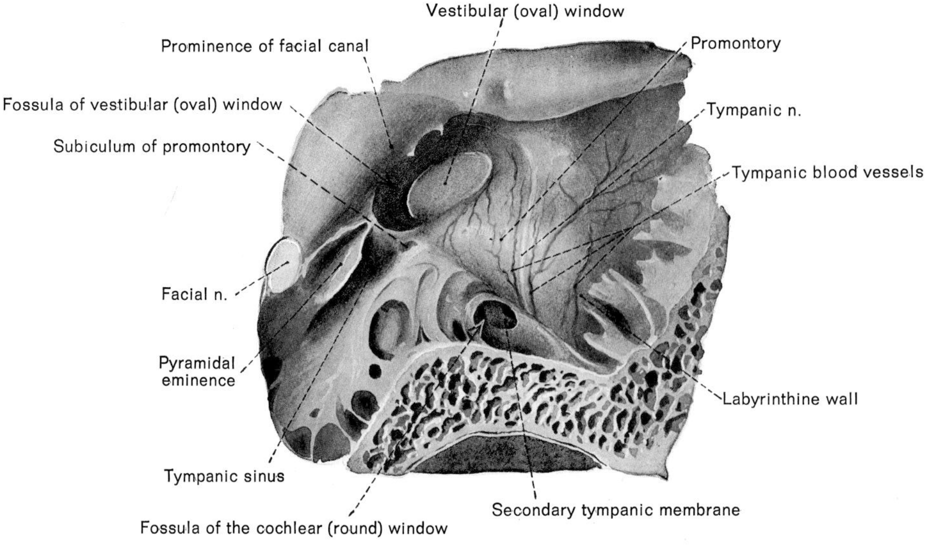
Vestibular (oval) window
Prominence of facial canal
Promontory
Fossula of vestibular (oval) window
Tympanic n.
Subiculum of promontory
Tympanic blood vessels
Facial n.
Pyramidal eminence
Labyrinthine wall
Tympanic sinus
Secondary tympanic membrane
Fossula of the cochlear (round) window

Fig. 255. Vestibular (oval) and cochlear (round) window seen from the right tympanic cavity. The pyramidal eminence has been opened, stapedius muscle and stapes have been removed. The bone has been dissected away so as to expose the round window with the secondary tympanic membrane and the adjacent mucosal folds. Blood vessels and tympanic nerve are seen through the mucosa of the promontory.

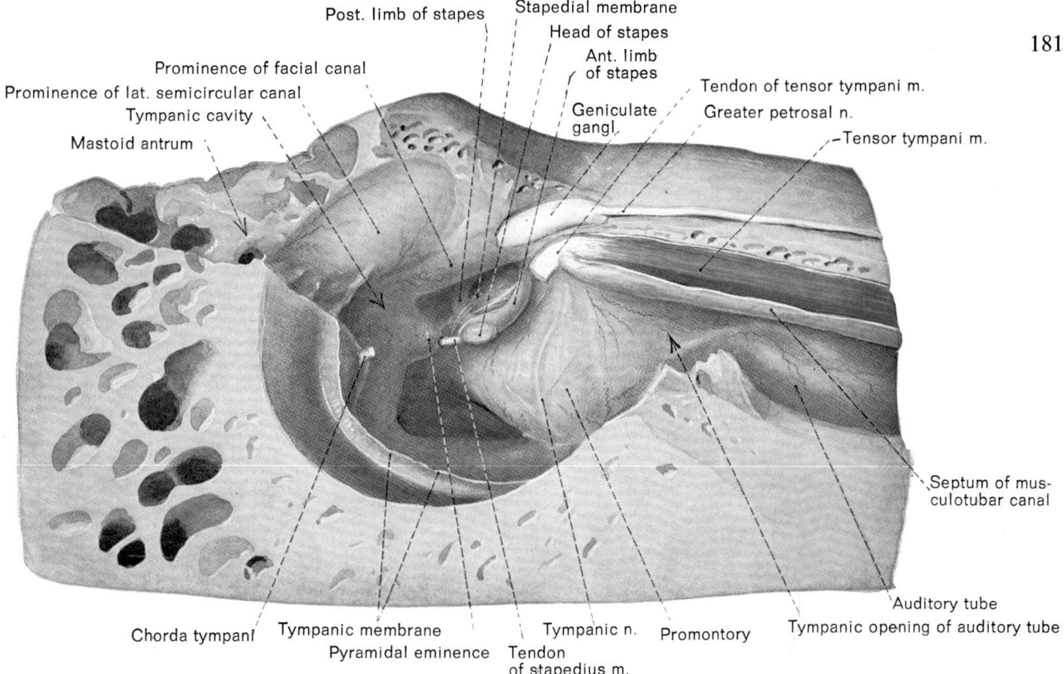
Post. limb of stapes
Stapedial membrane
Head of stapes
Ant. limb of stapes
Prominence of facial canal
Prominence of lat. semicircular canal
Tympanic cavity
Mastoid antrum
Geniculate gangl.
Tendon of tensor tympani m.
Greater petrosal n.
Tensor tympani m.
Septum of musculotubar canal
Auditory tube
Chorda tympani
Tympanic membrane
Pyramidal eminence
Tympanic n.
Tendon of stapedius m.
Promontory
Tympanic opening of auditory tube

Fig. 256. Medial (labyrinthine) wall of right tympanic cavity, lateral view. Preparation similar to the one in Fig. 254. The lateral and superior wall of the tympanic cavity, malleus and incus as well as the major portion of the external auditory meatus have been removed. A small rim of tympanic membrane has been retained. The chorda tympani has been severed where it enters the tympanic cavity through the tympanic orifice of its canaliculus. The septum of the musculotubar canal has been partially cut off in order to expose the tensor tympani muscle, the tendon of which is sectioned close to the cochleariform process. The facial nerve has been exposed for a short distance near the geniculate ganglion, and the greater petrosal nerve was dissected where it emerges from the hiatus of the facial canal and enters the middle cranial fossa.

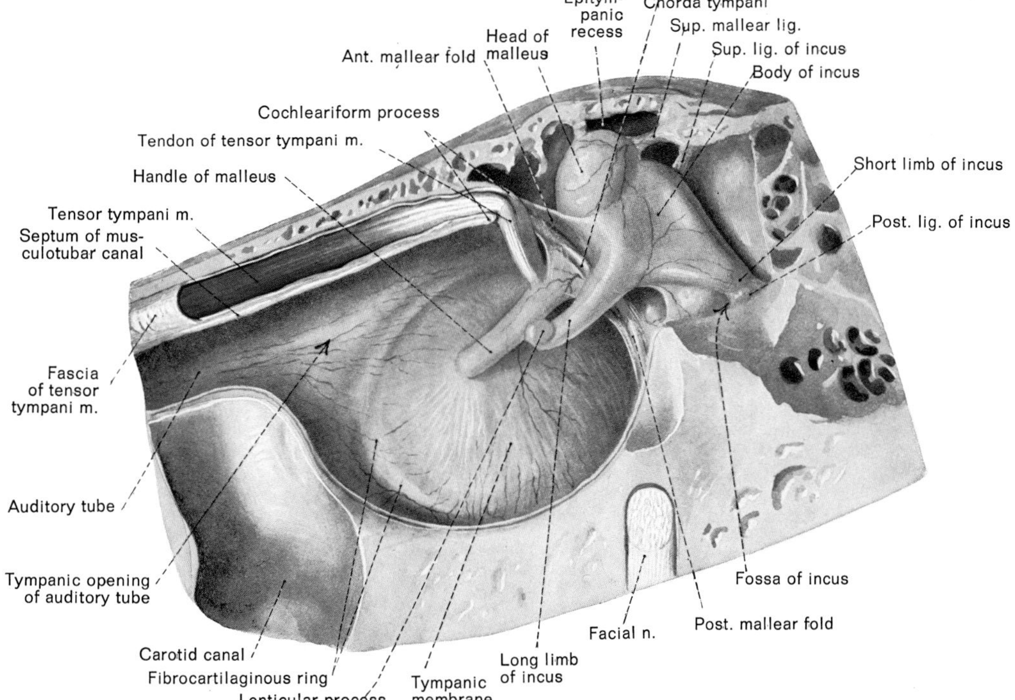
Epitympanic recess
Chorda tympani
Sup. mallear lig.
Sup. lig. of incus
Body of incus
Head of malleus
Ant. mallear fold
Cochleariform process
Tendon of tensor tympani m.
Handle of malleus
Tensor tympani m.
Septum of musculotubar canal
Short limb of incus
Post. lig. of incus
Fascia of tensor tympani m.
Auditory tube
Tympanic opening of auditory tube
Fossa of incus
Post. mallear fold
Facial n.
Carotid canal
Fibrocartilaginous ring
Lenticular process
Tympanic membrane
Long limb of incus

Fig. 257. Lateral (membranous) wall of the right tympanic cavity, medial view. The tensor tympani muscle is made visible by removal of the major portion of the septum of the musculotubar canal up to the cochleariform process. Note the insertion of the tendon of the muscle on the handle of the malleus and its course within a mucosal fold. The dense fascia surrounding the muscle has been partially retained. Compare with Fig. 260.

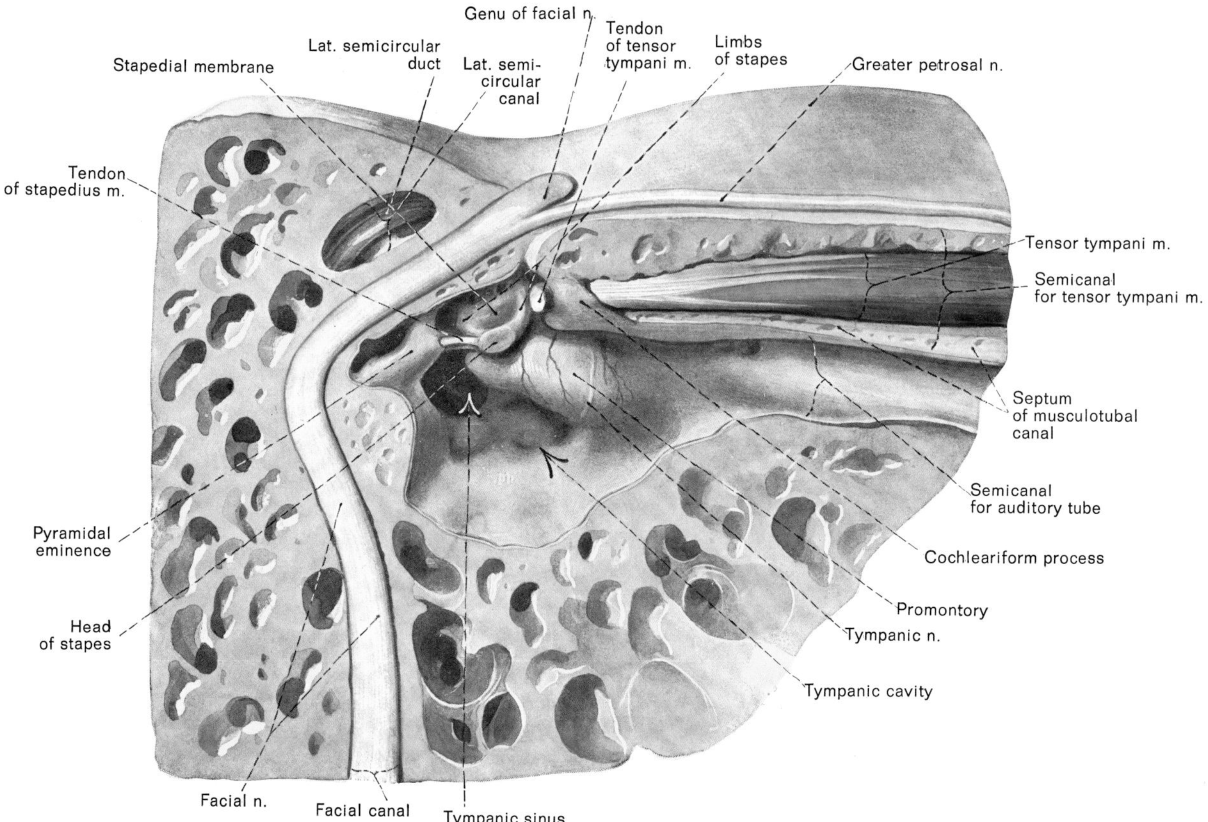
Genu of facial n.
Tendon of tensor tympani m.
Limbs of stapes
Lat. semicircular duct
Lat. semicircular canal
Stapedial membrane
Greater petrosal n.
Tendon of stapedius m.
Tensor tympani m.
Semicanal for tensor tympani m.
Septum of musculotubal canal
Semicanal for auditory tube
Cochleariform process
Pyramidal eminence
Promontory
Head of stapes
Tympanic n.
Tympanic cavity
Facial n.
Facial canal
Tympanic sinus

Fig. 258. Medial (labyrinthine) wall of the right tympanic cavity with stapes, lateral view. The facial canal has been opened from its hiatus to near the stylomastoid foramen in order to expose the facial nerve. The tympanic cavity has been divided by a section approximately parallel to the long axis of the petrous bone; the lateral wall including tympanic membrane, malleus and incus have been removed. The tendon of the tensor tympani muscle has been cut off near the cochleariform process; the musculotubar canal has been opened.

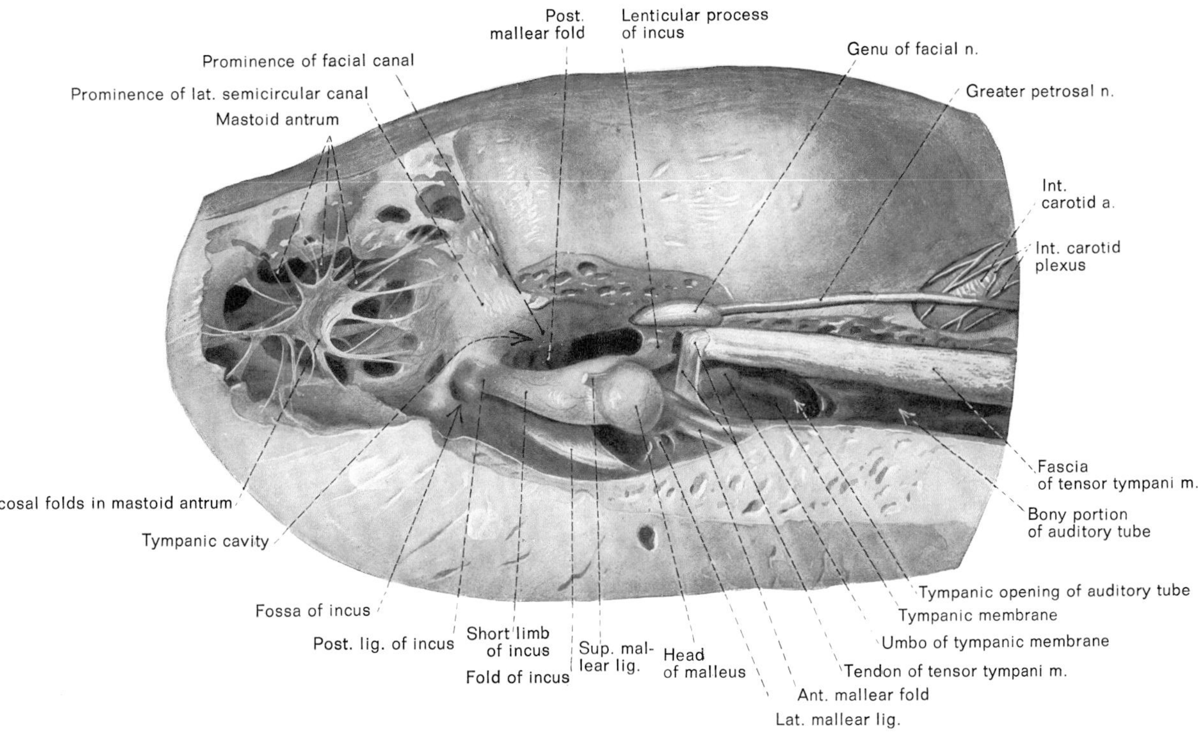
Post. mallear fold
Lenticular process of incus
Prominence of facial canal
Genu of facial n.
Prominence of lat. semicircular canal
Greater petrosal n.
Mastoid antrum
Int. carotid a.
Int. carotid plexus
Fascia of tensor tympani m.
ucosal folds in mastoid antrum
Bony portion of auditory tube
Tympanic cavity
Tympanic opening of auditory tube
Fossa of incus
Tympanic membrane
Post. lig. of incus
Short limb of incus
Sup. mal-lear lig.
Head of malleus
Umbo of tympanic membrane
Fold of incus
Tendon of tensor tympani m.
Ant. mallear fold
Lat. mallear lig.

Fig. 259. Right tympanic cavity opened from above. The roof (tegmen tympani), the upper wall of the musculotubal canal and the mastoid antrum have been removed. The facial nerve is exposed at its genu.

Note: There are three stories in the tympanic cavity.

Upper story: epitympanic recess with mastoid antrum extending to the neck of the malleus and the anterior and posterior mallear folds.

Middle story: area of the tympanic membrane and the tympanic opening of the auditory tube.

Lower story: hypotympanic recess extending to the jugular wall (floor) of the tympanic cavity.

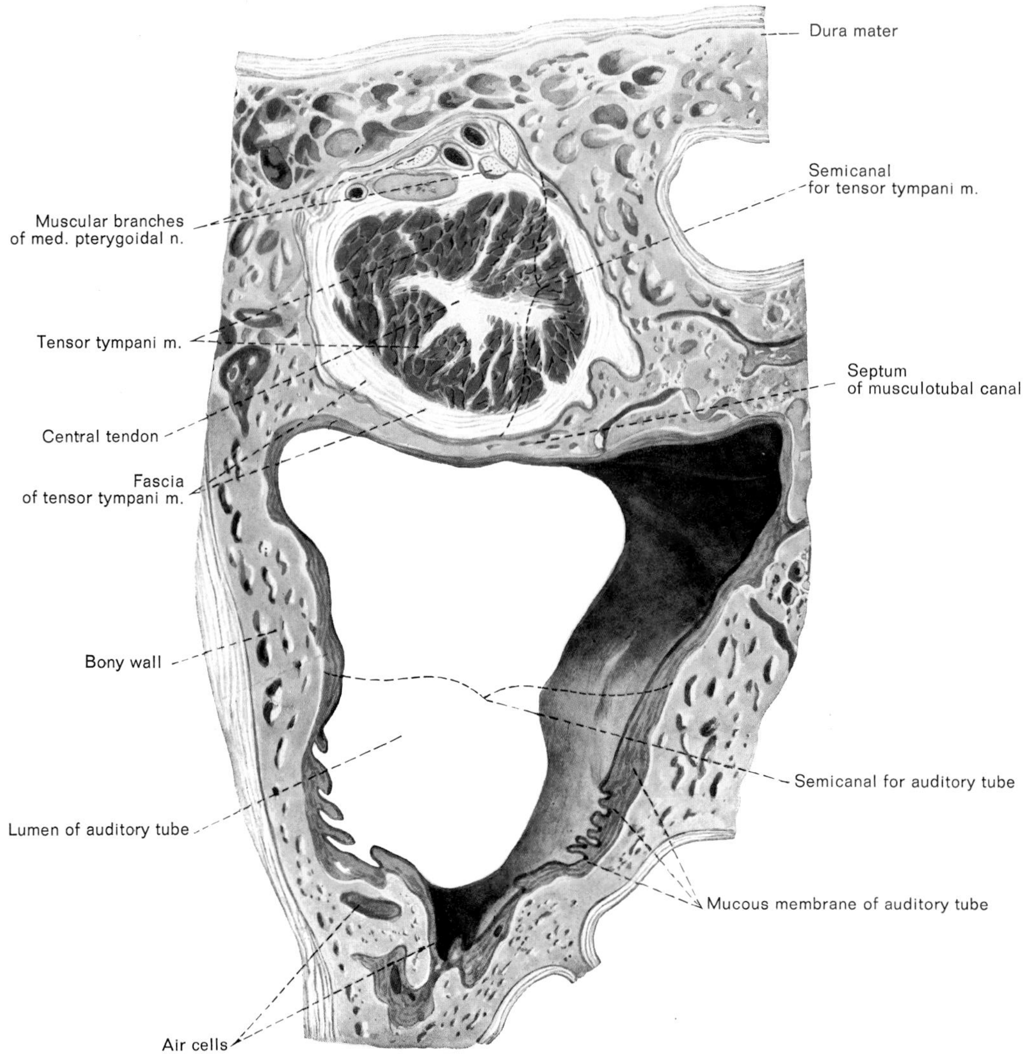
Dura mater
Muscular branches of med. pterygoidal n.
Semicanal for tensor tympani m.
Tensor tympani m.
Septum of musculotubal canal
Central tendon
Fascia of tensor tympani m.
Bony wall
Semicanal for auditory tube
Lumen of auditory tube
Mucous membrane of auditory tube
Air cells

Fig. 260. Cross section through musculotubar canal showing tensor tympani muscle and bony portion of auditory tube. Magnification 20×.

Fig. 261. Cartilage of right auditory tube in normal position at the cranial base.
Fig. 262. Cross section through the cartilaginous portion of the left auditory tube in the region of the isthmus (border between osseous and cartilaginous portion).
Fig. 263. Cross section through the cartilaginous portion of the left auditory tube near the pharyngeal opening.

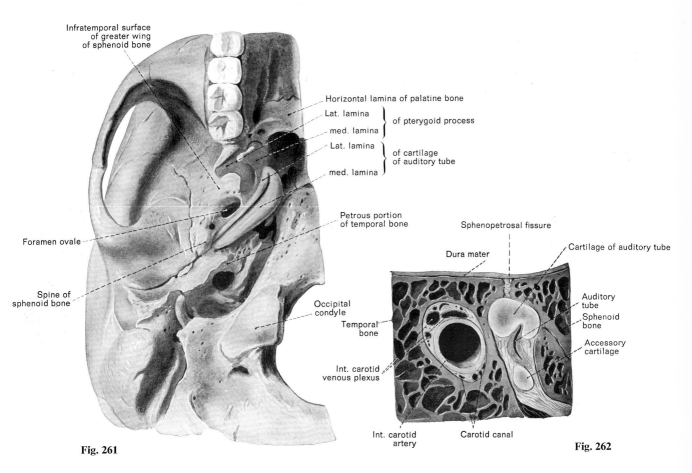

Infratemporal surface of greater wing of sphenoid bone

Horizontal lamina of palatine bone

Lat. lamina, med. lamina — of pterygoid process

Lat. lamina, med. lamina — of cartilage of auditory tube

Petrous portion of temporal bone

Foramen ovale

Spine of sphenoid bone

Occipital condyle

Fig. 261

Sphenopetrosal fissure

Dura mater

Cartilage of auditory tube

Auditory tube

Sphenoid bone

Accessory cartilage

Temporal bone

Int. carotid venous plexus

Int. carotid artery

Carotid canal

Fig. 262

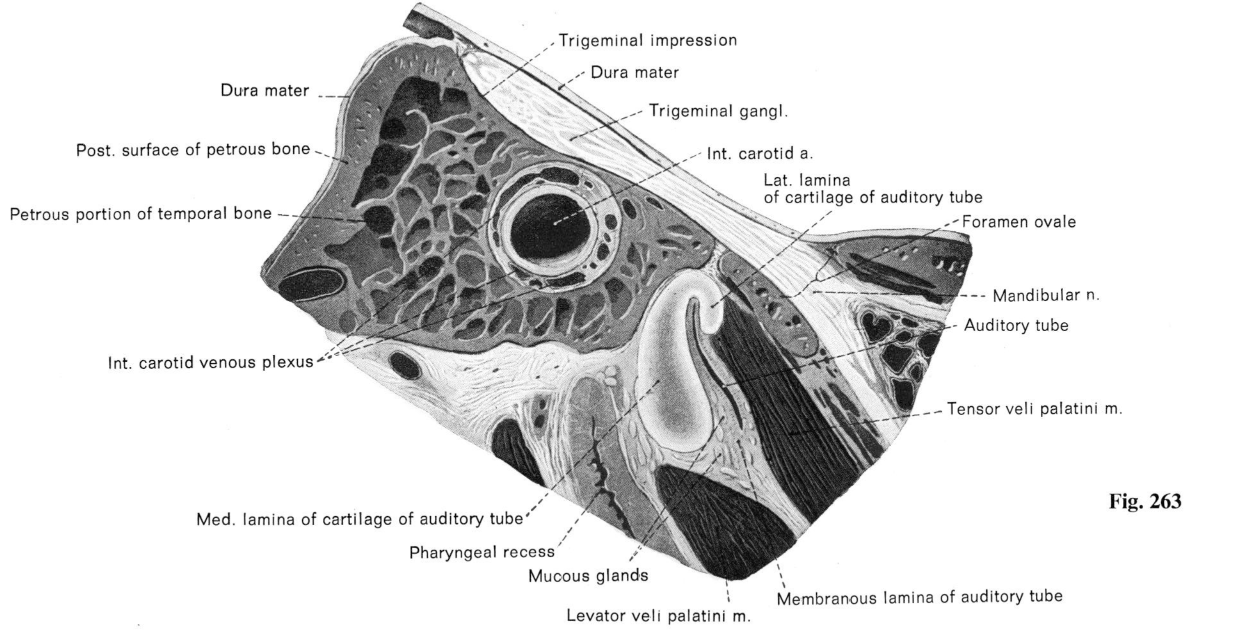

Trigeminal impression
Dura mater
Dura mater
Trigeminal gangl.
Post. surface of petrous bone
Int. carotid a.
Lat. lamina
of cartilage of auditory tube
Petrous portion of temporal bone
Foramen ovale
Mandibular n.
Auditory tube
Int. carotid venous plexus
Tensor veli palatini m.
Med. lamina of cartilage of auditory tube
Pharyngeal recess
Mucous glands
Membranous lamina of auditory tube
Levator veli palatini m.

Fig. 263

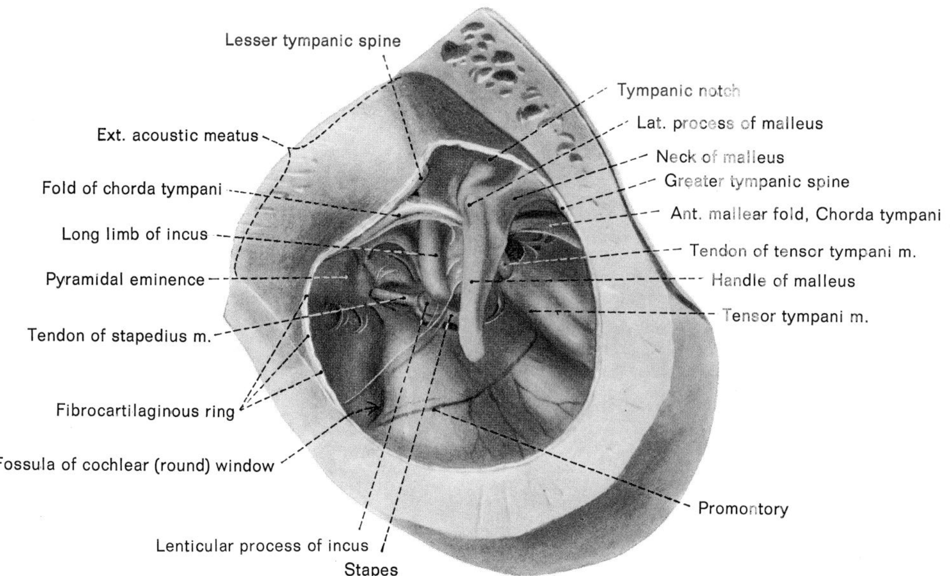
Lesser tympanic spine
Ext. acoustic meatus
Fold of chorda tympani
Long limb of incus
Pyramidal eminence
Tendon of stapedius m.
Fibrocartilaginous ring
Fossula of cochlear (round) window
Lenticular process of incus
Stapes
Tympanic notch
Lat. process of malleus
Neck of malleus
Greater tympanic spine
Ant. mallear fold, Chorda tympani
Tendon of tensor tympani m.
Handle of malleus
Tensor tympani m.
Promontory

Fig. 264. Right tympanic cavity after removal of the tympanic membrane, seen from the external acoustic meatus.

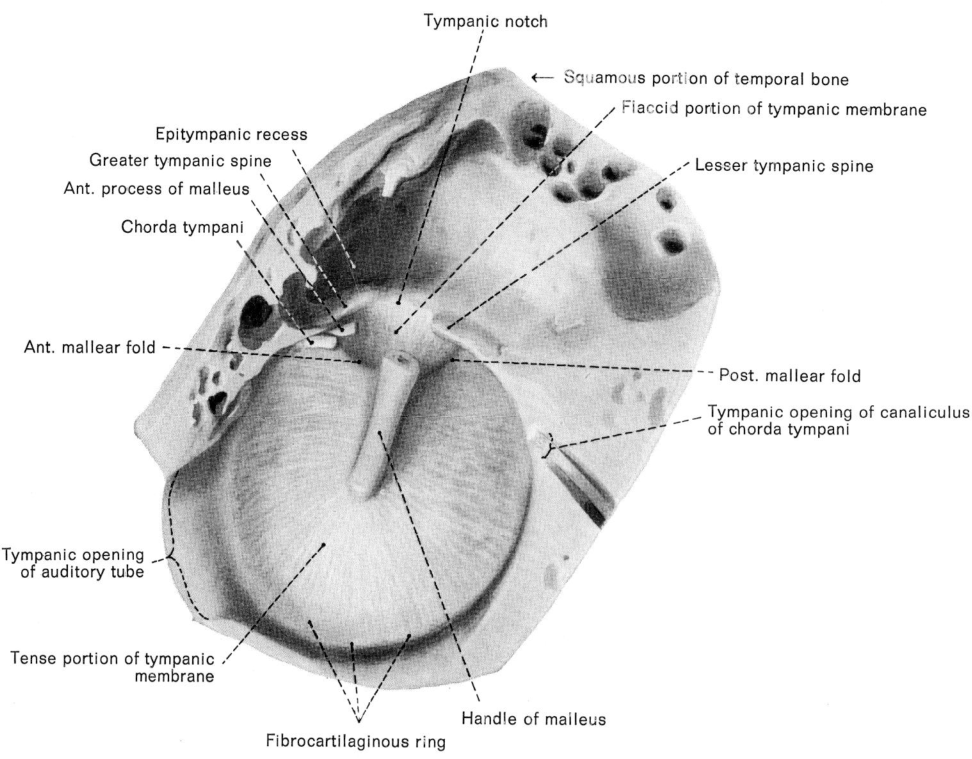
Tympanic notch
Squamous portion of temporal bone
Flaccid portion of tympanic membrane
Epitympanic recess
Greater tympanic spine
Ant. process of malleus
Lesser tympanic spine
Chorda tympani
Ant. mallear fold
Post. mallear fold
Tympanic opening of canaliculus of chorda tympani
Tympanic opening of auditory tube
Tense portion of tympanic membrane
Handle of malleus
Fibrocartilaginous ring

Fig. 265. Lateral (membranous) wall of the tympanic cavity and the tympanic surface of the tympanic membrane, medial view (from the tympanic cavity). The bone has been sectioned parallel to the tympanic membrane. The contents of the tympanic cavity including the mucous membrane have been removed. Only the handle of the malleus has been left in place on the tympanic membrane.

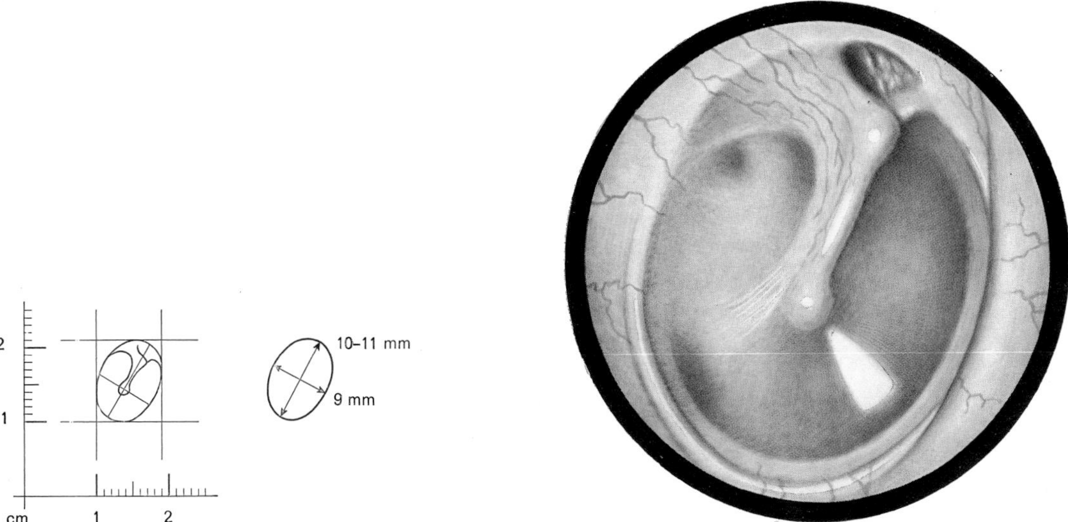
2
1
cm
1
2
10–11 mm
9 mm

Fig. 266. Natural size and orientation of right tympanic membrane.

Fig. 267. Right tympanic membrane as seen through an otoscope in a living person. Magnification about 6×.

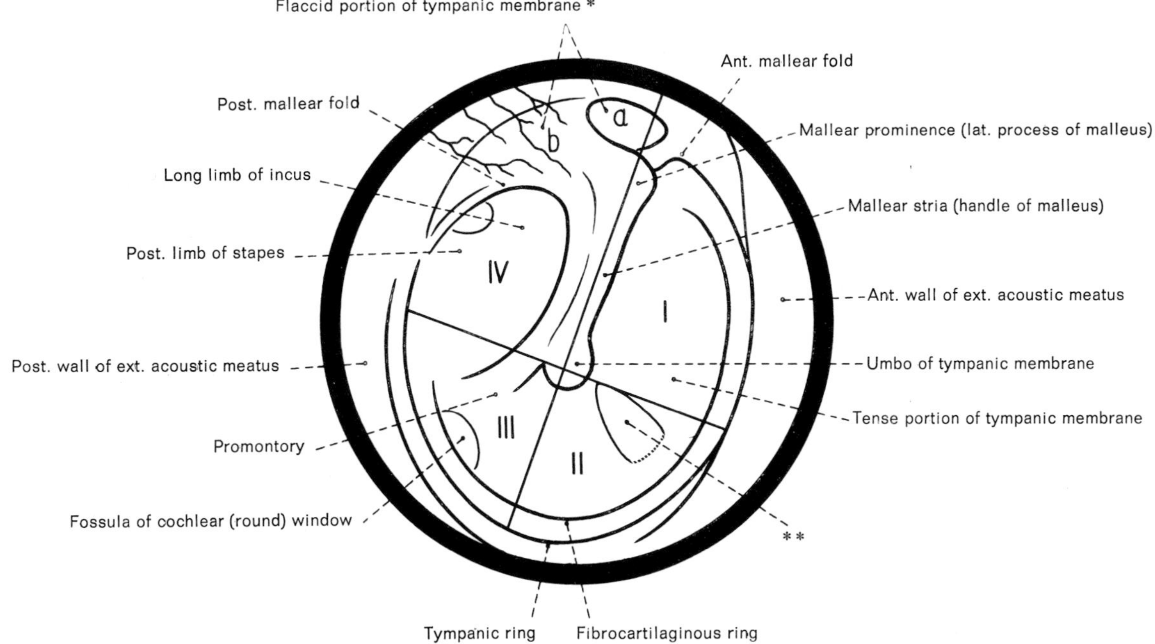
Flaccid portion of tympanic membrane *
Ant. mallear fold
Post. mallear fold
a
b
Mallear prominence (lat. process of malleus)
Long limb of incus
Mallear stria (handle of malleus)
Post. limb of stapes
IV
I
Ant. wall of ext. acoustic meatus
Post. wall of ext. acoustic meatus
Umbo of tympanic membrane
Tense portion of tympanic membrane
III
II
Promontory
Fossula of cochlear (round) window
**
Tympanic ring
Fibrocartilaginous ring

Fig. 268. Labeled line diagram for Figure 267. For practical reasons the surface of the tympanic membrane is subdivided into four quadrants (I–IV). In the otoscopic picture of the normal tympanic membrane a glistening light reflection extends from the umbo toward the second quadrant (**). * = *Shrapnell*'s membrane = flaccid portion of tympanic membrane.

Helix
Spine of helix
Scapha
Squamous portion of temporal bone
Anthelix
Notches of cartilaginous acoustic meatus
Lamina of tragus
Antitrago-helicine fissure
Tympanic portion of temporal bone
Tail of helix
Intertragic notch
Cartilage of ext. acoustic meatus
Styloid process
Mastoid process

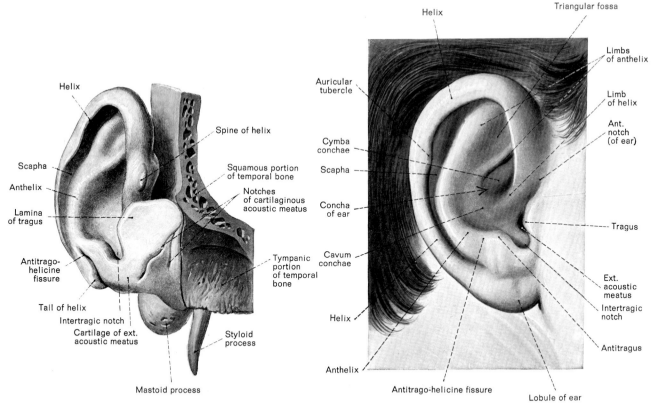

Fig. 269. Cartilage of right external ear, frontal view.

Helix
Triangular fossa
Limbs of anthelix
Auricular tubercle
Limb of helix
Ant. notch (of ear)
Cymba conchae
Scapha
Concha of ear
Tragus
Cavum conchae
Ext. acoustic meatus
Intertragic notch
Helix
Antitragus
Anthelix
Antitrago-helicine fissure
Lobule of ear

Fig. 270. Right external ear, lateral view.

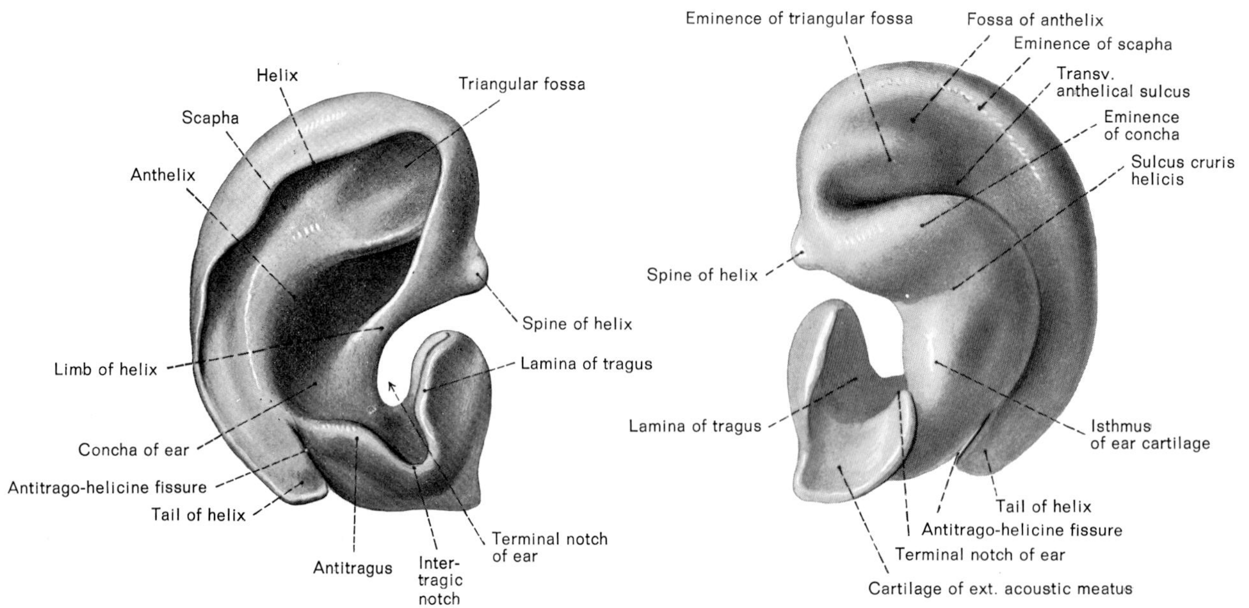
Helix
Triangular fossa
Scapha
Anthelix
Spine of helix
Limb of helix
Lamina of tragus
Concha of ear
Antitrago-helicine fissure
Tail of helix
Terminal notch of ear
Antitragus
Inter-tragic notch
Eminence of triangular fossa
Fossa of anthelix
Eminence of scapha
Transv. anthelical sulcus
Eminence of concha
Sulcus cruris helicis
Spine of helix
Lamina of tragus
Isthmus of ear cartilage
Tail of helix
Antitrago-helicine fissure
Terminal notch of ear
Cartilage of ext. acoustic meatus

Fig. 271. Cartilage of right external ear, lateral view.

Fig. 272. Cartilage of right external ear, medial view.

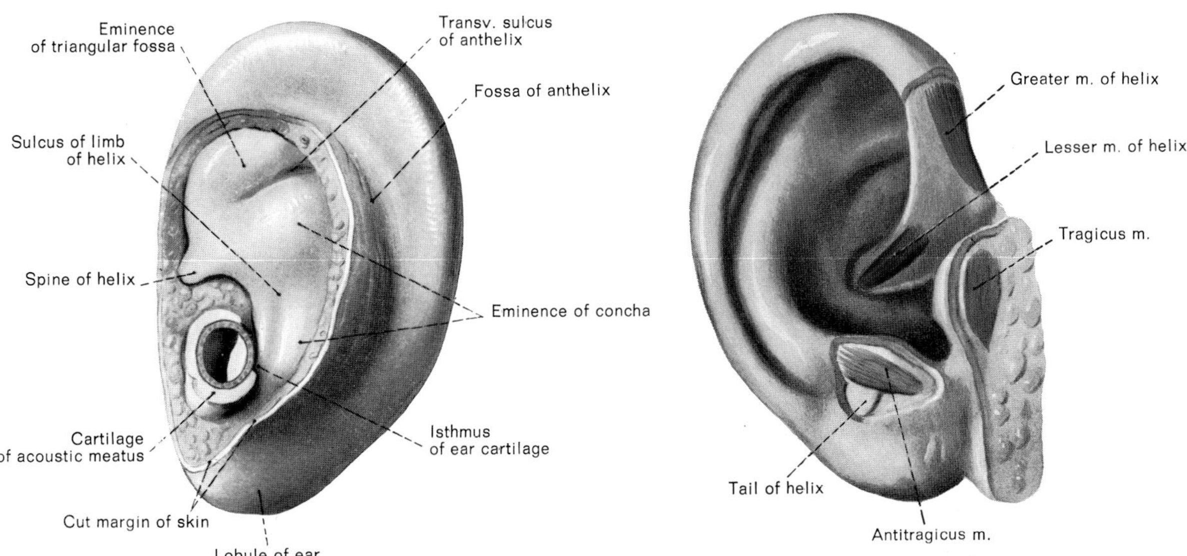
Eminence
of triangular fossa
Transv. sulcus
of anthelix
Fossa of anthelix
Sulcus of limb
of helix
Spine of helix
Eminence of concha
Cartilage
of acoustic meatus
Isthmus
of ear cartilage
Cut margin of skin
Lobule of ear
Greater m. of helix
Lesser m. of helix
Tragicus m.
Tail of helix
Antitragicus m.

Fig. 273. Right external ear, removed from head, medial view.

Fig. 274. Muscles of the lateral surface of the right external ear.

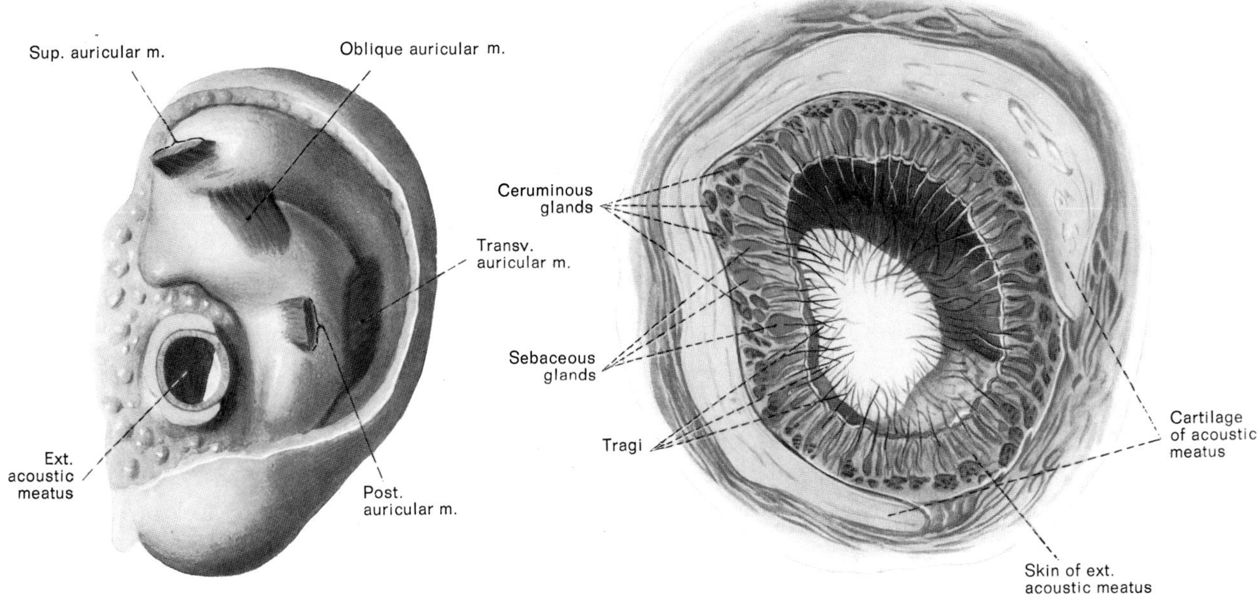
Sup. auricular m.
Oblique auricular m.
Transv.
auricular m.
Ext.
acoustic
meatus
Post.
auricular m.
Ceruminous
glands
Sebaceous
glands
Tragi
Cartilage
of acoustic
meatus
Skin of ext.
acoustic meatus

Fig. 275. Muscles of the medial surface of the right external ear. Ligaments may be present instead of superior and posterior auricular muscles.

Fig. 276. Cross section through cartilaginous portion of external acoustic meatus.

Sense Organs and Skin

Skin and Its Appendages

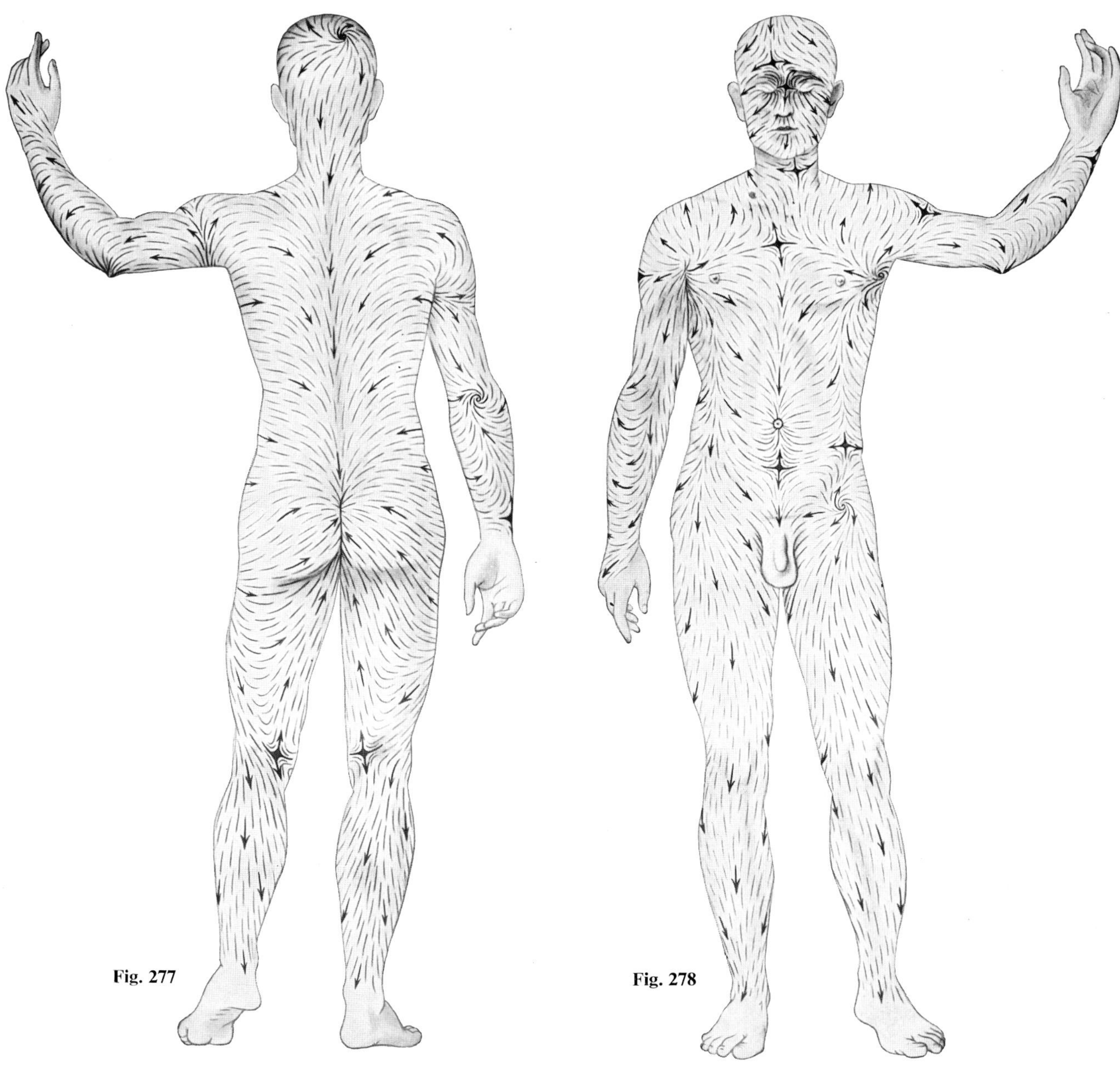

Fig. 277
Fig. 278

Figs. 277 and 278. Diagrams of hair streams and whorls on ventral and dorsal surfaces of the body. Fig. 277 = dorsal view, Fig. 278 = ventral view.

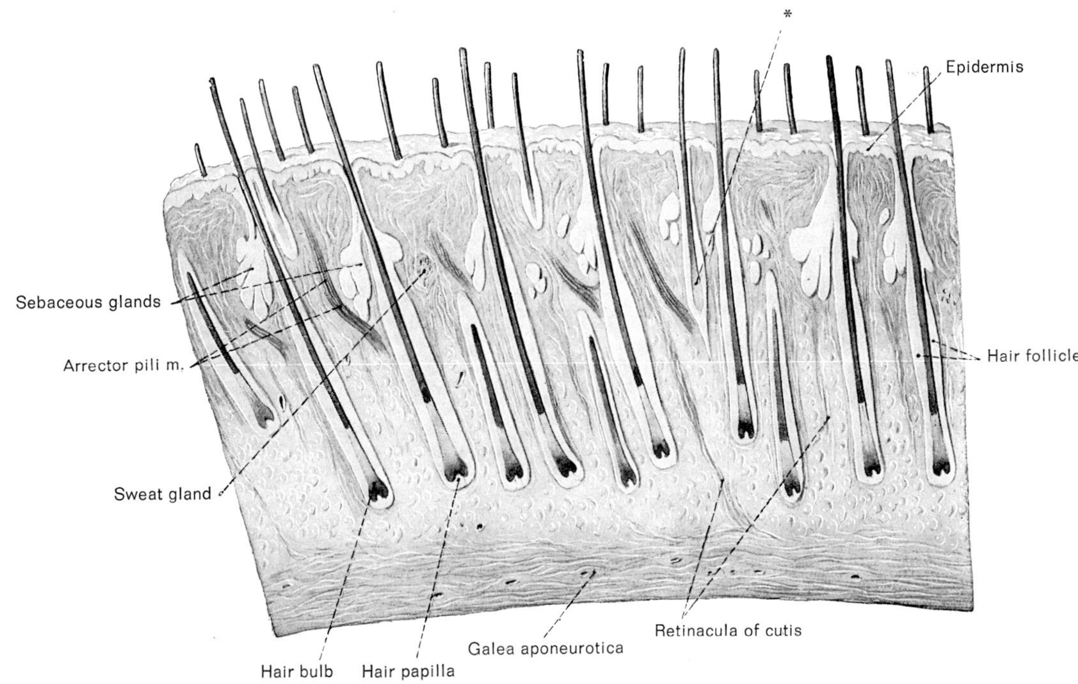
*
Epidermis
Sebaceous glands
Arrector pili m.
Hair follicle
Sweat gland
Retinacula of cutis
Galea aponeurotica
Hair bulb
Hair papilla

Fig. 279. Cross section through the scalp. * = so-called clubshaped hair.

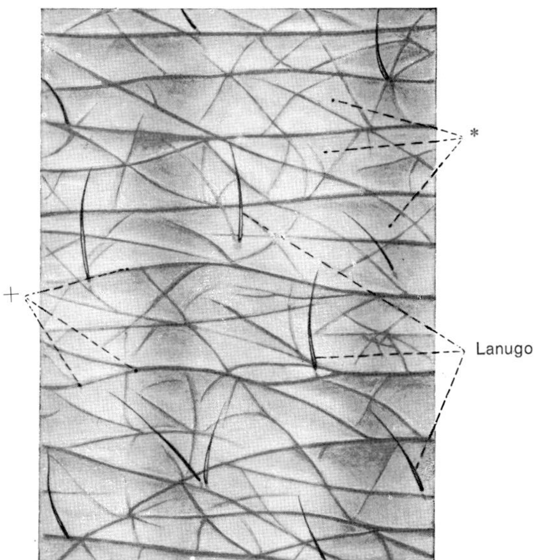
*
+
Lanugo

Fig. 280. Lanugo hairs of human skin. * = cutaneous areas, + = boundaries of cutaneous areas.

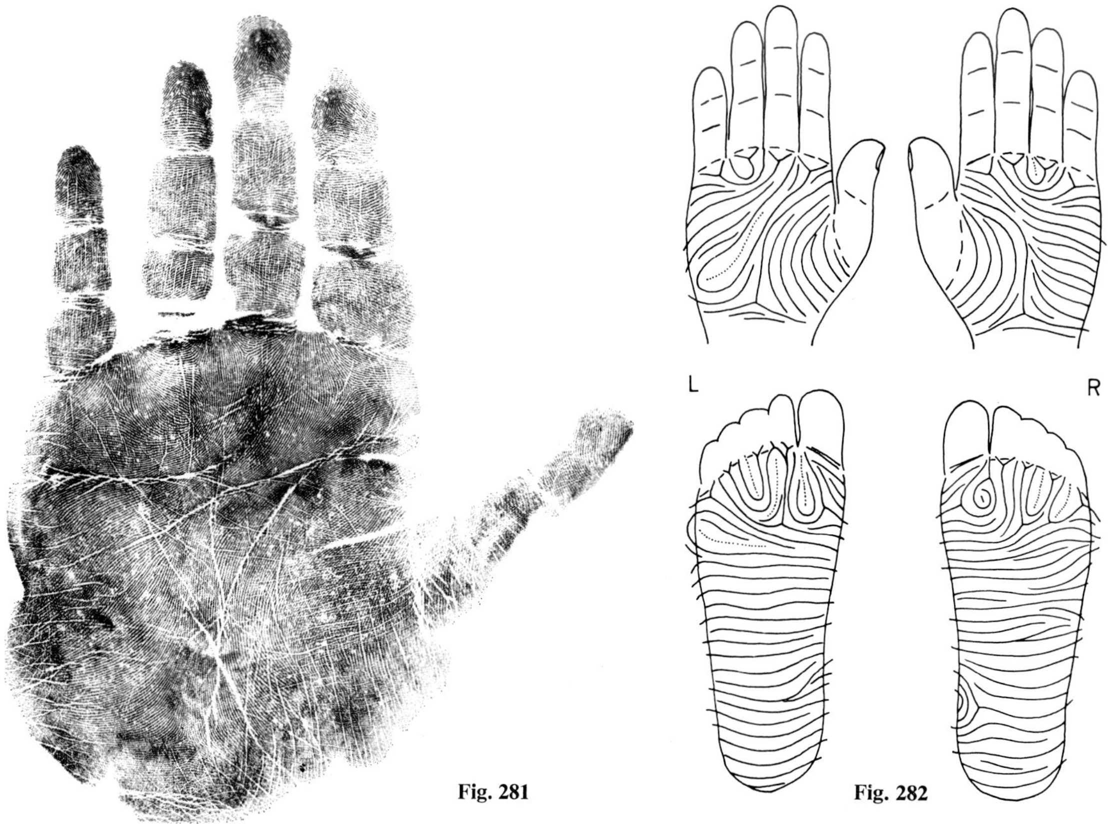
L
R
Fig. 281
Fig. 282

Fig. 281. Left palmar print of an adult man.

Fig. 282. Diagram of cutaneous ridges on palmar and plantar surfaces (from *H. Brehme* und *H. Baitsch:* Die Hautleistenmuster auf den Hand- und Fußflächen der höheren Primaten [Superfamilia Hominoidea] Studium Generale 17, 1964).

Note: The palmar surfaces of hands and fingers as well as the plantar surfaces of feet and toes are characterized by papillary ridges that begin to develop during the 3rd intrauterine month. These ridges form distinct patterns which are specific for the individual and remain unaltered throughout life (utilization of finger prints for purposes of identification). The main patterns are commonly termed arches, loops, and whorls including transitional and incidental forms. In phylogenetic view, the system of papillary ridges is species specific. The patterns of different plantar or palmar areas are correlated among each other and are subject to hereditary factors (analyses of zygosity and lineage). The relative frequencies of the patterns and their combinations differ from population to population. For clinical purposes the papillary ridge system may yield information, by more or less regular peculiarities, in patients with certain chromosomal aberrations and nonchromosomal genetic defects as well as constitutional anomalies (structural peculiarities of the ridges or percentually differing pattern frequencies as compared with normal persons). Compare *L. Loeffler:* Papillarleisten- und Hautfurchensystem. In *P. E. Becker* (ed.): Humangenetik. Ein kurzes Handbuch in fünf Bänden. Vol. I/2. Thieme, Stuttgart 1969.

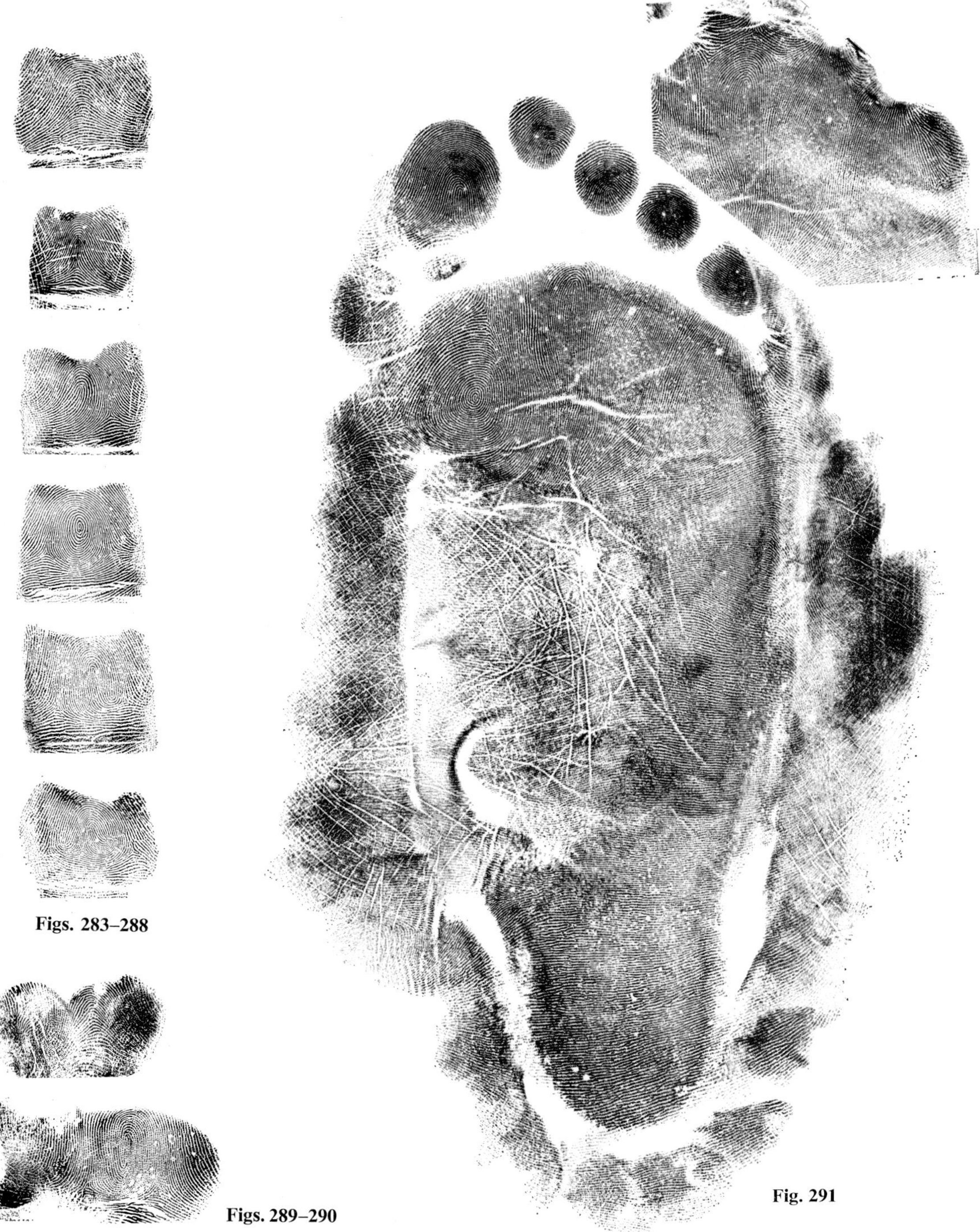

Figs. 283–288

Figs. 289–290

Fig. 291

Figs. 283–288. Various characteristic fingerprints.
Figs. 289–290. Various characteristic toeprints.
Fig. 291. Print of the right plantar surface of an adolescent, including the margins of the foot. Top right: print of the area of the base of the toes. Material for Figs. 281–291: *H. Brehme,* Institut für Humangenetik und Anthropologie der Universität Freiburg i. Br.

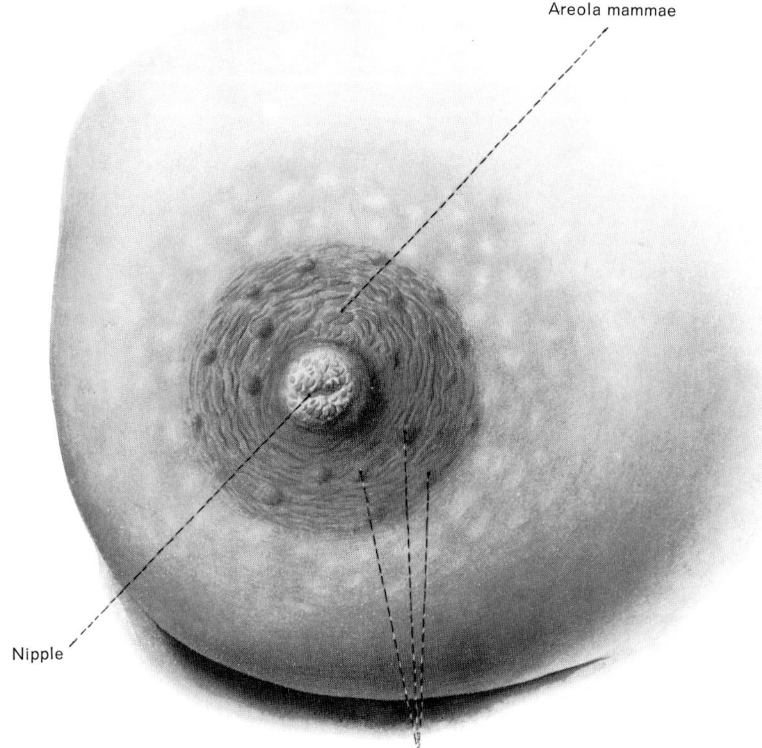
Areola mammae
Nipple
Areolar glands (Montgomery)

Fig. 292

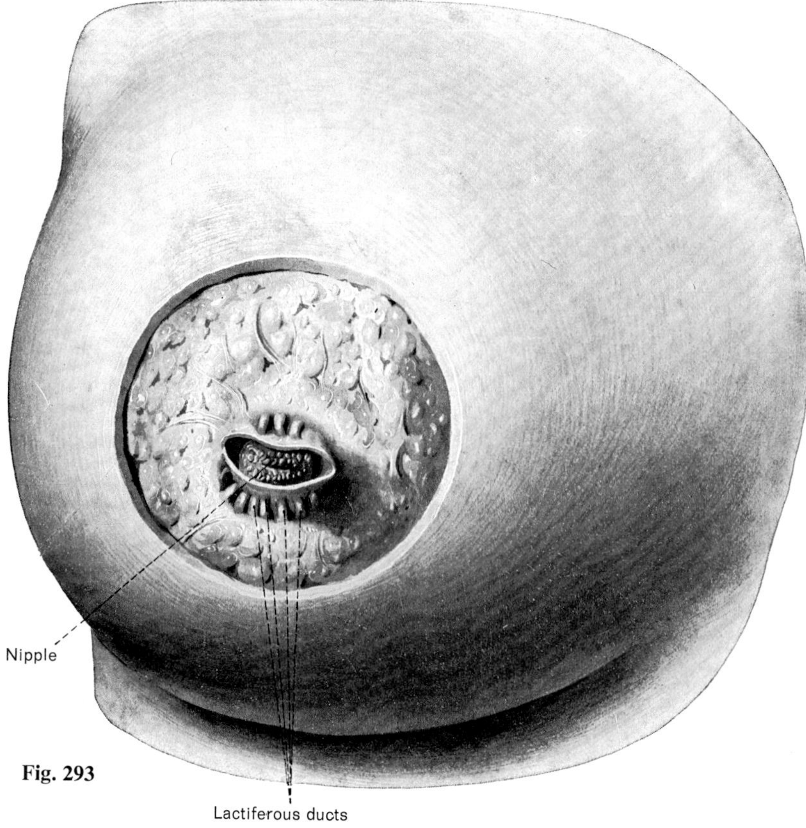
Nipple
Lactiferous ducts

Fig. 293

Fig. 292. Right breast of a pregnant woman.

Fig. 293. Right breast of a pregnant woman. A ring-shaped piece of skin surrounding the nipple has been removed. The margin of the skin near the nipple has been reflected in order to display the lactiferous ducts.

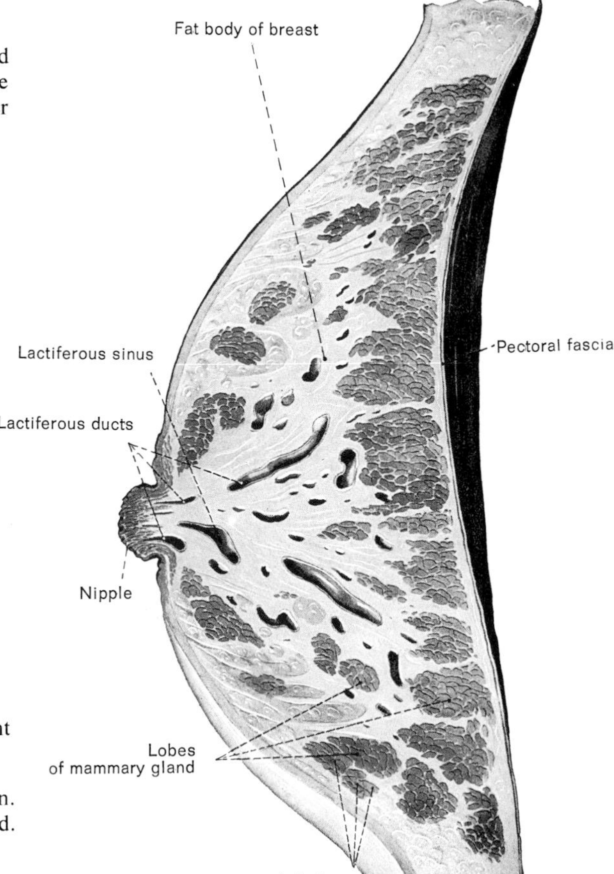
Fat body of breast
Pectoral fascia
Lactiferous sinus
Lactiferous ducts
Nipple
Lobes
of mammary gland
Lobules
of mammary gland

Fig. 294

Fig. 294. Sagittal section through the breast of a pregnant woman.

Fig. 295. Right mammary gland of a pregnant woman. Skin, except for nipple, and most of the fat have been removed.

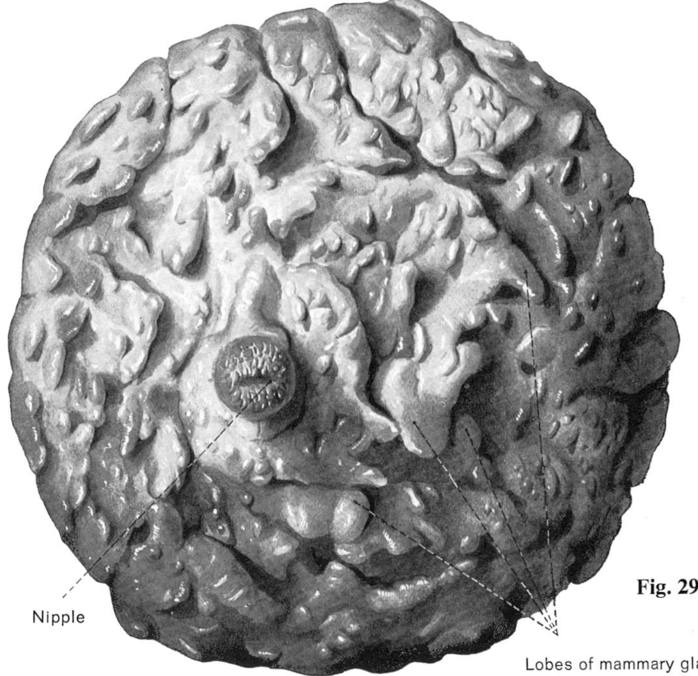
Nipple
Lobes of mammary gland

Fig. 295

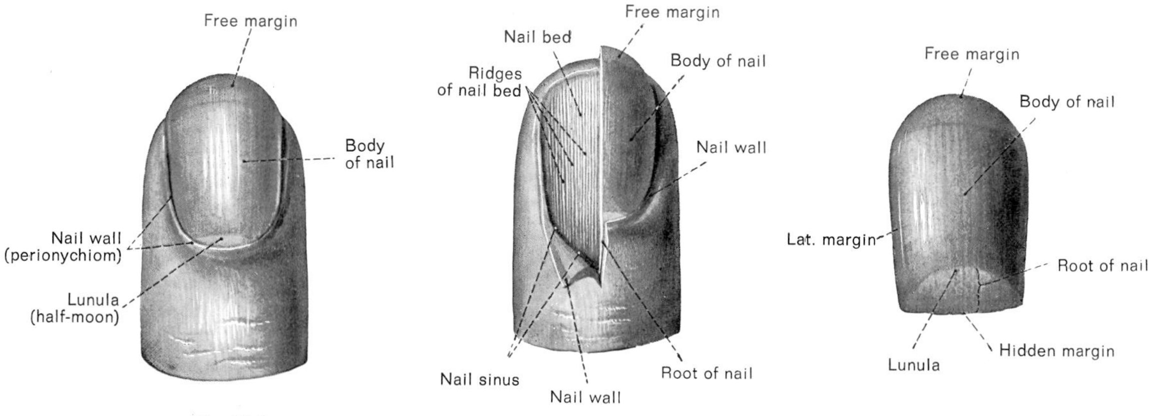
Free margin
Body
of nail
Nail wall
(perionychiom)
Lunula
(half-moon)
Free margin
Nail bed
Ridges
of nail bed
Body of nail
Nail wall
Nail sinus
Nail wall
Root of nail
Free margin
Body of nail
Lat. margin
Root of nail
Lunula
Hidden margin

Fig. 296　　Fig. 297　　Fig. 298

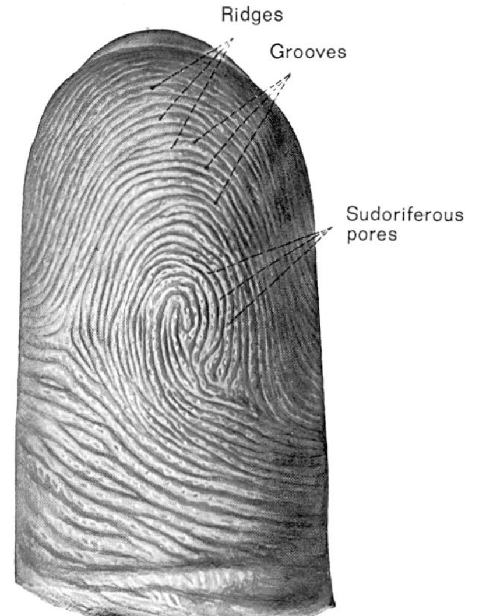
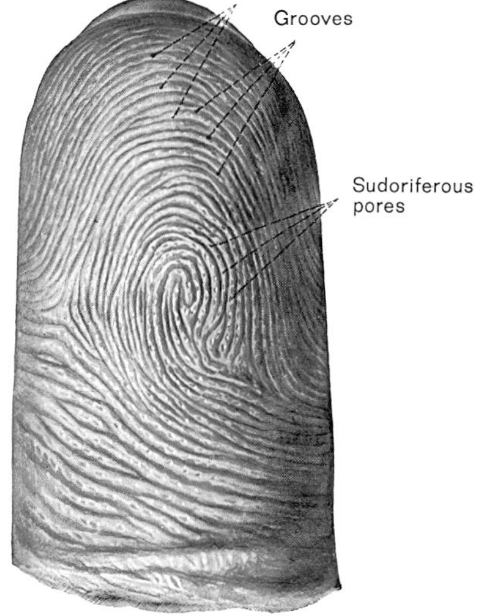
Ridges
Grooves
Sudoriferous
pores

Fig. 299

Fig. 296. Fingernail in its normal position, dorsal view.
Fig. 297. Dorsal view of finger nail, sectioned longitudinally to expose the nail bed on the left side.
Fig. 298. Body of nail, removed from nail bed; dorsal view.

Fig. 299. Grooves and ridges of palmar surface of finger tip.
Fig. 300. Nail bed of hallux, after removal of nail.
Fig. 301. Nail bed of hallux, after removal of nail and reflection of nail wall.

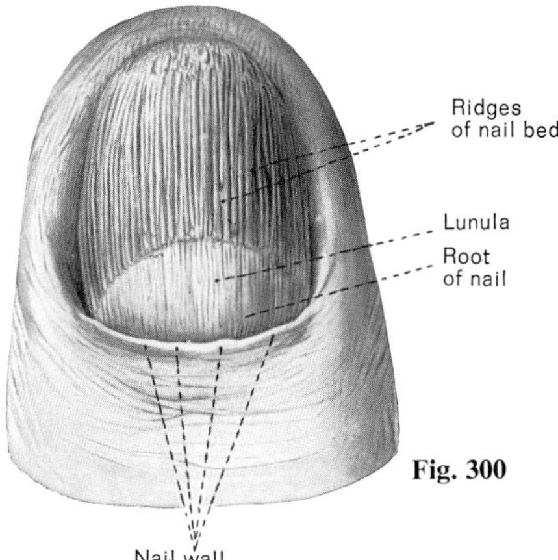
Ridges
of nail bed
Lunula
Root
of nail
Nail wall

Fig. 300

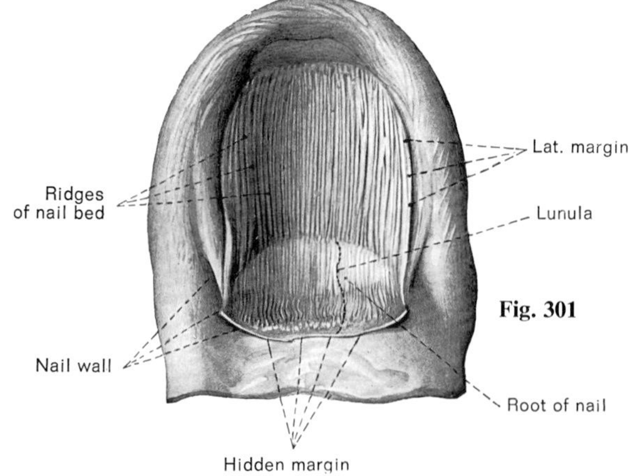
Lat. margin
Ridges
of nail bed
Lunula
Nail wall
Root of nail
Hidden margin

Fig. 301

Peripheral Nerves and Vessels

Nerves and Vessels of the Head

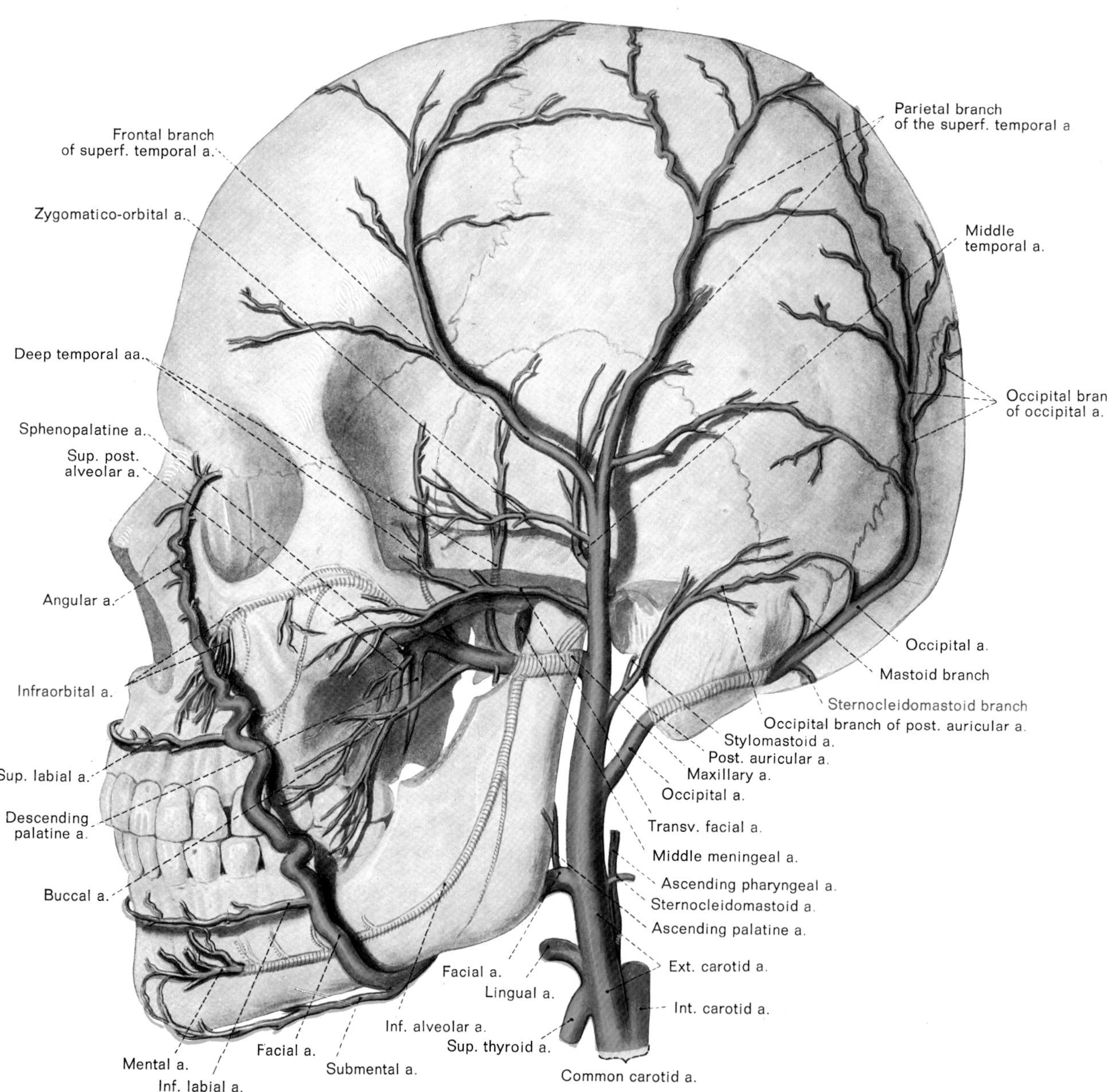
Frontal branch of superf. temporal a.
Zygomatico-orbital a.
Deep temporal aa.
Sphenopalatine a.
Sup. post. alveolar a.
Angular a.
Infraorbital a.
Sup. labial a.
Descending palatine a.
Buccal a.
Mental a.
Inf. labial a.
Facial a.
Submental a.
Inf. alveolar a.
Sup. thyroid a.
Common carotid a.
Lingual a.
Facial a.
Int. carotid a.
Ext. carotid a.
Ascending palatine a.
Sternocleidomastoid a.
Ascending pharyngeal a.
Middle meningeal a.
Transv. facial a.
Occipital a.
Maxillary a.
Post. auricular a.
Stylomastoid a.
Occipital branch of post. auricular a.
Sternocleidomastoid branch
Mastoid branch
Occipital a.
Occipital branches of occipital a.
Middle temporal a.
Parietal branch of the superf. temporal a

Fig. 302. Diagram of the external carotid artery and its branches.

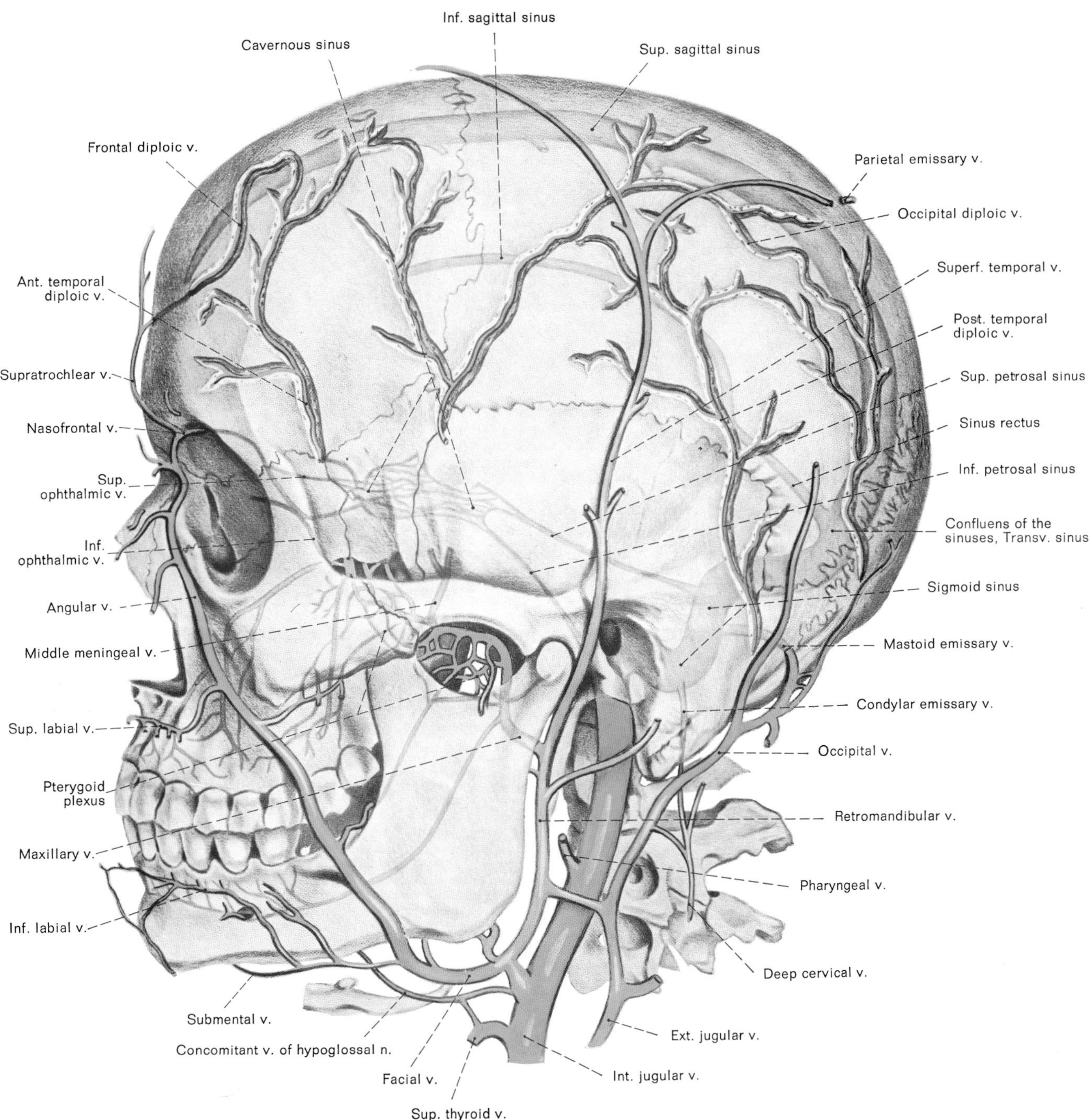
Inf. sagittal sinus
Cavernous sinus
Sup. sagittal sinus
Frontal diploic v.
Parietal emissary v.
Occipital diploic v.
Ant. temporal diploic v.
Superf. temporal v.
Post. temporal diploic v.
Supratrochlear v.
Sup. petrosal sinus
Nasofrontal v.
Sinus rectus
Sup. ophthalmic v.
Inf. petrosal sinus
Confluens of the sinuses, Transv. sinus
Inf. ophthalmic v.
Sigmoid sinus
Angular v.
Middle meningeal v.
Mastoid emissary v.
Condylar emissary v.
Sup. labial v.
Occipital v.
Pterygoid plexus
Retromandibular v.
Maxillary v.
Pharyngeal v.
Inf. labial v.
Deep cervical v.
Submental v.
Ext. jugular v.
Concomitant v. of hypoglossal n.
Facial v.
Int. jugular v.
Sup. thyroid v.

Fig. 303. Diploic veins and large veins of the head. Veins seen through bony structures and the venous sinuses of the dura mater are shown in lighter blue (from *Pernkopf/Ferner:* Atlas der topographischen und angewandten Anatomie des Menschen, vol. 1. Urban & Schwarzenberg, München–Berlin 1963).

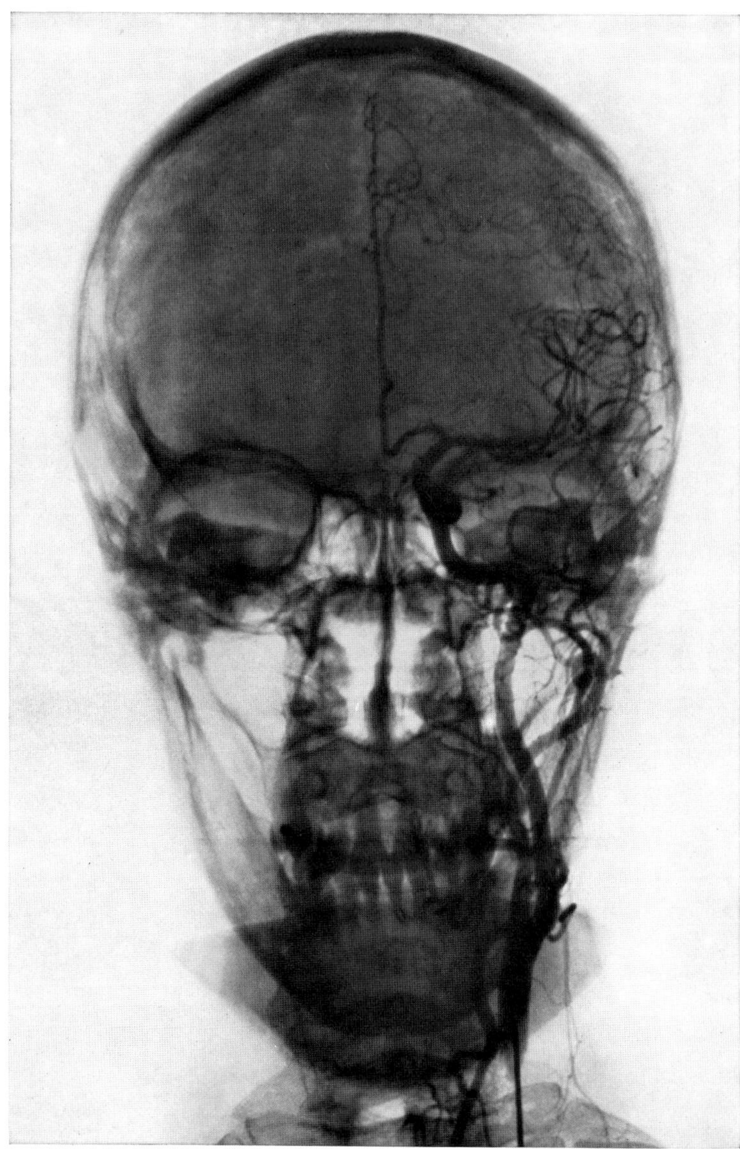

Fig. 304. Arteriogram of the left common carotid artery and its branches after injection of a contrast medium into the vessel. (A-P film: Dr. *H. Schmidt,* Pforzheim.)

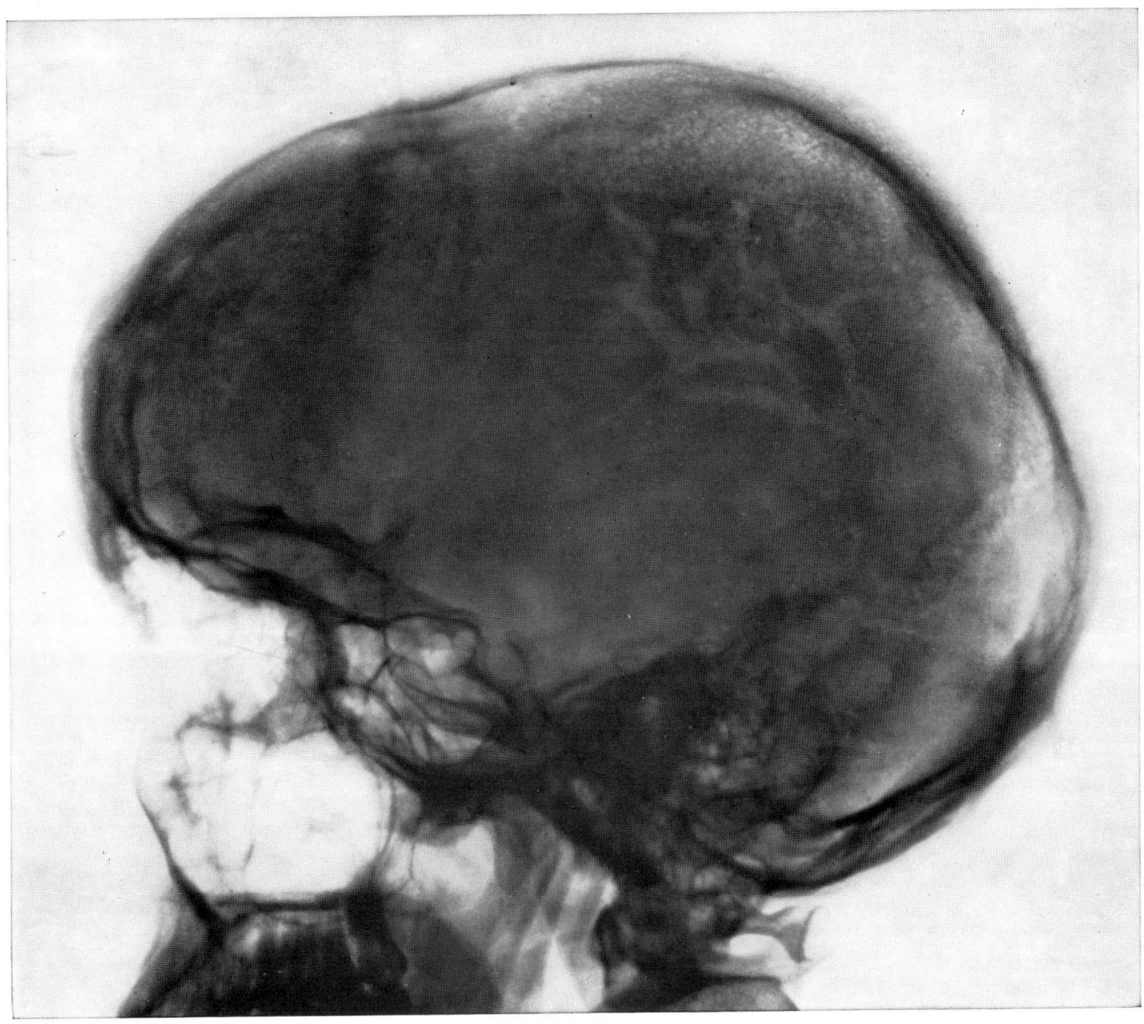

Fig. 305. Phlebogram of the diploic veins. Note especially the well recognizable temporal diploic veins. (Left lateral film: Prof. Dr. *R. Kautzky*, Hamburg.)

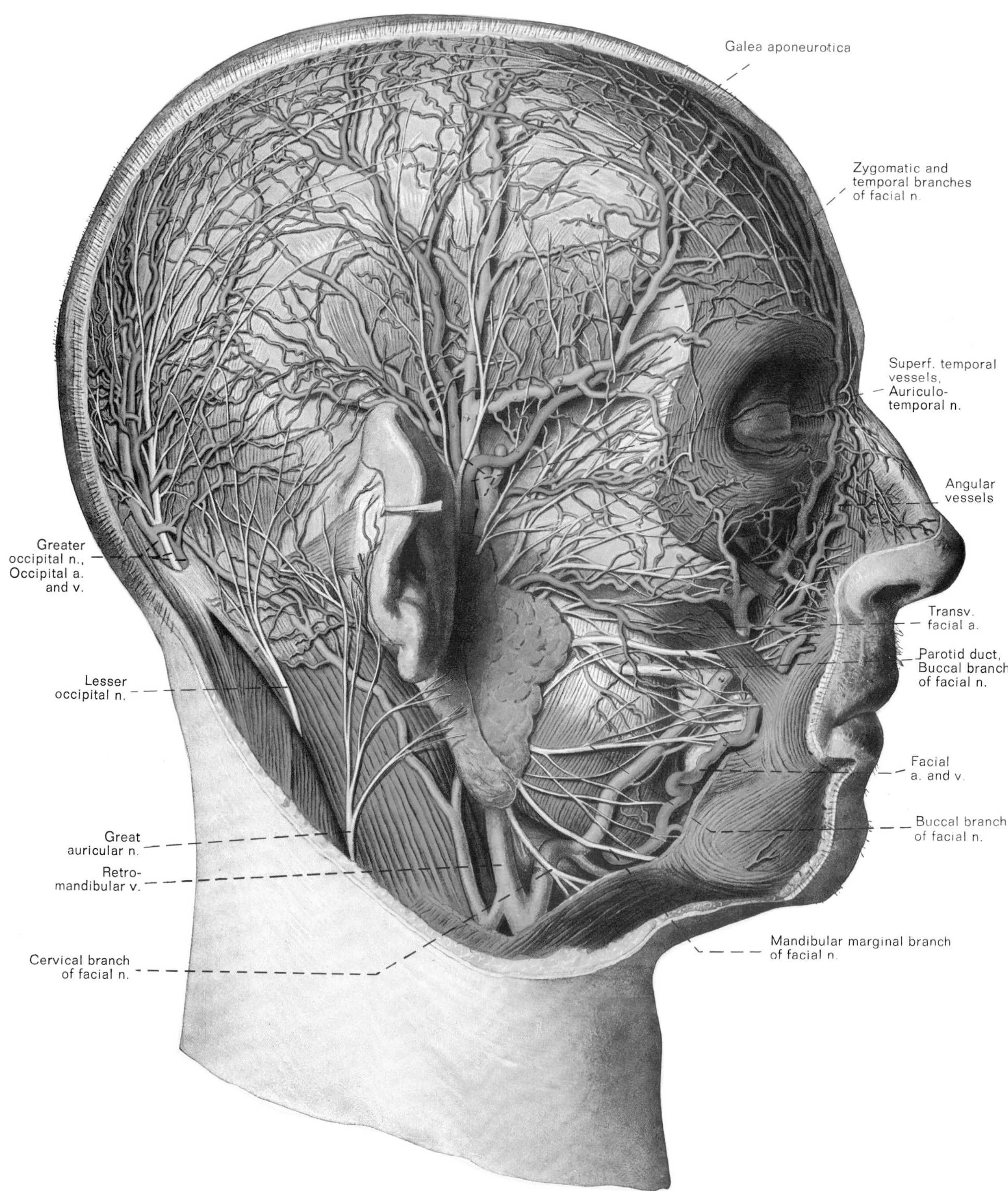
Galea aponeurotica
Zygomatic and temporal branches of facial n.
Superf. temporal vessels, Auriculo-temporal n.
Angular vessels
Greater occipital n., Occipital a. and v.
Transv. facial a.
Parotid duct, Buccal branch of facial n.
Lesser occipital n.
Facial a. and v.
Buccal branch of facial n.
Great auricular n.
Retro-mandibular v.
Mandibular marginal branch of facial n.
Cervical branch of facial n.

Fig. 306. Superficial nerves and vessels of head.

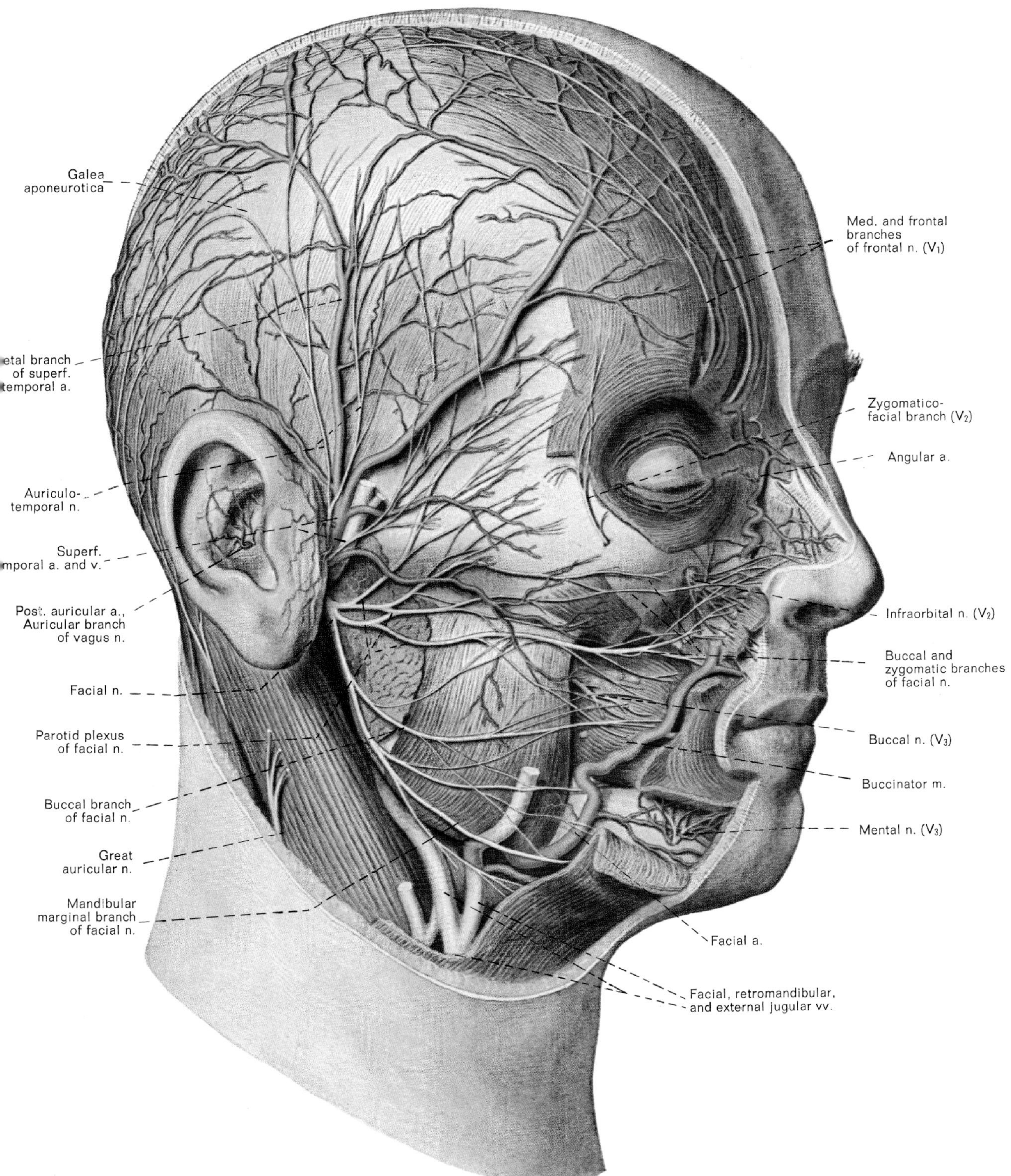
Galea aponeurotica
etal branch of superf. temporal a.
Auriculo-temporal n.
Superf. mporal a. and v.
Post. auricular a., Auricular branch of vagus n.
Facial n.
Parotid plexus of facial n.
Buccal branch of facial n.
Great auricular n.
Mandibular marginal branch of facial n.
Med. and frontal branches of frontal n. (V1)
Zygomatico-facial branch (V2)
Angular a.
Infraorbital n. (V2)
Buccal and zygomatic branches of facial n.
Buccal n. (V3)
Buccinator m.
Mental n. (V3)
Facial a.
Facial, retromandibular, and external jugular vv.

Fig. 307. Nerves and arteries of head, intermediate layer. Superficial portions of the parotid gland have been removed in order to expose the stem and the parotid plexus of the facial nerve.

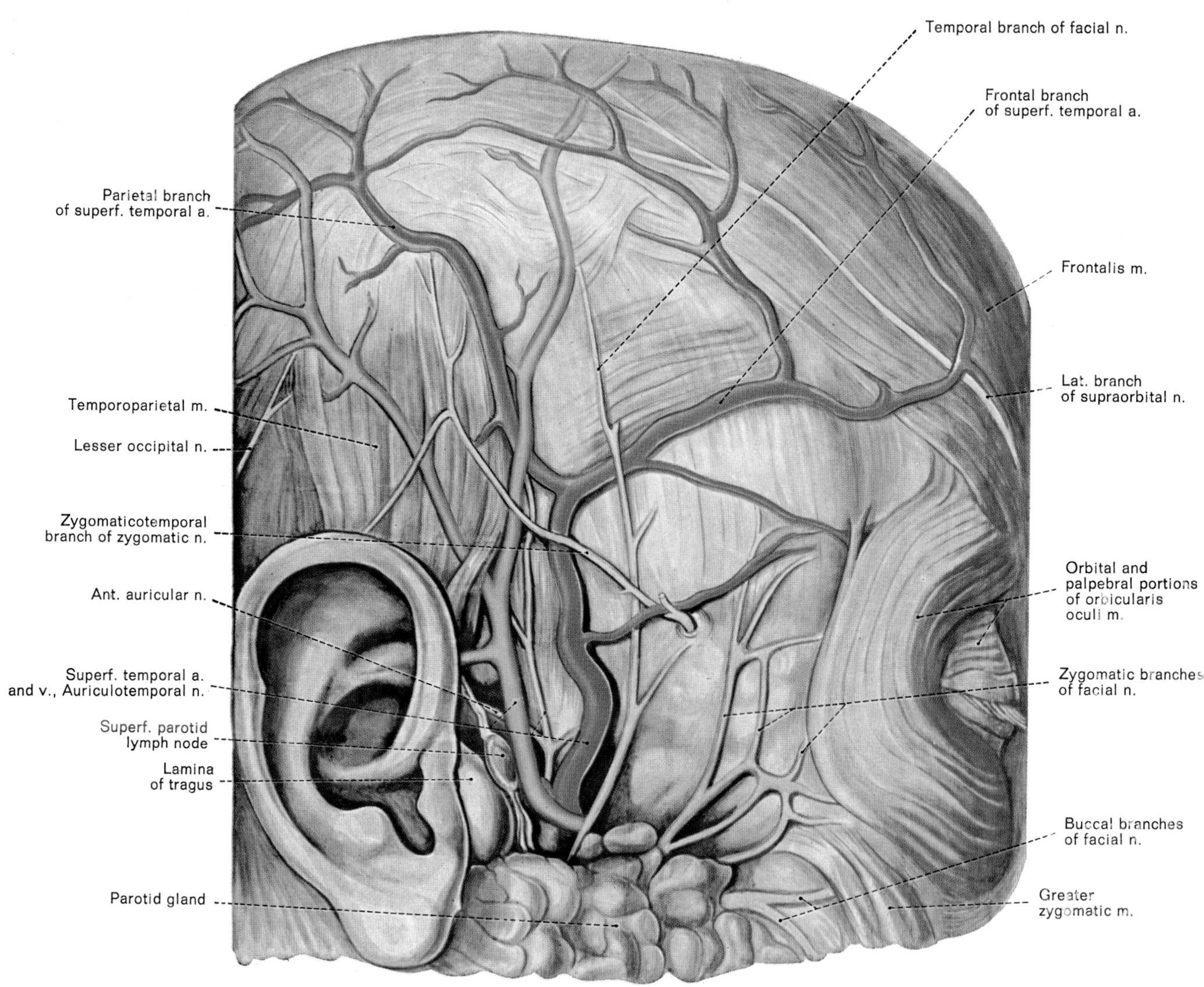

Temporal branch of facial n.
Frontal branch of superf. temporal a.
Parietal branch of superf. temporal a.
Frontalis m.
Lat. branch of supraorbital n.
Temporoparietal m.
Lesser occipital n.
Zygomaticotemporal branch of zygomatic n.
Orbital and palpebral portions of orbicularis oculi m.
Ant. auricular n.
Superf. temporal a. and v., Auriculotemporal n.
Zygomatic branches of facial n.
Superf. parotid lymph node
Lamina of tragus
Buccal branches of facial n.
Parotid gland
Greater zygomatic m.

Fig. 308. Superficial layer of the temporal region with superficial temporal artery, auriculotemporal nerve, branches of facial nerve, and zygomaticotemporal branch of zygomatic nerve.

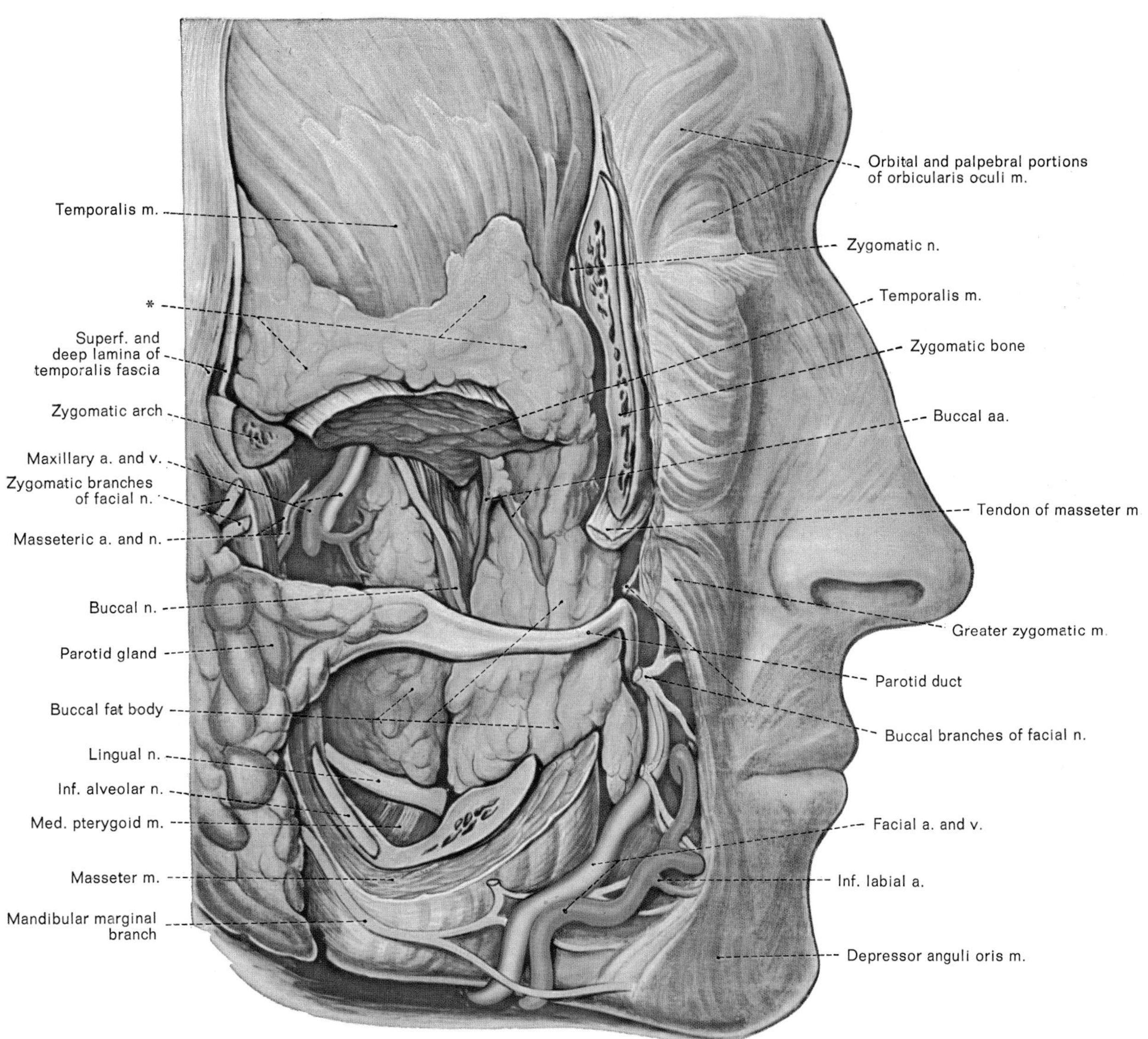
Orbital and palpebral portions of orbicularis oculi m.
Temporalis m.
Zygomatic n.
*
Temporalis m.
Superf. and deep lamina of temporalis fascia
Zygomatic bone
Zygomatic arch
Buccal aa.
Maxillary a. and v.
Zygomatic branches of facial n.
Tendon of masseter m
Masseteric a. and n.
Buccal n.
Greater zygomatic m.
Parotid gland
Parotid duct
Buccal fat body
Buccal branches of facial n.
Lingual n.
Inf. alveolar n.
Med. pterygoid m.
Facial a. and v.
Masseter m.
Inf. labial a.
Mandibular marginal branch
Depressor anguli oris m.

Fig. 309. Buccal region with parotid duct and buccal fat body *(Bichat)*. The zygomatic arch, mandibular ramus, temporalis and masseter muscles have been partially removed. * = fat body superficial to the temporalis muscle.

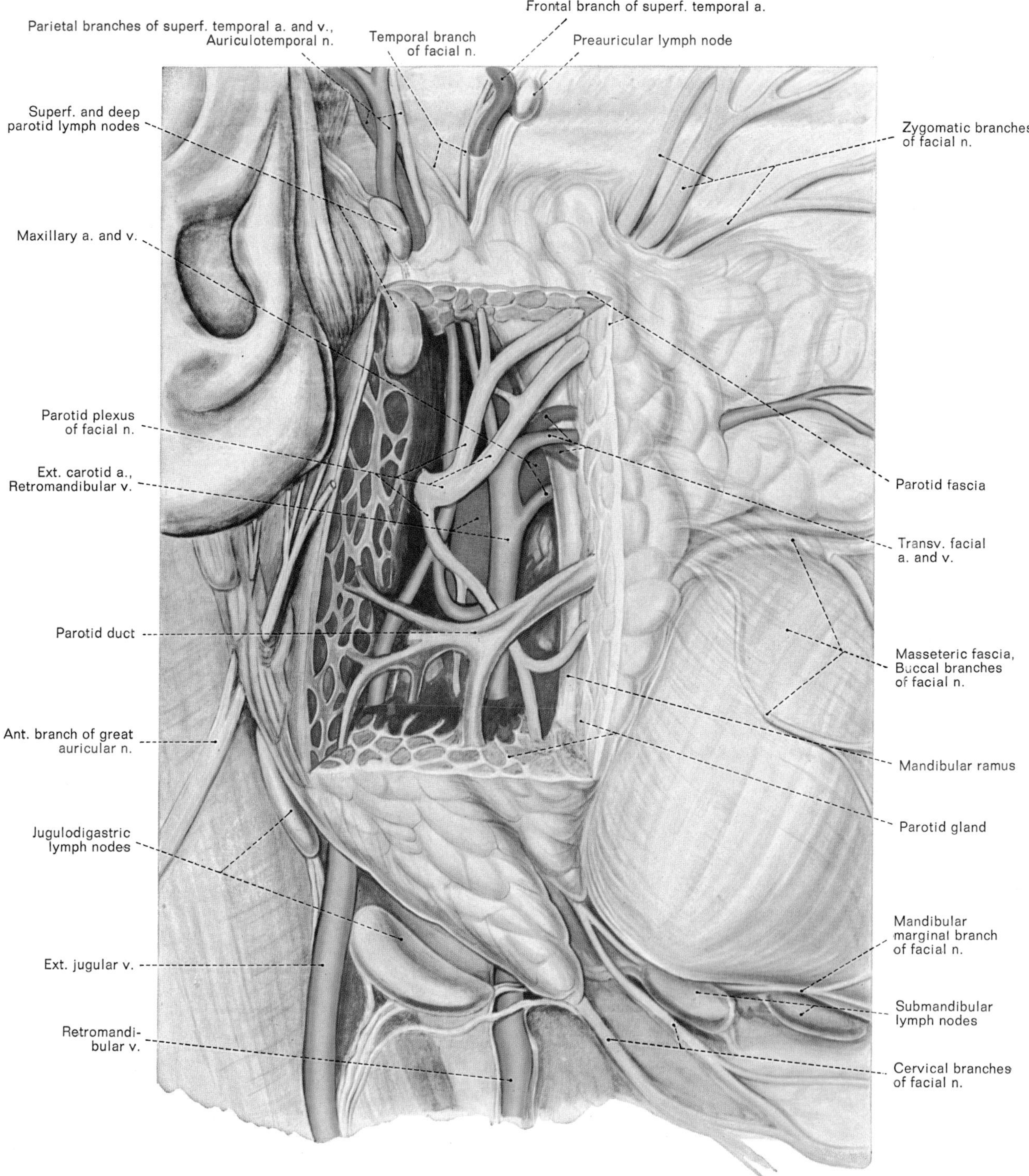

Frontal branch of superf. temporal a.
Parietal branches of superf. temporal a. and v.,
Auriculotemporal n.
Temporal branch
of facial n.
Preauricular lymph node
Superf. and deep
parotid lymph nodes
Zygomatic branches
of facial n.
Maxillary a. and v.
Parotid plexus
of facial n.
Ext. carotid a.,
Retromandibular v.
Parotid fascia
Transv. facial
a. and v.
Parotid duct
Masseteric fascia,
Buccal branches
of facial n.
Ant. branch of great
auricular n.
Mandibular ramus
Parotid gland
Jugulodigastric
lymph nodes
Mandibular
marginal branch
of facial n.
Ext. jugular v.
Submandibular
lymph nodes
Retromandi-
bular v.
Cervical branches
of facial n.

Fig. 310. Parotid region; parotid plexus of facial nerve, parotid duct. A window has been cut into the parotid gland.

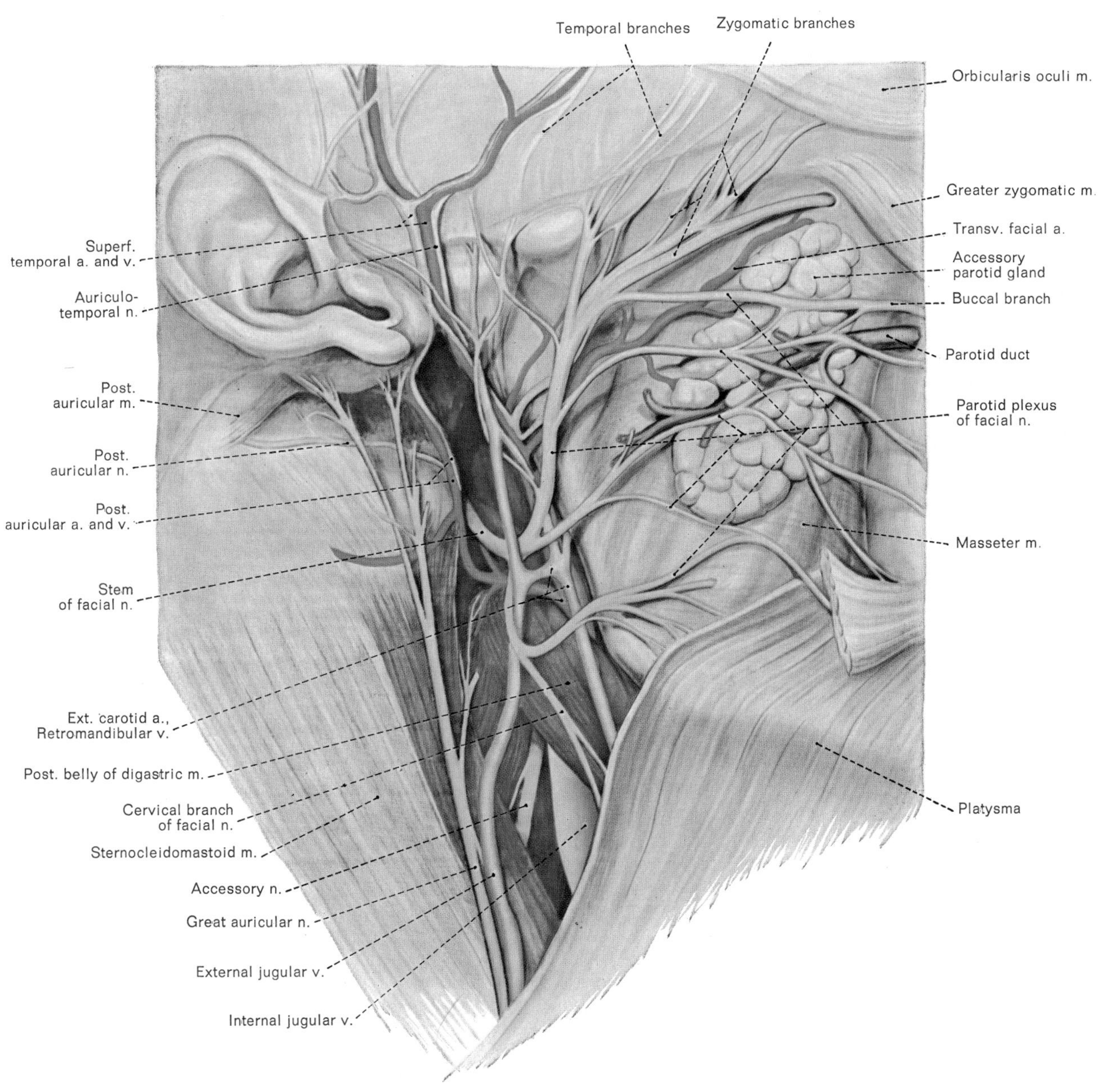
Temporal branches
Zygomatic branches
Orbicularis oculi m.
Greater zygomatic m.
Transv. facial a.
Accessory parotid gland
Buccal branch
Parotid duct
Parotid plexus of facial n.
Masseter m.
Platysma
Superf. temporal a. and v.
Auriculo-temporal n.
Post. auricular m.
Post. auricular n.
Post. auricular a. and v.
Stem of facial n.
Ext. carotid a., Retromandibular v.
Post. belly of digastric m.
Cervical branch of facial n.
Sternocleidomastoid m.
Accessory n.
Great auricular n.
External jugular v.
Internal jugular v.

Fig. 311. Nerves and vessels of the retromandibular fossa. Facial nerve and parotid plexus, parotid duct and accessory parotid gland.

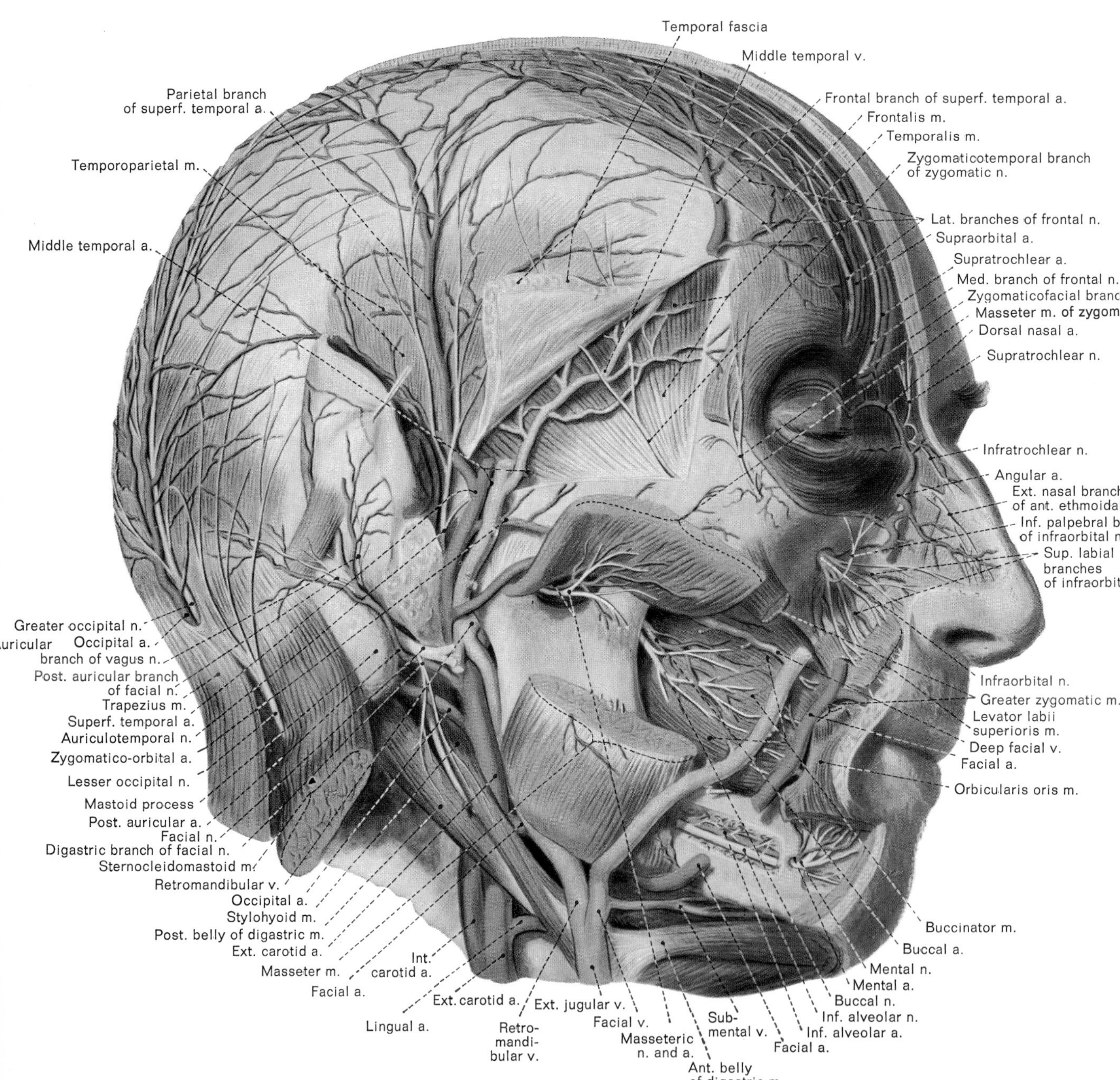
Temporal fascia
Middle temporal v.
Parietal branch of superf. temporal a.
Frontal branch of superf. temporal a.
Frontalis m.
Temporalis m.
Temporoparietal m.
Zygomaticotemporal branch of zygomatic n.
Lat. branches of frontal n.
Supraorbital a.
Middle temporal a.
Supratrochlear a.
Med. branch of frontal n.
Masseter m.
Dorsal nasal a.
Supratrochlear n.
Infratrochlear n.
Angular a.
Sup. labial
branches
Greater occipital n.
Occipital a.
branch of vagus n.
Post. auricular branch of facial n.
Trapezius m.
Superf. temporal a.
Auriculotemporal n.
Zygomatico-orbital a.
Lesser occipital n.
Mastoid process
Post. auricular a.
Facial n.
Digastric branch of facial n.
Sternocleidomastoid m.
Retromandibular v.
Occipital a.
Stylohyoid m.
Post. belly of digastric m.
Ext. carotid a.
Masseter m.
Int. carotid a.
Facial a.
Lingual a.
Ext. carotid a.
Retro-mandi-bular v.
Ext. jugular v.
Facial v.
Masseteric n. and a.
Sub-mental v.
Ant. belly of digastric m.
Facial a.
Inf. alveolar a.
Inf. alveolar n.
Buccal n.
Mental a.
Mental n.
Buccal a.
Buccinator m.
Infraorbital n.
Greater zygomatic m.
Levator labii superioris m.
Deep facial v.
Facial a.
Orbicularis oris m.

Fig. 312. Nerves and vessels of the right side of the head, third layer. The masseter muscle has been severed and reflected, both laminae of the temporal fascia have been reflected from the upper margin of the zygomatic arch, parotid gland and facial nerve have been removed, several facial muscles have been partially removed, the mandibular canal has been opened.

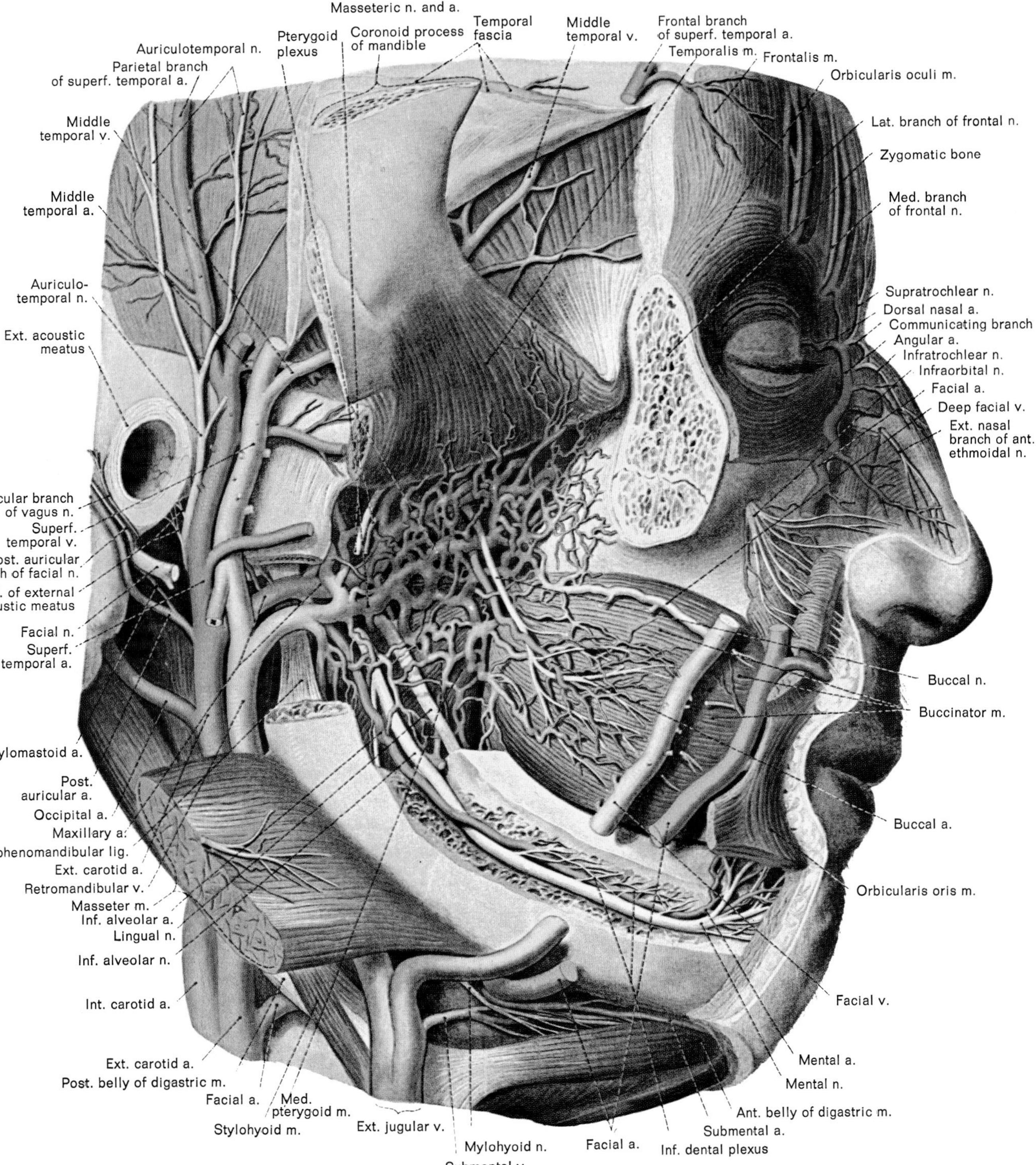
Masseteric n. and a.
Pterygoid plexus
Coronoid process of mandible
Temporal fascia
Middle temporal v.
Frontal branch of superf. temporal a.
Temporalis m.
Frontalis m.
Orbicularis oculi m.
Auriculotemporal n.
Parietal branch of superf. temporal a.
Middle temporal v.
Middle temporal a.
Auriculo-temporal n.
Ext. acoustic meatus
cular branch of vagus n.
Superf. temporal v.
ost. auricular h of facial n.
. of external ustic meatus
Facial n.
Superf. temporal a.
ylomastoid a.
Post. auricular a.
Occipital a.
Maxillary a.
phenomandibular lig.
Ext. carotid a.
Retromandibular v.
Masseter m.
Inf. alveolar a.
Lingual n.
Inf. alveolar n.
Int. carotid a.
Ext. carotid a.
Post. belly of digastric m.
Facial a.
Med. pterygoid m.
Stylohyoid m.
Ext. jugular v.
Mylohyoid n.
Submental v.
Facial a.
Inf. dental plexus
Submental a.
Ant. belly of digastric m.
Mental n.
Mental a.
Facial v.
Orbicularis oris m.
Buccal a.
Buccinator m.
Buccal n.
Lat. branch of frontal n.
Zygomatic bone
Med. branch of frontal n.
Supratrochlear n.
Dorsal nasal a.
Communicating branch
Angular a.
Infratrochlear n.
Infraorbital n.
Facial a.
Deep facial v.
Ext. nasal branch of ant. ethmoidal n.

Fig. 313. Nerves and vessels of the right side of the face, fourth layer. Zygomatic arch and neck of mandible have been removed, the mandibular canal has been opened, the temporalis muscle together with the coronoid process of the mandible have been reflected upward. Note the venous plexus between the pterygoid muscles.

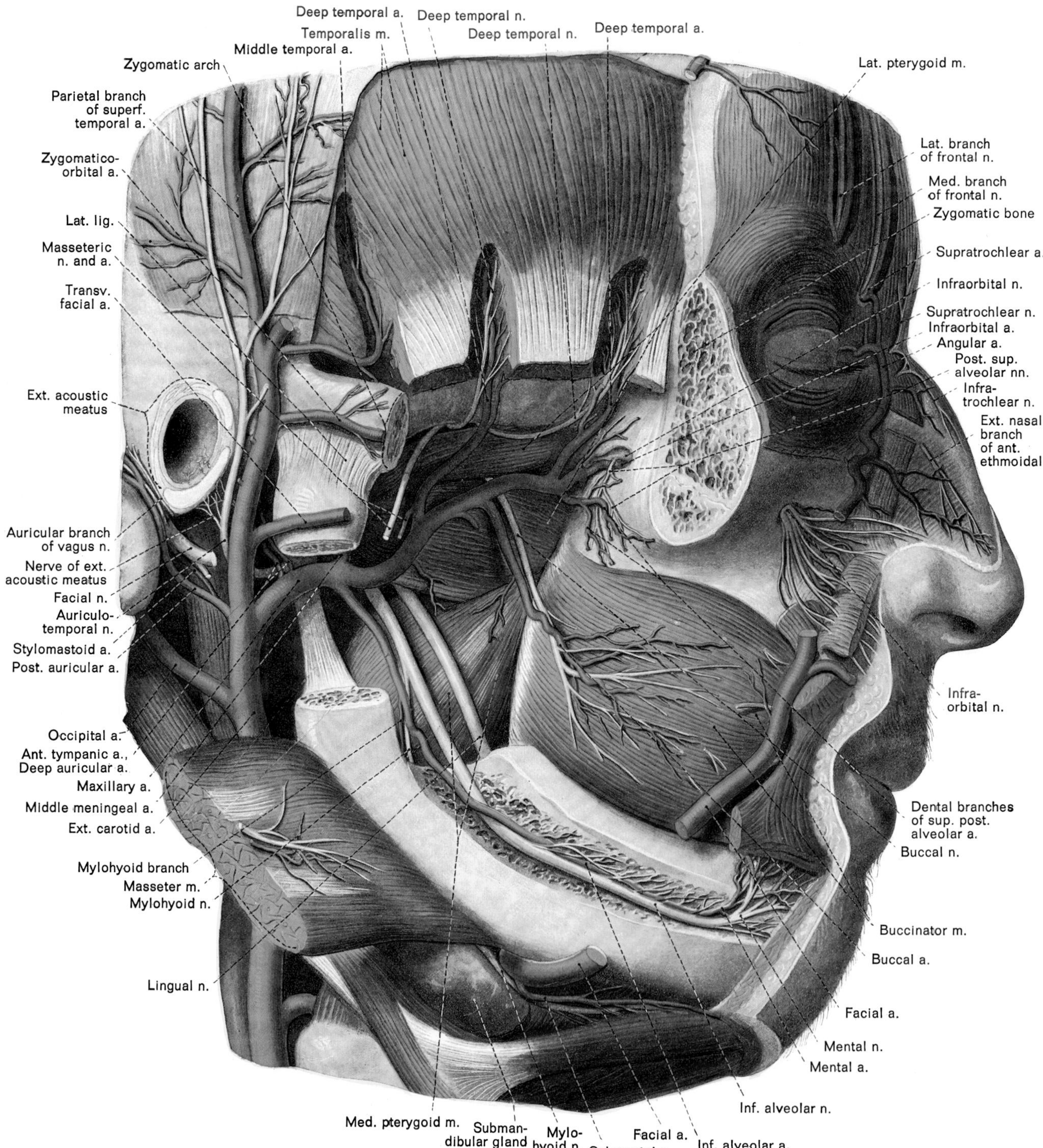

Deep temporal a.
Deep temporal n.
Temporalis m.
Deep temporal n.
Deep temporal a.
Middle temporal a.
Zygomatic arch
Lat. pterygoid m.
Parietal branch of superf. temporal a.
Zygomatico-orbital a.
Lat. branch of frontal n.
Med. branch of frontal n.
Zygomatic bone
Lat. lig.
Masseteric n. and a.
Supratrochlear a.
Infraorbital n.
Transv. facial a.
Supratrochlear n.
Infraorbital a.
Angular a.
Post. sup. alveolar nn.
Ext. acoustic meatus
Infra-trochlear n.
Ext. nasal branch of ant. ethmoidal n.
Auricular branch of vagus n.
Nerve of ext. acoustic meatus
Facial n.
Auriculo-temporal n.
Stylomastoid a.
Post. auricular a.
Infra-orbital n.
Occipital a.
Ant. tympanic a., Deep auricular a.
Maxillary a.
Middle meningeal a.
Ext. carotid a.
Dental branches of sup. post. alveolar a.
Buccal n.
Mylohyoid branch
Masseter m.
Mylohyoid n.
Buccinator m.
Buccal a.
Lingual n.
Facial a.
Mental n.
Mental a.
Inf. alveolar n.
Med. pterygoid m.
Submandibular gland
Mylohyoid n.
Submental a.
Facial a.
Inf. alveolar a.

Fig. 314. Nerves and vessels of the right side of the face, deep layer: maxillary artery and its branches. Preparation similar to the one in Fig. 313, but the insertion of the temporalis muscle together with the coronoid process of the mandible have been removed and the deep temporal arteries have been exposed.

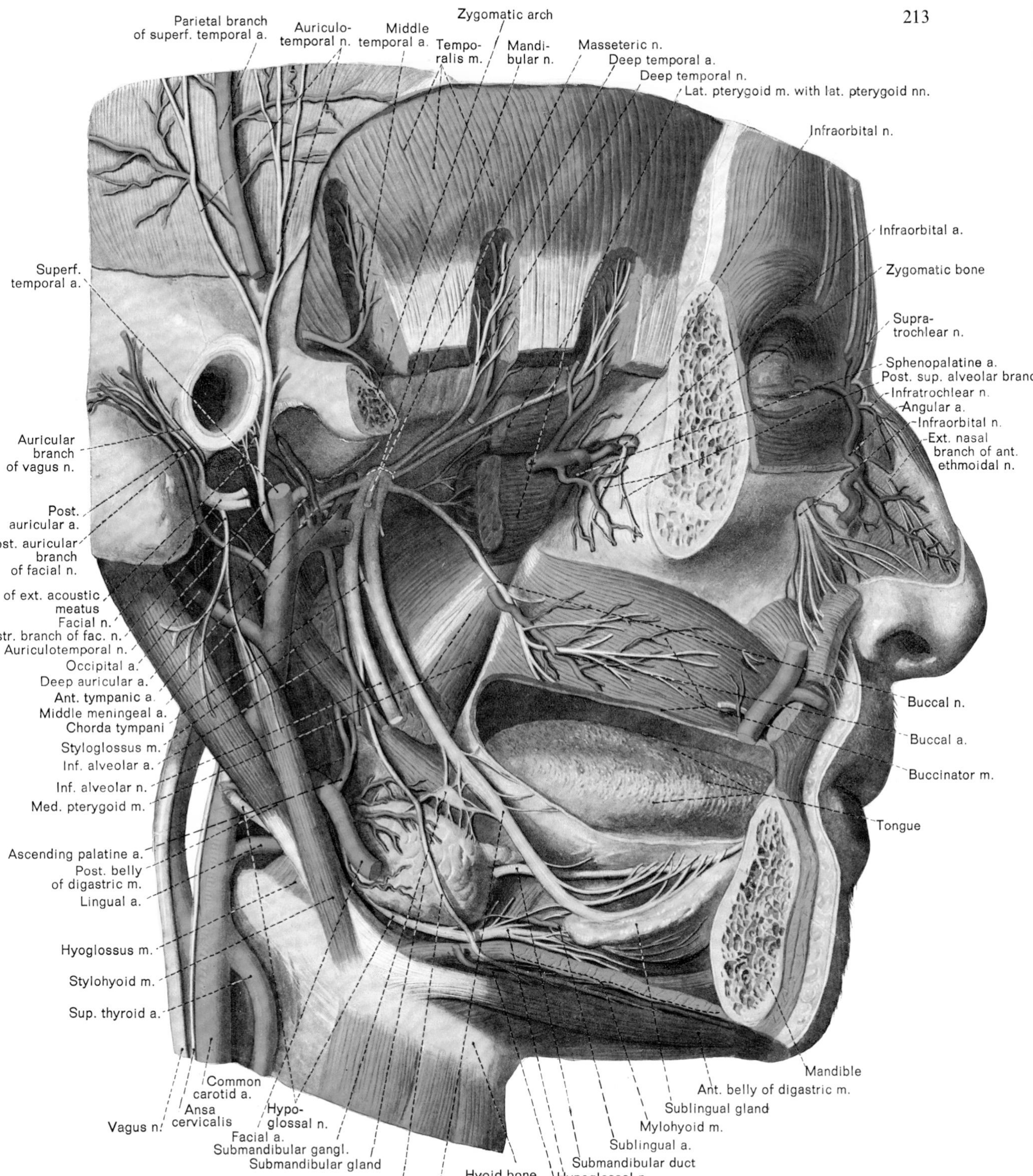
Parietal branch of superf. temporal a.
Auriculo-temporal n.
Middle temporal a.
Zygomatic arch
Tempo-ralis m.
Mandi-bular n.
Masseteric n.
Deep temporal a.
Deep temporal n.
Lat. pterygoid m. with lat. pterygoid nn.
Infraorbital n.
Infraorbital a.
Zygomatic bone
Supra-trochlear n.
Sphenopalatine a.
Post. sup. alveolar branches
Infratrochlear n.
Angular a.
Infraorbital n.
Ext. nasal branch of ant. ethmoidal n.
Superf. temporal a.
Auricular branch of vagus n.
Post. auricular a.
Post. auricular branch of facial n.
N. of ext. acoustic meatus
Facial n.
gastr. branch of fac. n.
Auriculotemporal n.
Occipital a.
Deep auricular a.
Ant. tympanic a.
Middle meningeal a.
Chorda tympani
Styloglossus m.
Inf. alveolar a.
Inf. alveolar n.
Med. pterygoid m.
Ascending palatine a.
Post. belly of digastric m.
Lingual a.
Hyoglossus m.
Stylohyoid m.
Sup. thyroid a.
Buccal n.
Buccal a.
Buccinator m.
Tongue
Mandible
Ant. belly of digastric m.
Sublingual gland
Mylohyoid m.
Sublingual a.
Submandibular duct
Hypoglossal n.
Submental a.
Lingual n.
Hyoid bone
Mylohyoid n.
Submandibular gland
Submandibular gangl.
Facial a.
Hypo-glossal n.
Ansa cervicalis
Vagus n.
Common carotid a.

Fig. 315. Nerves and vessels of the right side of the face, deep layer: mandibular nerve and its branches. Preparation similar to the one in Fig. 314, but the condylar process of the mandible has been disjointed and removed together with the rest of the right lower jaw. The lower half of the buccinator muscle and the underlying oral mucosa have been removed.
+ = maxillary artery.

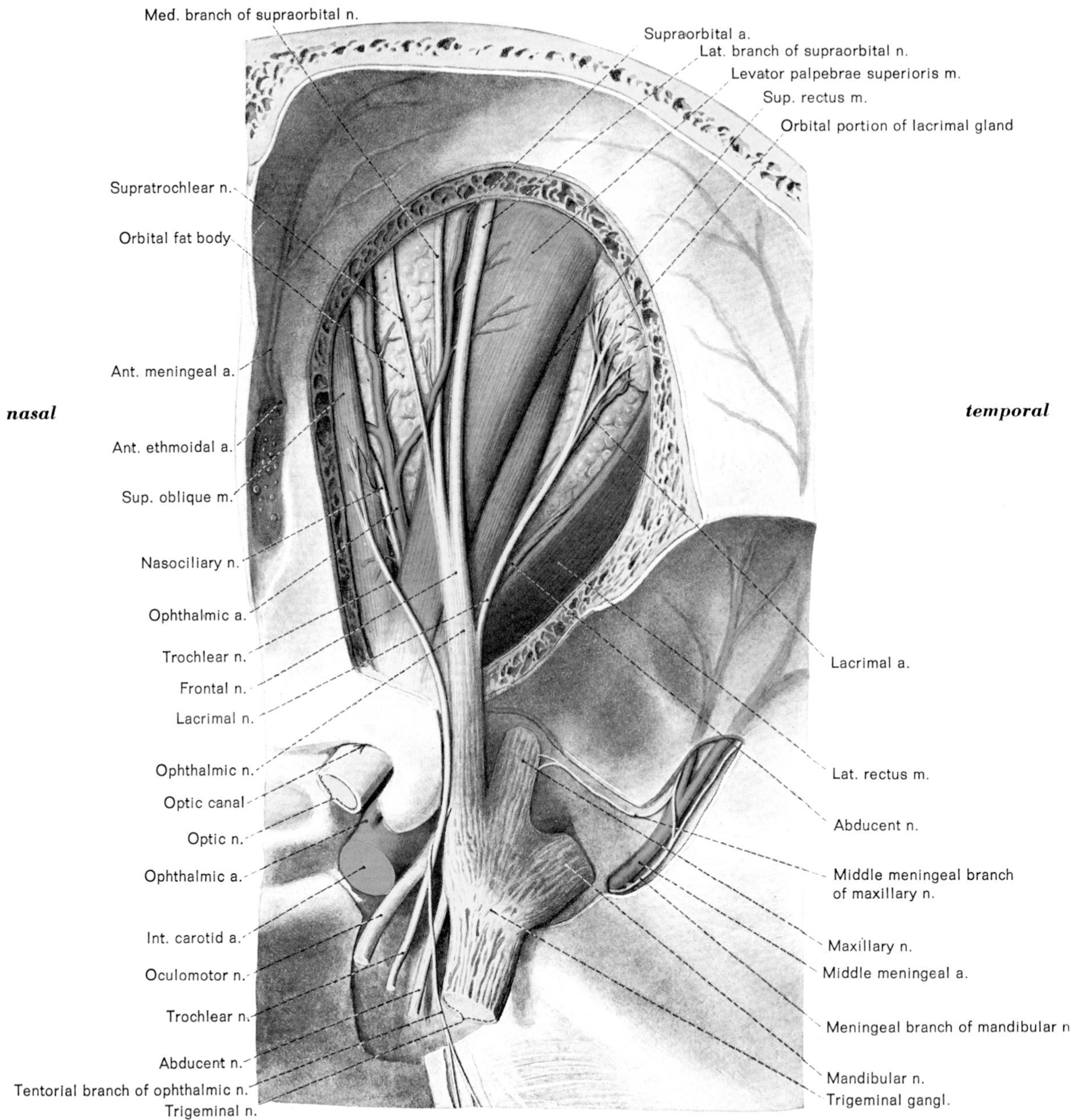
Med. branch of supraorbital n.
Supraorbital a.
Lat. branch of supraorbital n.
Levator palpebrae superioris m.
Sup. rectus m.
Orbital portion of lacrimal gland
Supratrochlear n.
Orbital fat body
Ant. meningeal a.
nasal
temporal
Ant. ethmoidal a.
Sup. oblique m.
Nasociliary n.
Ophthalmic a.
Trochlear n.
Frontal n.
Lacrimal n.
Lacrimal a.
Ophthalmic n.
Optic canal
Optic n.
Ophthalmic a.
Lat. rectus m.
Abducent n.
Middle meningeal branch
of maxillary n.
Int. carotid a.
Oculomotor n.
Maxillary n.
Middle meningeal a.
Trochlear n.
Meningeal branch of mandibular n
Abducent n.
Tentorial branch of ophthalmic n.
Trigeminal n.
Mandibular n.
Trigeminal gangl.

Fig. 316. Nerves and arteries of the right orbit, superficial layer. The roof of the orbit and the upper portion of its lateral wall as well as the periorbit have been removed. The dura mater has been split along the middle meningeal artery, and has been removed in the area of the trigeminal ganglion and the nerves for the extrinsic ocular muscles.

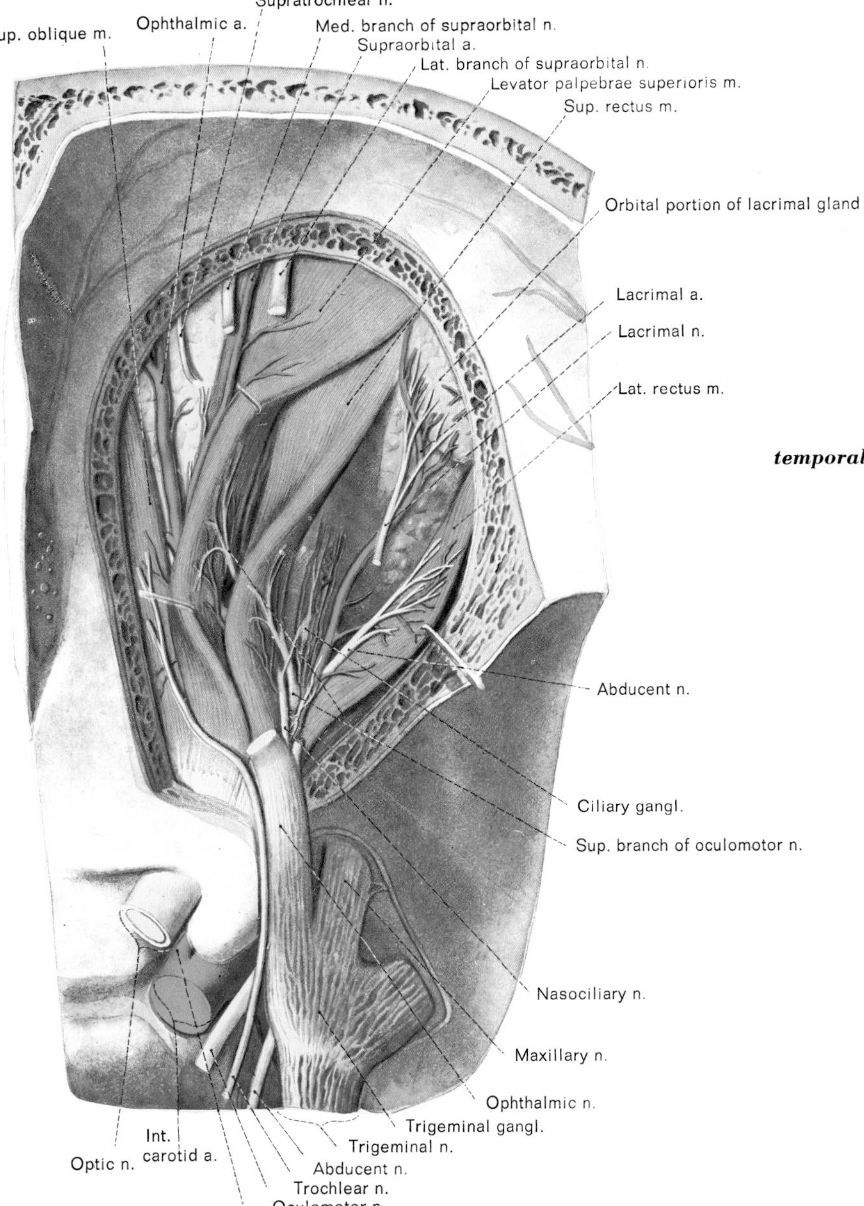
Supratrochlear n.
Sup. oblique m.
Ophthalmic a.
Med. branch of supraorbital n.
Supraorbital a.
Lat. branch of supraorbital n.
Levator palpebrae superioris m.
Sup. rectus m.
Orbital portion of lacrimal gland
Lacrimal a.
Lacrimal n.
Lat. rectus m.
nasal
temporal
Abducent n.
Ciliary gangl.
Sup. branch of oculomotor n.
Nasociliary n.
Maxillary n.
Ophthalmic n.
Trigeminal gangl.
Trigeminal n.
Abducent n.
Trochlear n.
Oculomotor n.
Ophthalmic a.
Int. carotid a.
Optic n.

Fig. 317. Nerves and arteries of the right orbit, second layer. Preparation similar to the one in Fig. 316. Major part of frontal nerve and a part of the temporal portion of the orbital fat body have been removed, the superior rectus muscle and the levator palpebrae superioris muscle have been pulled medially, the lateral rectus muscle laterally.

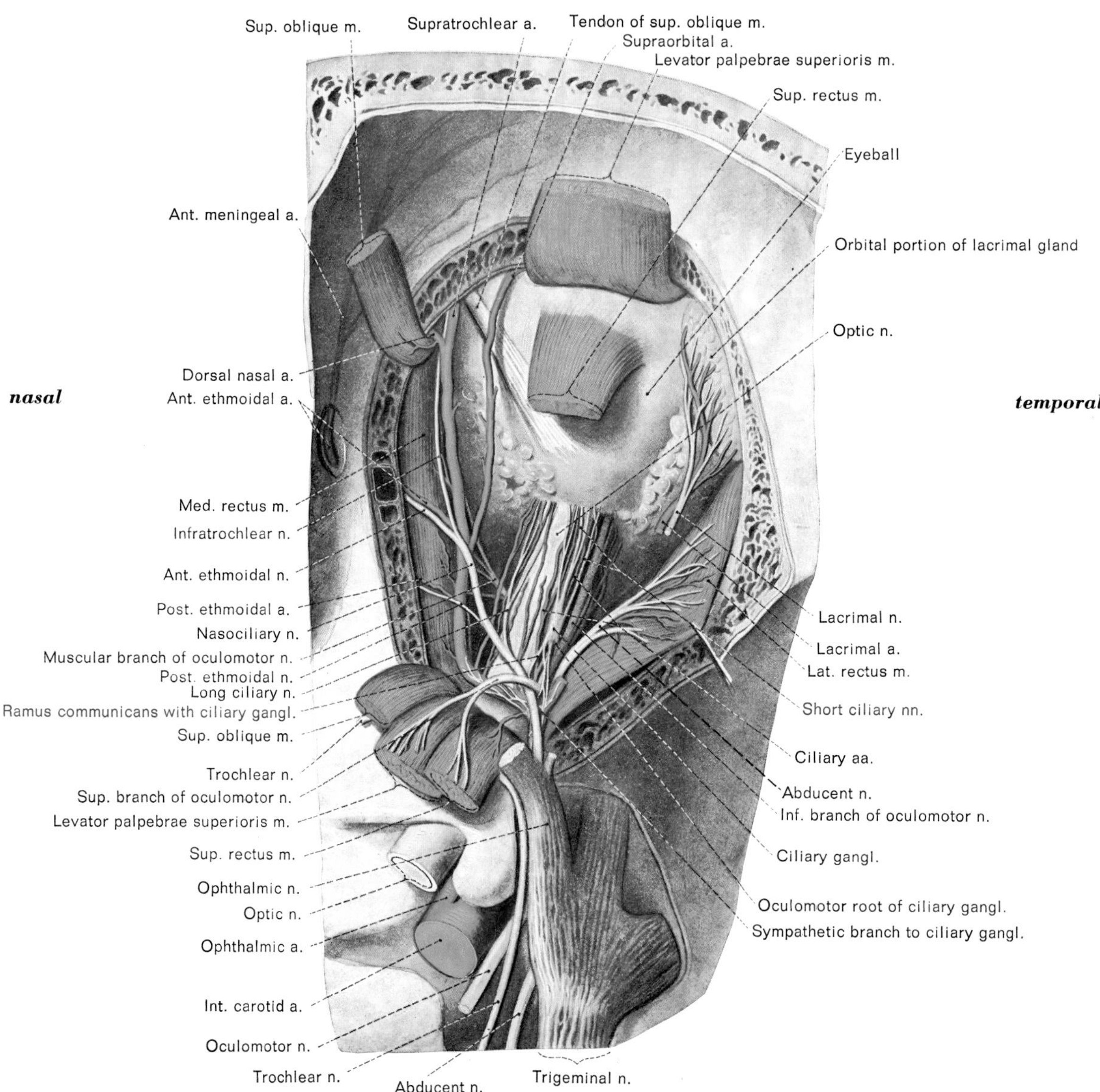
Sup. oblique m.
Supratrochlear a.
Tendon of sup. oblique m.
Supraorbital a.
Levator palpebrae superioris m.
Sup. rectus m.
Eyeball
Ant. meningeal a.
Orbital portion of lacrimal gland
Optic n.
Dorsal nasal a.
nasal
Ant. ethmoidal a.
temporal
Med. rectus m.
Infratrochlear n.
Ant. ethmoidal n.
Post. ethmoidal a.
Nasociliary n.
Muscular branch of oculomotor n.
Post. ethmoidal n.
Long ciliary n.
Ramus communicans with ciliary gangl.
Sup. oblique m.
Trochlear n.
Sup. branch of oculomotor n.
Levator palpebrae superioris m.
Sup. rectus m.
Ophthalmic n.
Optic n.
Ophthalmic a.
Int. carotid a.
Oculomotor n.
Trochlear n.
Abducent n.
Trigeminal n.
Lacrimal n.
Lacrimal a.
Lat. rectus m.
Short ciliary nn.
Ciliary aa.
Abducent n.
Inf. branch of oculomotor n.
Ciliary gangl.
Oculomotor root of ciliary gangl.
Sympathetic branch to ciliary gangl.

Fig. 318. Nerves and arteries of the right orbit, third layer. Preparation similar to the one in Fig. 317, but, in addition, the superior rectus, superior oblique and levator palpebrae superioris muscles have been sectioned and reflected.

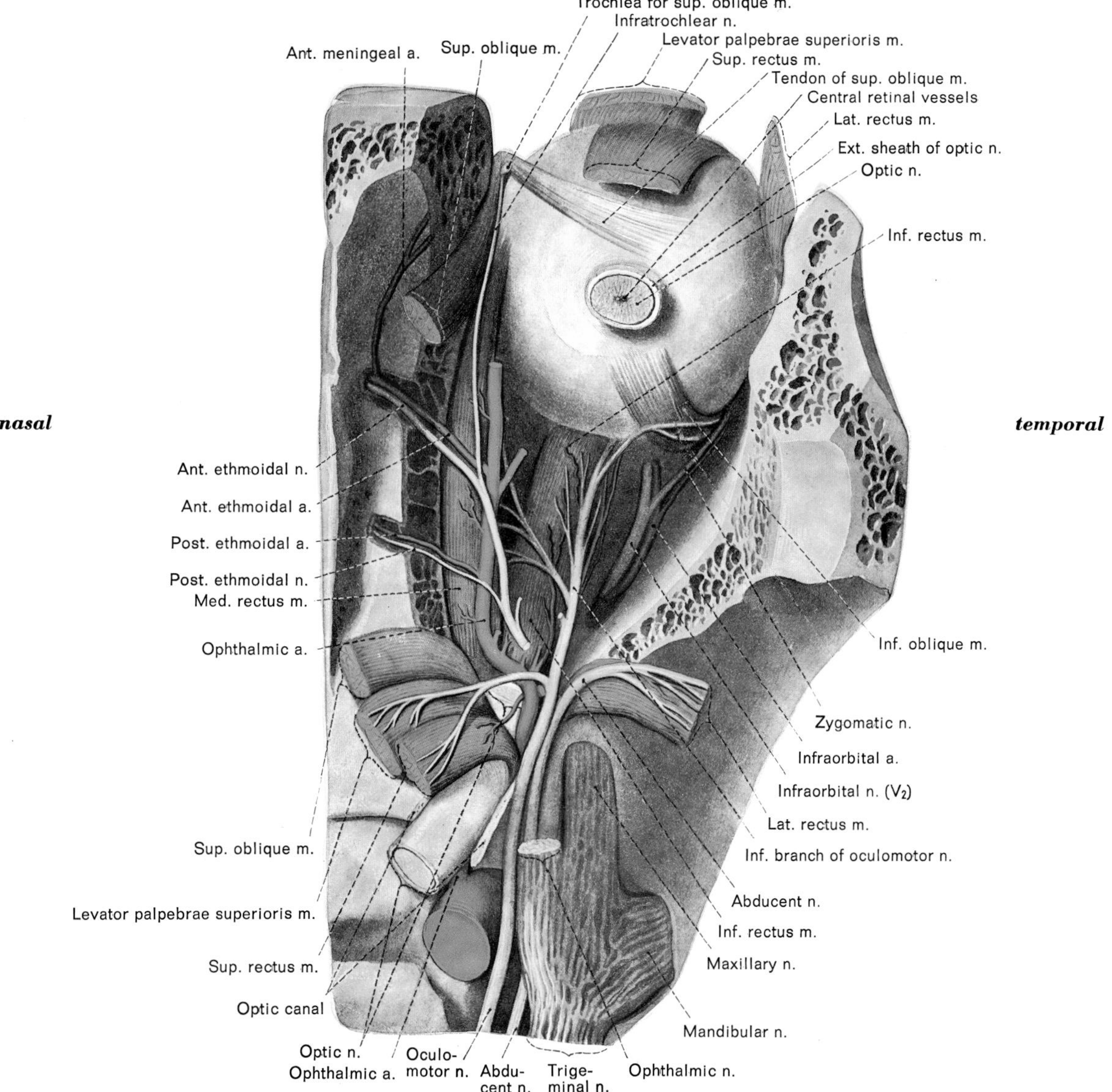
Trochlea for sup. oblique m.
Infratrochlear n.
Ant. meningeal a.
Sup. oblique m.
Levator palpebrae superioris m.
Sup. rectus m.
Tendon of sup. oblique m.
Central retinal vessels
Lat. rectus m.
Ext. sheath of optic n.
Optic n.
Inf. rectus m.
nasal
temporal
Ant. ethmoidal n.
Ant. ethmoidal a.
Post. ethmoidal a.
Post. ethmoidal n.
Med. rectus m.
Ophthalmic a.
Inf. oblique m.
Zygomatic n.
Infraorbital a.
Infraorbital n. (V2)
Lat. rectus m.
Inf. branch of oculomotor n.
Sup. oblique m.
Abducent n.
Levator palpebrae superioris m.
Inf. rectus m.
Sup. rectus m.
Maxillary n.
Optic canal
Mandibular n.
Optic n.
Ophthalmic a.
Oculo-motor n.
Abdu-cent n.
Trige-minal n.
Ophthalmic n.

Fig. 319. Nerves and arteries of the right orbit, fourth layer. Preparation similar to the one in Fig. 318, but the lateral rectus muscle, the optic nerve, and the ophthalmic artery have been sectioned additionally. The eyeball with the stump of the optic nerve has been rotated forward in order to expose the ramification of the lower branch of the oculomotor nerve. The optic canal as well as the anterior and posterior ethmoidal foramina have been opened.

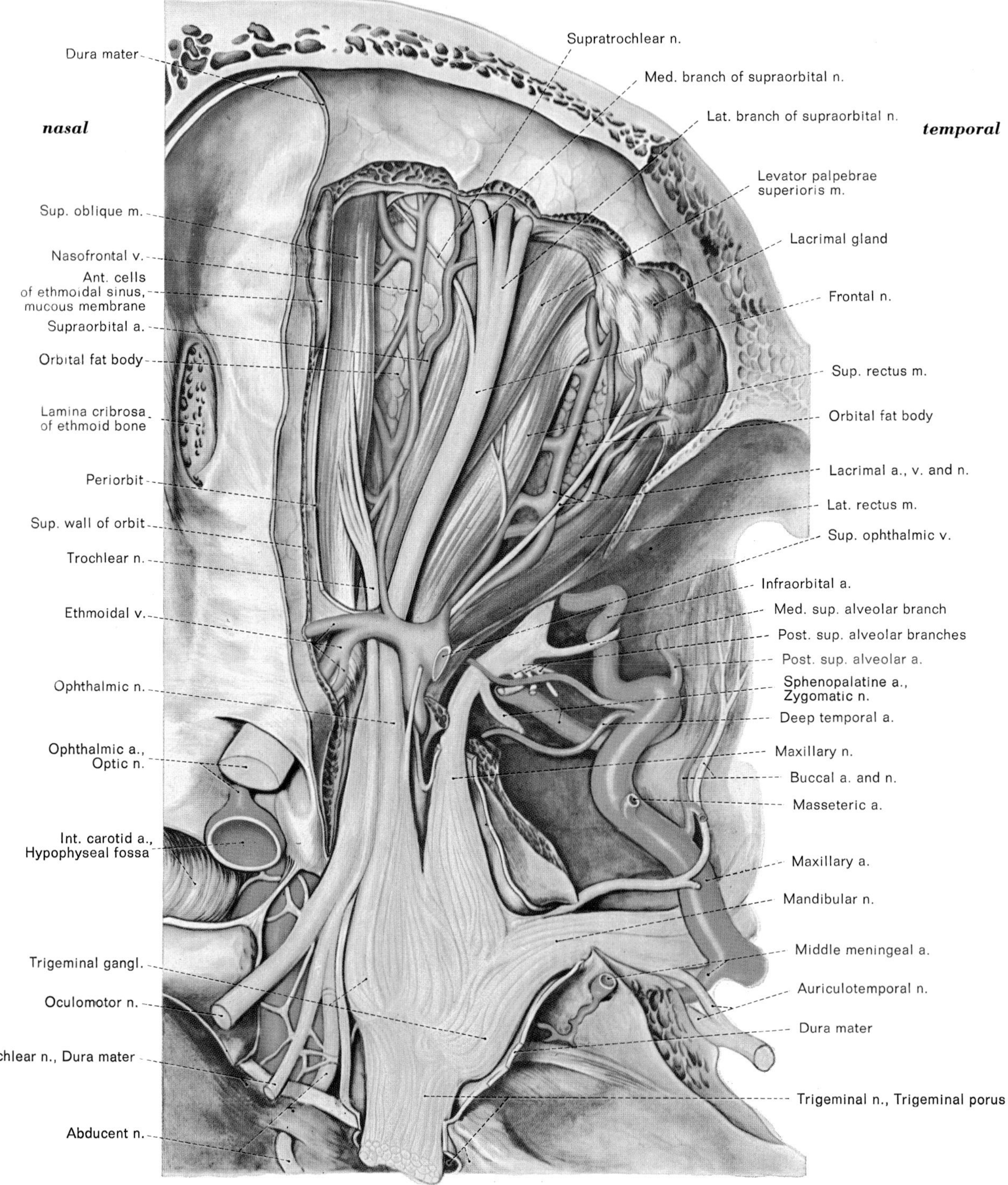
nasal
temporal
Dura mater
Supratrochlear n.
Med. branch of supraorbital n.
Lat. branch of supraorbital n.
Levator palpebrae superioris m.
Lacrimal gland
Frontal n.
Sup. rectus m.
Orbital fat body
Lacrimal a., v. and n.
Lat. rectus m.
Sup. ophthalmic v.
Infraorbital a.
Med. sup. alveolar branch
Post. sup. alveolar branches
Post. sup. alveolar a.
Sphenopalatine a., Zygomatic n.
Deep temporal a.
Maxillary n.
Buccal a. and n.
Masseteric a.
Maxillary a.
Mandibular n.
Middle meningeal a.
Auriculotemporal n.
Dura mater
Trigeminal n., Trigeminal porus
Sup. oblique m.
Nasofrontal v.
Ant. cells of ethmoidal sinus, mucous membrane
Supraorbital a.
Orbital fat body
Lamina cribrosa of ethmoid bone
Periorbit
Sup. wall of orbit
Trochlear n.
Ethmoidal v.
Ophthalmic n.
Ophthalmic a., Optic n.
Int. carotid a., Hypophyseal fossa
Trigeminal gangl.
Oculomotor n.
Trochlear n., Dura mater
Abducent n.

Fig. 320. Right orbit opened from above. The superior orbital wall and periorbit have been removed to expose the superficial layer. The trigeminal ganglion with its three main branches has been exposed by removal of the dural covering. The cavernous sinus with internal carotid artery, oculomotor, trochlear and abducent nerves has been opened. After partial removal of the bone in the area of the middle cranial fossa the infratemporal fossa with the maxillary artery has been exposed.

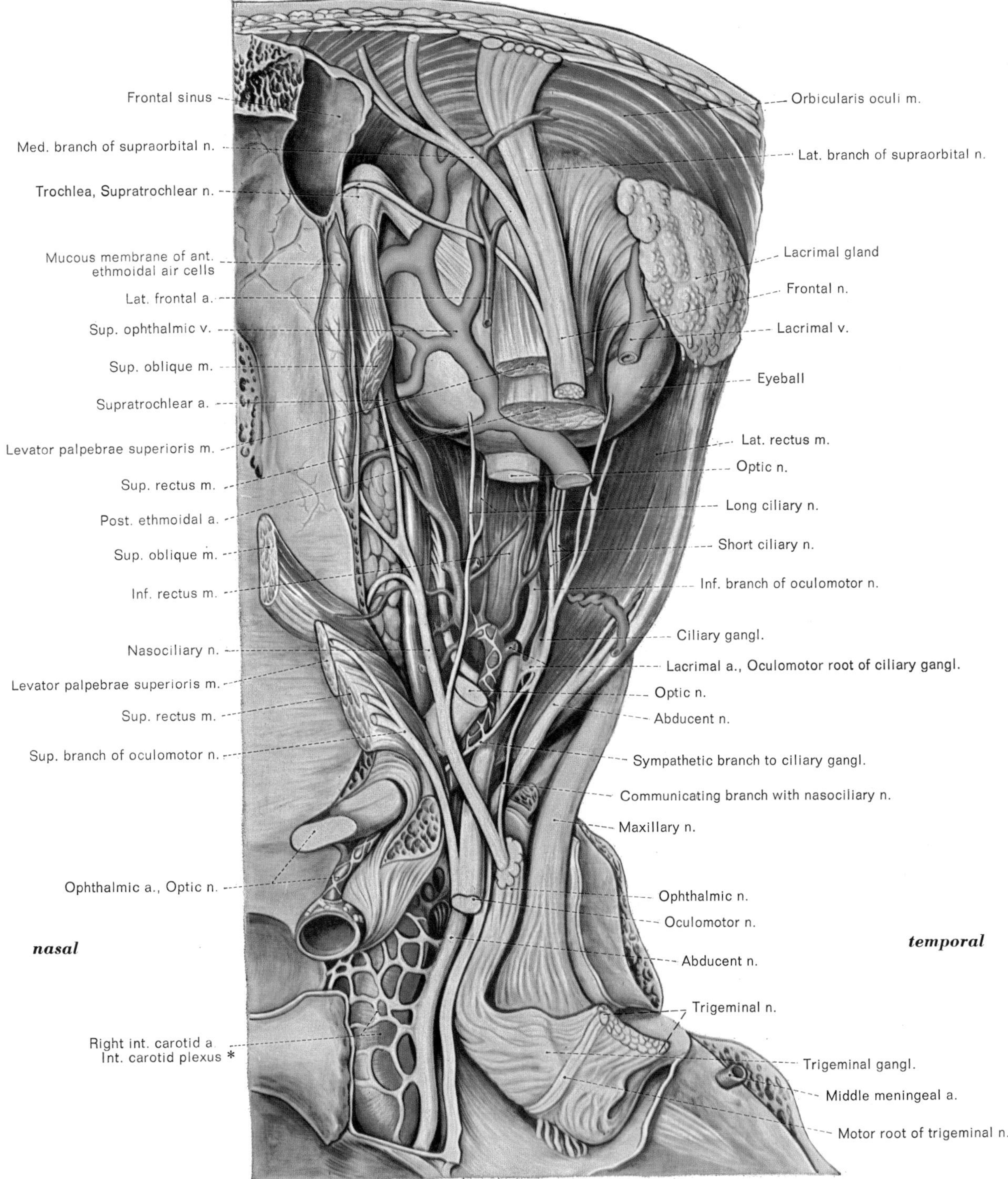
Frontal sinus
Med. branch of supraorbital n.
Trochlea, Supratrochlear n.
Mucous membrane of ant. ethmoidal air cells
Lat. frontal a.
Sup. ophthalmic v.
Sup. oblique m.
Supratrochlear a.
Levator palpebrae superioris m.
Sup. rectus m.
Post. ethmoidal a.
Sup. oblique m.
Inf. rectus m.
Nasociliary n.
Levator palpebrae superioris m.
Sup. rectus m.
Sup. branch of oculomotor n.
Ophthalmic a., Optic n.
nasal
Right int. carotid a.
Int. carotid plexus *
Orbicularis oculi m.
Lat. branch of supraorbital n.
Lacrimal gland
Frontal n.
Lacrimal v.
Eyeball
Lat. rectus m.
Optic n.
Long ciliary n.
Short ciliary n.
Inf. branch of oculomotor n.
Ciliary gangl.
Lacrimal a., Oculomotor root of ciliary gangl.
Optic n.
Abducent n.
Sympathetic branch to ciliary gangl.
Communicating branch with nasociliary n.
Maxillary n.
Ophthalmic n.
Oculomotor n.
temporal
Abducent n.
Trigeminal n.
Trigeminal gangl.
Middle meningeal a.
Motor root of trigeminal n.

Fig. 321. Right orbit, opened from above. The superior orbital wall and the frontal squama have been removed to expose the ramification of the first trigeminal branch. Trigeminal nerve and ganglion have been elevated.
* = sympathetic fiber bundles from the internal carotid plexus within the cavernous sinus connecting to the abducent nerve.

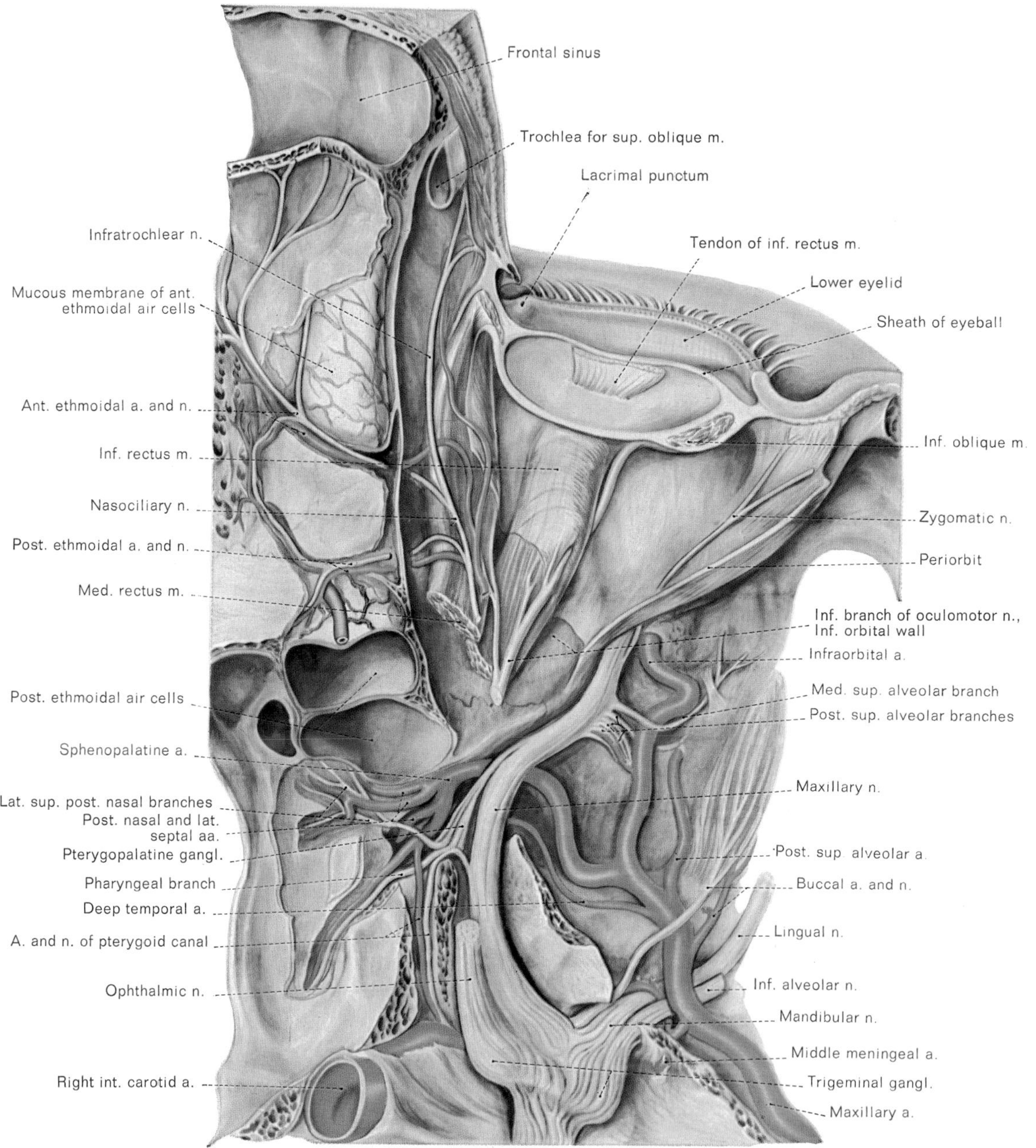

Frontal sinus
Trochlea for sup. oblique m.
Lacrimal punctum
Infratrochlear n.
Tendon of inf. rectus m.
Lower eyelid
Mucous membrane of ant. ethmoidal air cells
Sheath of eyeball
Ant. ethmoidal a. and n.
Inf. oblique m.
Inf. rectus m.
Nasociliary n.
Zygomatic n.
Post. ethmoidal a. and n.
Periorbit
Med. rectus m.
Inf. branch of oculomotor n.,
Inf. orbital wall
Infraorbital a.
Post. ethmoidal air cells
Med. sup. alveolar branch
Post. sup. alveolar branches
Sphenopalatine a.
Maxillary n.
Lat. sup. post. nasal branches
Post. nasal and lat. septal aa.
Pterygopalatine gangl.
Post. sup. alveolar a.
Pharyngeal branch
Buccal a. and n.
Deep temporal a.
A. and n. of pterygoid canal
Lingual n.
Ophthalmic n.
Inf. alveolar n.
Mandibular n.
Middle meningeal a.
Right int. carotid a.
Trigeminal gangl.
Maxillary a.

Fig. 322. Floor of the right orbit after removal of the eyeball and optic nerve as well as the extrinsic ocular muscles with the exception of the medial and inferior rectus muscles. After partial removal of the cranial base the infratemporal fossa with the maxillary artery has been exposed. The posterior ethmoidal cells have been opened and the anterior and posterior ethmoidal arteries and nerves have been displayed.

Fig. 323. Connection between zygomatic and lacrimal nerves in the orbit. The orbit is opened from medial and its contents have been removed with the exception of the lacrimal gland and the nerves mentioned. ▶

Fig. 324. Right orbit opened from lateral to show the position and connections of the ciliary ganglion. Lateral rectus, superior rectus and levator palpebrae superioris muscles have been partially removed.

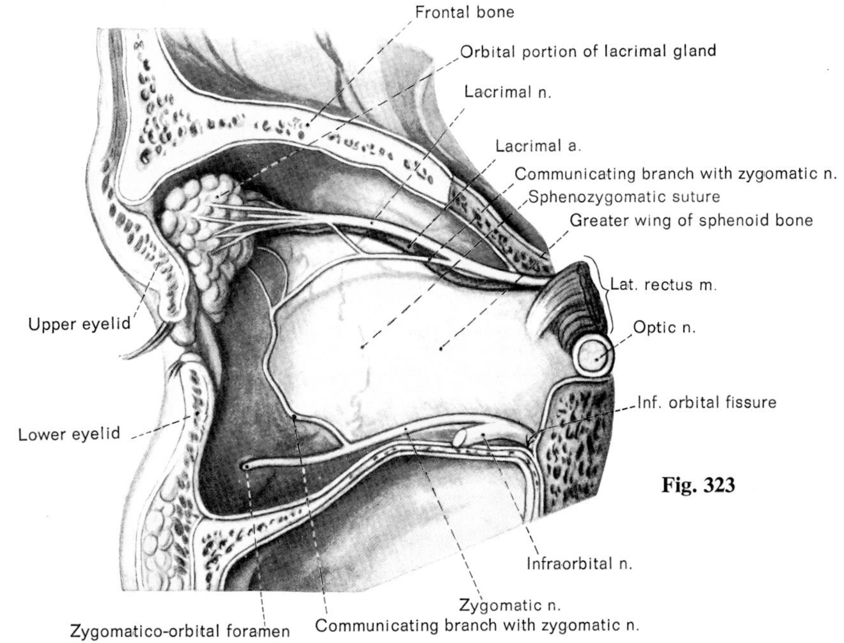
Frontal bone
Orbital portion of lacrimal gland
Lacrimal n.
Lacrimal a.
Communicating branch with zygomatic n.
Sphenozygomatic suture
Greater wing of sphenoid bone
Lat. rectus m.
Optic n.
Upper eyelid
Inf. orbital fissure
Lower eyelid
Infraorbital n.
Zygomatic n.
Zygomatico-orbital foramen
Communicating branch with zygomatic n.

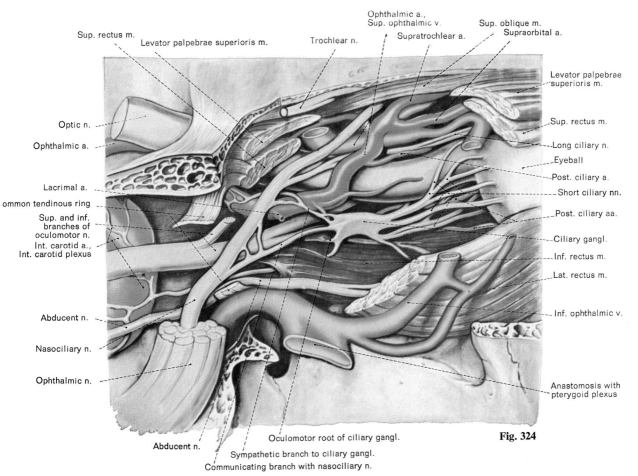

Fig. 323

Ophthalmic a.,
Sup. ophthalmic v.
Sup. oblique m.
Supraorbital a.
Sup. rectus m.
Supratrochlear a.
Levator palpebrae superioris m.
Trochlear n.
Levator palpebrae superioris m.
Optic n.
Sup. rectus m.
Ophthalmic a.
Long ciliary n.
Eyeball
Post. ciliary a.
Lacrimal a.
Short ciliary nn.
ommon tendinous ring
Post. ciliary aa.
Sup. and inf. branches of oculomotor n.
Ciliary gangl.
Int. carotid a., Int. carotid plexus
Inf. rectus m.
Lat. rectus m.
Abducent n.
Inf. ophthalmic v.
Nasociliary n.
Ophthalmic n.
Anastomosis with pterygoid plexus
Oculomotor root of ciliary gangl.
Abducent n.
Sympathetic branch to ciliary gangl.
Communicating branch with nasociliary n.

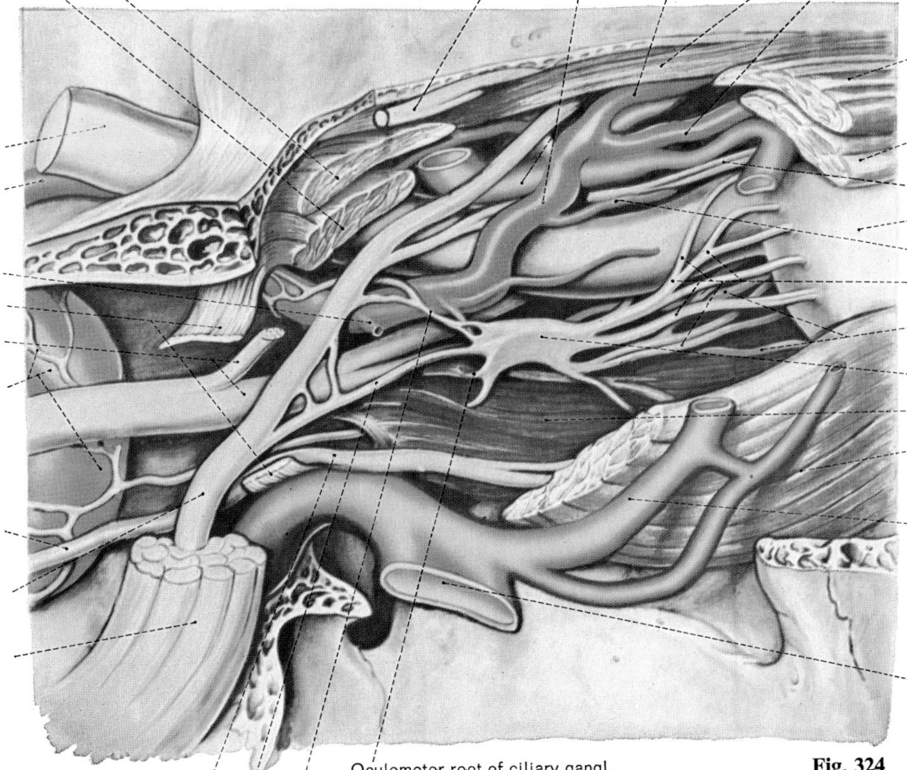

Fig. 324

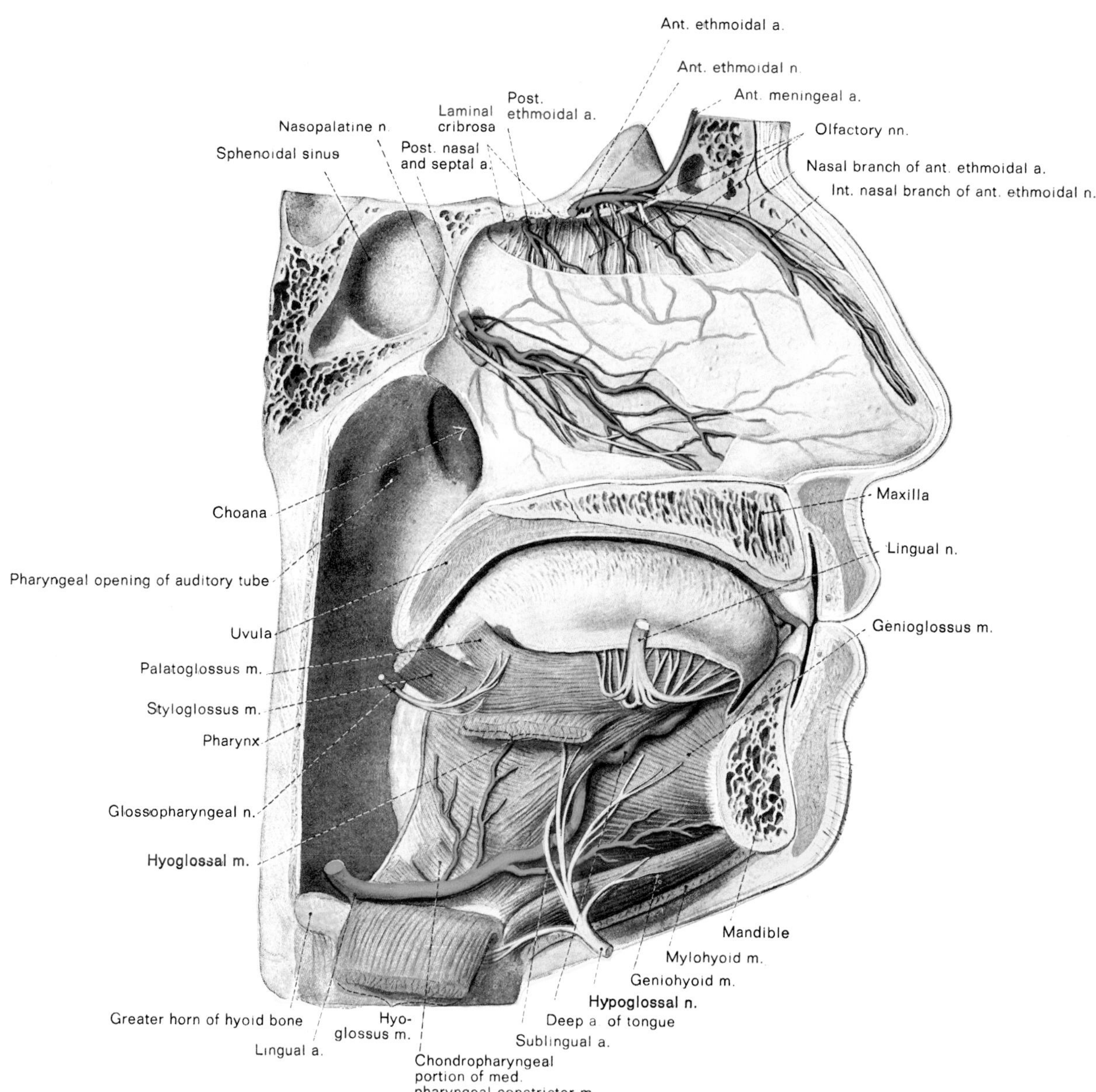
Ant. ethmoidal a.
Ant. ethmoidal n.
Ant. meningeal a.
Post. ethmoidal a.
Laminal cribrosa
Nasopalatine n.
Sphenoidal sinus
Post. nasal and septal a.
Olfactory nn.
Nasal branch of ant. ethmoidal a.
Int. nasal branch of ant. ethmoidal n.
Choana
Pharyngeal opening of auditory tube
Uvula
Palatoglossus m.
Styloglossus m.
Pharynx
Glossopharyngeal n.
Hyoglossal m.
Maxilla
Lingual n.
Genioglossus m.
Mandible
Mylohyoid m.
Geniohyoid m.
Hypoglossal n.
Deep a. of tongue
Sublingual a.
Greater horn of hyoid bone
Lingual a.
Hyo-glossus m.
Chondropharyngeal portion of med. pharyngeal constrictor m.

Fig. 325. Nerves and arteries of nasal septum and tongue.

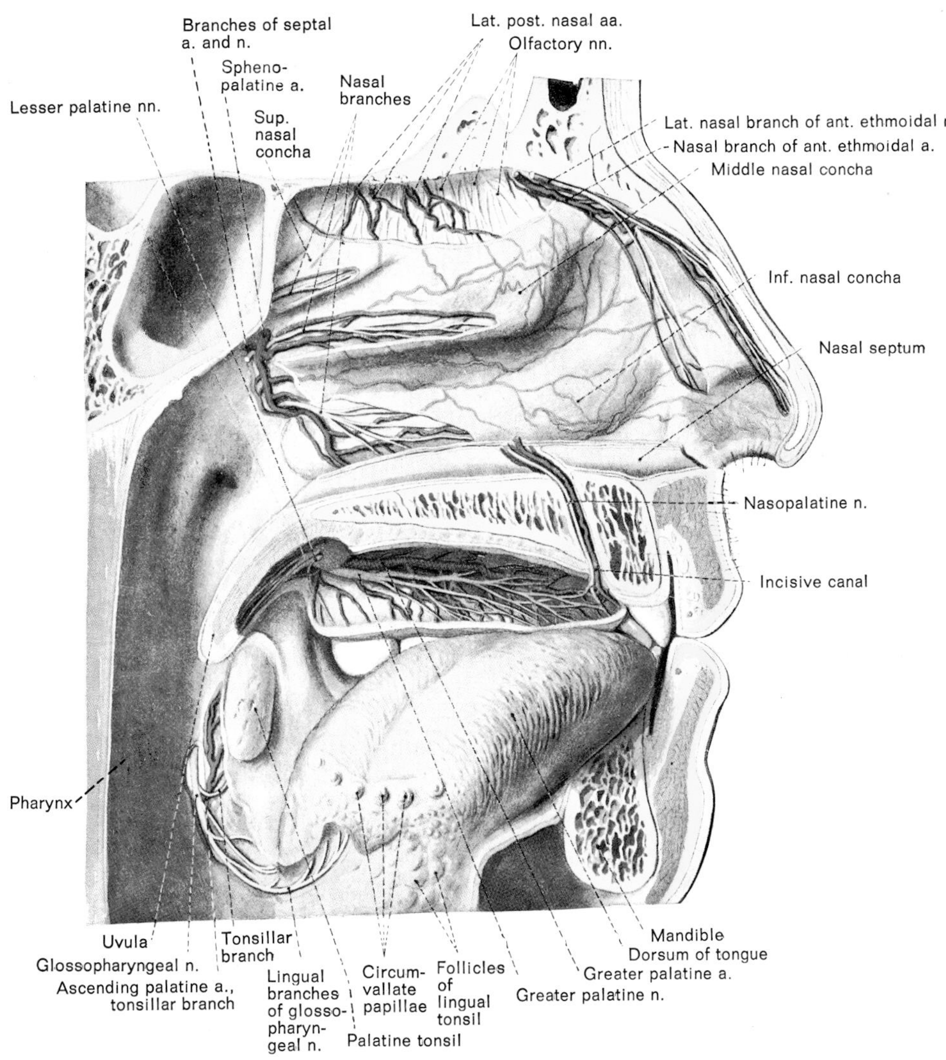
Branches of septal a. and n.
Spheno-palatine a.
Nasal branches
Lat. post. nasal aa.
Olfactory nn.
Lesser palatine nn.
Sup. nasal concha
Lat. nasal branch of ant. ethmoidal n.
Nasal branch of ant. ethmoidal a.
Middle nasal concha
Inf. nasal concha
Nasal septum
Nasopalatine n.
Incisive canal
Pharynx
Uvula
Glossopharyngeal n.
Ascending palatine a., tonsillar branch
Tonsillar branch
Lingual branches of glosso-pharyn-geal n.
Circum-vallate papillae
Palatine tonsil
Follicles of lingual tonsil
Greater palatine n.
Greater palatine a.
Dorsum of tongue
Mandible

Fig. 326. Nerves and arteries of lateral nasal wall and palate, superficial layer. The root of the tongue is pulled forward; the nasal septum has been removed with the exception of its lower portion; the mucous membrane of the isthmus of the fauces has been split along the glossopharyngeal nerve and the ascending palatine artery.

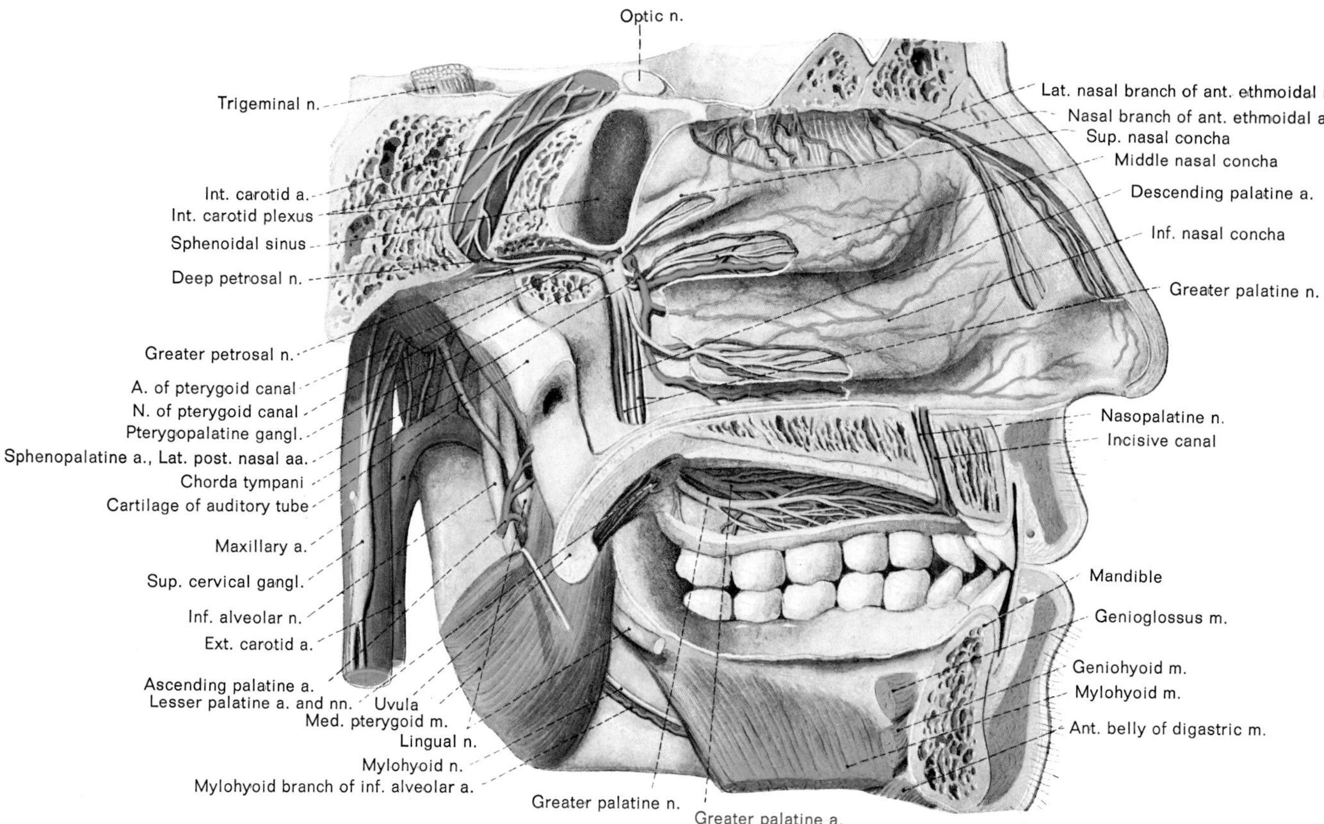
Optic n.
Trigeminal n.
Int. carotid a.
Int. carotid plexus
Sphenoidal sinus
Deep petrosal n.
Greater petrosal n.
A. of pterygoid canal
N. of pterygoid canal
Pterygopalatine gangl.
Sphenopalatine a., Lat. post. nasal aa.
Chorda tympani
Cartilage of auditory tube
Maxillary a.
Sup. cervical gangl.
Inf. alveolar n.
Ext. carotid a.
Ascending palatine a.
Lesser palatine a. and nn.
Uvula
Med. pterygoid m.
Lingual n.
Mylohyoid n.
Mylohyoid branch of inf. alveolar a.
Greater palatine n.
Greater palatine a.
Lat. nasal branch of ant. ethmoidal n
Nasal branch of ant. ethmoidal a.
Sup. nasal concha
Middle nasal concha
Descending palatine a.
Inf. nasal concha
Greater palatine n.
Nasopalatine n.
Incisive canal
Mandible
Genioglossus m.
Geniohyoid m.
Mylohyoid m.
Ant. belly of digastric m.

Fig. 327. Nerves and arteries of the lateral nasal wall, deeper layer, pterygopalatine ganglion. The carotid, pterygopalatine and pterygoid canals have been opened; the temporal bone has been sectioned obliquely; the tongue has been removed.

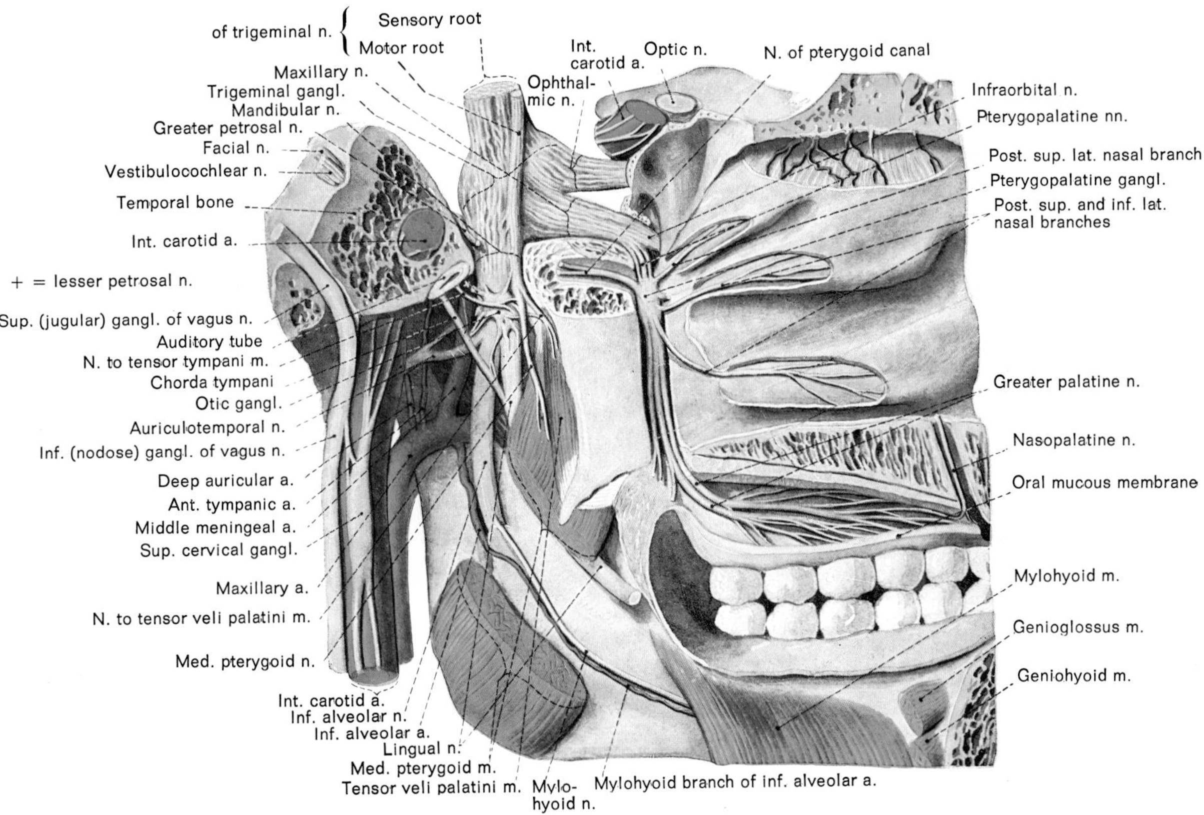
of trigeminal n.
Sensory root
Motor root
Maxillary n.
Trigeminal gangl.
Mandibular n.
Greater petrosal n.
Facial n.
Vestibulocochlear n.
Temporal bone
Int. carotid a.
+ = lesser petrosal n.
Sup. (jugular) gangl. of vagus n.
Auditory tube
N. to tensor tympani m.
Chorda tympani
Otic gangl.
Auriculotemporal n.
Inf. (nodose) gangl. of vagus n.
Deep auricular a.
Ant. tympanic a.
Middle meningeal a.
Sup. cervical gangl.
Maxillary a.
N. to tensor veli palatini m.
Med. pterygoid n.
Int. carotid a.
Inf. alveolar n.
Inf. alveolar a.
Lingual n.
Med. pterygoid m.
Tensor veli palatini m.
Mylo-hyoid n.
Mylohyoid branch of inf. alveolar a.
Int. carotid a.
Optic n.
Ophthal-mic n.
N. of pterygoid canal
Infraorbital n.
Pterygopalatine nn.
Post. sup. lat. nasal branch
Pterygopalatine gangl.
Post. sup. and inf. lat. nasal branches
Greater palatine n.
Nasopalatine n.
Oral mucous membrane
Mylohyoid m.
Genioglossus m.
Geniohyoid m.

Fig. 328. Trigeminal, otic and pterygopalatine ganglia. Nasal and palatine branches of maxillary nerve. Preparation similar to the one in Fig. 327, but the major part of the body of the sphenoid bone has been removed; the oval and greater palatine foramina have been opened; the temporal bone has been sectioned.

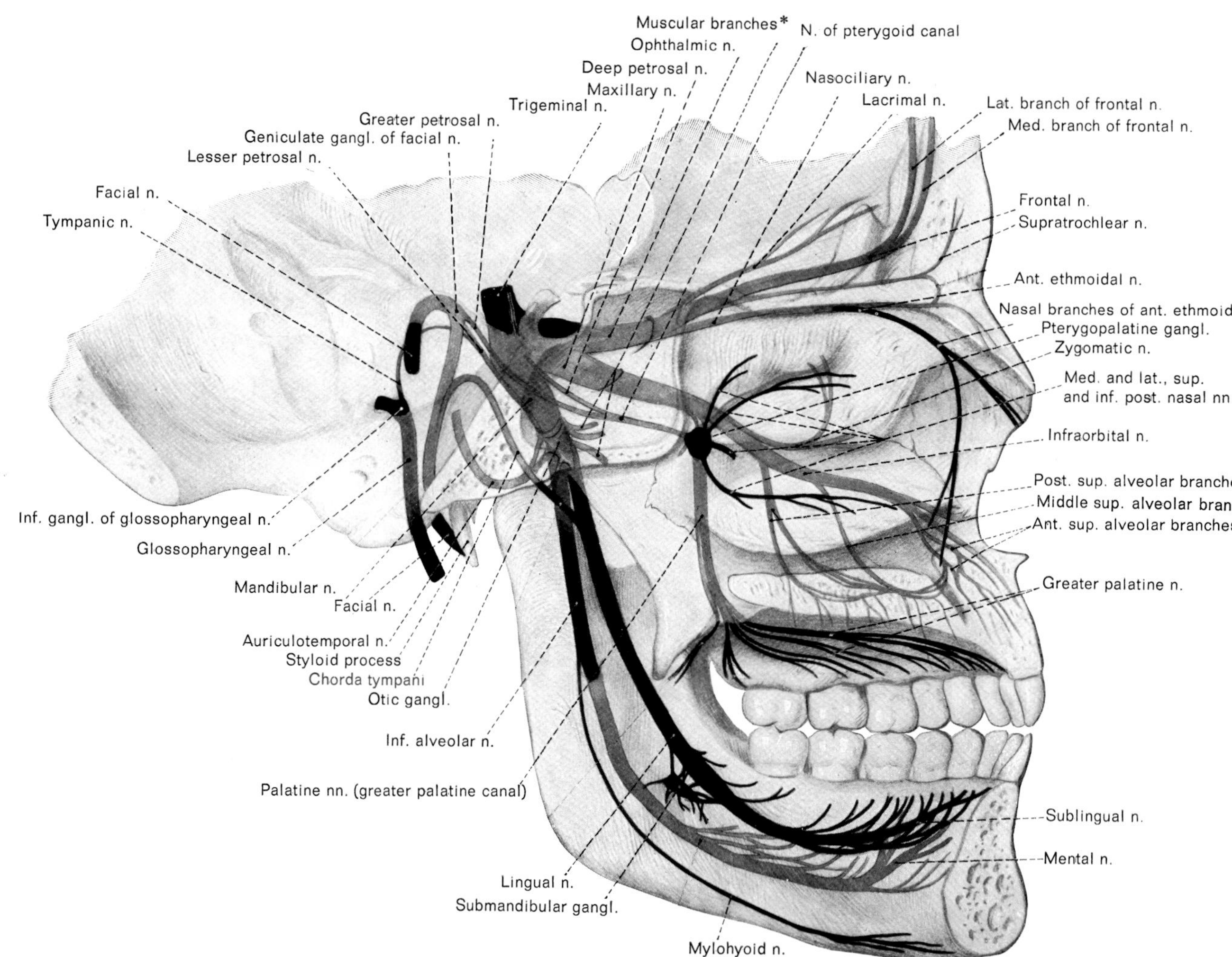

Muscular branches*
N. of pterygoid canal
Ophthalmic n.
Deep petrosal n.
Nasociliary n.
Maxillary n.
Lacrimal n.
Trigeminal n.
Lat. branch of frontal n.
Med. branch of frontal n.
Greater petrosal n.
Geniculate gangl. of facial n.
Lesser petrosal n.
Facial n.
Frontal n.
Tympanic n.
Supratrochlear n.
Ant. ethmoidal n.
Nasal branches of ant. ethmoidal
Pterygopalatine gangl.
Zygomatic n.
Med. and lat., sup. and inf. post. nasal nn.
Infraorbital n.
Post. sup. alveolar branches
Middle sup. alveolar branc
Inf. gangl. of glossopharyngeal n.
Ant. sup. alveolar branches
Glossopharyngeal n.
Mandibular n.
Greater palatine n.
Facial n.
Auriculotemporal n.
Styloid process
Chorda tympani
Otic gangl.
Inf. alveolar n.
Palatine nn. (greater palatine canal)
Sublingual n.
Mental n.
Lingual n.
Submandibular gangl.
Mylohyoid n.

Fig. 329. Diagram of the ramifications of the trigeminal nerve and its connections with the facial and glossopharyngeal nerves (projected onto a median section of the skull). Black: exposed portions of nerves, gray: portions covered by bone. * = previously called masticatory nerve.

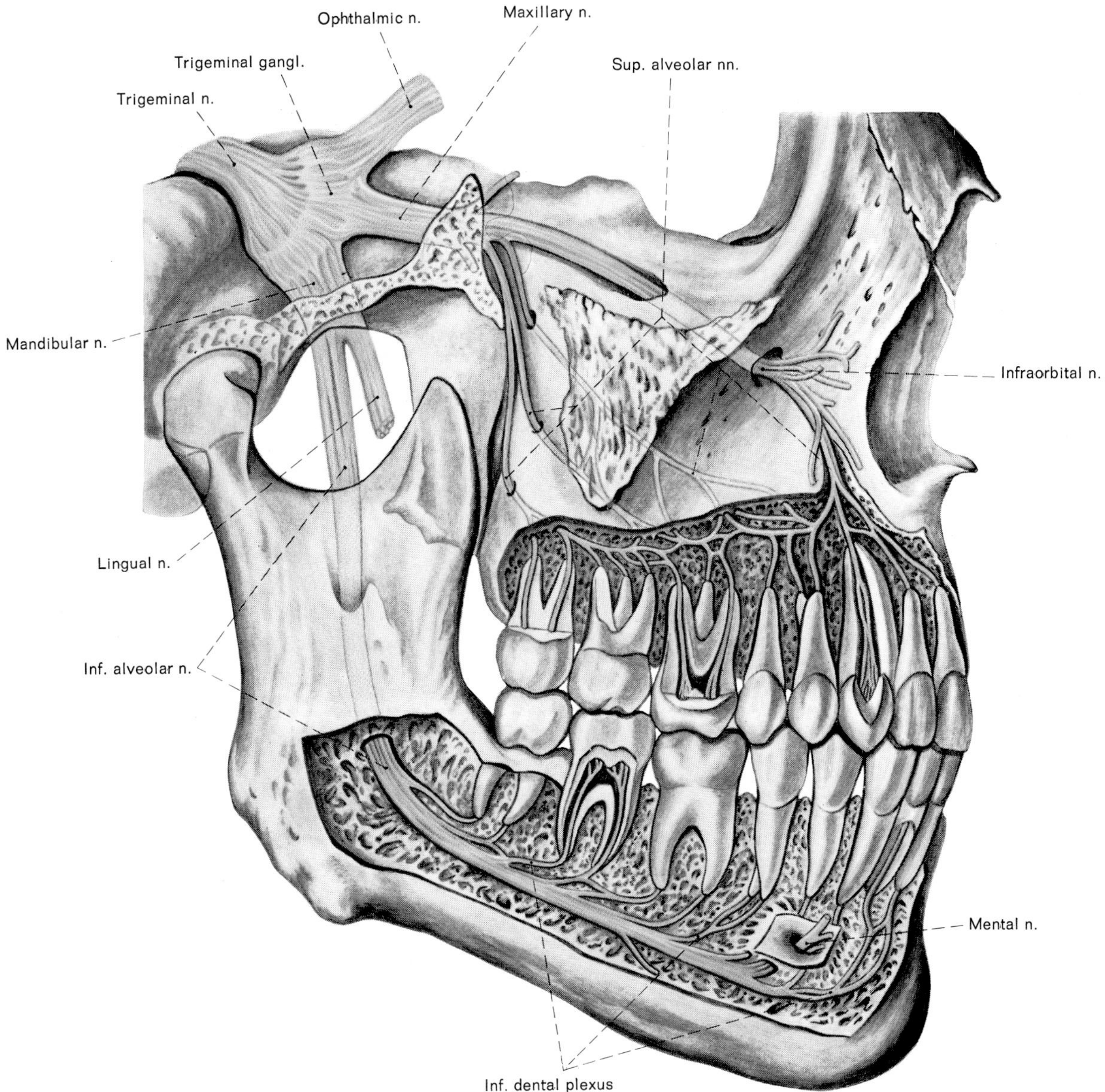
Ophthalmic n.
Maxillary n.
Trigeminal gangl.
Sup. alveolar nn.
Trigeminal n.
Mandibular n.
Infraorbital n.
Lingual n.
Inf. alveolar n.
Mental n.
Inf. dental plexus

Fig. 330. Innervation of the teeth by the second and third branch of the trigeminal nerve.

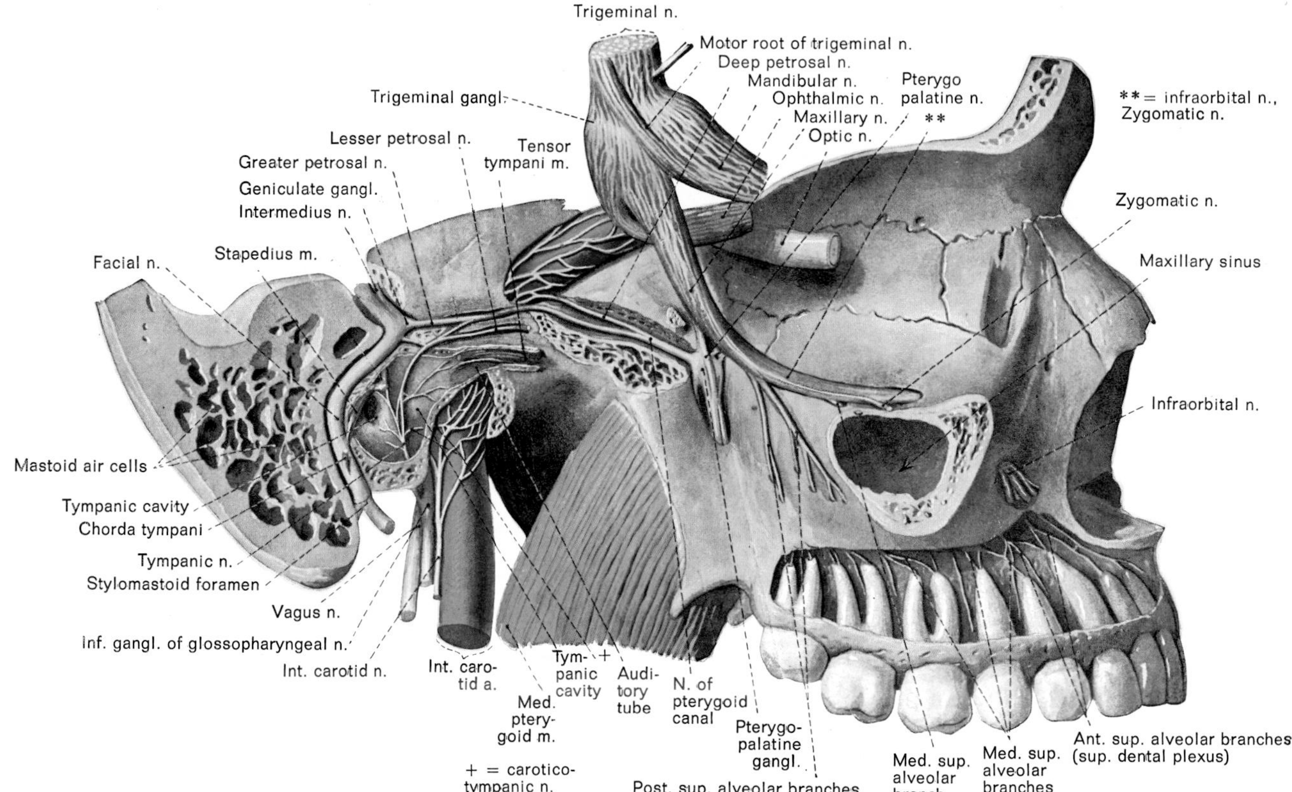
Trigeminal n.
Motor root of trigeminal n.
Deep petrosal n.
Mandibular n.
Pterygo palatine n.
Ophthalmic n.
Maxillary n.
**
Optic n.
** = infraorbital n., Zygomatic n.
Trigeminal gangl.
Lesser petrosal n.
Tensor tympani m.
Greater petrosal n.
Geniculate gangl.
Intermedius n.
Zygomatic n.
Facial n.
Stapedius m.
Maxillary sinus
Infraorbital n.
Mastoid air cells
Tympanic cavity
Chorda tympani
Tympanic n.
Stylomastoid foramen
Vagus n.
Inf. gangl. of glossopharyngeal n.
Int. carotid n.
Int. carotid a.
Tympanic cavity
+
Med. pterygoid m.
Auditory tube
N. of pterygoid canal
Pterygopalatine gangl.
+ = caroticotympanic n.
Post. sup. alveolar branches
Med. sup. alveolar branch
Med. sup. alveolar branches
Ant. sup. alveolar branches (sup. dental plexus)

Fig. 331. Maxillary nerve, pterygopalatine ganglion, intracranial portion of facial nerve and tympanic nerve. The orbit has been opened laterally and its contents have been removed. The pterygoid canal, tympanic cavity and facial canals have been opened, the temporal bone has been sectioned obliquely and the trigeminal ganglion has been pulled upward. The labyrinthine wall of the tympanic cavity is exposed.

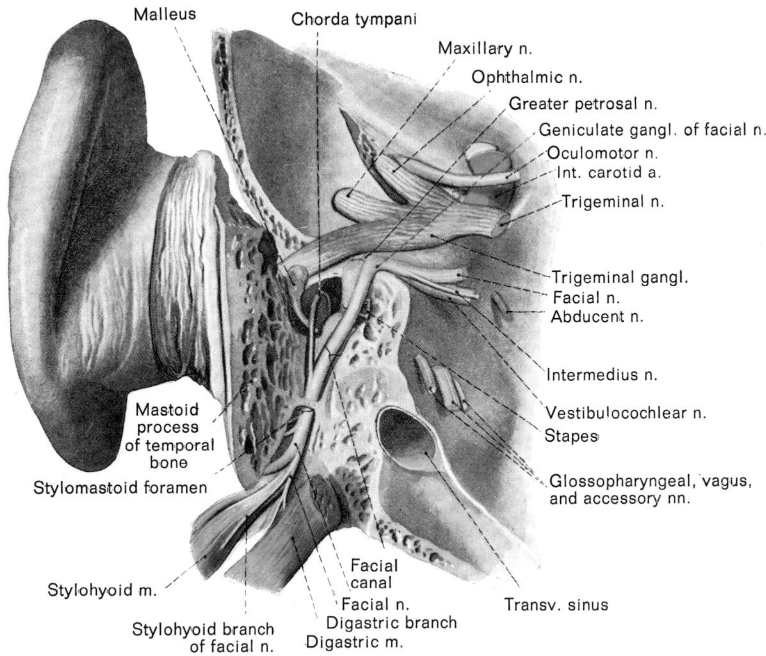
Malleus
Chorda tympani
Maxillary n.
Ophthalmic n.
Greater petrosal n.
Geniculate gangl. of facial n.
Oculomotor n.
Int. carotid a.
Trigeminal n.
Trigeminal gangl.
Facial n.
Abducent n.
Intermedius n.
Vestibulocochlear n.
Stapes
Glossopharyngeal, vagus, and accessory nn.
Mastoid process of temporal bone
Stylomastoid foramen
Stylohyoid m.
Facial canal
Facial n.
Transv. sinus
Stylohyoid branch of facial n.
Digastric branch
Digastric m.

Fig. 332. Intracranial extent of facial nerve. Facial canal and tympanic cavity have been opened from behind.

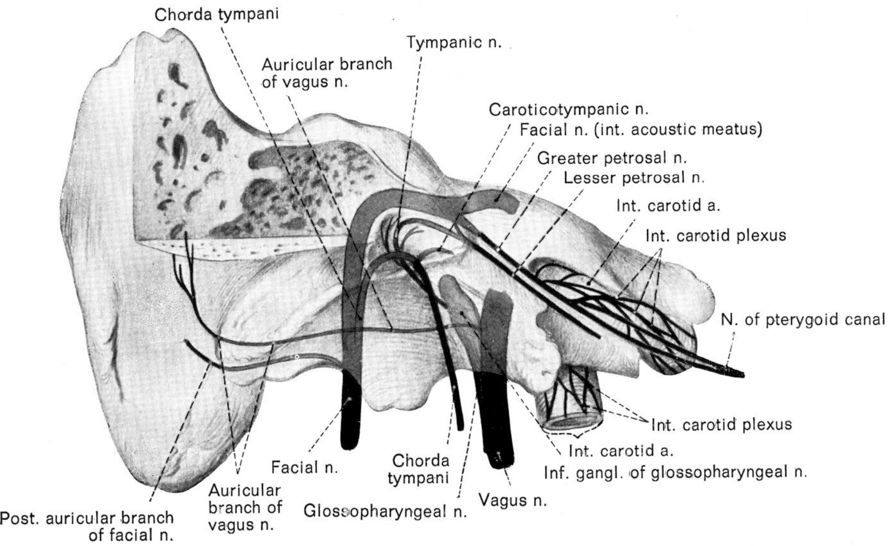
Chorda tympani
Tympanic n.
Auricular branch of vagus n.
Caroticotympanic n.
Facial n. (int. acoustic meatus)
Greater petrosal n.
Lesser petrosal n.
Int. carotid a.
Int. carotid plexus
N. of pterygoid canal
Int. carotid plexus
Int. carotid a.
Inf. gangl. of glossopharyngeal n.
Facial n.
Chorda tympani
Vagus n.
Auricular branch of vagus n.
Glossopharyngeal n.
Post. auricular branch of facial n.

Fig. 333. Intracranial course of the facial nerve and its connections, projected onto the temporal bone (compare with Fig. 83, *Sobotta-Figge,* vol. 1, 9th edition).

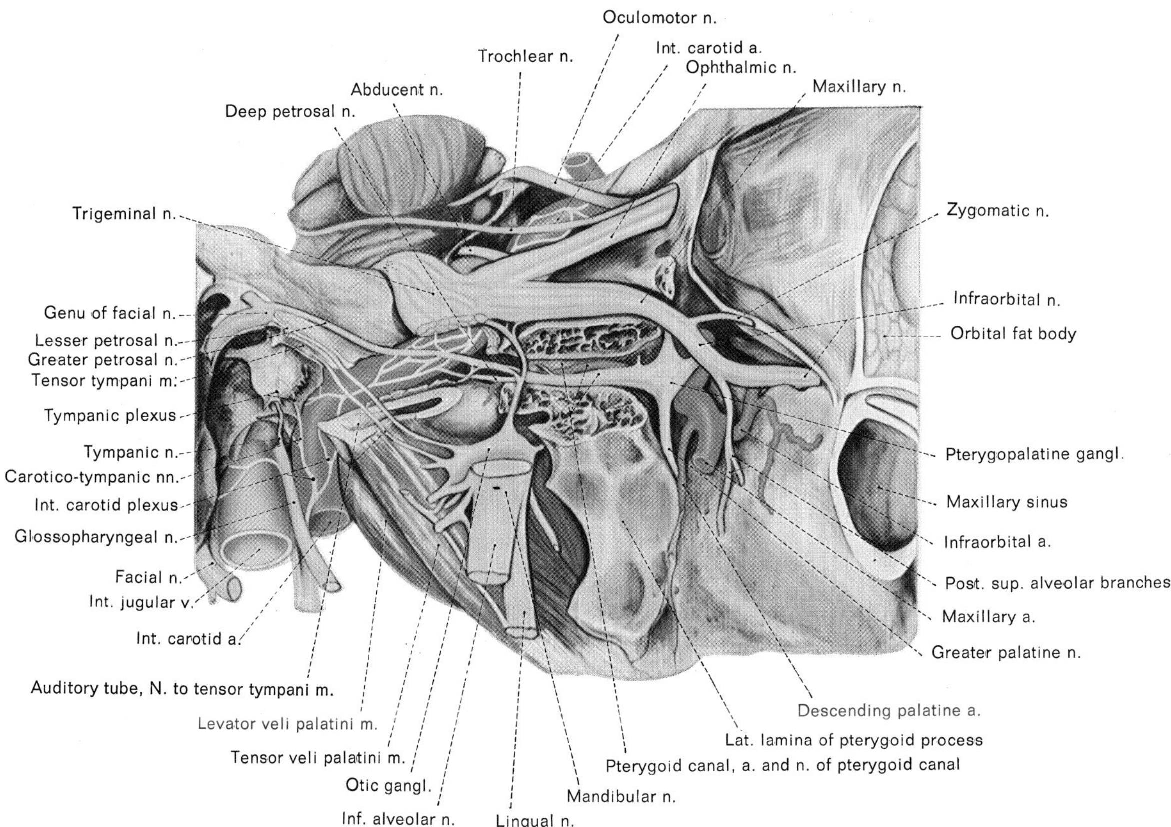
Oculomotor n.
Int. carotid a.
Ophthalmic n.
Trochlear n.
Maxillary n.
Abducent n.
Deep petrosal n.
Trigeminal n.
Zygomatic n.
Infraorbital n.
Genu of facial n.
Orbital fat body
Lesser petrosal n.
Greater petrosal n.
Tensor tympani m.
Tympanic plexus
Tympanic n.
Pterygopalatine gangl.
Carotico-tympanic nn.
Int. carotid plexus
Maxillary sinus
Glossopharyngeal n.
Infraorbital a.
Facial n.
Int. jugular v.
Post. sup. alveolar branches
Maxillary a.
Int. carotid a.
Greater palatine n.
Auditory tube, N. to tensor tympani m.
Descending palatine a.
Levator veli palatini m.
Lat. lamina of pterygoid process
Tensor veli palatini m.
Pterygoid canal, a. and n. of pterygoid canal
Otic gangl.
Mandibular n.
Inf. alveolar n.
Lingual n.

Fig. 334. Middle cranial fossa and pterygo-palatine fossa; trigeminal, pterygopalatine, and otic ganglia and their connections. The pterygoid canal has been opened. Lateral view.

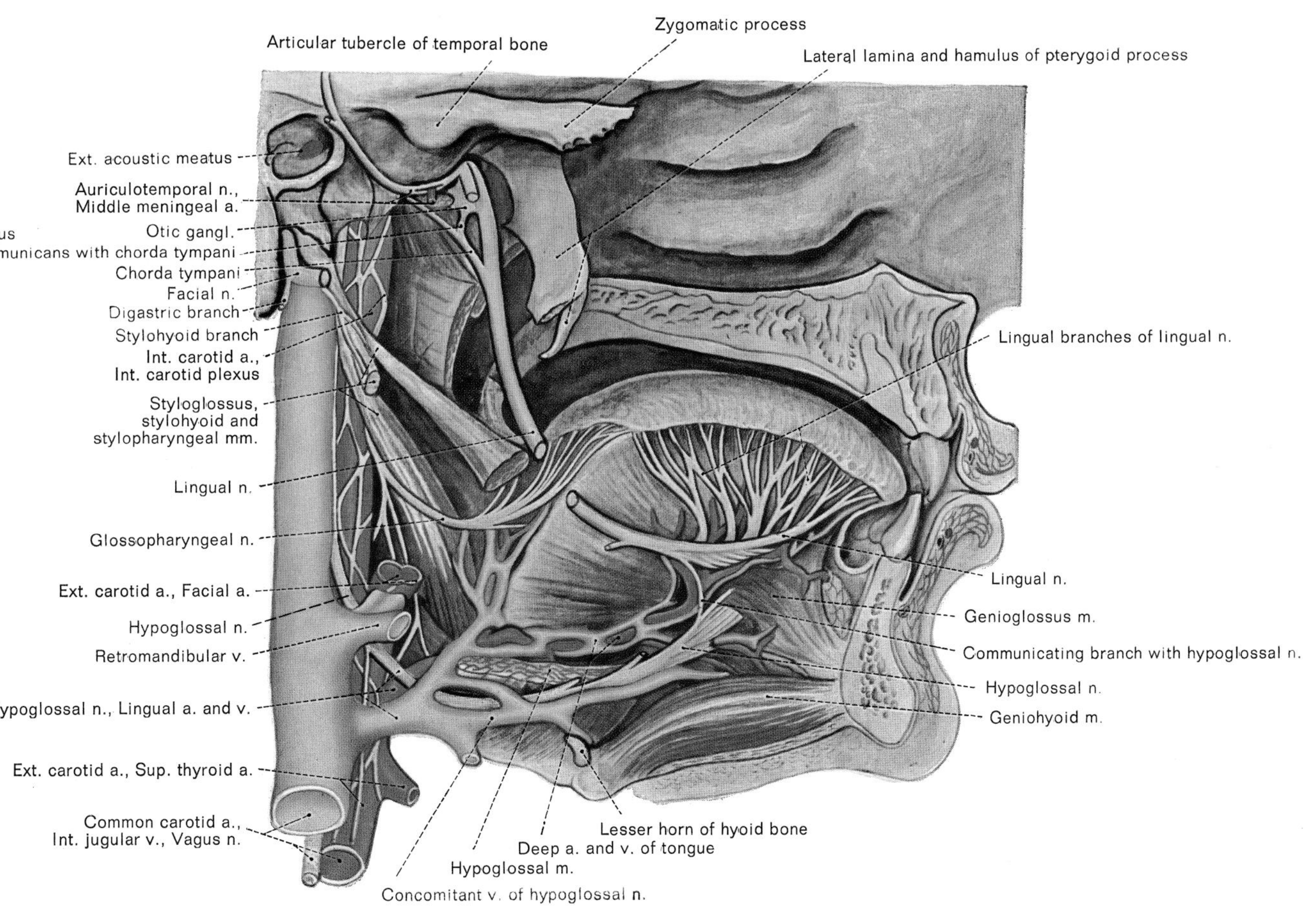
Zygomatic process
Articular tubercle of temporal bone
Lateral lamina and hamulus of pterygoid process
Ext. acoustic meatus
Auriculotemporal n.,
Middle meningeal a.
mus
Otic gangl.
mmunicans with chorda tympani
Chorda tympani
Facial n.
Digastric branch
Stylohyoid branch
Int. carotid a.,
Int. carotid plexus
Lingual branches of lingual n.
Styloglossus,
stylohyoid and
stylopharyngeal mm.
Lingual n.
Glossopharyngeal n.
Lingual n.
Ext. carotid a., Facial a.
Genioglossus m.
Hypoglossal n.
Communicating branch with hypoglossal n.
Retromandibular v.
Hypoglossal n.
Hypoglossal n., Lingual a. and v.
Geniohyoid m.
Ext. carotid a., Sup. thyroid a.
Common carotid a.,
Int. jugular v., Vagus n.
Lesser horn of hyoid bone
Deep a. and v. of tongue
Hypoglossal m.
Concomitant v. of hypoglossal n.

Fig. 335. Nerves and vessels of the tongue; otic ganglion, chorda tympani. Mucous membrane and muscles of tongue as well as mandible have been partially removed.

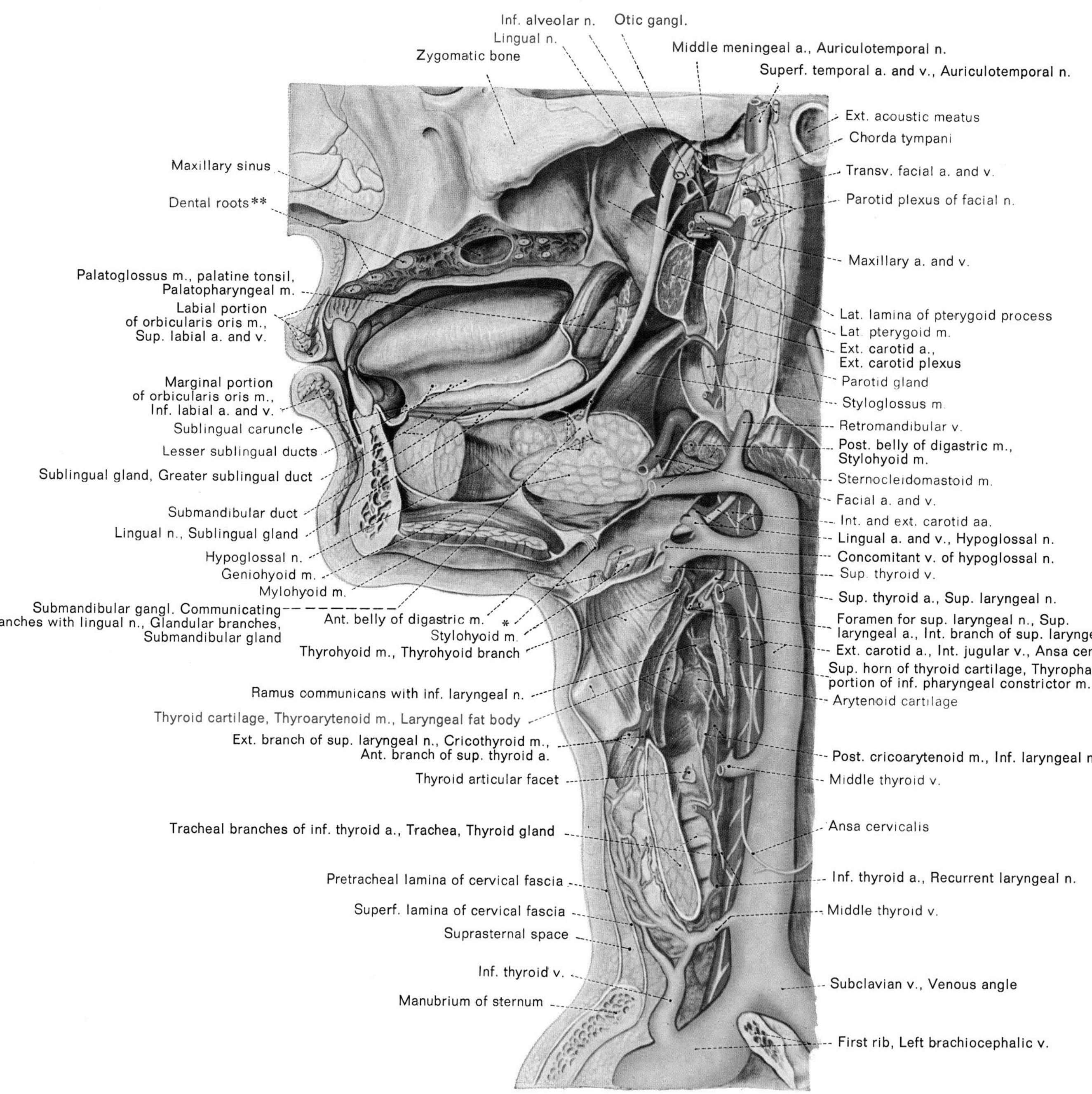

Inf. alveolar n.
Otic gangl.
Lingual n.
Zygomatic bone
Middle meningeal a., Auriculotemporal n.
Superf. temporal a. and v., Auriculotemporal n.
Ext. acoustic meatus
Chorda tympani
Transv. facial a. and v.
Parotid plexus of facial n.
Maxillary a. and v.
Lat. lamina of pterygoid process
Lat. pterygoid m.
Ext. carotid a., Ext. carotid plexus
Parotid gland
Styloglossus m.
Retromandibular v.
Post. belly of digastric m., Stylohyoid m.
Sternocleidomastoid m.
Facial a. and v.
Int. and ext. carotid aa.
Lingual a. and v., Hypoglossal n.
Concomitant v. of hypoglossal n.
Sup. thyroid v.
Sup. thyroid a., Sup. laryngeal n.
Foramen for sup. laryngeal n., Sup. laryngeal a., Int. branch of sup. laryngea
Ext. carotid a., Int. jugular v., Ansa cervi
Sup. horn of thyroid cartilage, Thyrophary portion of inf. pharyngeal constrictor m.
Arytenoid cartilage
Post. cricoarytenoid m., Inf. laryngeal n.
Middle thyroid v.
Ansa cervicalis
Inf. thyroid a., Recurrent laryngeal n.
Middle thyroid v.
Subclavian v., Venous angle
First rib, Left brachiocephalic v.
Maxillary sinus
Dental roots**
Palatoglossus m., palatine tonsil, Palatopharyngeal m.
Labial portion of orbicularis oris m., Sup. labial a. and v.
Marginal portion of orbicularis oris m., Inf. labial a. and v.
Sublingual caruncle
Lesser sublingual ducts
Sublingual gland, Greater sublingual duct
Submandibular duct
Lingual n., Sublingual gland
Hypoglossal n.
Geniohyoid m.
Mylohyoid m.
Submandibular gangl. Communicating branches with lingual n., Glandular branches, Submandibular gland
Ant. belly of digastric m.
*
Stylohyoid m.
Thyrohyoid m., Thyrohyoid branch
Ramus communicans with inf. laryngeal n.
Thyroid cartilage, Thyroarytenoid m., Laryngeal fat body
Ext. branch of sup. laryngeal n., Cricothyroid m., Ant. branch of sup. thyroid a.
Thyroid articular facet
Tracheal branches of inf. thyroid a., Trachea, Thyroid gland
Pretracheal lamina of cervical fascia
Superf. lamina of cervical fascia
Suprasternal space
Inf. thyroid v.
Manubrium of sternum

Fig. 338. Oral cavity, salivary glands, larynx, thyroid gland. Parasagittal section. The maxilla has been sectioned horizontally at the level of the dental roots and the lower pole of the maxillary sinus. The left half of the mandible has been removed.
* = ligamentous loop for the fixation of the intermediate tendon of the digastric muscle to the hyoid bone.
** = the roots of the following teeth (from medial to lateral) can be seen: first incisor, second incisor, canine tooth, first premolar, second and third molar. Note the close topographical relationship between the inferior recess of the maxillary sinus and the root of premolar and molar teeth.

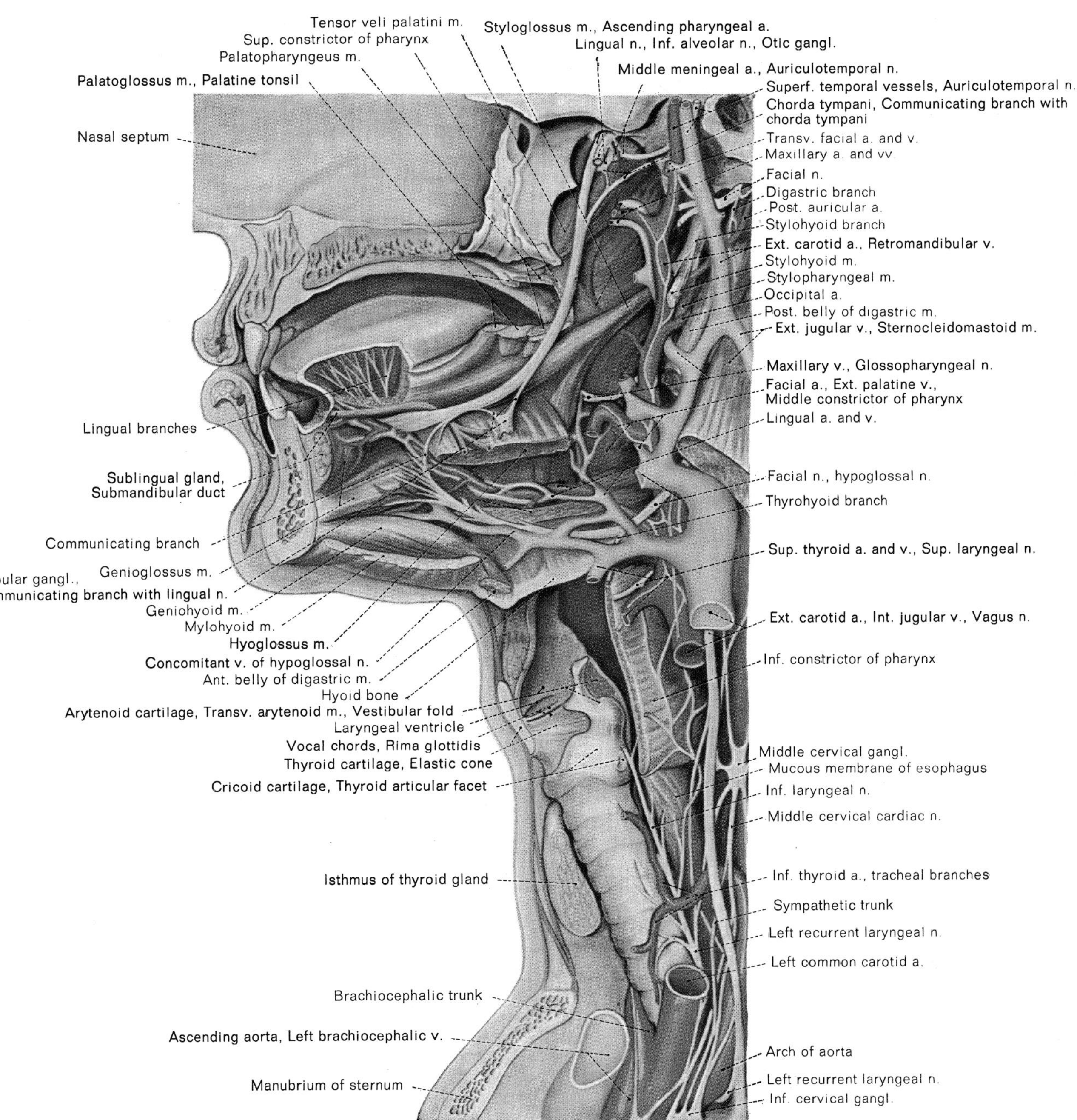
Tensor veli palatini m.
Sup. constrictor of pharynx
Palatopharyngeus m.
Palatoglossus m., Palatine tonsil
Styloglossus m., Ascending pharyngeal a.
Lingual n., Inf. alveolar n., Otic gangl.
Middle meningeal a., Auriculotemporal n.
Superf. temporal vessels, Auriculotemporal n.
Chorda tympani, Communicating branch with chorda tympani
Nasal septum
Transv. facial a. and v.
Maxillary a. and vv.
Facial n.
Digastric branch
Post. auricular a.
Stylohyoid branch
Ext. carotid a., Retromandibular v.
Stylohyoid m.
Stylopharyngeal m.
Occipital a.
Post. belly of digastric m.
Ext. jugular v., Sternocleidomastoid m.
Maxillary v., Glossopharyngeal n.
Facial a., Ext. palatine v.,
Middle constrictor of pharynx
Lingual branches
Lingual a. and v.
Sublingual gland,
Submandibular duct
Facial n., hypoglossal n.
Thyrohyoid branch
Communicating branch
Sup. thyroid a. and v., Sup. laryngeal n.
dibular gangl.,
Genioglossus m.
ommunicating branch with lingual n.
Geniohyoid m.
Mylohyoid m.
Ext. carotid a., Int. jugular v., Vagus n.
Hyoglossus m.
Concomitant v. of hypoglossal n.
Inf. constrictor of pharynx
Ant. belly of digastric m.
Hyoid bone
Arytenoid cartilage, Transv. arytenoid m., Vestibular fold
Laryngeal ventricle
Vocal chords, Rima glottidis
Middle cervical gangl.
Thyroid cartilage, Elastic cone
Mucous membrane of esophagus
Cricoid cartilage, Thyroid articular facet
Inf. laryngeal n.
Middle cervical cardiac n.
Isthmus of thyroid gland
Inf. thyroid a., tracheal branches
Sympathetic trunk
Left recurrent laryngeal n.
Left common carotid a.
Brachiocephalic trunk
Ascending aorta, Left brachiocephalic v.
Arch of aorta
Left recurrent laryngeal n.
Manubrium of sternum
Inf. cervical gangl.

Fig. 339. Same preparation as in Fig. 338 but, in addition, the maxilla has been removed to the sagittal plane. The parotid and submandibular glands have been removed, the palatine arches and palatine tonsil have been partially retained. The larynx has been opened. The lingual artery, hypoglossal nerve, vagus nerve and portions of the cervical sympathetic trunk have been exposed.

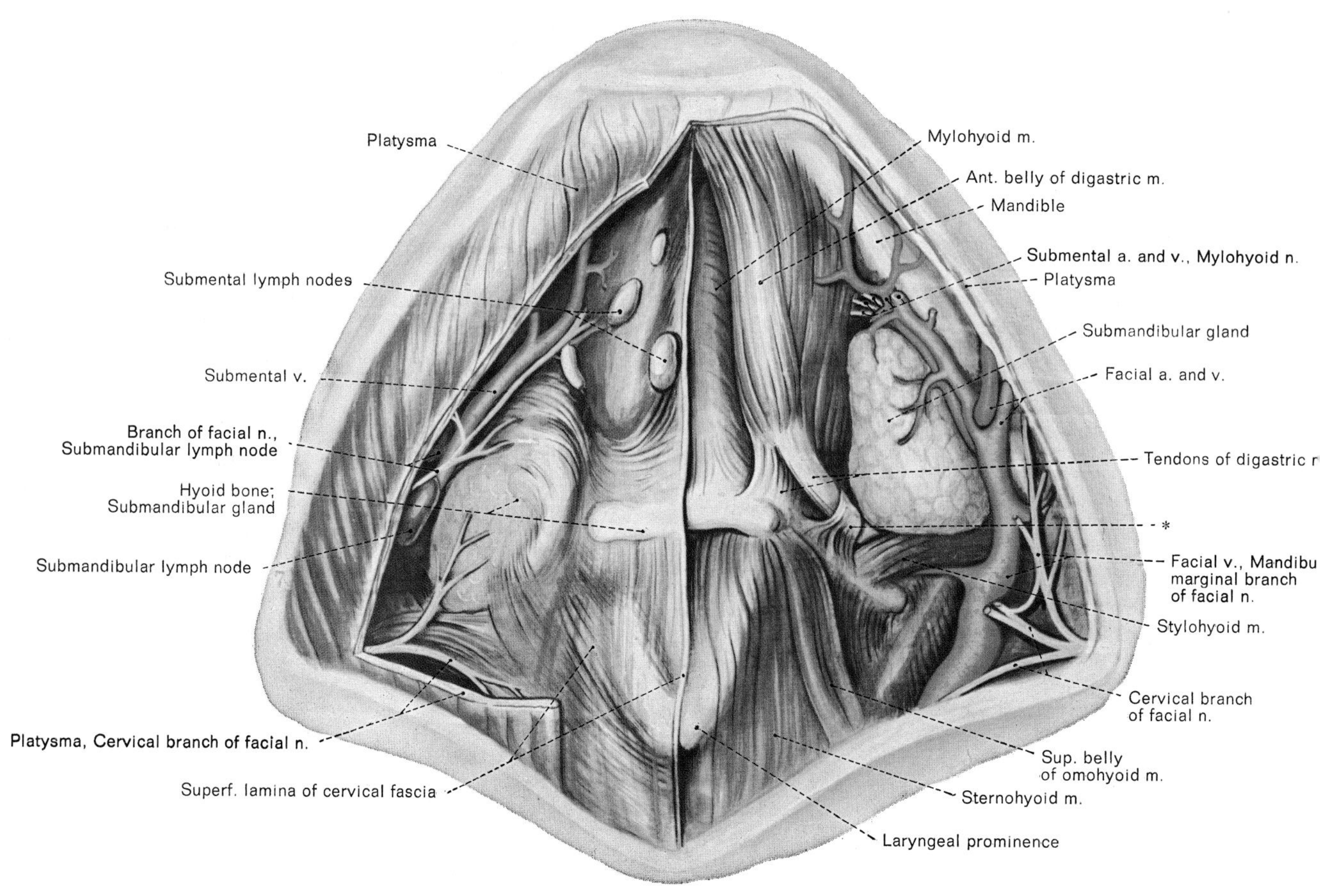
Platysma
Mylohyoid m.
Ant. belly of digastric m.
Mandible
Submental a. and v., Mylohyoid n.
Platysma
Submental lymph nodes
Submandibular gland
Facial a. and v.
Submental v.
Branch of facial n.,
Submandibular lymph node
Tendons of digastric r
Hyoid bone;
Submandibular gland
*
Submandibular lymph node
Facial v., Mandibu
marginal branch
of facial n.
Stylohyoid m.
Cervical branch
of facial n.
Platysma, Cervical branch of facial n.
Sup. belly
of omohyoid m.
Superf. lamina of cervical fascia
Sternohyoid m.
Laryngeal prominence

Fig. 340. Submandibular and submental area seen from below. On the right side of the picture, the superficial lamina of the cervical fascia together with the niche for the submandibular gland has been removed.
* = ligamentous loop for the fixation of the intermediate tendon of the digastric muscle to the hyoid bone.

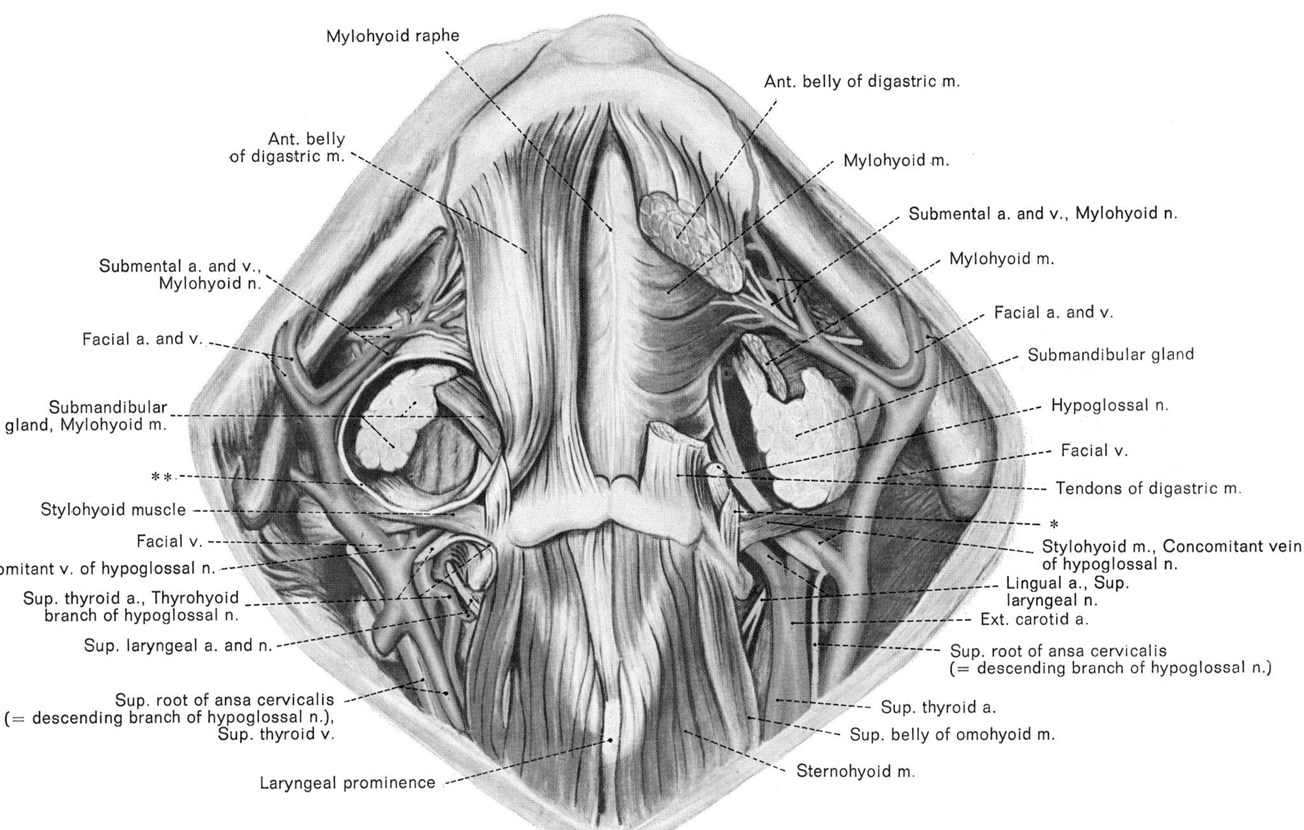
Mylohyoid raphe
Ant. belly of digastric m.
Ant. belly of digastric m.
Mylohyoid m.
Submental a. and v., Mylohyoid n.
Submental a. and v., Mylohyoid n.
Mylohyoid m.
Facial a. and v.
Facial a. and v.
Submandibular gland
Submandibular gland, Mylohyoid m.
Hypoglossal n.
Facial v.
**
Tendons of digastric m.
Stylohyoid muscle
*
Facial v.
Stylohyoid m., Concomitant vein of hypoglossal n.
ncomitant v. of hypoglossal n.
Lingual a., Sup. laryngeal n.
Sup. thyroid a., Thyrohyoid branch of hypoglossal n.
Ext. carotid a.
Sup. laryngeal a. and n.
Sup. root of ansa cervicalis (= descending branch of hypoglossal n.)
Sup. root of ansa cervicalis (= descending branch of hypoglossal n.), Sup. thyroid v.
Sup. thyroid a.
Sup. belly of omohyoid m.
Sternohyoid m.
Laryngeal prominence

Fig. 341. Submandibular and submental region seen from below after removal of the superficial lamina of the cervical fascia. On the right side of the picture, the anterior belly of the digastric muscle and the mylohyoid muscle have been partially removed in order to expose the hypoglossal nerve. On the left side of the picture, the niche for the submandibular gland is shown.
* = ligamentous loop for the fixation of the intermediate tendon of the digastric muscle to the hyoid bone.
** = capsule of the submandibular gland.

Peripheral Nerves and Vessels

Nerves and Vessels of the Neck

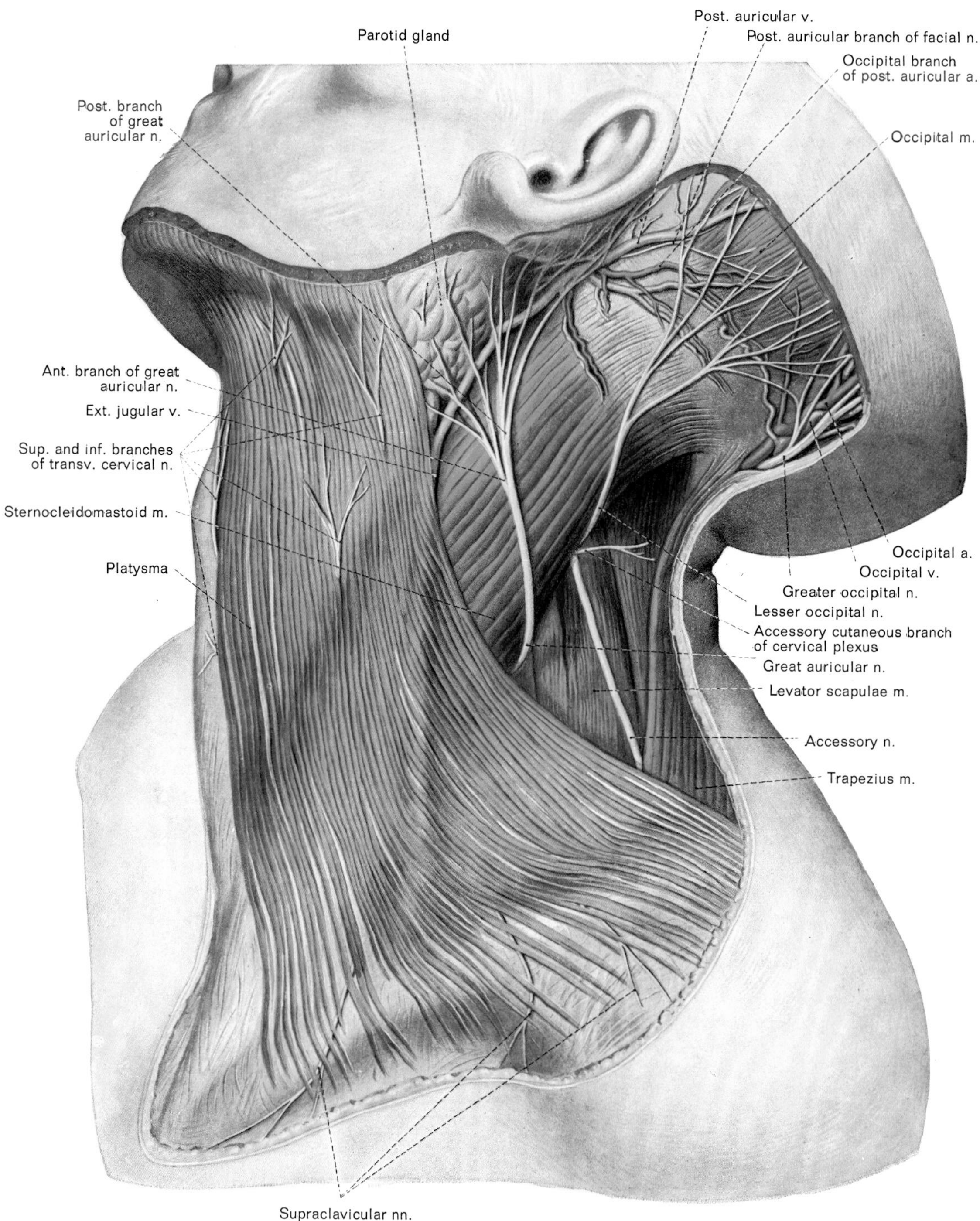
Post. auricular v.
Post. auricular branch of facial n.
Parotid gland
Occipital branch
of post. auricular a.
Post. branch
of great
auricular n.
Occipital m.
Ant. branch of great
auricular n.
Ext. jugular v.
Sup. and inf. branches
of transv. cervical n.
Sternocleidomastoid m.
Platysma
Occipital a.
Occipital v.
Greater occipital n.
Lesser occipital n.
Accessory cutaneous branch
of cervical plexus
Great auricular n.
Levator scapulae m.
Accessory n.
Trapezius m.
Supraclavicular nn.

Fig. 342. Cutaneous branches of the cervical plexus, left side.

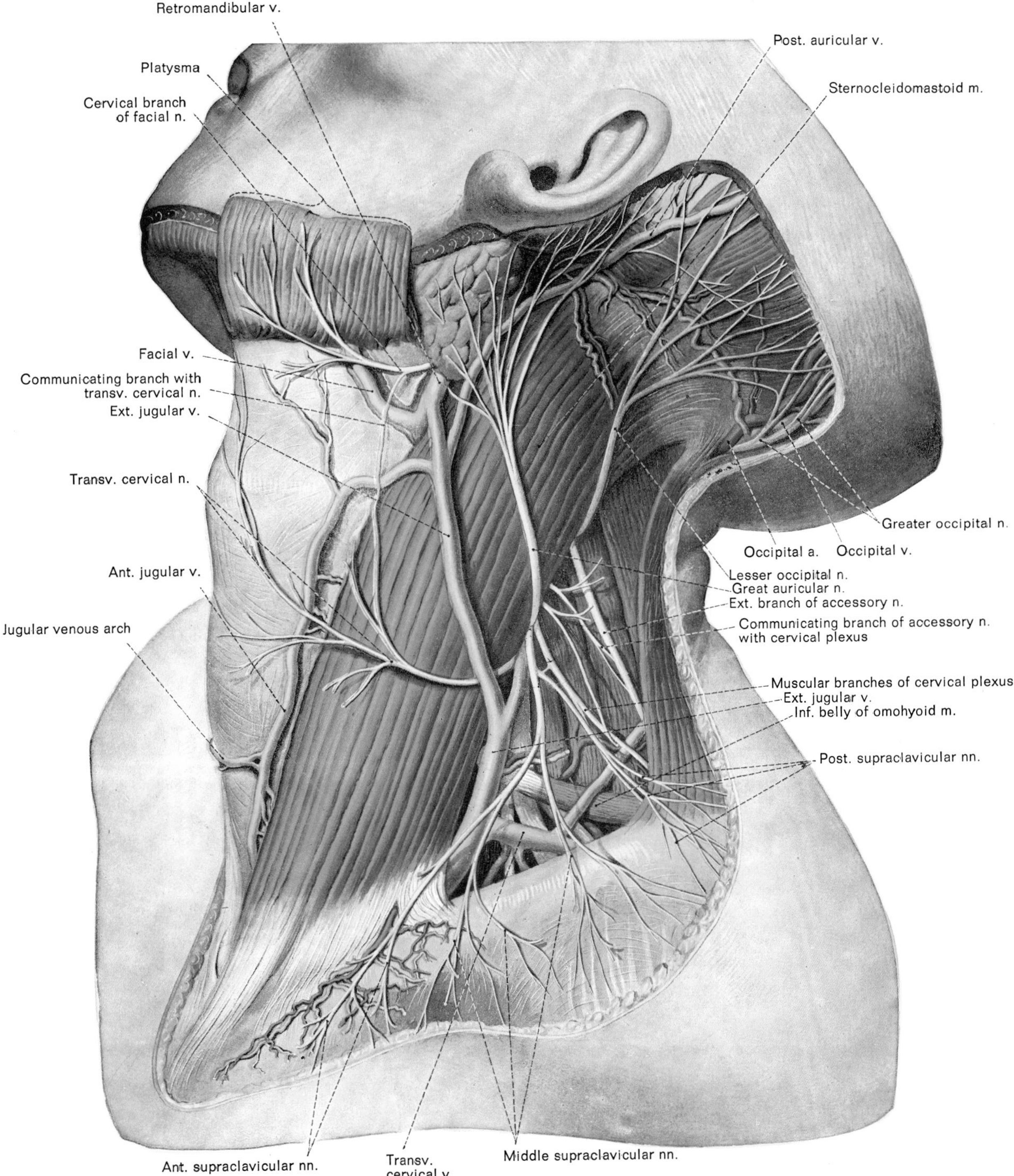
Retromandibular v.
Platysma
Cervical branch of facial n.
Post. auricular v.
Sternocleidomastoid m.
Facial v.
Communicating branch with transv. cervical n.
Ext. jugular v.
Transv. cervical n.
Greater occipital n.
Occipital a.
Occipital v.
Ant. jugular v.
Lesser occipital n.
Great auricular n.
Ext. branch of accessory n.
Jugular venous arch
Communicating branch of accessory n. with cervical plexus
Muscular branches of cervical plexus
Ext. jugular v.
Inf. belly of omohyoid m.
Post. supraclavicular nn.
Ant. supraclavicular nn.
Transv. cervical v.
Middle supraclavicular nn.

Fig. 343. Cutaneous and muscular branches of the cervical plexus, superficial veins on the left side of the neck. Platysma partially removed, its upper portion reflected upward. Superficial lamina of cervical fascia anterior to the sternocleidomastoid muscle has been retained and split along the facial vein.

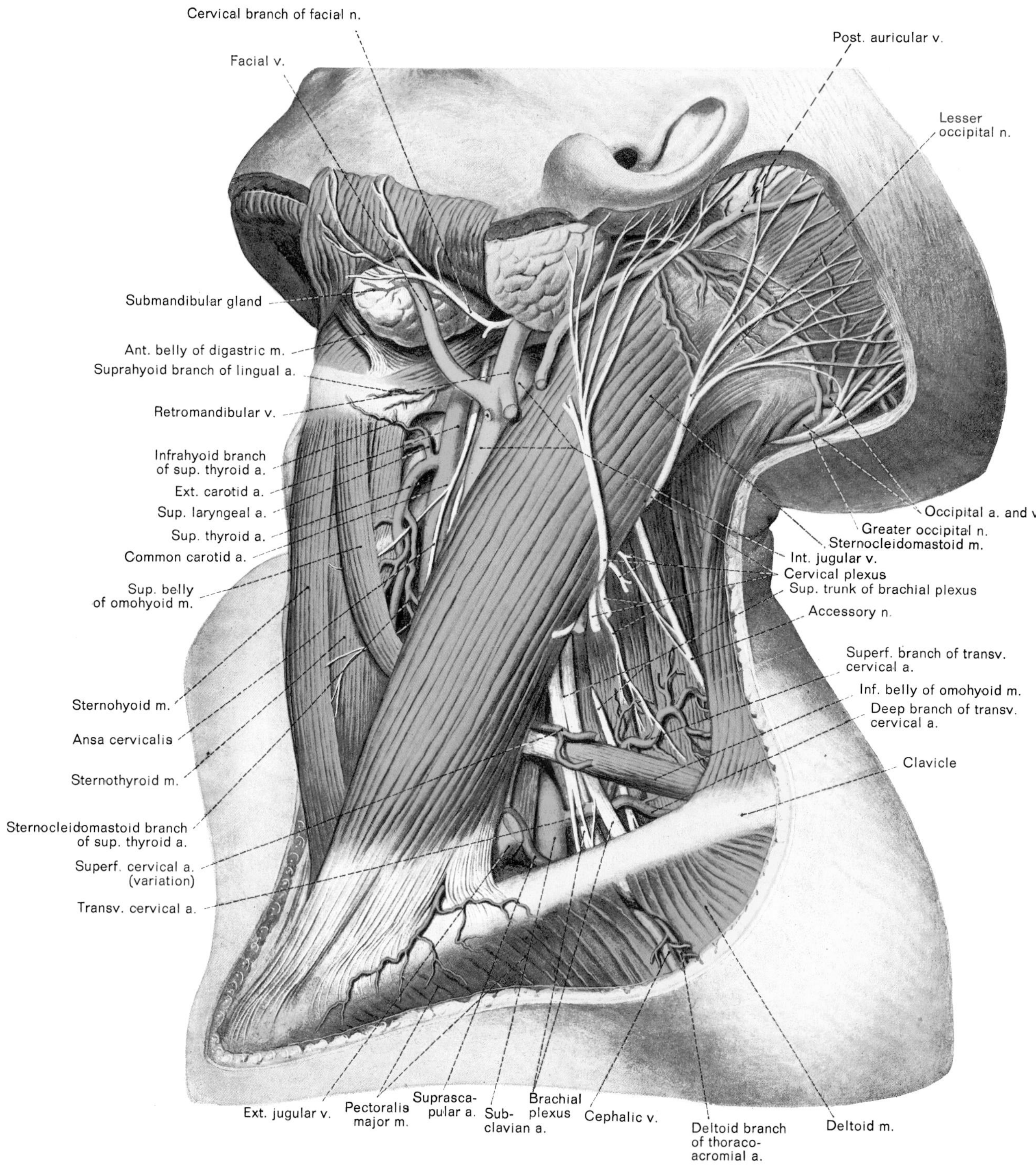
Cervical branch of facial n.
Facial v.
Post. auricular v.
Lesser occipital n.
Submandibular gland
Ant. belly of digastric m.
Suprahyoid branch of lingual a.
Retromandibular v.
Infrahyoid branch of sup. thyroid a.
Ext. carotid a.
Sup. laryngeal a.
Sup. thyroid a.
Common carotid a.
Sup. belly of omohyoid m.
Occipital a. and v.
Greater occipital n.
Sternocleidomastoid m.
Int. jugular v.
Cervical plexus
Sup. trunk of brachial plexus
Accessory n.
Superf. branch of transv. cervical a.
Inf. belly of omohyoid m.
Deep branch of transv. cervical a.
Clavicle
Sternohyoid m.
Ansa cervicalis
Sternothyroid m.
Sternocleidomastoid branch of sup. thyroid a.
Superf. cervical a. (variation)
Transv. cervical a.
Ext. jugular v.
Pectoralis major m.
Suprascapular a.
Subclavian a.
Brachial plexus
Cephalic v.
Deltoid branch of thoracoacromial a.
Deltoid m.

Fig. 344. Nerves and vessels of the medial and lateral cervical triangle. Superficial lamina of cervical fascia and superficial veins have been removed.

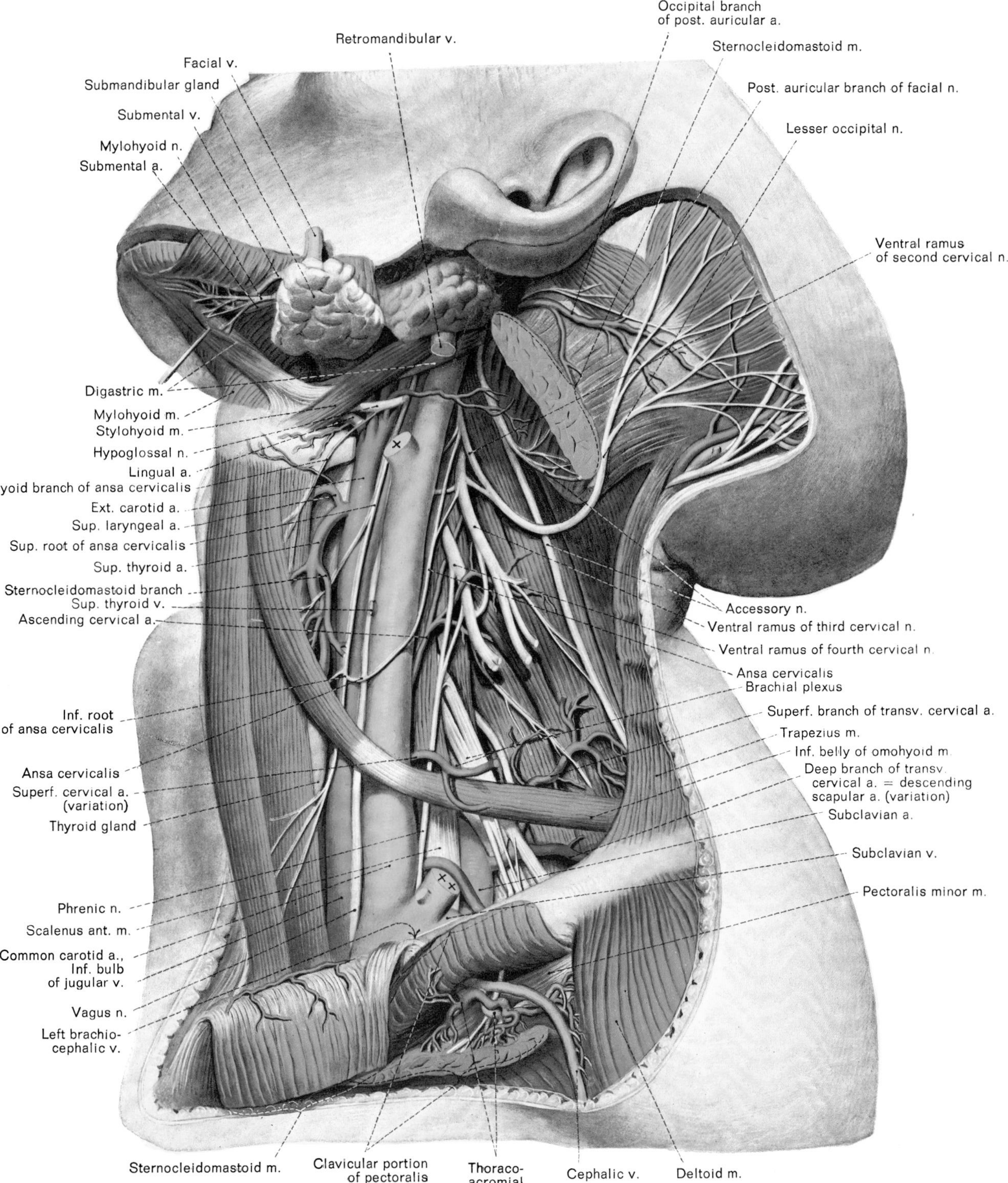
Occipital branch
of post. auricular a.
Retromandibular v.
Sternocleidomastoid m.
Facial v.
Submandibular gland
Post. auricular branch of facial n.
Submental v.
Lesser occipital n.
Mylohyoid n.
Submental a.
Ventral ramus
of second cervical n.
Digastric m.
Mylohyoid m.
Stylohyoid m.
Hypoglossal n.
Lingual a.
ohyoid branch of ansa cervicalis
Ext. carotid a.
Sup. laryngeal a.
Sup. root of ansa cervicalis
Sup. thyroid a.
Sternocleidomastoid branch
Sup. thyroid v.
Ascending cervical a.
Accessory n.
Ventral ramus of third cervical n.
Ventral ramus of fourth cervical n.
Ansa cervicalis
Brachial plexus
Inf. root
of ansa cervicalis
Superf. branch of transv. cervical a.
Trapezius m.
Inf. belly of omohyoid m.
Ansa cervicalis
Deep branch of transv.
cervical a. = descending
scapular a. (variation)
Superf. cervical a.
(variation)
Thyroid gland
Subclavian a.
Subclavian v.
Pectoralis minor m.
Phrenic n.
Scalenus ant. m.
Common carotid a.,
Inf. bulb
of jugular v.
Vagus n.
Left brachio-
cephalic v.
Sternocleidomastoid m.
Clavicular portion
of pectoralis
major m.
Thoraco-
acromial
a. and v.
Cephalic v.
Deltoid m.

Fig. 345. Deeper layer of nerves and vessels of the left side of the neck. The sternocleidomastoid muscle has been sectioned and mostly removed. The superficial veins have been removed, the nerves of the cervical plexus (with the exception of the lesser occipital nerve, phrenic nerve and muscular branches) have been cut off. ×, ×× = external jugular vein.

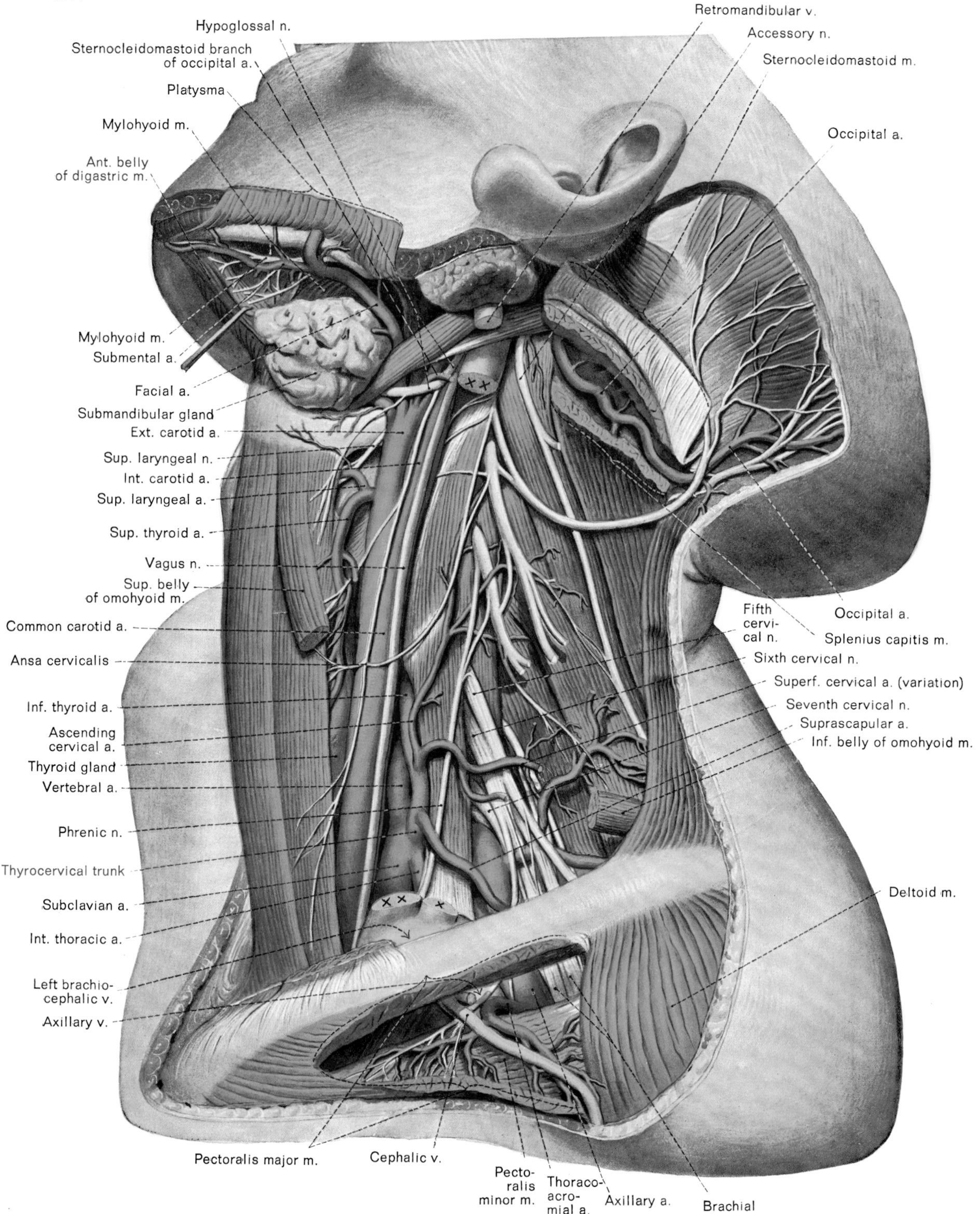

Hypoglossal n.
Sternocleidomastoid branch of occipital a.
Platysma
Mylohyoid m.
Ant. belly of digastric m.
Mylohyoid m.
Submental a.
Facial a.
Submandibular gland
Ext. carotid a.
Sup. laryngeal n.
Int. carotid a.
Sup. laryngeal a.
Sup. thyroid a.
Vagus n.
Sup. belly of omohyoid m.
Common carotid a.
Ansa cervicalis
Inf. thyroid a.
Ascending cervical a.
Thyroid gland
Vertebral a.
Phrenic n.
Thyrocervical trunk
Subclavian a.
Int. thoracic a.
Left brachiocephalic v.
Axillary v.
Retromandibular v.
Accessory n.
Sternocleidomastoid m.
Occipital a.
Fifth cervical n.
Occipital a.
Splenius capitis m.
Sixth cervical n.
Superf. cervical a. (variation)
Seventh cervical n.
Suprascapular a.
Inf. belly of omohyoid m.
Deltoid m.
Pectoralis major m.
Cephalic v.
Pectoralis minor m.
Thoracoacromial a.
Axillary a.
Brachial plexus

Fig. 346. Intermediate layer of nerves and arteries of the left side of the neck; nerves and vessels of the deltoideopectoral triangle. × = external jugular vein, × × = internal jugular vein.

Fig. 347. Deep layers of nerves and vessels of neck and axilla. The clavicle has been removed from the sternoclavicular joint to the insertion of the trapezius muscle. Strap muscles, sternocleidomastoid muscle and major cervical vessels have been mostly removed. × = first rib.

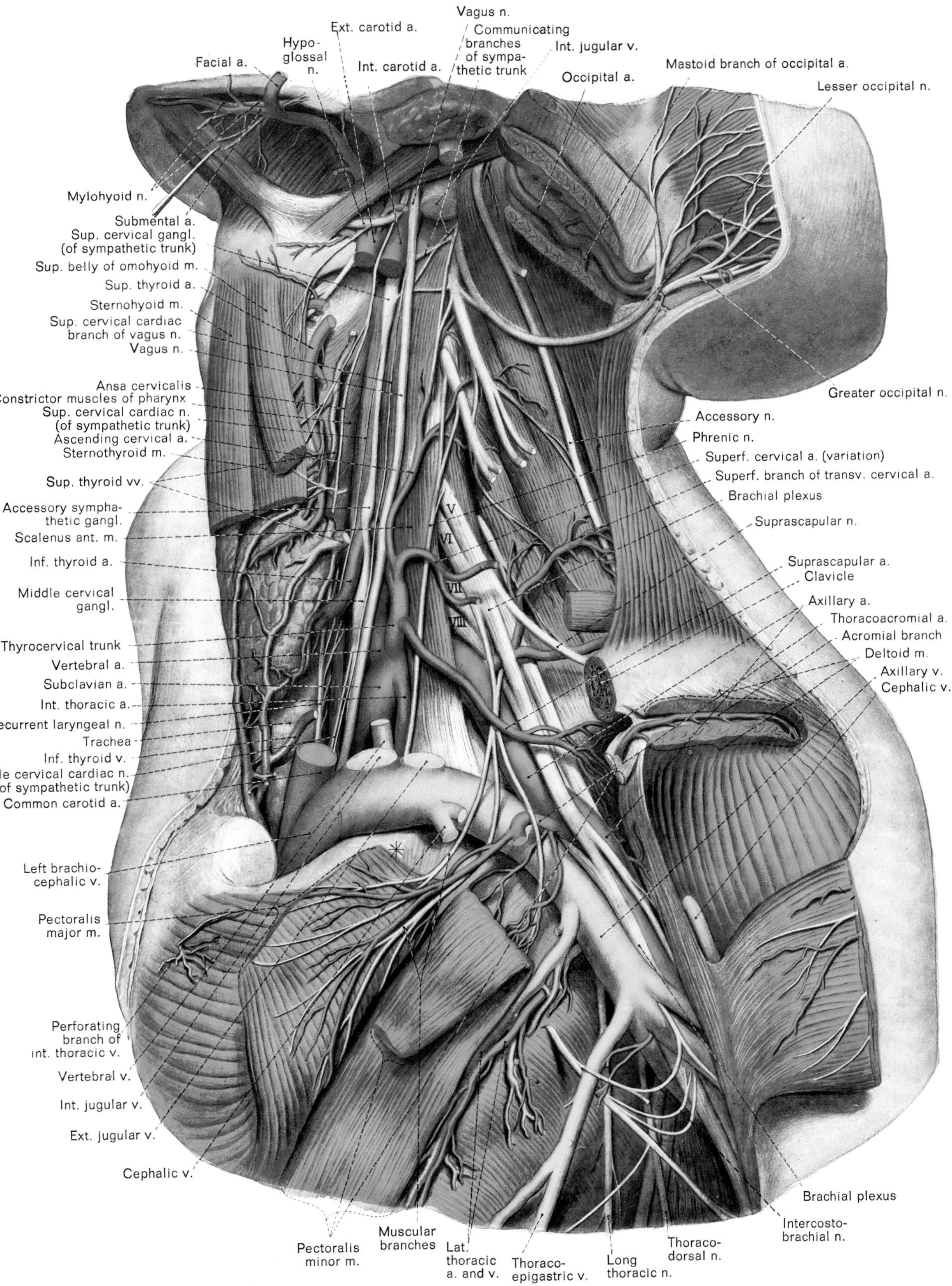
Vagus n.
Ext. carotid a.
Communicating branches of sympathetic trunk
Hypoglossal n.
Int. jugular v.
Facial a.
Int. carotid a.
Mastoid branch of occipital a.
Occipital a.
Lesser occipital n.
Mylohyoid n.
Submental a.
Sup. cervical gangl. (of sympathetic trunk)
Sup. belly of omohyoid m.
Sup. thyroid a.
Sternohyoid m.
Sup. cervical cardiac branch of vagus n.
Vagus n.
Ansa cervicalis
Constrictor muscles of pharynx
Sup. cervical cardiac n. (of sympathetic trunk)
Ascending cervical a.
Sternothyroid m.
Sup. thyroid vv.
Accessory sympathetic gangl.
Scalenus ant. m.
Inf. thyroid a.
Middle cervical gangl.
Thyrocervical trunk
Vertebral a.
Subclavian a.
Int. thoracic a.
Recurrent laryngeal n.
Trachea
Inf. thyroid v.
Middle cervical cardiac n. (of sympathetic trunk)
Common carotid a.
Left brachiocephalic v.
Pectoralis major m.
Perforating branch of int. thoracic v.
Vertebral v.
Int. jugular v.
Ext. jugular v.
Cephalic v.
Greater occipital n.
Accessory n.
Phrenic n.
Superf. cervical a. (variation)
Superf. branch of transv. cervical a.
Brachial plexus
Suprascapular n.
Suprascapular a.
Clavicle
Axillary a.
Thoracoacromial a.
Acromial branch
Deltoid m.
Axillary v.
Cephalic v.
V
VI
VII
VIII
*
Brachial plexus
Intercostobrachial n.
Thoracodorsal n.
Long thoracic n.
Thoracoepigastric v.
Lat. thoracic a. and v.
Muscular branches
Pectoralis minor m.

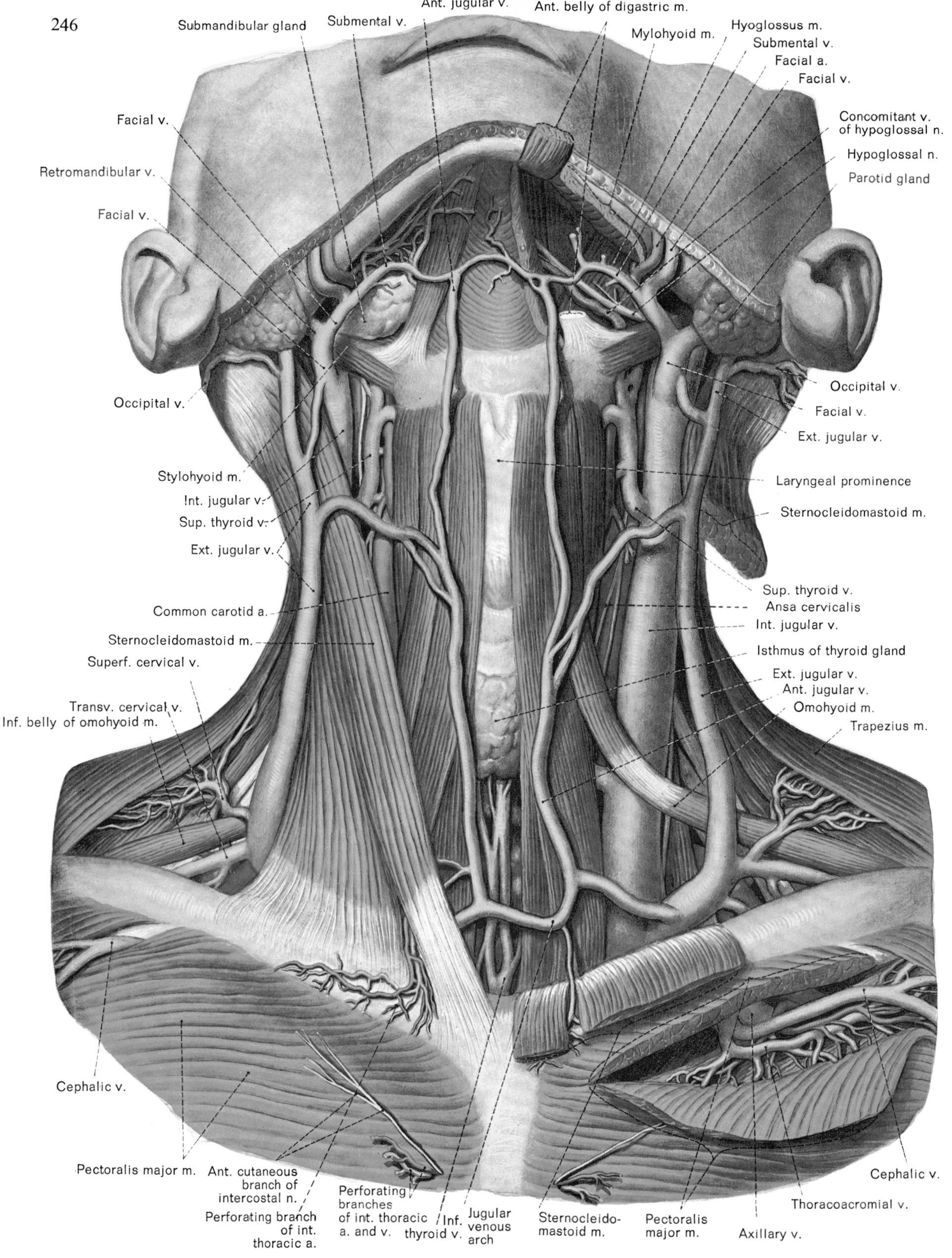

Submandibular gland
Submental v.
Ant. jugular v.
Ant. belly of digastric m.
Mylohyoid m.
Hyoglossus m.
Submental v.
Facial a.
Facial v.
Facial v.
Concomitant v. of hypoglossal n.
Hypoglossal n.
Parotid gland
Retromandibular v.
Facial v.
Occipital v.
Occipital v.
Facial v.
Ext. jugular v.
Stylohyoid m.
Laryngeal prominence
Int. jugular v.
Sternocleidomastoid m.
Sup. thyroid v.
Ext. jugular v.
Sup. thyroid v.
Ansa cervicalis
Common carotid a.
Int. jugular v.
Sternocleidomastoid m.
Isthmus of thyroid gland
Superf. cervical v.
Ext. jugular v.
Ant. jugular v.
Transv. cervical v.
Omohyoid m.
Inf. belly of omohyoid m.
Trapezius m.
Cephalic v.
Pectoralis major m.
Ant. cutaneous branch of intercostal n.
Perforating branches of int. thoracic a. and v.
Perforating branch of int. thoracic a.
Inf. thyroid v.
Jugular venous arch
Sternocleido-mastoid m.
Pectoralis major m.
Axillary v.
Thoracoacromial v.
Cephalic v.

Fig. 348. Superficial veins of neck and infraclavicular fossa; ventral view. The major portion of the left sternocleidomastoid muscle has been removed; the anterior belly of the digastric muscle and the mylohyoid muscle have been sectioned. The veins are maximally filled.

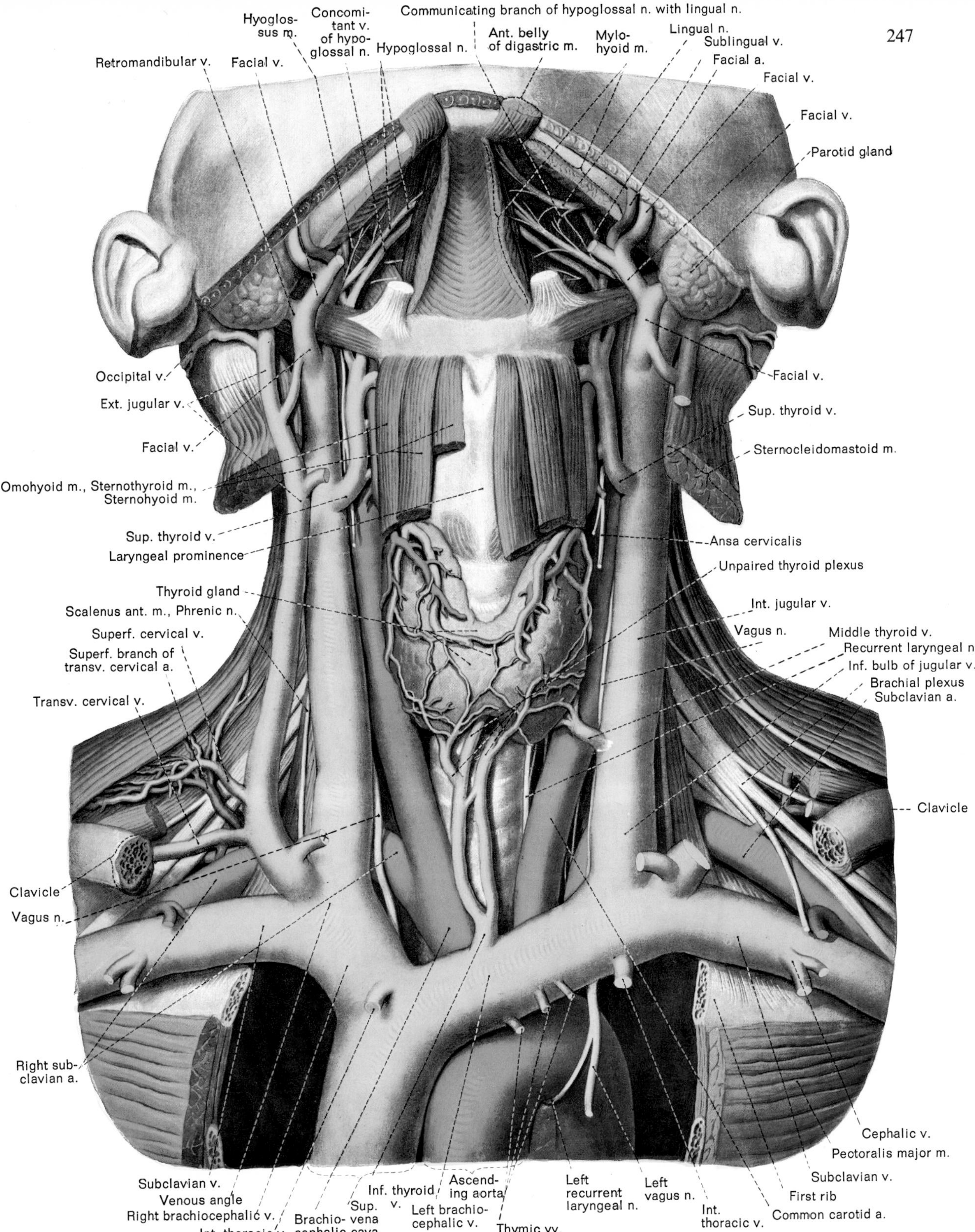
Hyoglossus m.
Concomitant v. of hypoglossal n.
Communicating branch of hypoglossal n. with lingual n.
Ant. belly of digastric m.
Mylohyoid m.
Lingual n.
Sublingual v.
Facial a.
Facial v.
Retromandibular v.
Facial v.
Hypoglossal n.
Facial v.
Parotid gland
Occipital v.
Ext. jugular v.
Facial v.
Omohyoid m., Sternothyroid m., Sternohyoid m.
Sup. thyroid v.
Laryngeal prominence
Thyroid gland
Scalenus ant. m., Phrenic n.
Superf. cervical v.
Superf. branch of transv. cervical a.
Transv. cervical v.
Clavicle
Vagus n.
Right subclavian a.
Facial v.
Sup. thyroid v.
Sternocleidomastoid m.
Ansa cervicalis
Unpaired thyroid plexus
Int. jugular v.
Vagus n.
Middle thyroid v.
Recurrent laryngeal n.
Inf. bulb of jugular v.
Brachial plexus
Subclavian a.
Clavicle
Cephalic v.
Pectoralis major m.
Subclavian v.
First rib
Common carotid a.
Subclavian v.
Venous angle
Right brachiocephalic v.
Int. thoracic v.
Sup.
Brachiocephalic trunk
Inf. thyroid v.
vena cava
Ascending aorta
Left brachiocephalic v.
Thymic vv.
Left recurrent laryngeal n.
Left vagus n.
Int. thoracic v.

Fig. 349. Nerves and vessels of the deep cervical region and upper thoracic aperture. Sternocleidomastoid muscles and strap muscles partially removed. Mylohyoid and digastric muscles sectioned. Sternum and anterior portions of first and second rib removed. Veins maximally filled. × = anterior jugular vein.

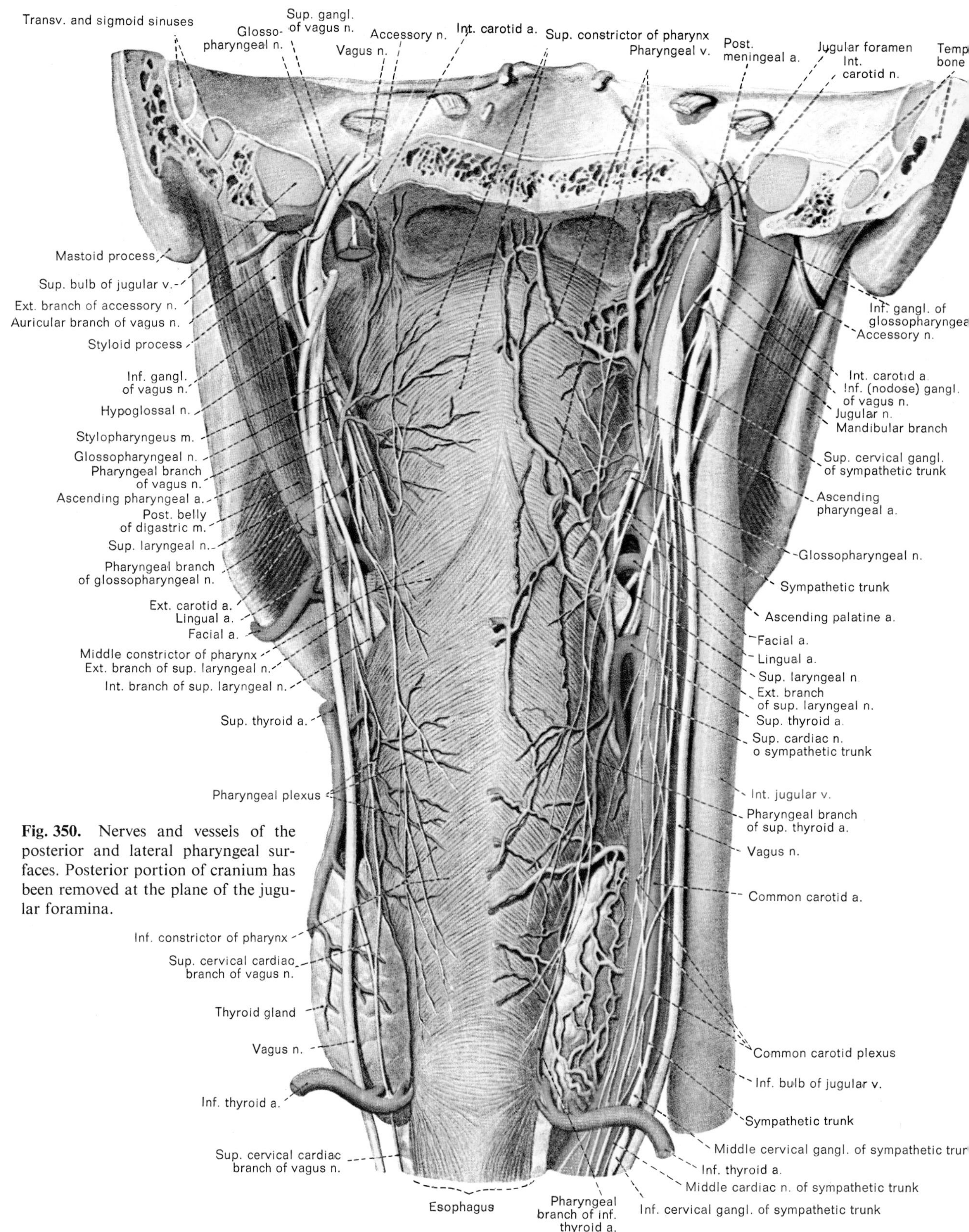

Transv. and sigmoid sinuses
Glosso-pharyngeal n.
Sup. gangl. of vagus n.
Vagus n.
Accessory n.
Int. carotid a.
Sup. constrictor of pharynx
Pharyngeal v.
Post. meningeal a.
Jugular foramen
Int. carotid n.
Temp bone
Mastoid process
Sup. bulb of jugular v.
Ext. branch of accessory n.
Auricular branch of vagus n.
Styloid process
Inf. gangl. of vagus n.
Hypoglossal n.
Stylopharyngeus m.
Glossopharyngeal n.
Pharyngeal branch of vagus n.
Ascending pharyngeal a.
Post. belly of digastric m.
Sup. laryngeal n.
Pharyngeal branch of glossopharyngeal n.
Ext. carotid a.
Lingual a.
Facial a.
Middle constrictor of pharynx
Ext. branch of sup. laryngeal n.
Int. branch of sup. laryngeal n.
Sup. thyroid a.
Pharyngeal plexus
Inf. constrictor of pharynx
Sup. cervical cardiac branch of vagus n.
Thyroid gland
Vagus n.
Inf. thyroid a.
Sup. cervical cardiac branch of vagus n.
Esophagus
Pharyngeal branch of inf. thyroid a.
Inf. gangl. of glossopharynge
Accessory n.
Int. carotid a.
Inf. (nodose) gangl. of vagus n.
Jugular n.
Mandibular branch
Sup. cervical gangl. of sympathetic trunk
Ascending pharyngeal a.
Glossopharyngeal n.
Sympathetic trunk
Ascending palatine a.
Facial a.
Lingual a.
Sup. laryngeal n
Ext. branch of sup. laryngeal n.
Sup. thyroid a.
Sup. cardiac n. o sympathetic trunk
Int. jugular v.
Pharyngeal branch of sup. thyroid a.
Vagus n.
Common carotid a.
Common carotid plexus
Inf. bulb of jugular v.
Sympathetic trunk
Middle cervical gangl. of sympathetic trur
Inf. thyroid a.
Middle cardiac n. of sympathetic trunk
Inf. cervical gangl. of sympathetic trunk

Fig. 350. Nerves and vessels of the posterior and lateral pharyngeal surfaces. Posterior portion of cranium has been removed at the plane of the jugular foramina.

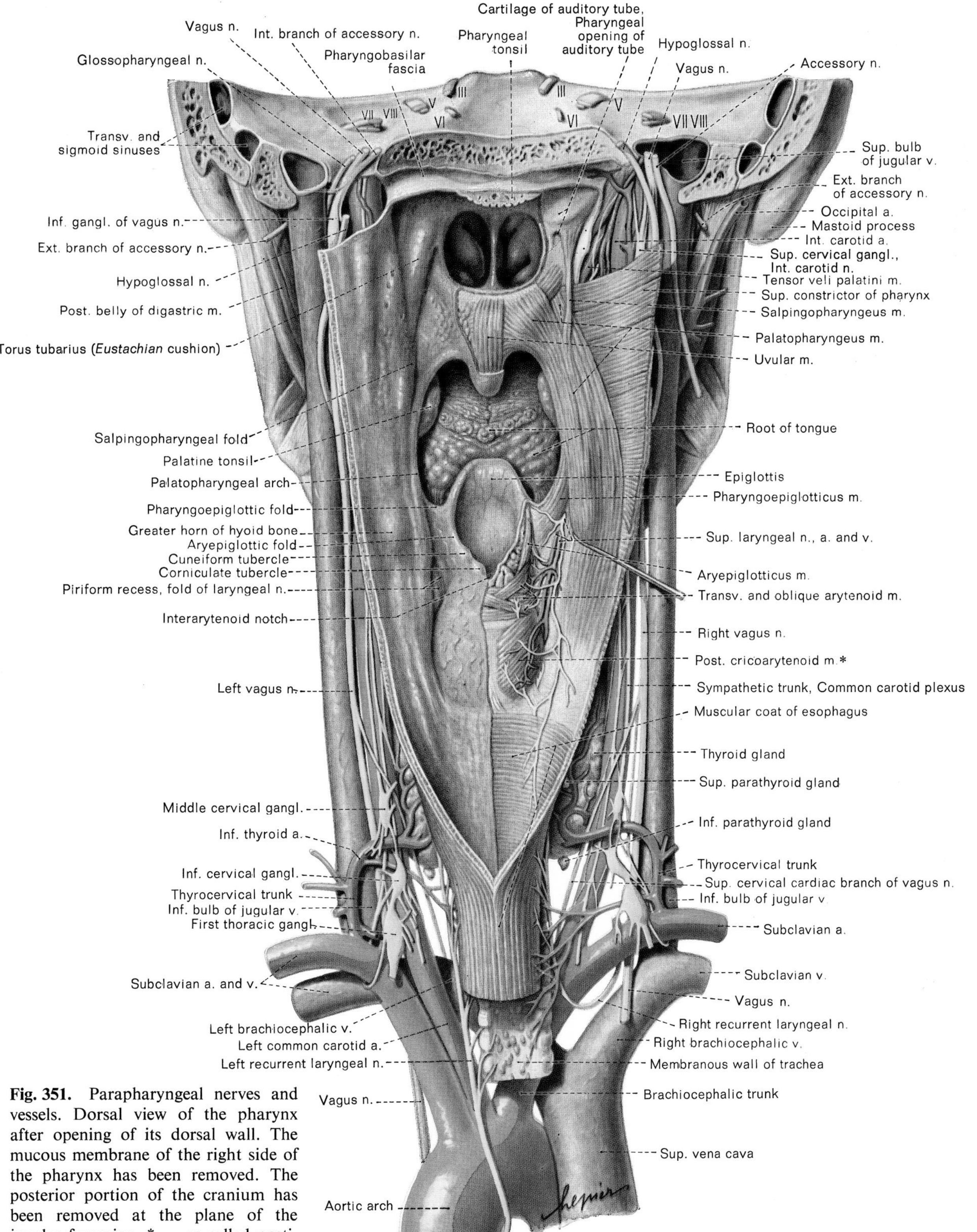

Vagus n.
Int. branch of accessory n.
Cartilage of auditory tube, Pharyngeal opening of auditory tube
Pharyngeal tonsil
Hypoglossal n.
Glossopharyngeal n.
Pharyngobasilar fascia
Vagus n.
Accessory n.
III
V
VI
VII VIII
Transv. and sigmoid sinuses
Sup. bulb of jugular v.
Ext. branch of accessory n.
Occipital a.
Inf. gangl. of vagus n.
Mastoid process
Int. carotid a.
Ext. branch of accessory n.
Sup. cervical gangl., Int. carotid n.
Hypoglossal n.
Tensor veli palatini m.
Sup. constrictor of pharynx
Post. belly of digastric m.
Salpingopharyngeus m.
Torus tubarius (Eustachian cushion)
Palatopharyngeus m.
Uvular m.
Root of tongue
Salpingopharyngeal fold
Palatine tonsil
Epiglottis
Palatopharyngeal arch
Pharyngoepiglotticus m.
Pharyngoepiglottic fold
Greater horn of hyoid bone
Sup. laryngeal n., a. and v.
Aryepiglottic fold
Cuneiform tubercle
Corniculate tubercle
Aryepiglotticus m.
Piriform recess, fold of laryngeal n.
Transv. and oblique arytenoid m.
Interarytenoid notch
Right vagus n.
Post. cricoarytenoid m.*
Left vagus n.
Sympathetic trunk, Common carotid plexus
Muscular coat of esophagus
Thyroid gland
Sup. parathyroid gland
Middle cervical gangl.
Inf. parathyroid gland
Inf. thyroid a.
Thyrocervical trunk
Inf. cervical gangl.
Sup. cervical cardiac branch of vagus n.
Thyrocervical trunk
Inf. bulb of jugular v.
Inf. bulb of jugular v.
First thoracic gangl.
Subclavian a.
Subclavian v.
Subclavian a. and v.
Vagus n.
Right recurrent laryngeal n.
Left brachiocephalic v.
Right brachiocephalic v.
Left common carotid a.
Left recurrent laryngeal n.
Membranous wall of trachea
Brachiocephalic trunk
Vagus n.
Sup. vena cava
Aortic arch

Fig. 351. Parapharyngeal nerves and vessels. Dorsal view of the pharynx after opening of its dorsal wall. The mucous membrane of the right side of the pharynx has been removed. The posterior portion of the cranium has been removed at the plane of the jugular foramina. * = so-called posticus muscle.

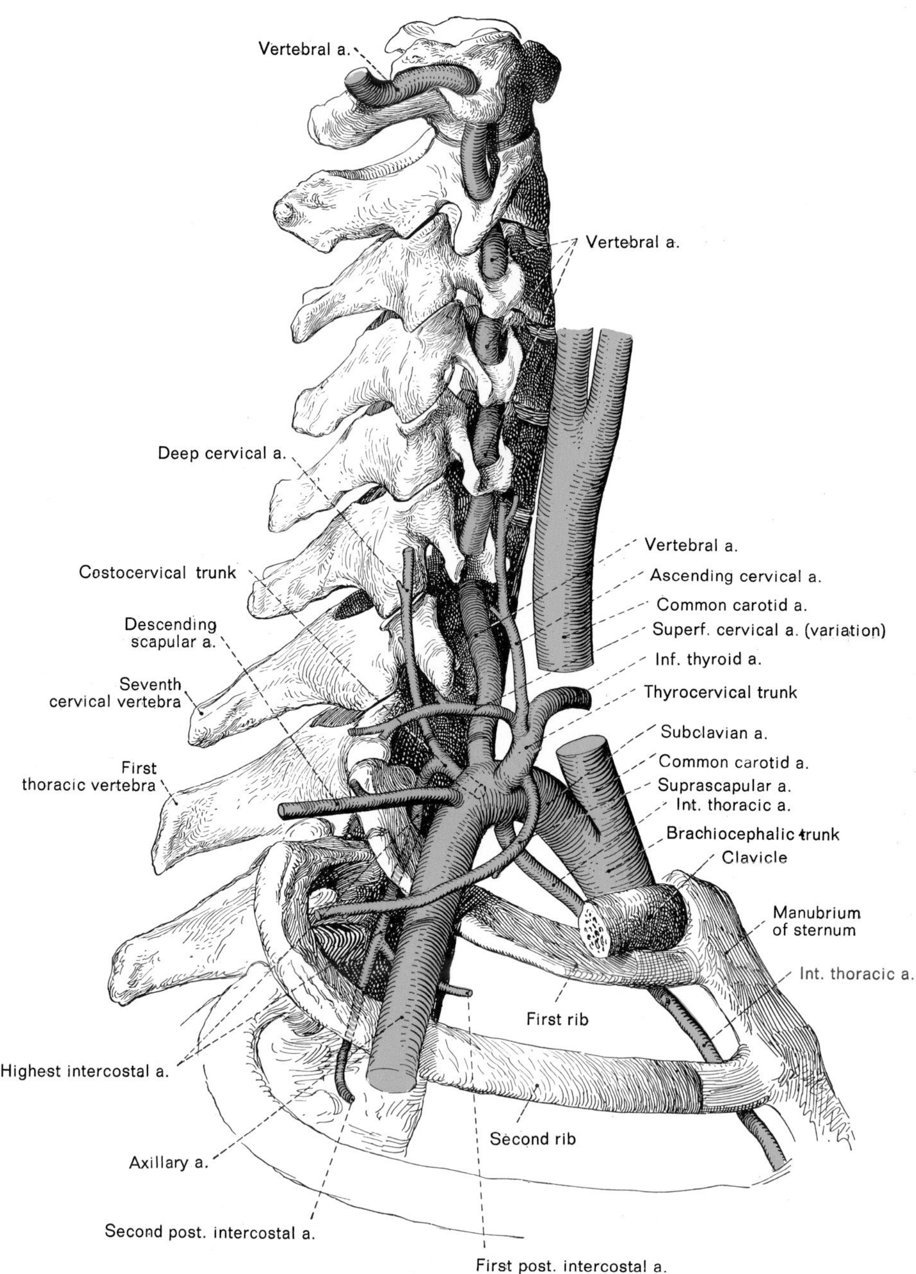

Vertebral a.
Vertebral a.
Deep cervical a.
Costocervical trunk
Descending scapular a.
Seventh cervical vertebra
First thoracic vertebra
Vertebral a.
Ascending cervical a.
Common carotid a.
Superf. cervical a. (variation)
Inf. thyroid a.
Thyrocervical trunk
Subclavian a.
Common carotid a.
Suprascapular a.
Int. thoracic a.
Brachiocephalic trunk
Clavicle
Manubrium of sternum
Int. thoracic a.
First rib
Highest intercostal a.
Second rib
Axillary a.
Second post. intercostal a.
First post. intercostal a.

Fig. 352. Diagram of the subclavian artery and its branches and the course of the vertebral artery.

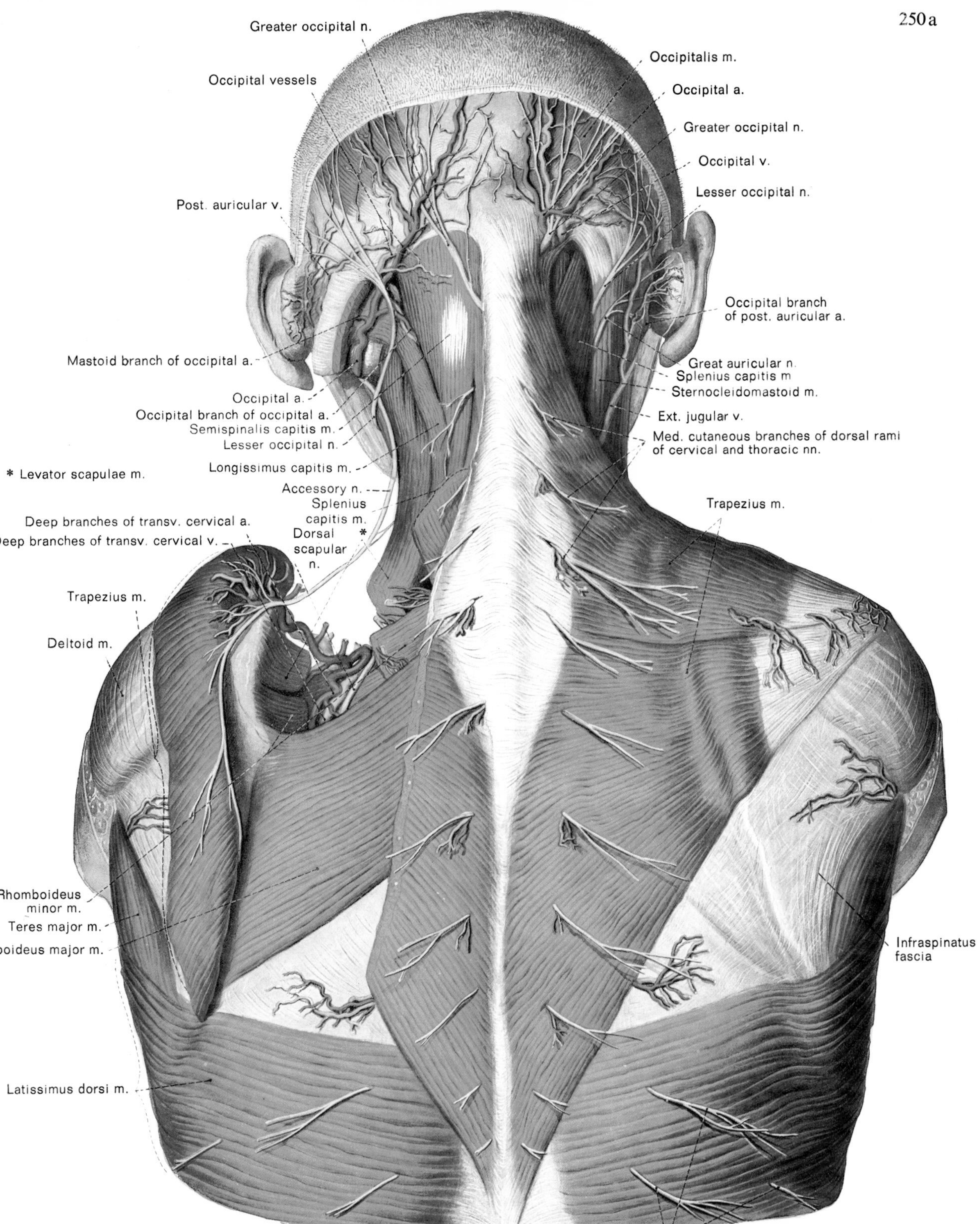
Greater occipital n.
Occipital vessels
Post. auricular v.
Mastoid branch of occipital a.
Occipital a.
Occipital branch of occipital a.
Semispinalis capitis m.
Lesser occipital n.
* Levator scapulae m.
Longissimus capitis m.
Accessory n.
Splenius capitis m.
Deep branches of transv. cervical a.
Deep branches of transv. cervical v.
Dorsal scapular n.
*
Trapezius m.
Deltoid m.
Rhomboideus minor m.
Teres major m.
mboideus major m.
Latissimus dorsi m.
Occipitalis m.
Occipital a.
Greater occipital n.
Occipital v.
Lesser occipital n.
Occipital branch of post. auricular a.
Great auricular n.
Splenius capitis m
Sternocleidomastoid m.
Ext. jugular v.
Med. cutaneous branches of dorsal rami of cervical and thoracic nn.
Trapezius m.
Infraspinatus fascia
Lat. cutaneous branches of dorsal rami of thoracic nn.

Fig. 352a. Superficial and middle layer of nerves and vessels of the upper back and neck. On the left side, the trapezius, sternocleidomastoid, splenius capitis and levator scapulae muscles were divided.

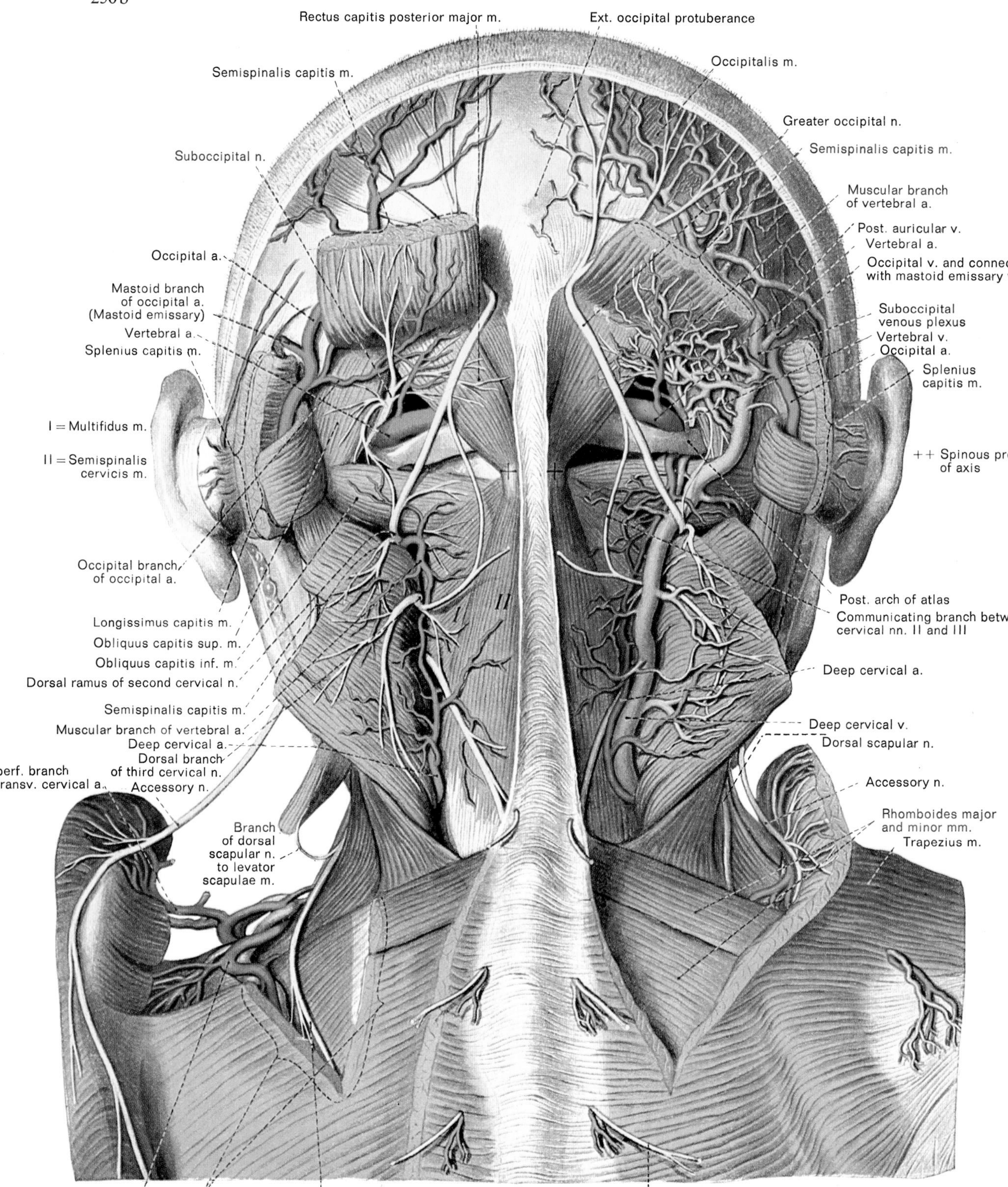
Rectus capitis posterior major m.
Ext. occipital protuberance
Semispinalis capitis m.
Occipitalis m.
Greater occipital n.
Semispinalis capitis m.
Suboccipital n.
Muscular branch of vertebral a.
Post. auricular v.
Vertebral a.
Occipital a.
Occipital v. and connecti with mastoid emissary v.
Mastoid branch of occipital a. (Mastoid emissary)
Suboccipital venous plexus
Vertebral v.
Vertebral a.
Occipital a.
Splenius capitis m.
Splenius capitis m.
I = Multifidus m.
II = Semispinalis cervicis m.
++ Spinous proc of axis
Occipital branch of occipital a.
Post. arch of atlas
Communicating branch betwe cervical nn. II and III
Longissimus capitis m.
Obliquus capitis sup. m.
Obliquus capitis inf. m.
Dorsal ramus of second cervical n.
Deep cervical a.
Semispinalis capitis m.
Muscular branch of vertebral a.
Deep cervical v.
Deep cervical a.
Dorsal scapular n.
Dorsal branch of third cervical n.
Superf. branch of transv. cervical a.
Accessory n.
Accessory n.
Rhomboides major and minor mm.
Trapezius m.
Branch of dorsal scapular n. to levator scapulae m.
Deep branch of transv. cervical a.
Rhomboideus major and minor mm.
Dorsal scapular n.
Med. cutaneous branch of dorsal ramus of thoracic n.

Fig. 352b. Deeper layer of nerves and vessels of upper back, neck and suboccipital triangle. Both semispinalis capitis muscles were divided and the suboccipital triangle was exposed. On the right side, the veins were preserved and the trapezius muscle was notched by a deep incision. On the left side, the trapezius was removed and the rhomboid muscles were notched.

Peripheral Nerves and Vessels

Nerves and Vessels of the Trunk

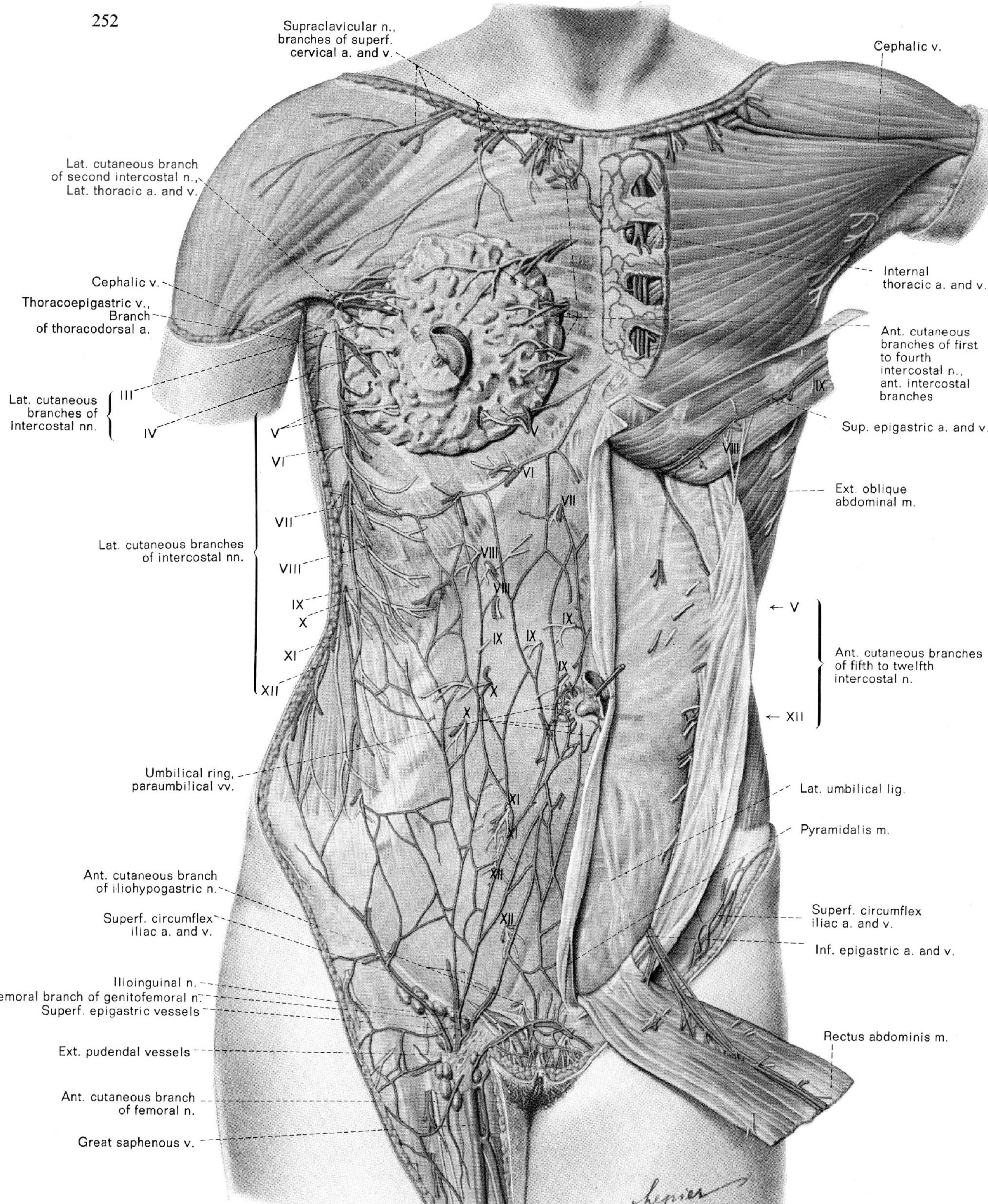
Supraclavicular n.,
branches of superf.
cervical a. and v.
Cephalic v.
Lat. cutaneous branch
of second intercostal n.,
Lat. thoracic a. and v.
Internal
thoracic a. and v.
Cephalic v.
Thoracoepigastric v.,
Branch
of thoracodorsal a.
Ant. cutaneous
branches of first
to fourth
intercostal n.,
ant. intercostal
branches
Lat. cutaneous
branches of
intercostal nn.
III
IV
V
V
IX
Sup. epigastric a. and v.
VIII
VI
VI
Ext. oblique
abdominal m.
VII
VII
Lat. cutaneous branches
of intercostal nn.
VIII
VIII
VIII
IX
X
V
IX
IX
IX
XI
Ant. cutaneous branches
of fifth to twelfth
intercostal n.
IX
XII
X
X
XII
Umbilical ring,
paraumbilical vv.
Lat. umbilical lig.
XI
XI
Pyramidalis m.
Ant. cutaneous branch
of iliohypogastric n.
XII
Superf. circumflex
iliac a. and v.
XII
Superf. circumflex
iliac a. and v.
Inf. epigastric a. and v.
Ilioinguinal n.
Femoral branch of genitofemoral n.
Superf. epigastric vessels
Rectus abdominis m.
Ext. pudendal vessels
Ant. cutaneous branch
of femoral n.
Great saphenous v.

Fig. 353. Nerves and vessels of the anterior thoracic and abdominal wall. Superficial layer on the left side of the picture.

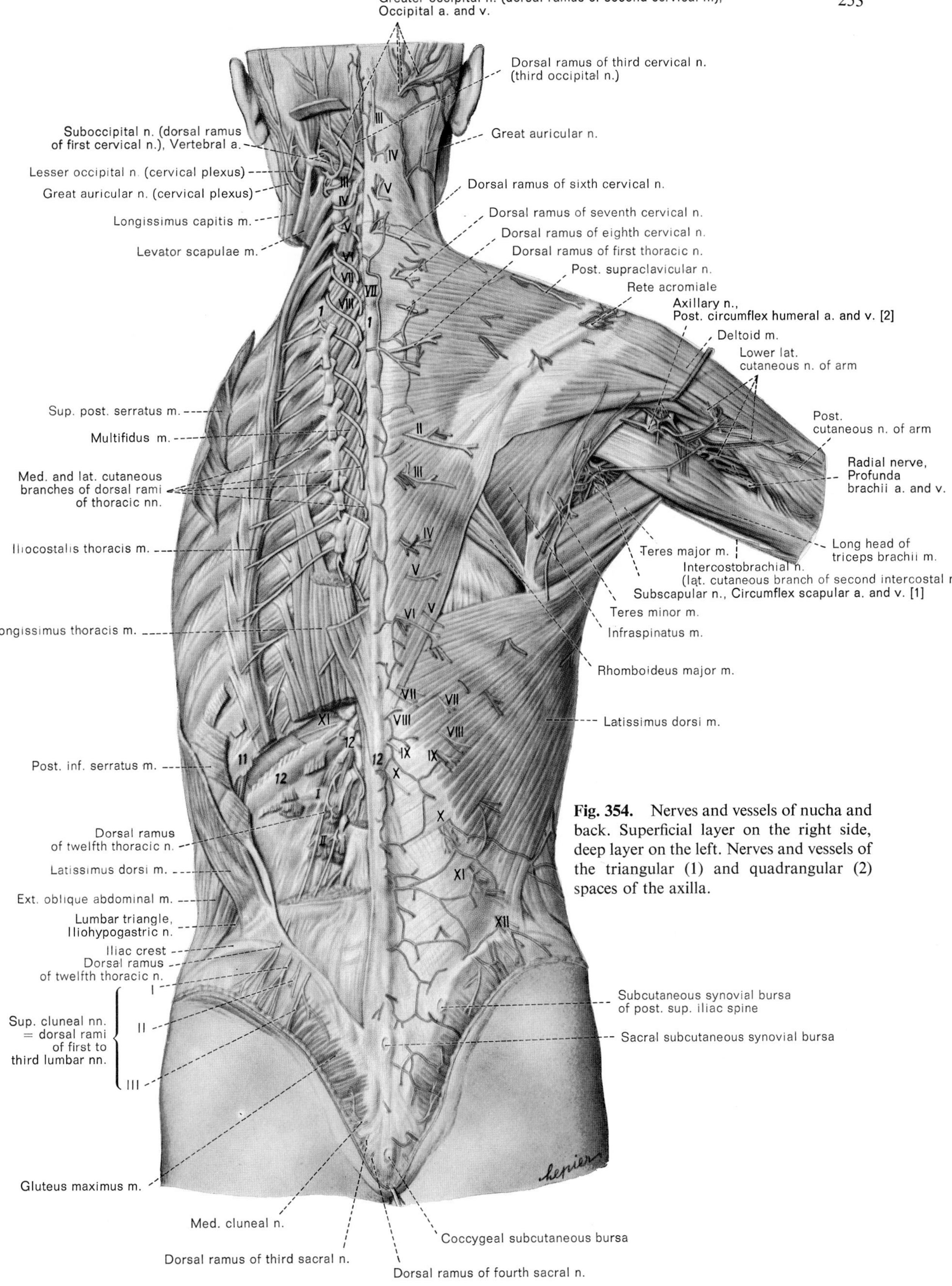
Greater occipital n. (dorsal ramus of second cervical n.),
Occipital a. and v.
Dorsal ramus of third cervical n.
(third occipital n.)
Suboccipital n. (dorsal ramus
of first cervical n.), Vertebral a.
Great auricular n.
Lesser occipital n. (cervical plexus)
Great auricular n. (cervical plexus)
Dorsal ramus of sixth cervical n.
Longissimus capitis m.
Dorsal ramus of seventh cervical n.
Dorsal ramus of eighth cervical n.
Levator scapulae m.
Dorsal ramus of first thoracic n.
Post. supraclavicular n.
Rete acromiale
Axillary n.,
Post. circumflex humeral a. and v. [2]
Deltoid m.
Lower lat.
cutaneous n. of arm
Sup. post. serratus m.
Post.
cutaneous n. of arm
Multifidus m.
Radial nerve,
Profunda
brachii a. and v.
Med. and lat. cutaneous
branches of dorsal rami
of thoracic nn.
Iliocostalis thoracis m.
Teres major m.
Long head of
triceps brachii m.
Intercostobrachial n.
(lat. cutaneous branch of second intercostal n.)
Subscapular n., Circumflex scapular a. and v. [1]
Teres minor m.
Longissimus thoracis m.
Infraspinatus m.
Rhomboideus major m.
Latissimus dorsi m.
Post. inf. serratus m.
Dorsal ramus
of twelfth thoracic n.
Latissimus dorsi m.
Ext. oblique abdominal m.
Lumbar triangle,
Iliohypogastric n.
Iliac crest
Dorsal ramus
of twelfth thoracic n.
Sup. cluneal nn.
= dorsal rami
of first to
third lumbar nn.
I
II
III
Subcutaneous synovial bursa
of post. sup. iliac spine
Sacral subcutaneous synovial bursa
Gluteus maximus m.
Med. cluneal n.
Coccygeal subcutaneous bursa
Dorsal ramus of third sacral n.
Dorsal ramus of fourth sacral n.

Fig. 354. Nerves and vessels of nucha and back. Superficial layer on the right side, deep layer on the left. Nerves and vessels of the triangular (1) and quadrangular (2) spaces of the axilla.

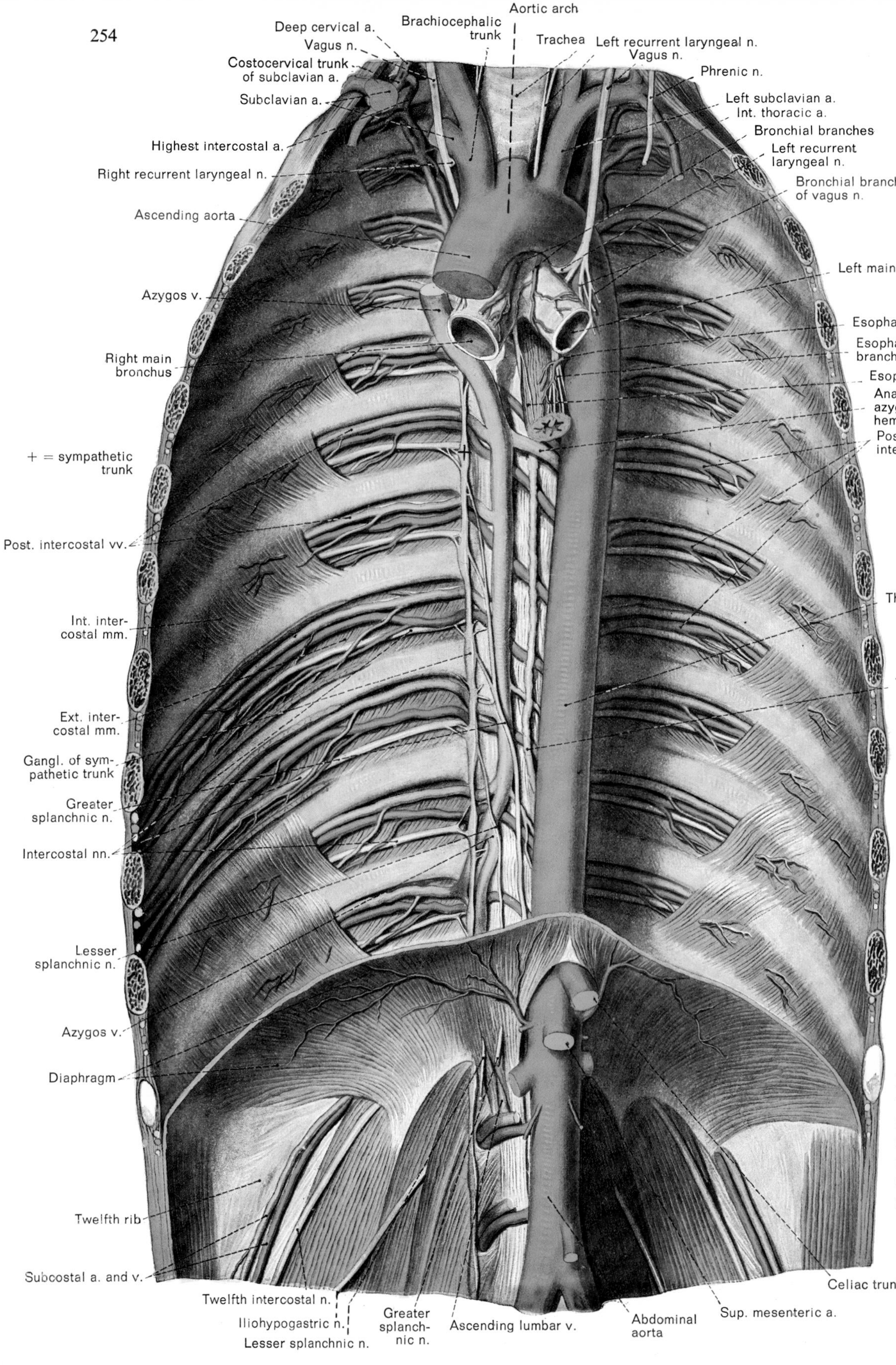

Deep cervical a.
Vagus n.
Costocervical trunk of subclavian a.
Subclavian a.
Highest intercostal a.
Right recurrent laryngeal n.
Ascending aorta
Azygos v.
Right main bronchus
+ = sympathetic trunk
Post. intercostal vv.
Int. intercostal mm.
Ext. intercostal mm.
Gangl. of sympathetic trunk
Greater splanchnic n.
Intercostal nn.
Lesser splanchnic n.
Azygos v.
Diaphragm
Twelfth rib
Subcostal a. and v.
Twelfth intercostal n.
Iliohypogastric n.
Lesser splanchnic n.
Greater splanchnic n.
Ascending lumbar v.
Abdominal aorta
Sup. mesenteric a.
Celiac trunk
Brachiocephalic trunk
Aortic arch
Trachea
Left recurrent laryngeal n.
Vagus n.
Phrenic n.
Left subclavian a.
Int. thoracic a.
Bronchial branches
Left recurrent laryngeal n.
Bronchial branches of vagus n.
Left main bronchus
Esophageal branches
Esophageal branches of vagus n.
Esophagus
Anastomosis between azygos and hemiazygos vv.
Post. intercostal aa.
Thoracic aorta
Thoracic duct

Fig. 355. Nerves vessels of interco spaces and poster mediastinum. T racic and abdomi aorta. Sympath trunk. Ventral vi

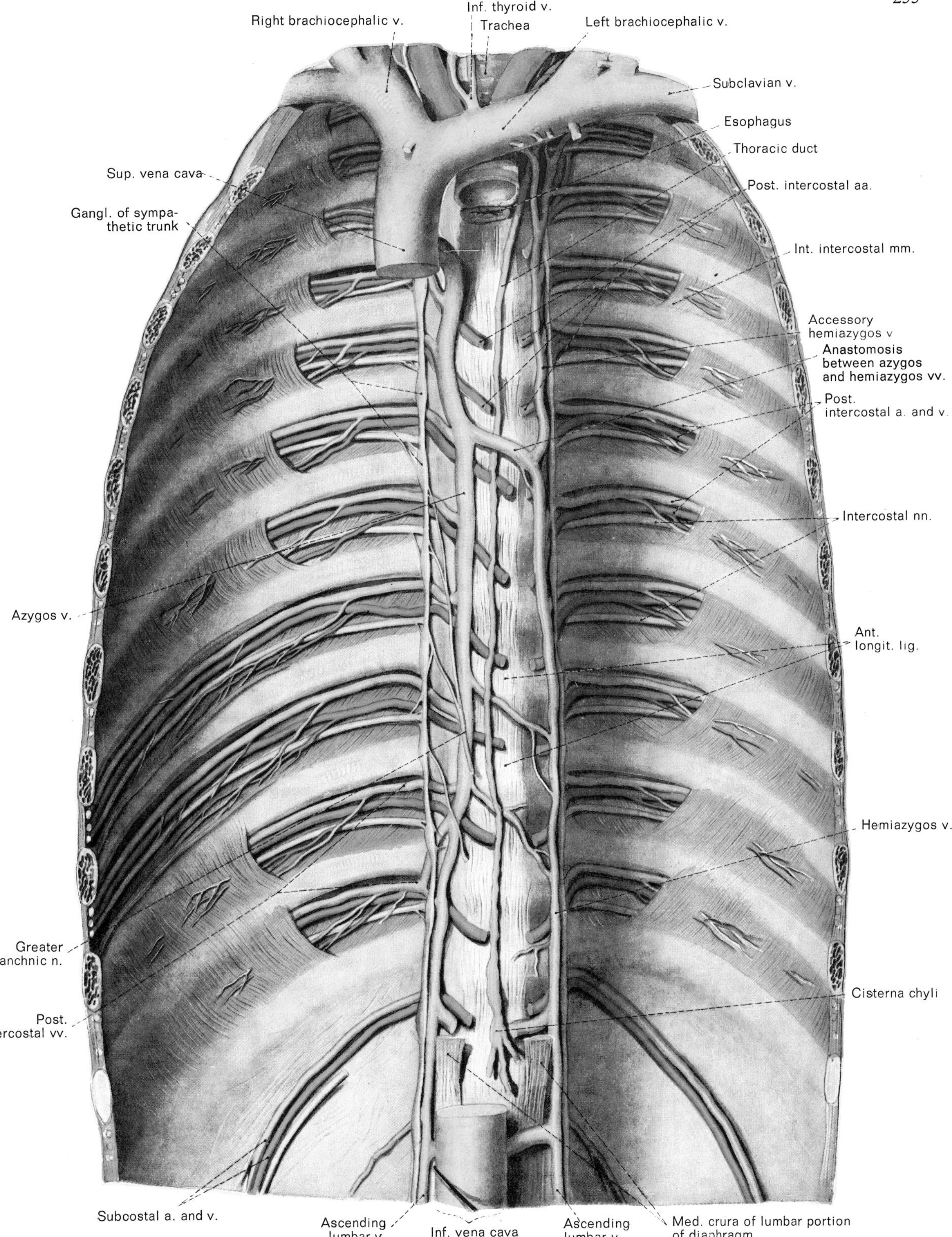
Inf. thyroid v.
Right brachiocephalic v.
Trachea
Left brachiocephalic v.
Subclavian v.
Esophagus
Thoracic duct
Sup. vena cava
Post. intercostal aa.
Gangl. of sympathetic trunk
Int. intercostal mm.
Accessory hemiazygos v
Anastomosis between azygos and hemiazygos vv.
Post. intercostal a. and v.
Intercostal nn.
Azygos v.
Ant. longit. lig.
Hemiazygos v.
Greater splanchnic n.
Cisterna chyli
Post. intercostal vv.
Subcostal a. and v.
Ascending lumbar v.
Inf. vena cava
Ascending lumbar v.
Med. crura of lumbar portion of diaphragm

Fig. 356. Nerves and vessels of the intercostal spaces; thoracic duct. The aorta has been removed, the superior and inferior vena cava have been cut off at the entry into the pericardial sac and caudal to the diaphragm, respectively.

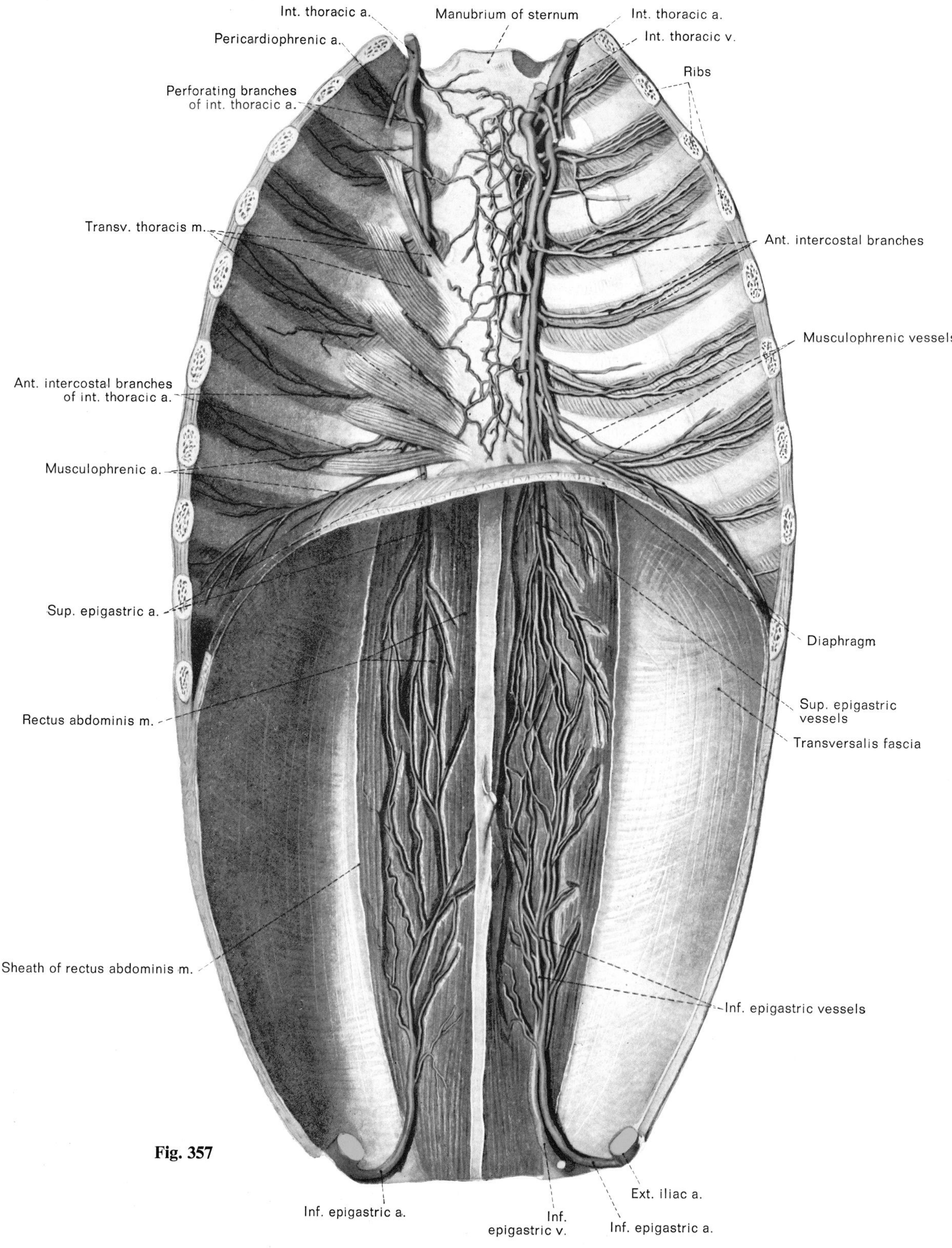
Int. thoracic a.
Manubrium of sternum
Int. thoracic a.
Pericardiophrenic a.
Int. thoracic v.
Ribs
Perforating branches of int. thoracic a.
Transv. thoracis m.
Ant. intercostal branches
Musculophrenic vessels
Ant. intercostal branches of int. thoracic a.
Musculophrenic a.
Sup. epigastric a.
Diaphragm
Rectus abdominis m.
Sup. epigastric vessels
Transversalis fascia
Sheath of rectus abdominis m.
Inf. epigastric vessels
Ext. iliac a.
Inf. epigastric a.
Inf. epigastric v.
Inf. epigastric a.

Fig. 357

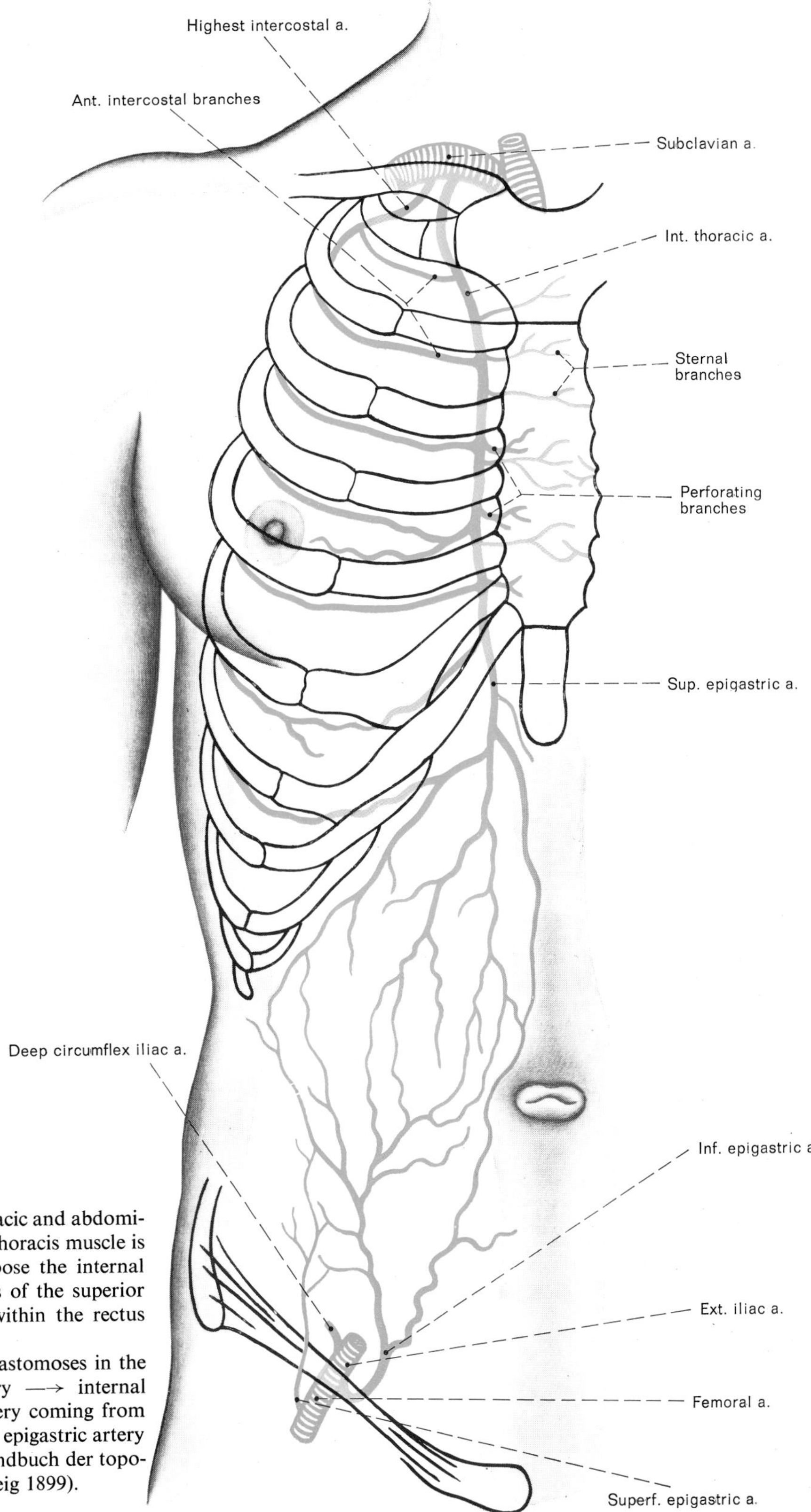
Highest intercostal a.
Ant. intercostal branches
Subclavian a.
Int. thoracic a.
Sternal branches
Perforating branches
Sup. epigastric a.
Deep circumflex iliac a.
Inf. epigastric a.
Ext. iliac a.
Femoral a.
Superf. epigastric a.

◀ **Fig. 357.** Blood vessels of the anterior thoracic and abdominal wall seen from behind. The transversus thoracis muscle is removed on the right side in order to expose the internal thoracic vessels. Branches and anastomoses of the superior and inferior epigastric vessels are shown within the rectus abdominis muscle.

Fig. 358. Diagram showing the arterial anastomoses in the abdominal wall between subclavian artery ⟶ internal thoracic artery ⟶ superior epigastric artery coming from above, and external iliac artery ⟶ inferior epigastric artery coming from below (after *F. R. Merkel:* Handbuch der topographischen Anatomie. Vieweg, Braunschweig 1899).

Peripheral Nerves and Vessels

Nerves and Vessels of Abdominal and Pelvic Cavities, of Perineum and Genital Organs

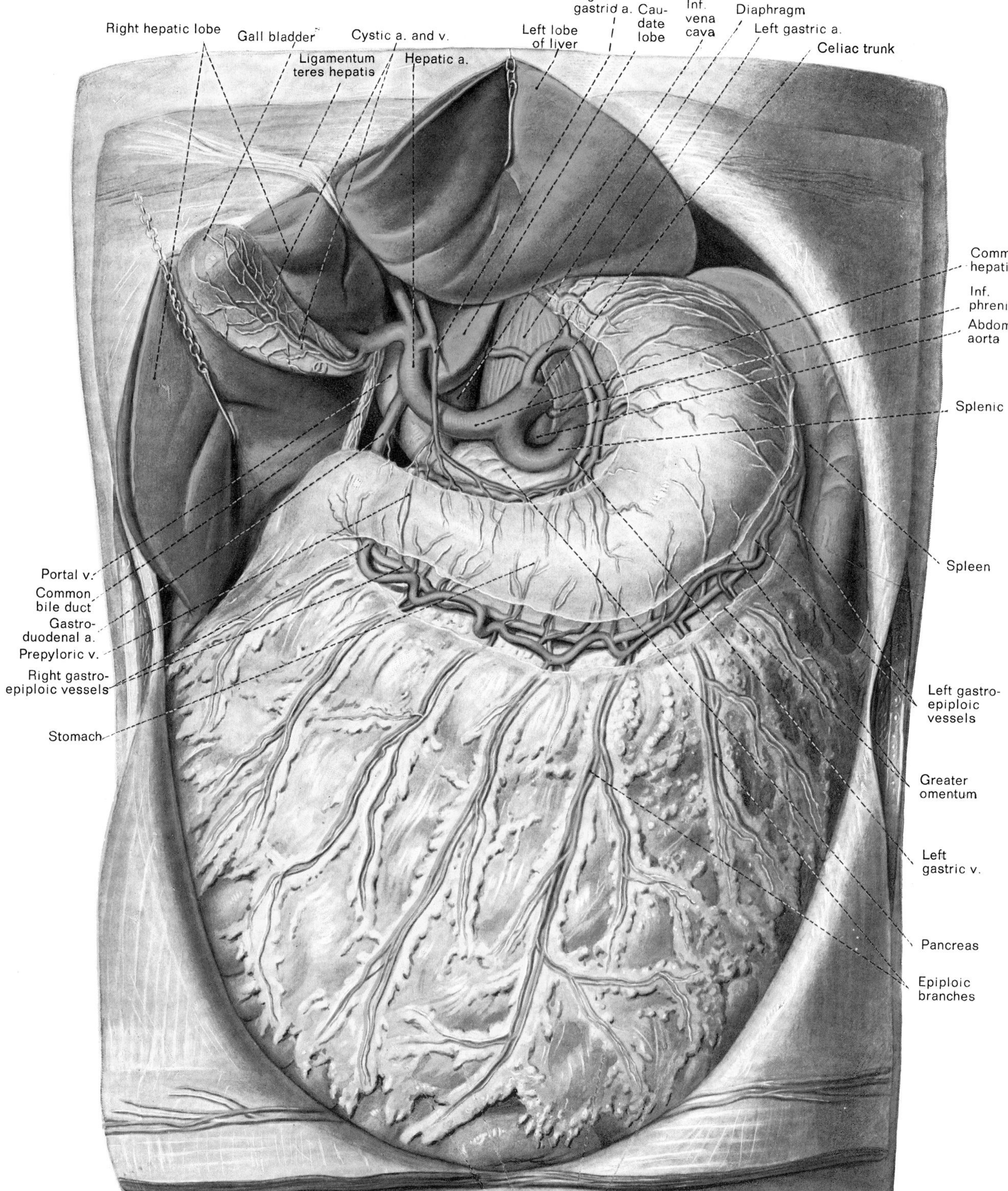

Right hepatic lobe
Gall bladder
Cystic a. and v.
Ligamentum teres hepatis
Hepatic a.
Left lobe of liver
Right gastric a.
Caudate lobe
Inf. vena cava
Diaphragm
Left gastric a.
Celiac trunk
Common hepatic
Inf. phrenic
Abdominal aorta
Splenic a.
Spleen
Left gastro-epiploic vessels
Greater omentum
Left gastric v.
Pancreas
Epiploic branches
Portal v.
Common bile duct
Gastro-duodenal a.
Prepyloric v.
Right gastro-epiploic vessels
Stomach

Fig. 359. Blood vessels of stomach and liver. The celiac trunk has been exposed; the ventral plate of the greater omentum has been opened along the greater curvature of the stomach in order to expose the gastroepiploic vessels; the lesser omentum and peritoneal membrane in the region of the vestibule to the omental bursa have been removed.

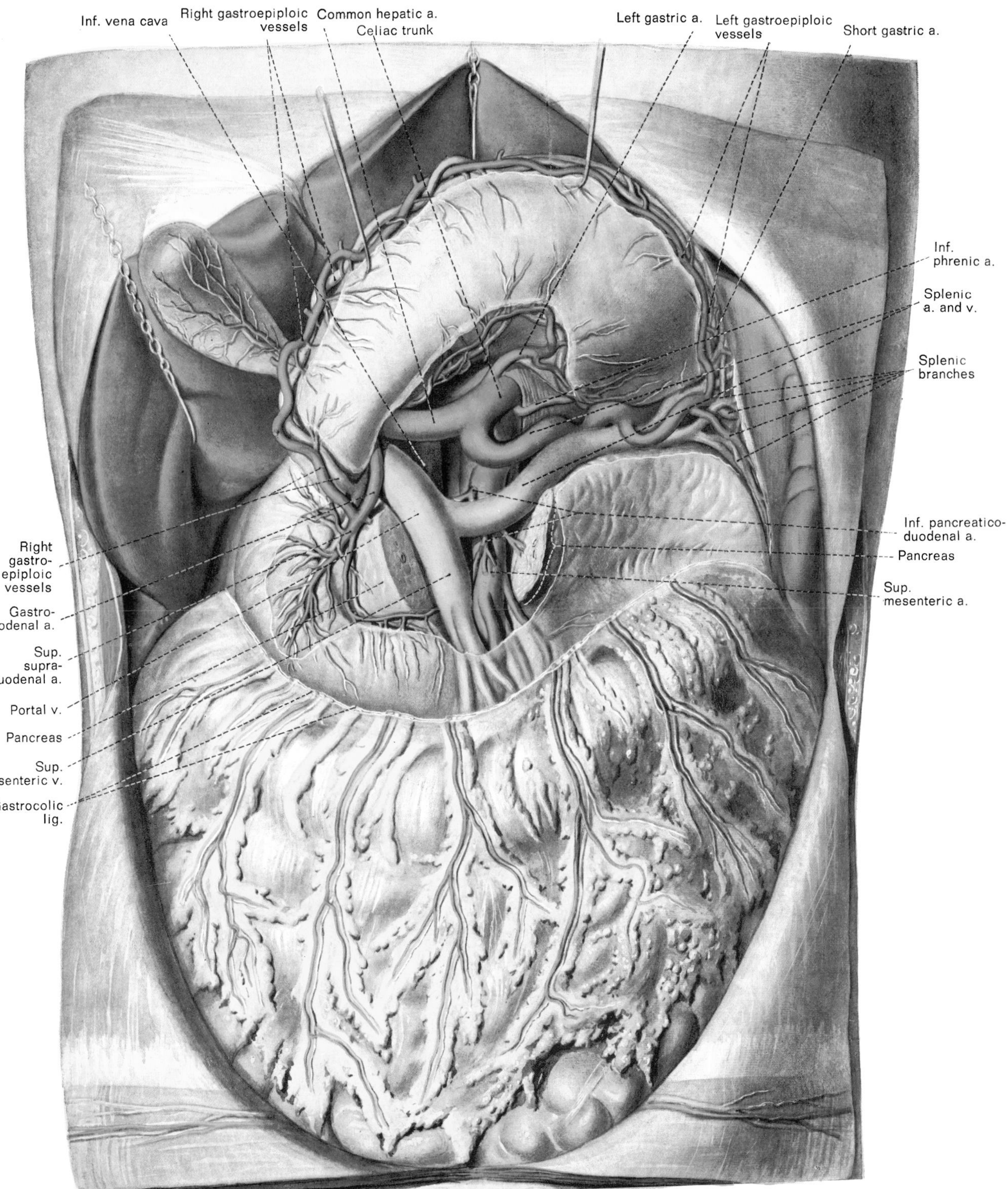
Inf. vena cava
Right gastroepiploic vessels
Common hepatic a.
Celiac trunk
Left gastric a.
Left gastroepiploic vessels
Short gastric a.
Inf. phrenic a.
Splenic a. and v.
Splenic branches
Inf. pancreatico-duodenal a.
Pancreas
Sup. mesenteric a.
Right gastro-epiploic vessels
Gastro-duodenal a.
Sup. supra-duodenal a.
Portal v.
Pancreas
Sup. mesenteric v.
Gastrocolic lig.

Fig. 360. Blood vessels of the stomach, tributaries to the portal vein, branches of the celiac trunk. The greater omentum has been sectioned and the stomach pulled upward so as to expose its posterior wall. A portion of the pancreas has been removed in order to expose the superior mesenteric artery and vein.

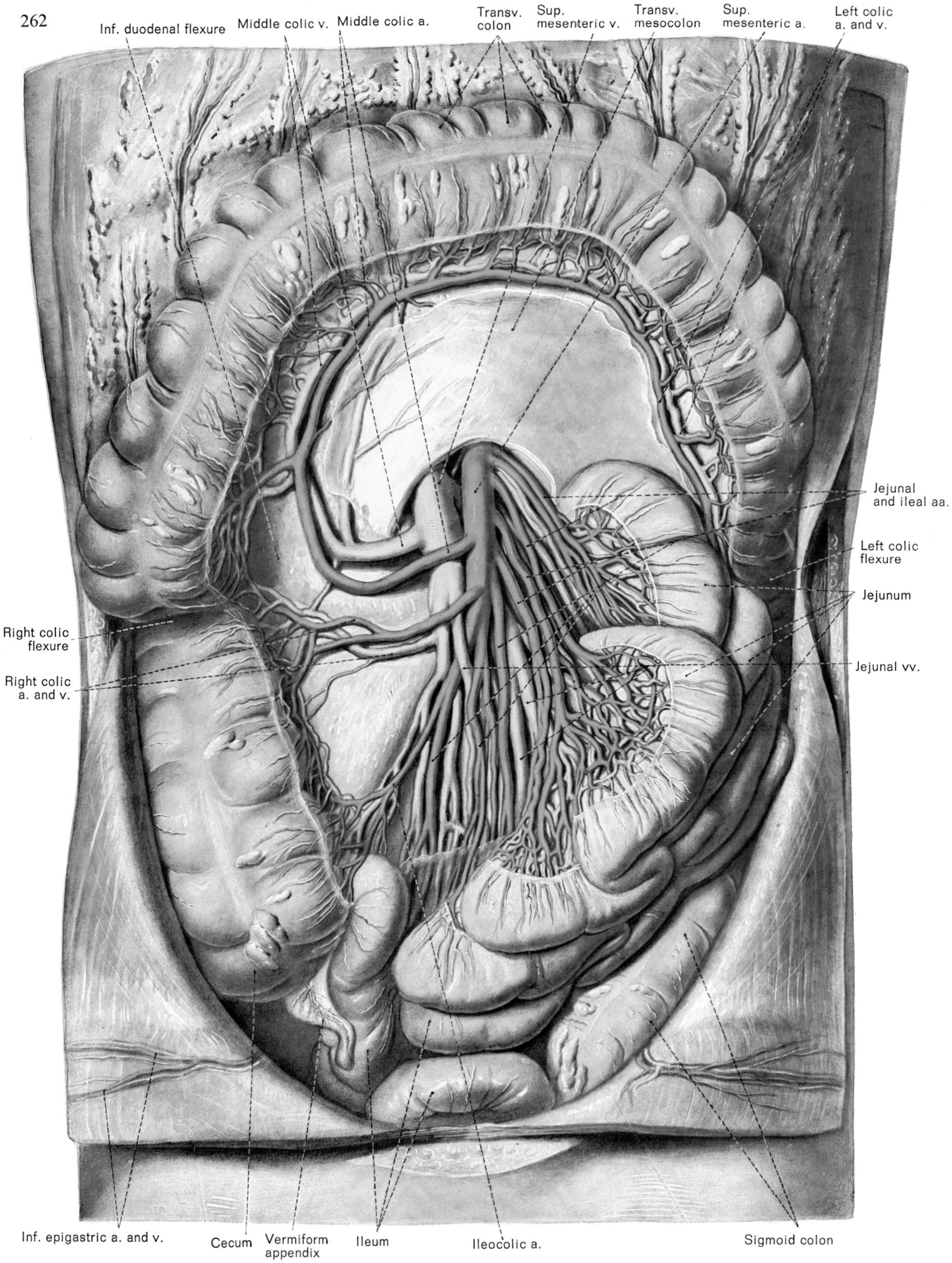

Inf. duodenal flexure
Middle colic v.
Middle colic a.
Transv. colon
Sup. mesenteric v.
Transv. mesocolon
Sup. mesenteric a.
Left colic a. and v.
Jejunal and ileal aa.
Left colic flexure
Jejunum
Jejunal vv.
Right colic flexure
Right colic a. and v.
Inf. epigastric a. and v.
Cecum
Vermiform appendix
Ileum
Ileocolic a.
Sigmoid colon

Fig. 361. Superior mesenteric artery and vein. The transverse colon with the greater omentum has been reflected upward, the loops of the small intestine have been moved toward the left. The parietal peritoneal membrane has been partially removed in order to expose the blood vessels.

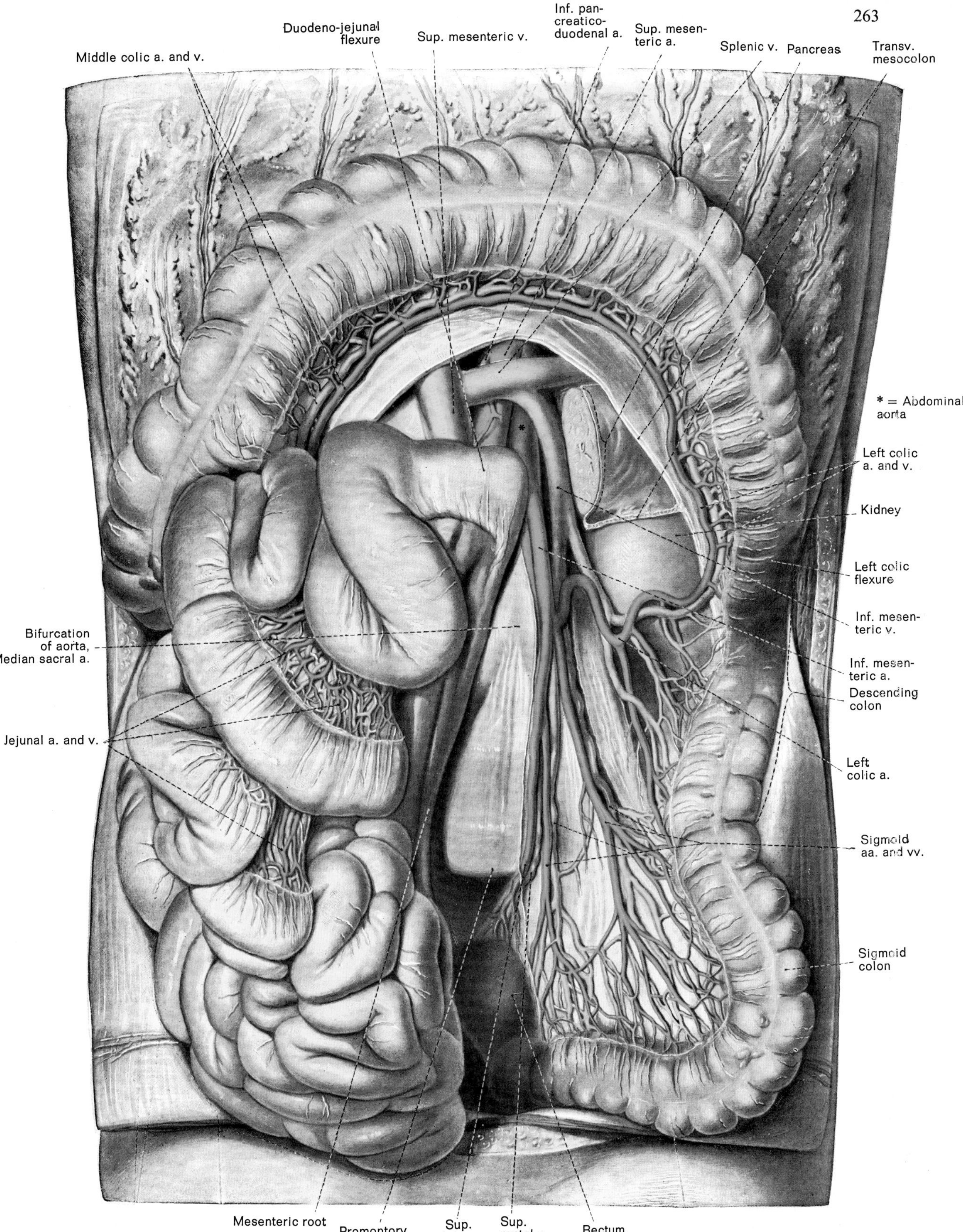

Middle colic a. and v.
Duodeno-jejunal flexure
Sup. mesenteric v.
Inf. pancreatico-duodenal a.
Sup. mesenteric a.
Splenic v.
Pancreas
Transv. mesocolon
* = Abdominal aorta
Left colic a. and v.
Kidney
Left colic flexure
Inf. mesenteric v.
Inf. mesenteric a.
Descending colon
Left colic a.
Sigmoid aa. and vv.
Sigmoid colon
Bifurcation of aorta, Median sacral a.
Jejunal a. and v.
Mesenteric root
Promontory
Sup. rectal a.
Sup. rectal v.
Rectum

Fig. 362. Inferior mesenteric artery and vein. Preparation similar to the one in Fig. 361, but the loops of the small intestine have been moved toward the right.

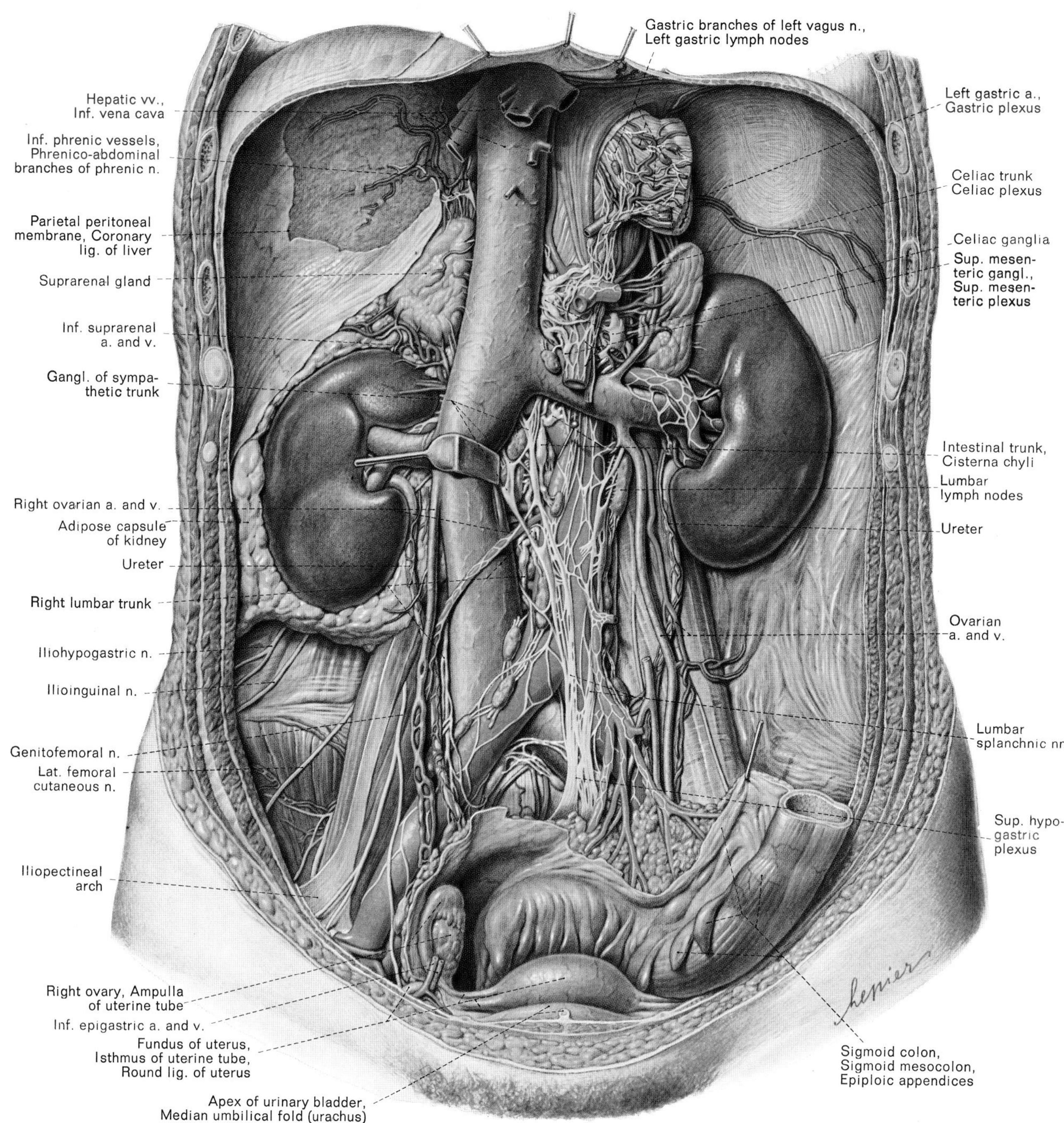
Gastric branches of left vagus n., Left gastric lymph nodes
Hepatic vv., Inf. vena cava
Inf. phrenic vessels, Phrenico-abdominal branches of phrenic n.
Parietal peritoneal membrane, Coronary lig. of liver
Suprarenal gland
Inf. suprarenal a. and v.
Gangl. of sympathetic trunk
Right ovarian a. and v.
Adipose capsule of kidney
Ureter
Right lumbar trunk
Iliohypogastric n.
Ilioinguinal n.
Genitofemoral n.
Lat. femoral cutaneous n.
Iliopectineal arch
Right ovary, Ampulla of uterine tube
Inf. epigastric a. and v.
Fundus of uterus, Isthmus of uterine tube, Round lig. of uterus
Apex of urinary bladder, Median umbilical fold (urachus)
Left gastric a., Gastric plexus
Celiac trunk Celiac plexus
Celiac ganglia
Sup. mesenteric gangl., Sup. mesenteric plexus
Intestinal trunk, Cisterna chyli
Lumbar lymph nodes
Ureter
Ovarian a. and v.
Lumbar splanchnic nn.
Sup. hypogastric plexus
Sigmoid colon, Sigmoid mesocolon, Epiploic appendices
Lepier

Fig. 363. Nerves, blood vessels and lymphatics of the posterior abdominal wall. The peritoneal membrane has been mostly removed and is retained only in the lesser pelvis, in the left iliac fossa and in the area of the coronary ligament of the liver. The adipose capsule of the left kidney is removed entirely, that of the right partially. Compare Fig. 165 relative to the abdominal and pelvic portions of the sympathetic trunk.

Fig. 364. Nerves and blood vessels of the posterior abdominal wall, lumbar plexus. The right psoas major muscle and portions of the common iliac vessels have been removed. × × = internal iliac vessels.

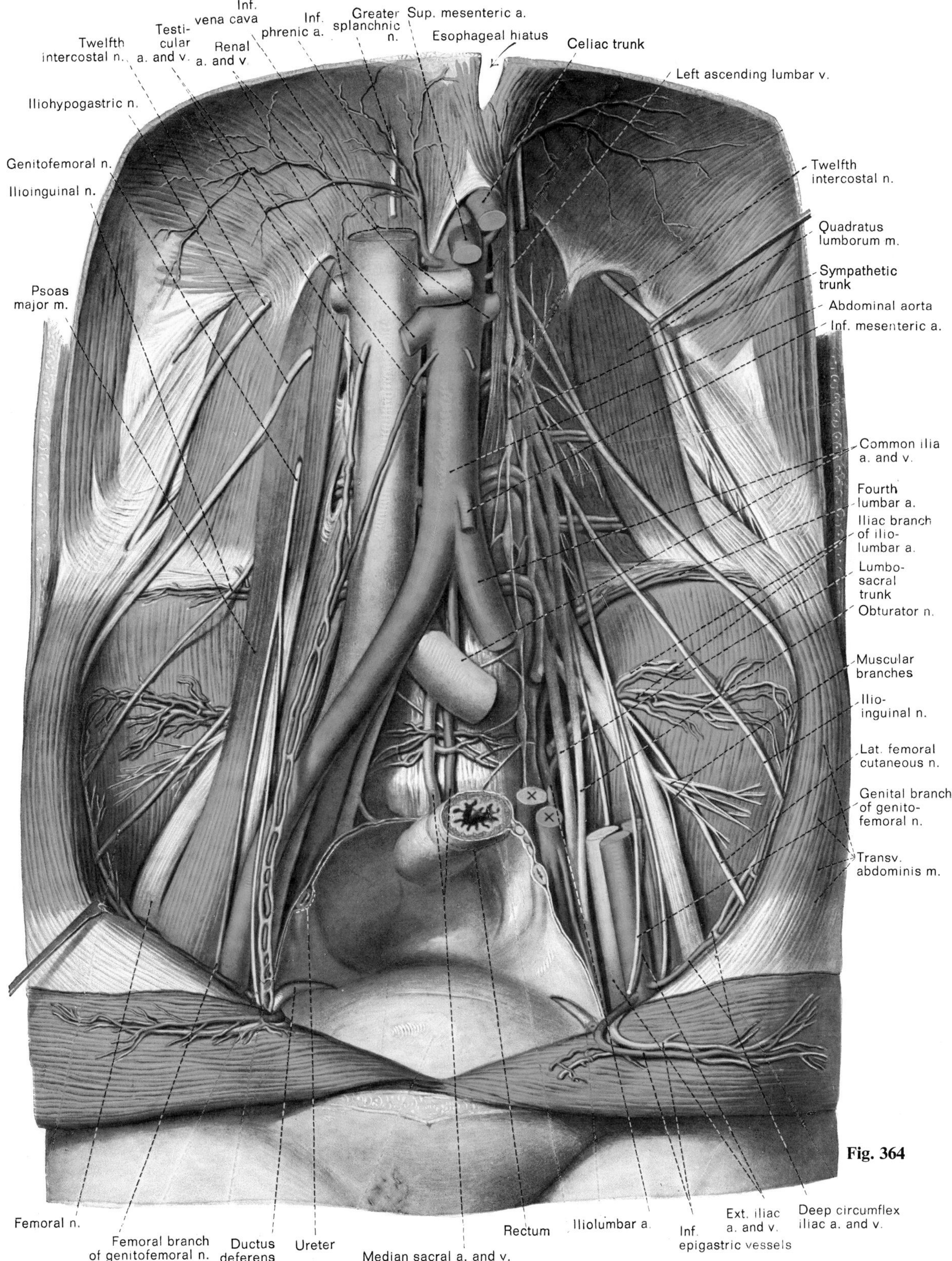

Inf. vena cava
Testicular a. and v.
Twelfth intercostal n.
Renal a. and v.
Inf. phrenic a.
Greater splanchnic n.
Sup. mesenteric a.
Esophageal hiatus
Celiac trunk
Left ascending lumbar v.
Iliohypogastric n.
Genitofemoral n.
Ilioinguinal n.
Psoas major m.
Twelfth intercostal n.
Quadratus lumborum m.
Sympathetic trunk
Abdominal aorta
Inf. mesenteric a.
Common ilia a. and v.
Fourth lumbar a.
Iliac branch of iliolumbar a.
Lumbosacral trunk
Obturator n.
Muscular branches
Ilioinguinal n.
Lat. femoral cutaneous n.
Genital branch of genitofemoral n.
Transv. abdominis m.
Femoral n.
Femoral branch of genitofemoral n.
Ductus deferens
Ureter
Median sacral a. and v.
Rectum
Iliolumbar a.
Inf. epigastric vessels
Ext. iliac a. and v.
Deep circumflex iliac a. and v.

Fig. 364

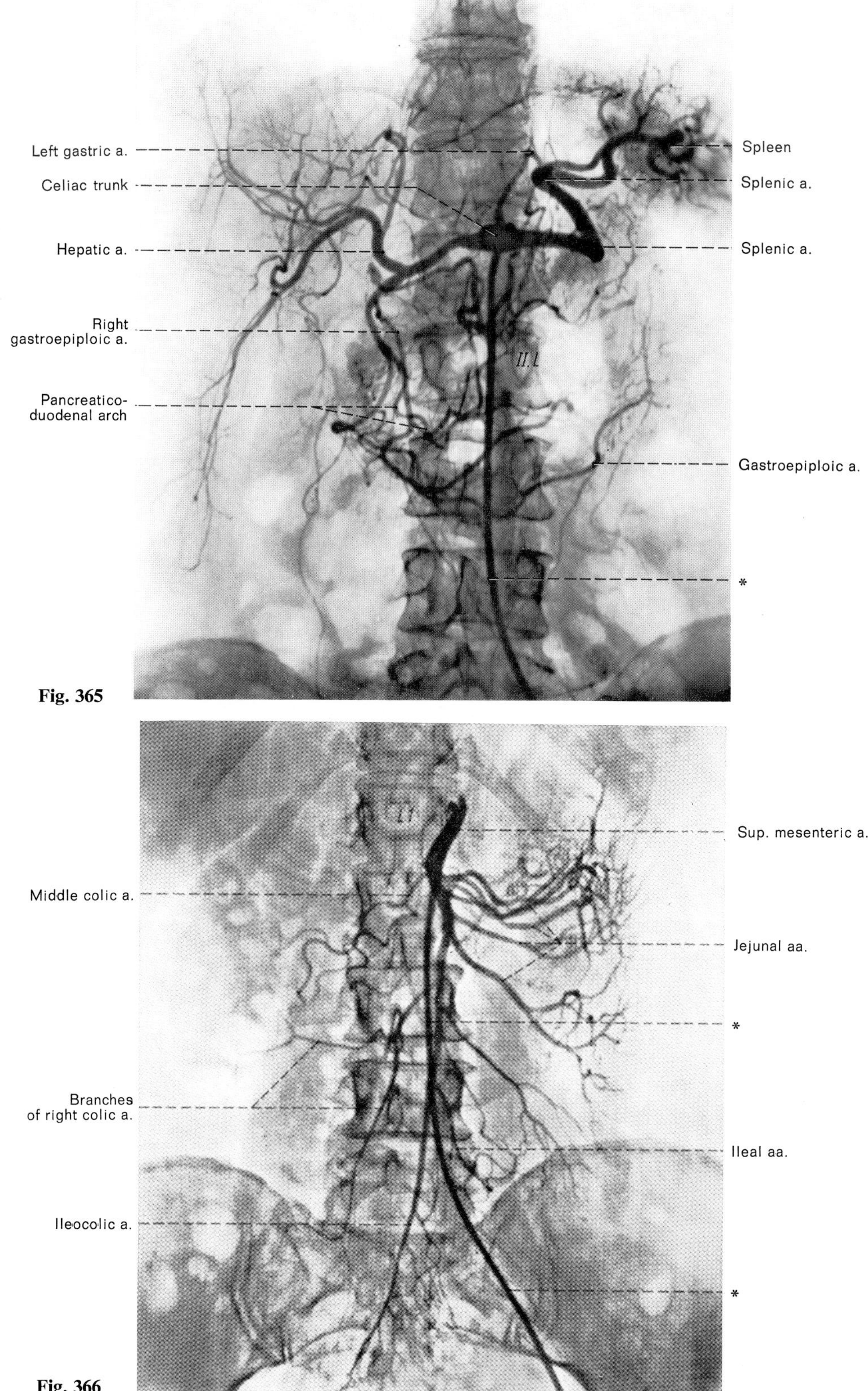
Left gastric a.
Celiac trunk
Hepatic a.
Right gastroepiploic a.
Pancreatico-duodenal arch
Spleen
Splenic a.
Splenic a.
Gastroepiploic a.
*
Sup. mesenteric a.
Middle colic a.
Jejunal aa.
*
Branches of right colic a.
Ileal aa.
Ileocolic a.
*

Fig. 365

Fig. 366

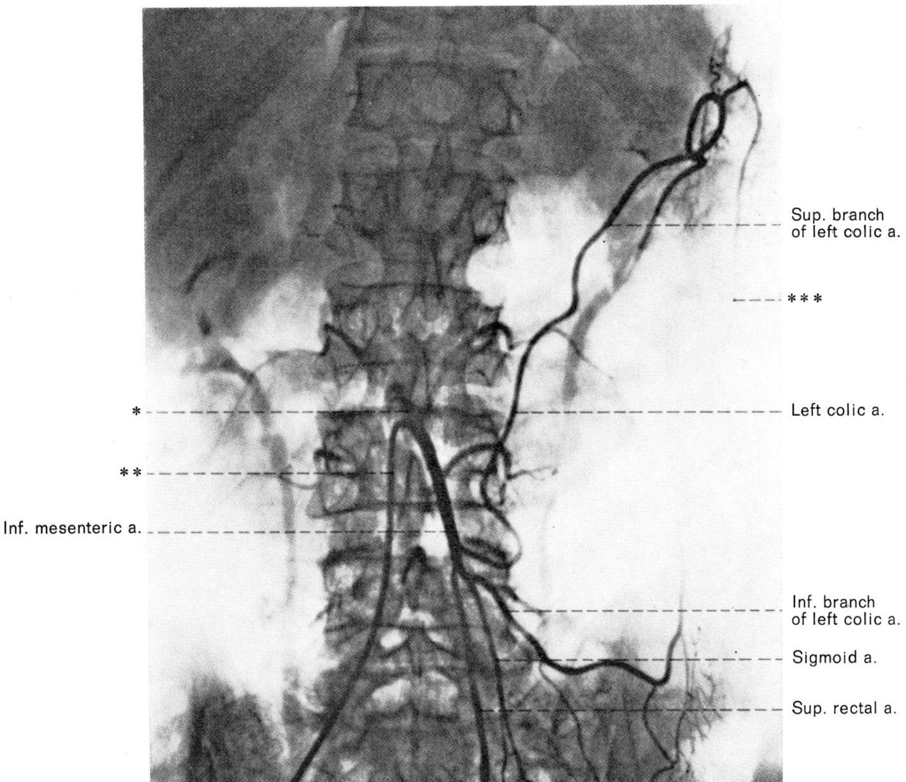
Sup. branch
of left colic a.
***
*
Left colic a.
**
Inf. mesenteric a.
Inf. branch
of left colic a.
Sigmoid a.
Sup. rectal a.

Fig. 367. Arteriogram of the inferior mesenteric artery. * = origin of the inferior mesenteric artery; ** = catheter; *** = anastomosis along the descending colon.

Fig. 365. Normal arteriogram of the branches of the celiac trunk. * = catheter in the aorta with its tip at the origin of the celiac trunk (Figs. 365–367 from *Benninghoff/Goerttler*, Lehrbuch der Anatomie des Menschen, vol. 2. Urban & Schwarzenberg, München–Berlin–Wien 1971).

Fig. 366. Arteriogram of the superior mesenteric artery. * = catheter in the abdominal aorta.

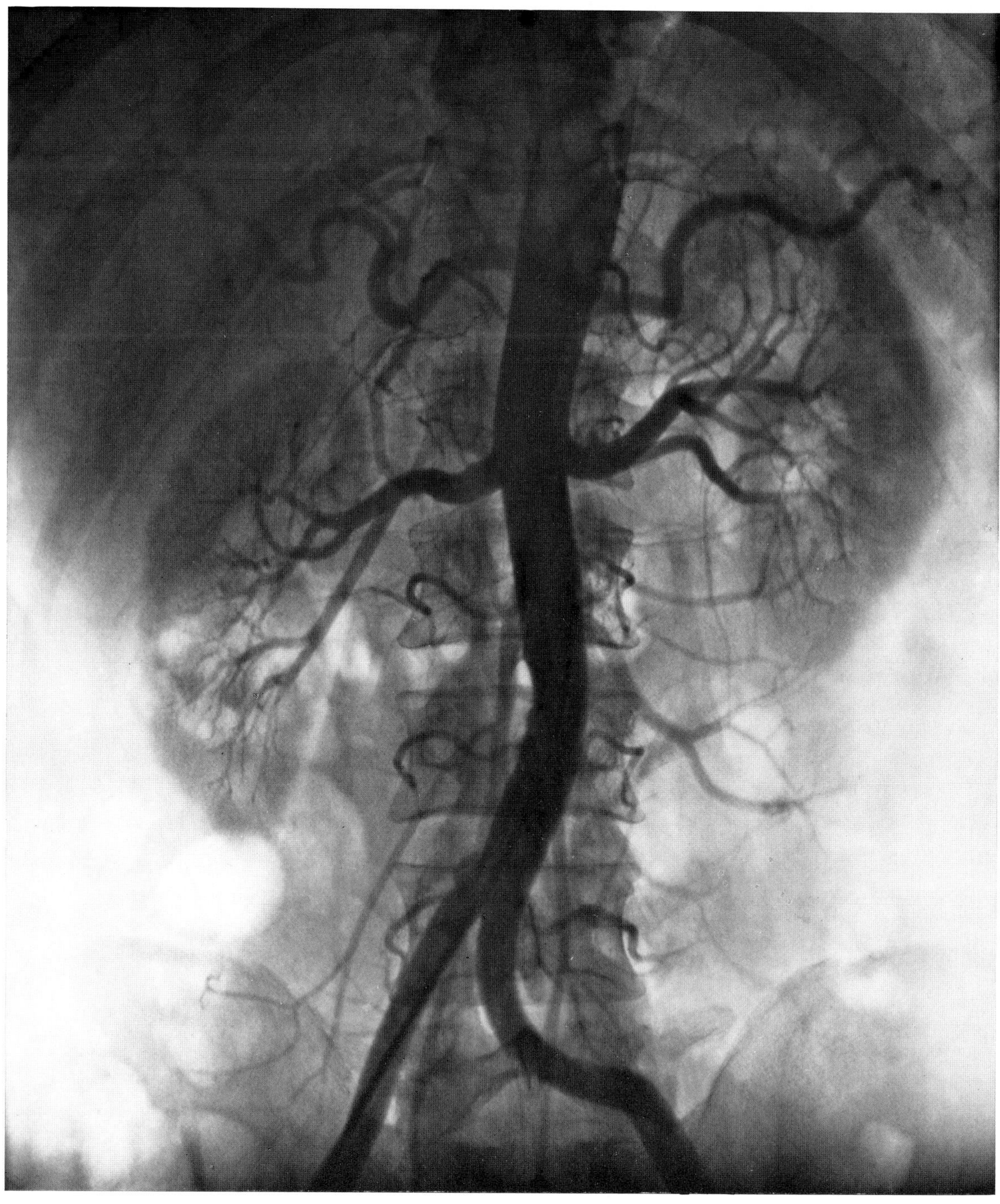

Fig. 368. Arteriogram of the abdominal aorta and of both renal arteries. Injection of the contrast medium was performed via a *Seldinger*-catheter which was introduced through the femoral artery and the tip of which had come to rest immediately above the origin of the renal arteries. (Sagittal film by Dr. *H. Schmid,* Pforzheim.)

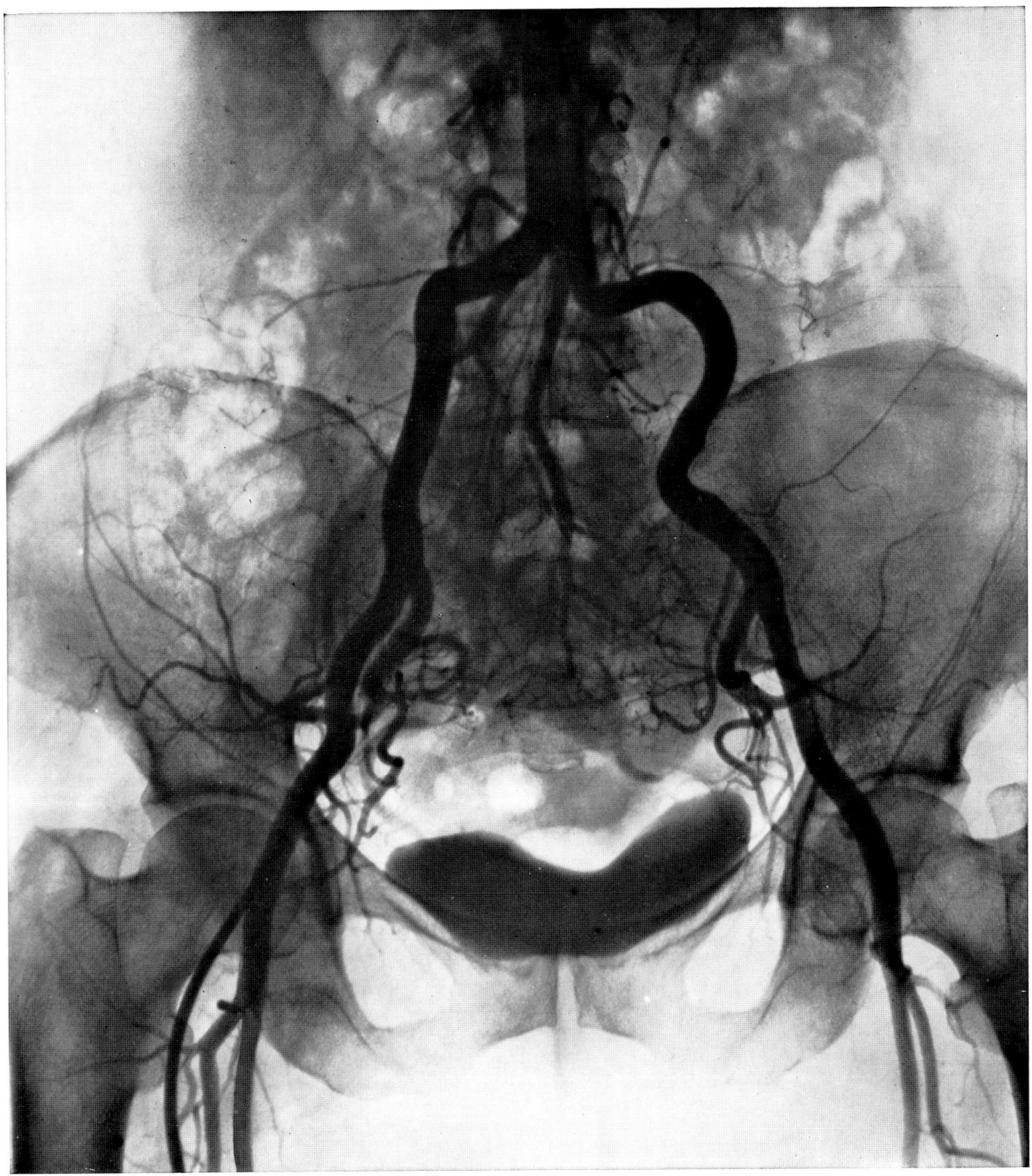

Fig. 369. Arteriogram of the lower abdominal aorta, iliac arteries and their branches. Observe the course of the median sacral artery and its branches. Contrast medium that has been eliminated by the kidneys can be seen in the urinary bladder. (Sagittal film by Dr. *H. Schmid,* Pforzheim.)

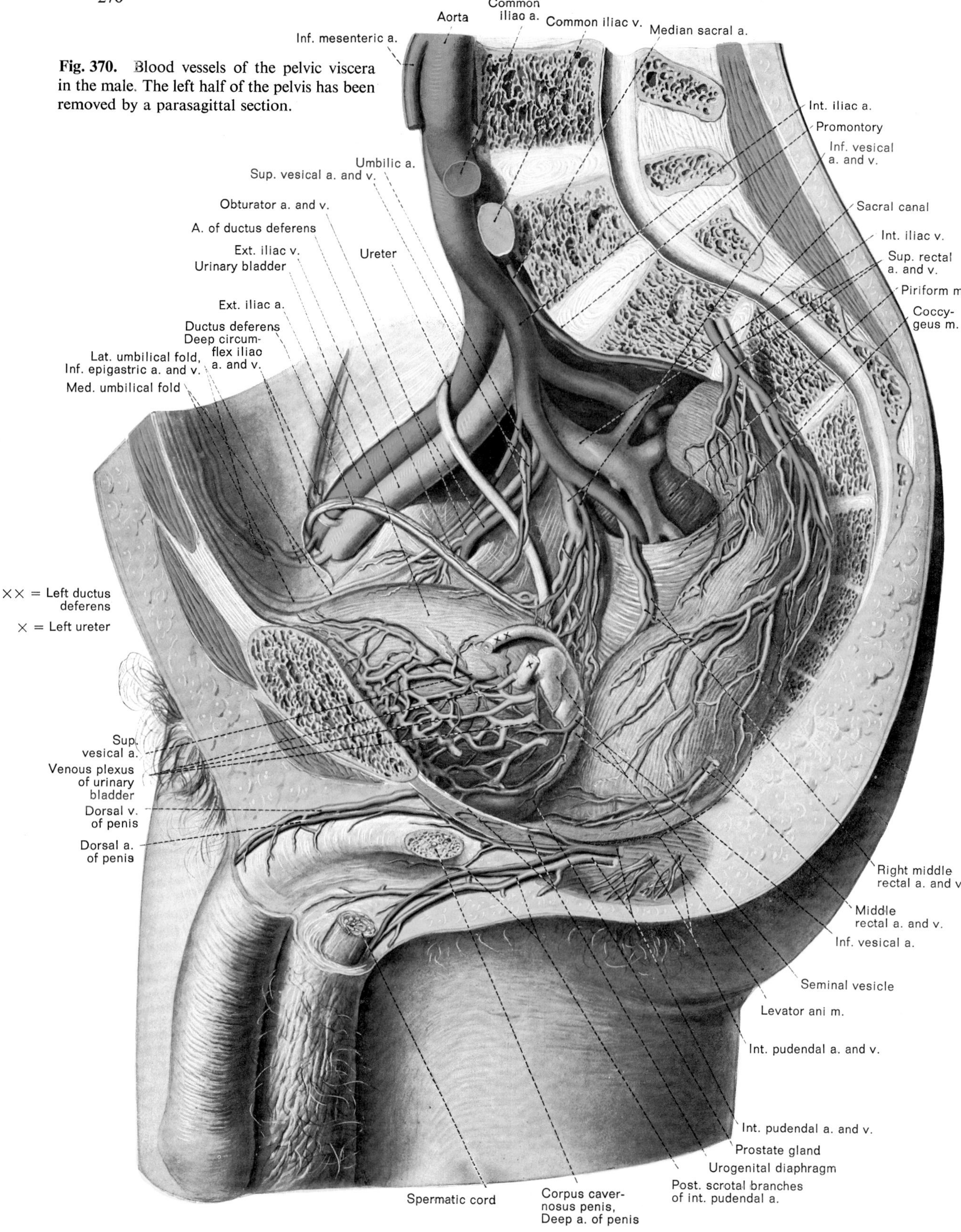
Aorta
Common iliac a.
Common iliac v.
Median sacral a.
Inf. mesenteric a.
Int. iliac a.
Promontory
Inf. vesical a. and v.
Umbilic a.
Sup. vesical a. and v.
Obturator a. and v.
Sacral canal
A. of ductus deferens
Int. iliac v.
Ext. iliac v.
Ureter
Sup. rectal a. and v.
Urinary bladder
Piriform m.
Ext. iliac a.
Coccygeus m.
Ductus deferens
Deep circumflex iliac a. and v.
Lat. umbilical fold,
Inf. epigastric a. and v.
Med. umbilical fold
XX = Left ductus deferens
X = Left ureter
Sup. vesical a.
Venous plexus of urinary bladder
Dorsal v. of penis
Dorsal a. of penis
Right middle rectal a. and v.
Middle rectal a. and v.
Inf. vesical a.
Seminal vesicle
Levator ani m.
Int. pudendal a. and v.
Int. pudendal a. and v.
Prostate gland
Urogenital diaphragm
Post. scrotal branches of int. pudendal a.
Spermatic cord
Corpus cavernosus penis,
Deep a. of penis

Fig. 370. Blood vessels of the pelvic viscera in the male. The left half of the pelvis has been removed by a parasagittal section.

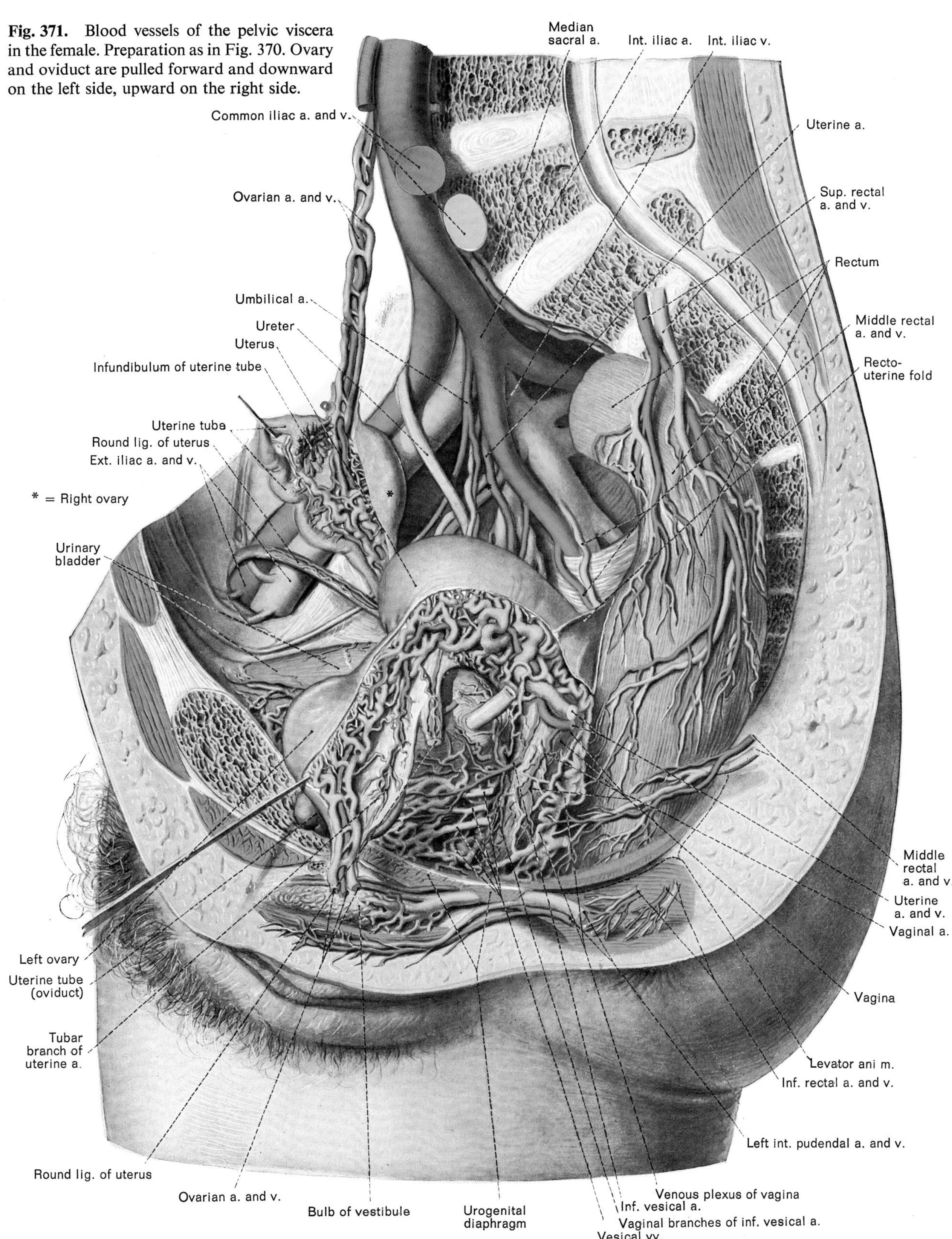

Median sacral a.
Int. iliac a.
Int. iliac v.
Common iliac a. and v.
Uterine a.
Ovarian a. and v.
Sup. rectal a. and v.
Rectum
Umbilical a.
Middle rectal a. and v.
Ureter
Uterus
Recto-uterine fold
Infundibulum of uterine tube
Uterine tube
Round lig. of uterus
Ext. iliac a. and v.
* = Right ovary
Urinary bladder
Middle rectal a. and v.
Uterine a. and v.
Vaginal a.
Left ovary
Uterine tube (oviduct)
Vagina
Tubar branch of uterine a.
Levator ani m.
Inf. rectal a. and v.
Left int. pudendal a. and v.
Round lig. of uterus
Venous plexus of vagina
Ovarian a. and v.
Inf. vesical a.
Bulb of vestibule
Urogenital diaphragm
Vaginal branches of inf. vesical a.
Vesical vv.

Fig. 371. Blood vessels of the pelvic viscera in the female. Preparation as in Fig. 370. Ovary and oviduct are pulled forward and downward on the left side, upward on the right side.

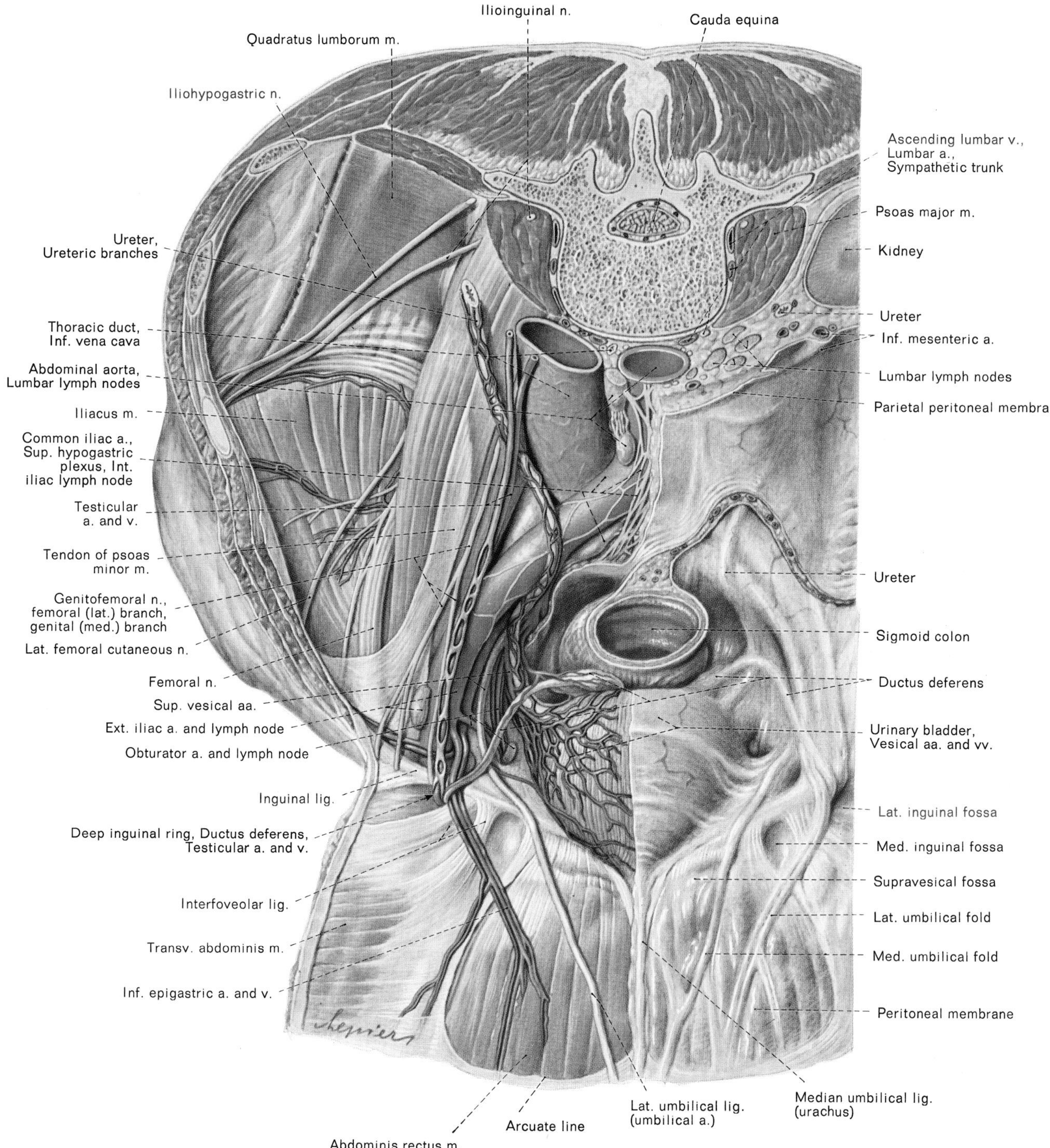
Ilioinguinal n.
Cauda equina
Quadratus lumborum m.
Iliohypogastric n.
Ascending lumbar v.,
Lumbar a.,
Sympathetic trunk
Psoas major m.
Kidney
Ureter,
Ureteric branches
Ureter
Thoracic duct,
Inf. vena cava
Inf. mesenteric a.
Abdominal aorta,
Lumbar lymph nodes
Lumbar lymph nodes
Parietal peritoneal membrane
Iliacus m.
Common iliac a.,
Sup. hypogastric
plexus, Int.
iliac lymph node
Testicular
a. and v.
Tendon of psoas
minor m.
Ureter
Genitofemoral n.,
femoral (lat.) branch,
genital (med.) branch
Sigmoid colon
Lat. femoral cutaneous n.
Femoral n.
Ductus deferens
Sup. vesical aa.
Ext. iliac a. and lymph node
Urinary bladder,
Vesical aa. and vv.
Obturator a. and lymph node
Inguinal lig.
Lat. inguinal fossa
Deep inguinal ring, Ductus deferens,
Testicular a. and v.
Med. inguinal fossa
Supravesical fossa
Interfoveolar lig.
Lat. umbilical fold
Transv. abdominis m.
Med. umbilical fold
Inf. epigastric a. and v.
Peritoneal membrane
Lepier
Lat. umbilical lig.
(umbilical a.)
Median umbilical lig.
(urachus)
Arcuate line
Abdominis rectus m.

Fig. 372. Nerves and vessels of posterior abdominal wall, pelvis and anterior abdominal wall. The anterior abdominal wall has been deflected downward, the peritoneal membrane has been removed on the right side.

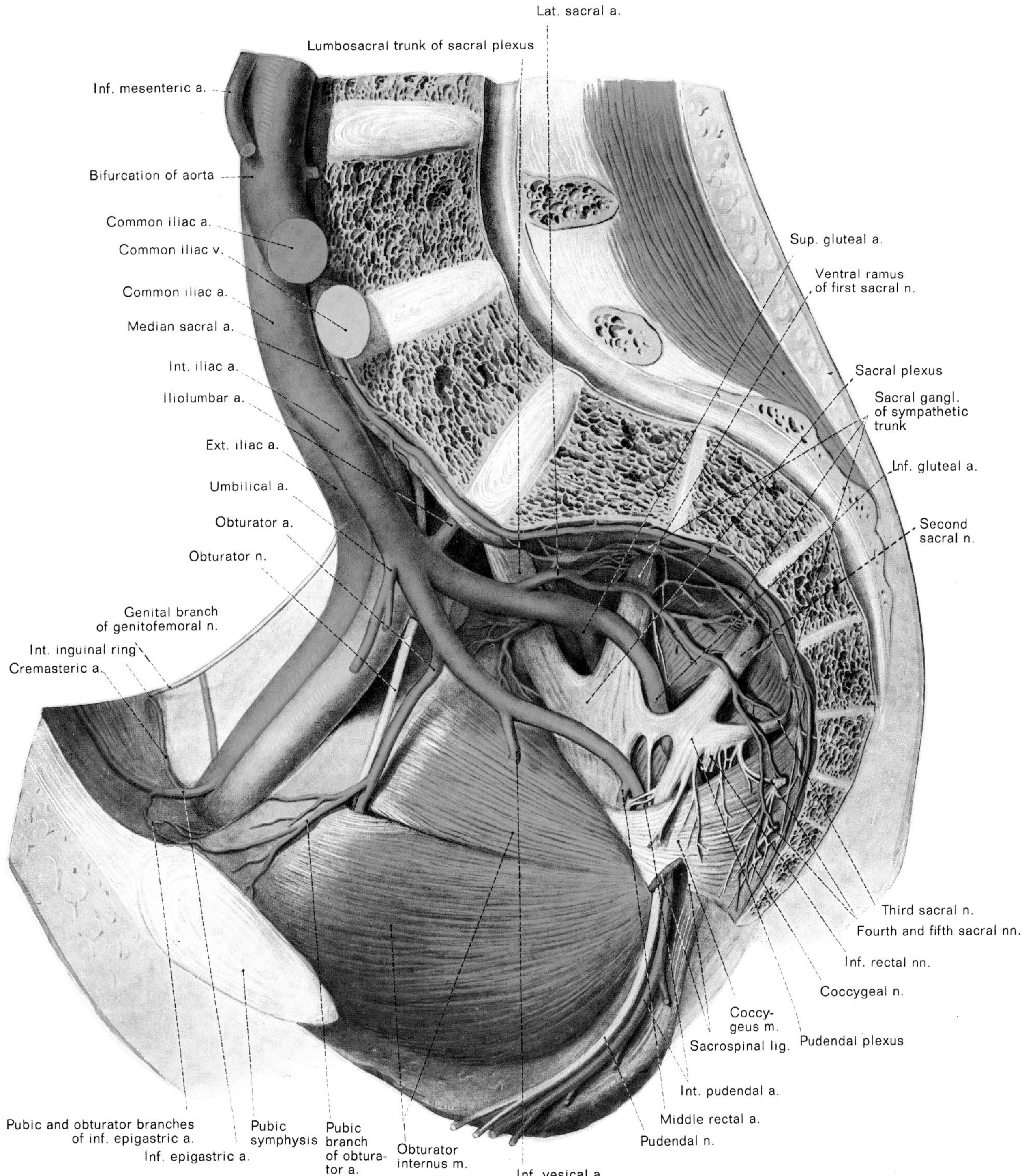
Lat. sacral a.
Lumbosacral trunk of sacral plexus
Inf. mesenteric a.
Bifurcation of aorta
Common iliac a.
Common iliac v.
Common iliac a.
Median sacral a.
Int. iliac a.
Iliolumbar a.
Ext. iliac a.
Umbilical a.
Obturator a.
Obturator n.
Genital branch of genitofemoral n.
Int. inguinal ring
Cremasteric a.
Sup. gluteal a.
Ventral ramus of first sacral n.
Sacral plexus
Sacral gangl. of sympathetic trunk
Inf. gluteal a.
Second sacral n.
Third sacral n.
Fourth and fifth sacral nn.
Inf. rectal nn.
Coccygeal n.
Coccygeus m.
Sacrospinal lig.
Pudendal plexus
Int. pudendal a.
Middle rectal a.
Pudendal n.
Pubic and obturator branches of inf. epigastric a.
Inf. epigastric a.
Pubic symphysis
Pubic branch of obturator a.
Obturator internus m.
Inf. vesical a.

Fig. 373. Blood vessels and nerves of the right pelvic wall. Pelvis has been divided in the sagittal plane and pelvic viscera have been removed.

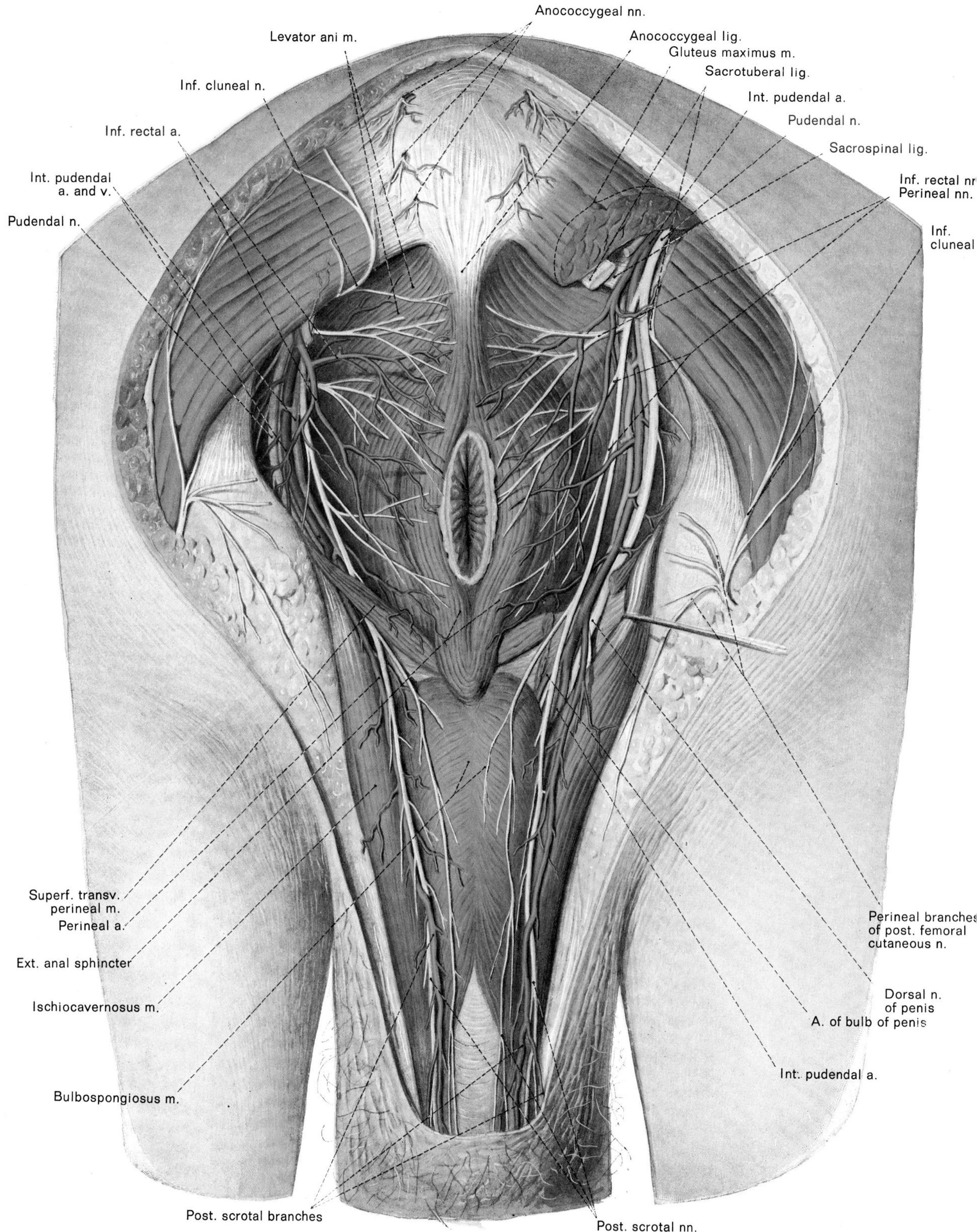

Anococcygeal nn.
Levator ani m.
Anococcygeal lig.
Gluteus maximus m.
Sacrotuberal lig.
Inf. cluneal n.
Int. pudendal a.
Pudendal n.
Inf. rectal a.
Sacrospinal lig.
Int. pudendal
a. and v.
Inf. rectal nr
Perineal nn.
Pudendal n.
Inf.
cluneal
Superf. transv.
perineal m.
Perineal a.
Ext. anal sphincter
Ischiocavernosus m.
Bulbospongiosus m.
Perineal branches
of post. femoral
cutaneous n.
Dorsal n.
of penis
A. of bulb of penis
Int. pudendal a.
Post. scrotal branches
Post. scrotal nn.

Fig. 374

Fig. 374. Nerves and vessels of the male perineum. Superficial perineal muscles are shown on the left side, fat of the ischiorectal fossa has been removed, nerves and vessels are exposed by incisions into the musculature on the right side.

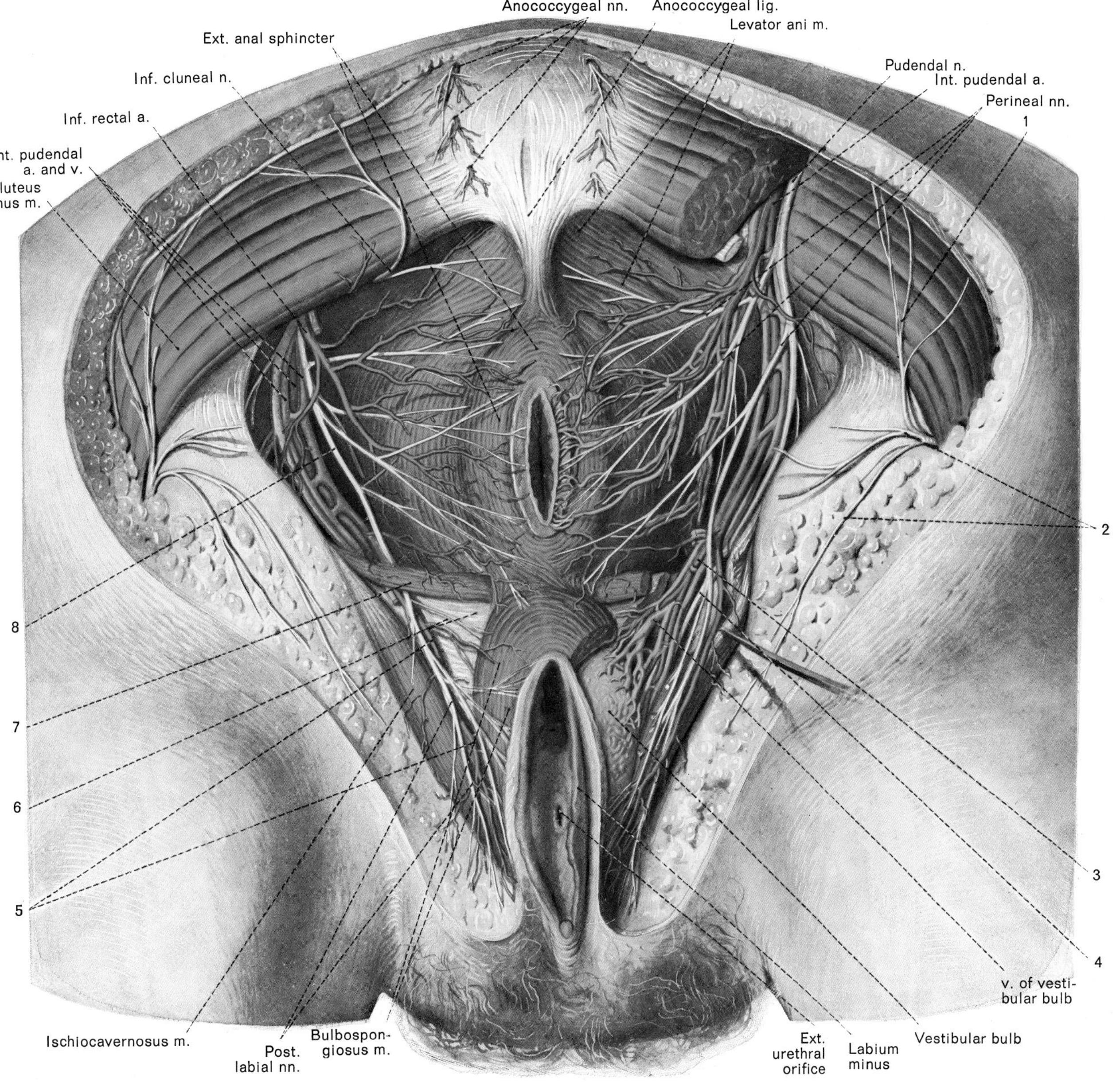

Anococcygeal nn.
Anococcygeal lig.
Levator ani m.
Ext. anal sphincter
Inf. cluneal n.
Inf. rectal a.
Int. pudendal a. and v.
Gluteus ximus m.
Pudendal n.
Int. pudendal a.
Perineal nn.
1
2
3
4
5
6
7
8
v. of vestibular bulb
Vestibular bulb
Labium minus
Ext. urethral orifice
Bulbospongiosus m.
Post. labial nn.
Ischiocavernosus m.

Fig. 375. Nerves and vessels of the female perineum. On the right side the bulbocavernosus muscle has been partially removed in order to expose the vestibular bulb. Nerves and vessels have been exposed by incisions into the musculature.

1 Inf. cluneal n.
2 Perineal branches of post. femoral cutaneous n.
3 Int. pudendal a.
4 Dorsal n. of clitoris
5 Post. labial branches of int. pudendal a.
6 Urogenital diaphragm
7 Superf. transv. perineal m.
8 Perineal nn.

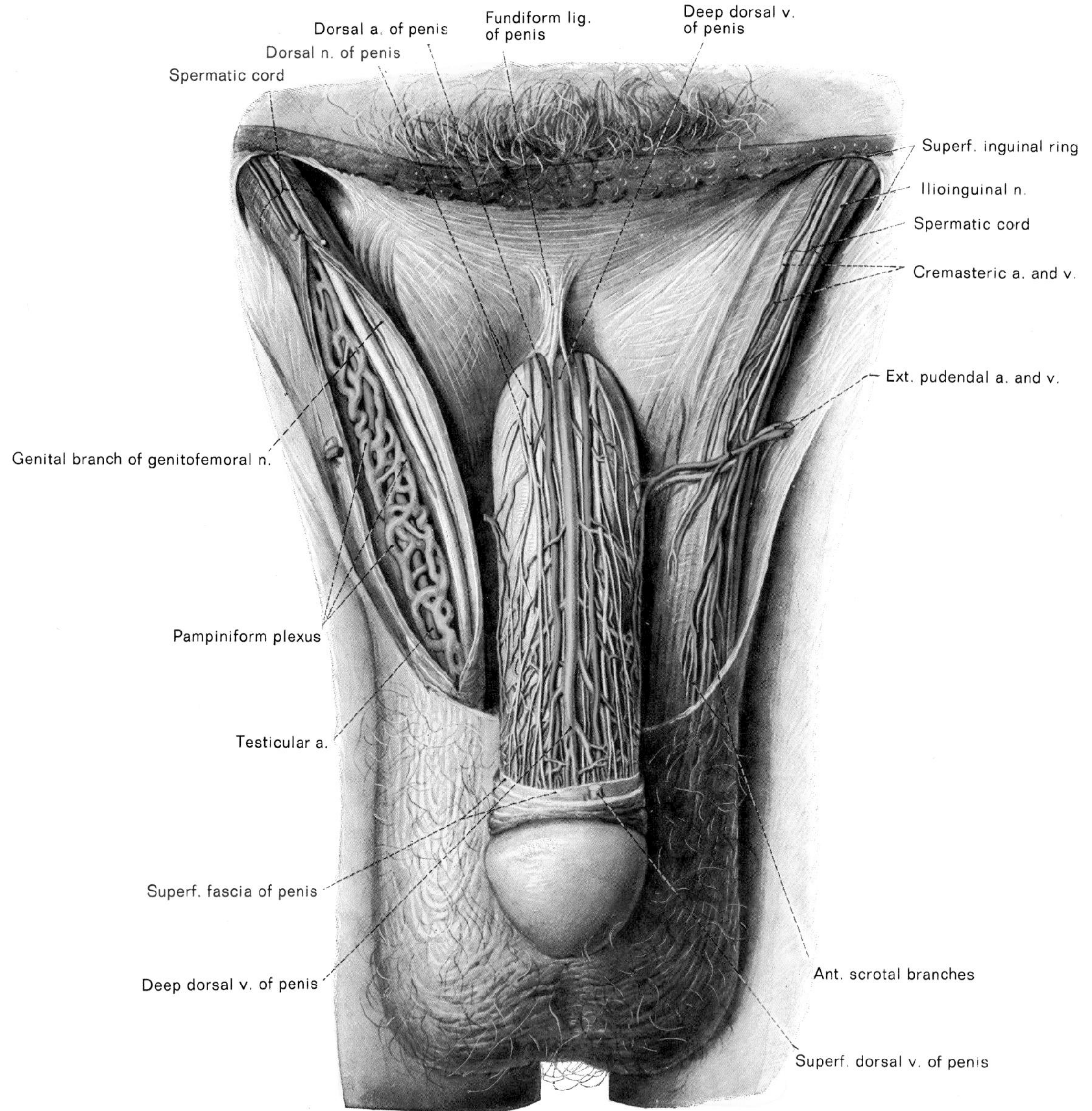
Dorsal a. of penis
Fundiform lig. of penis
Deep dorsal v. of penis
Dorsal n. of penis
Spermatic cord
Superf. inguinal ring
Ilioinguinal n.
Spermatic cord
Cremasteric a. and v.
Ext. pudendal a. and v.
Genital branch of genitofemoral n.
Pampiniform plexus
Testicular a.
Superf. fascia of penis
Deep dorsal v. of penis
Ant. scrotal branches
Superf. dorsal v. of penis

Fig. 376. Nerves and vessels of the external male genitalia. Skin and fascia of the penis have been removed. The right spermatic cord has been opened in order to expose the testicular artery and the pampiniform plexus.

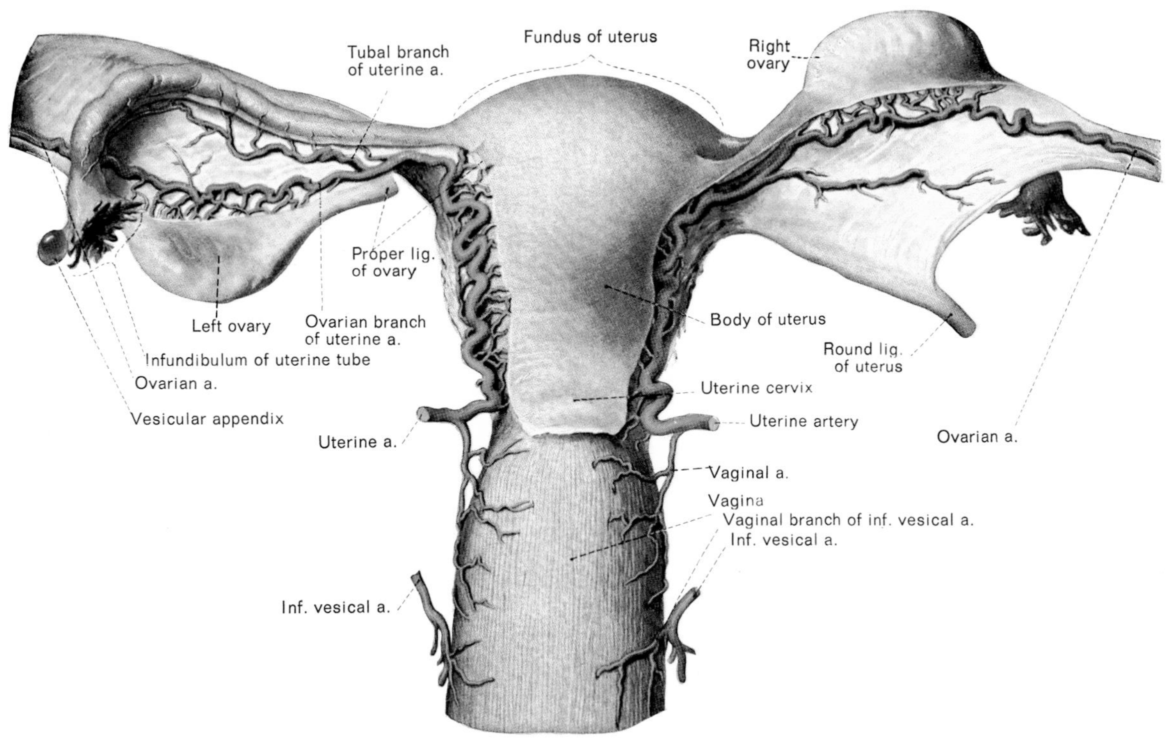
Fundus of uterus
Tubal branch of uterine a.
Right ovary
Proper lig. of ovary
Left ovary
Ovarian branch of uterine a.
Infundibulum of uterine tube
Ovarian a.
Vesicular appendix
Body of uterus
Round lig. of uterus
Uterine cervix
Uterine artery
Uterine a.
Ovarian a.
Vaginal a.
Vagina
Vaginal branch of inf. vesical a.
Inf. vesical a.
Inf. vesical a.

Fig. 377. Arteries of the internal female genitalia, dorsal view. The caudal portion of the broad ligament has been removed, the left proper ovarian ligament has been cut, the peritoneal covering of the mesosalpinx has been removed along the vessels.

Peripheral Nerves and Vessels

Nerves and Vessels of the Upper Extremity

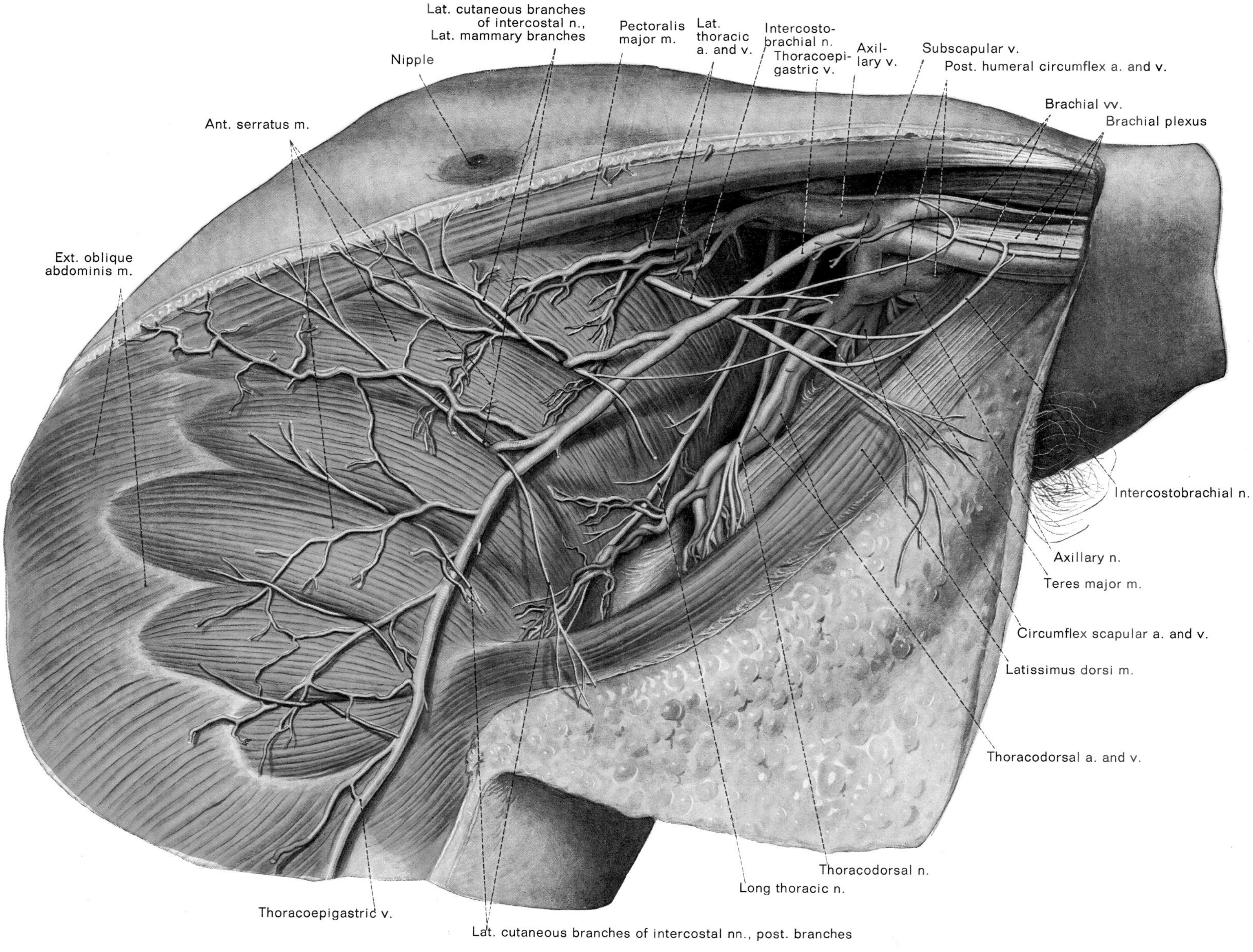
Lat. cutaneous branches of intercostal n., Lat. mammary branches
Nipple
Pectoralis major m.
Lat. thoracic a. and v.
Intercosto-brachial n.
Thoracoepi-gastric v.
Axil-lary v.
Subscapular v.
Post. humeral circumflex a. and v.
Brachial vv.
Brachial plexus
Ant. serratus m.
Ext. oblique abdominis m.
Intercostobrachial n.
Axillary n.
Teres major m.
Circumflex scapular a. and v.
Latissimus dorsi m.
Thoracodorsal a. and v.
Thoracodorsal n.
Long thoracic n.
Thoracoepigastric v.
Lat. cutaneous branches of intercostal nn., post. branches

Fig. 378. Superficial nerves and vessels of the left axilla. Skin and subcutaneous fat have been reflected, the superficial fascia removed.

Thyro-cervical trunk
Ant. scalenus m.
Phrenic n.
Inf. belly of omohyoid m.
Common carotid a.
Verte-bral a.
Brachial plexus
Subclavian a.
Transv. cervical a.
Inf. root of ansa cervicalis
Axillary v.
Vagus n.
Axillary a.
Left brachiocephalic v.
Brachial plexus
Sternocleidomastoid m.
Pectoral branches
Acromial branch
of thoraco-acromial a.
Deltoid m.
Pectoralis major m.
Cephalic v.
Ant. cutaneous branches of intercostal nn.,
Perforating branches of int. thoracic a. and v.
+ = Clavicle
Pectoralis major m.
Axillary a.
Axillary v.
Pectoralis minor m.
Intercostobrachial n.
Thoracodorsal n.
Lat. thoracic a. and v.
Thoracodorsal a. and v.
Long thoracic n.
Post. branch of lat. cutaneous branch of fourth intercostal n.
Ext. oblique abdominis m.
Ant. serratus m.
Lat. mammary branches of lat. cutaneous branches of intercostal nn.
Thoraco-epigastric v.
Latissimus dorsi m.

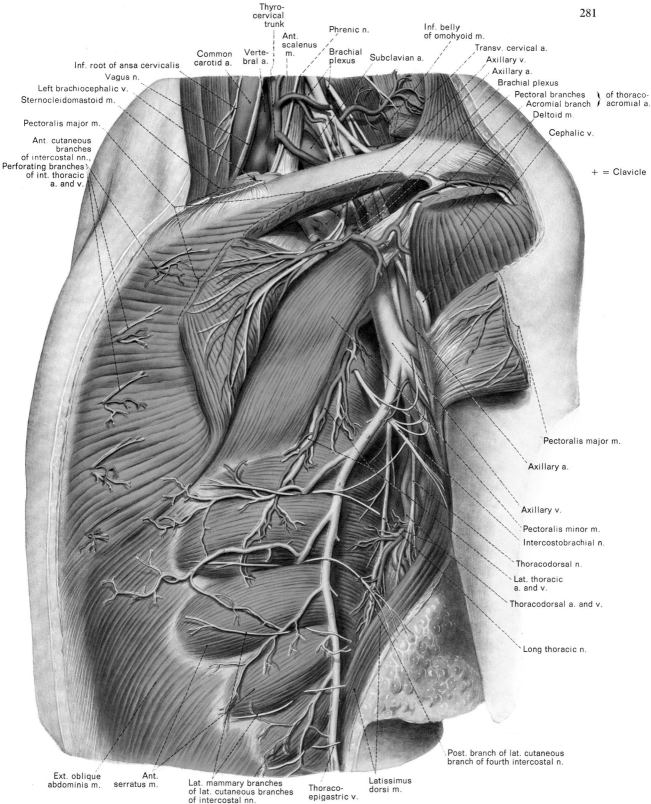

Fig. 379. Deeper nerves and vessels of the left axilla. Pectoralis major muscle cut and reflected.

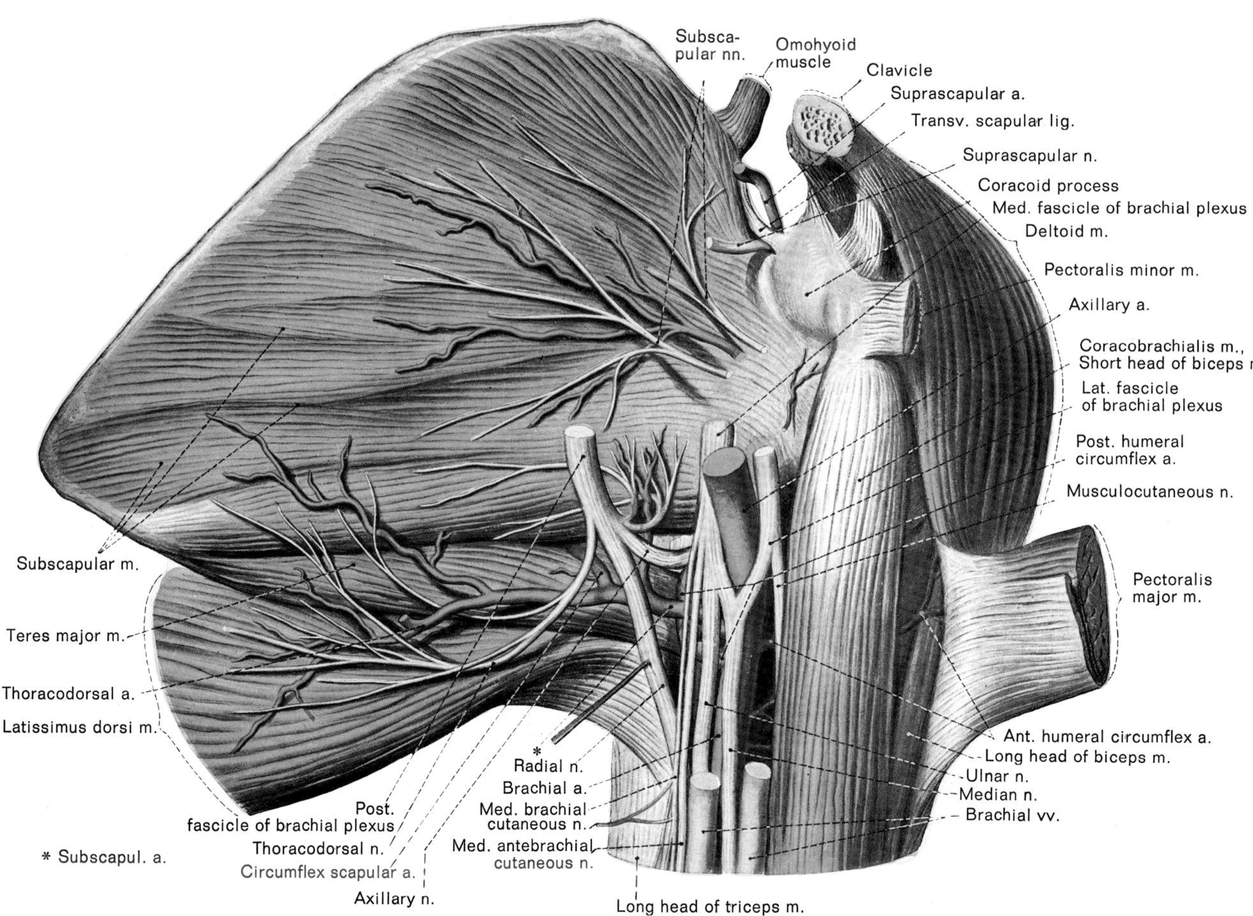
Subsca-
pular nn.
Omohyoid
muscle
Clavicle
Suprascapular a.
Transv. scapular lig.
Suprascapular n.
Coracoid process
Med. fascicle of brachial plexus
Deltoid m.
Pectoralis minor m.
Axillary a.
Coracobrachialis m.,
Short head of biceps m
Lat. fascicle
of brachial plexus
Post. humeral
circumflex a.
Musculocutaneous n.
Pectoralis
major m.
Ant. humeral circumflex a.
Long head of biceps m.
Ulnar n.
Median n.
Brachial vv.
Long head of triceps m.
Med. antebrachial
cutaneous n.
Med. brachial
cutaneous n.
Brachial a.
Radial n.
*
Axillary n.
Circumflex scapular a.
Thoracodorsal n.
Post.
fascicle of brachial plexus
* Subscapul. a.
Latissimus dorsi m.
Thoracodorsal a.
Teres major m.
Subscapular m.

Fig. 380. Nerves and vessels of the left shoulder region, ventral view.

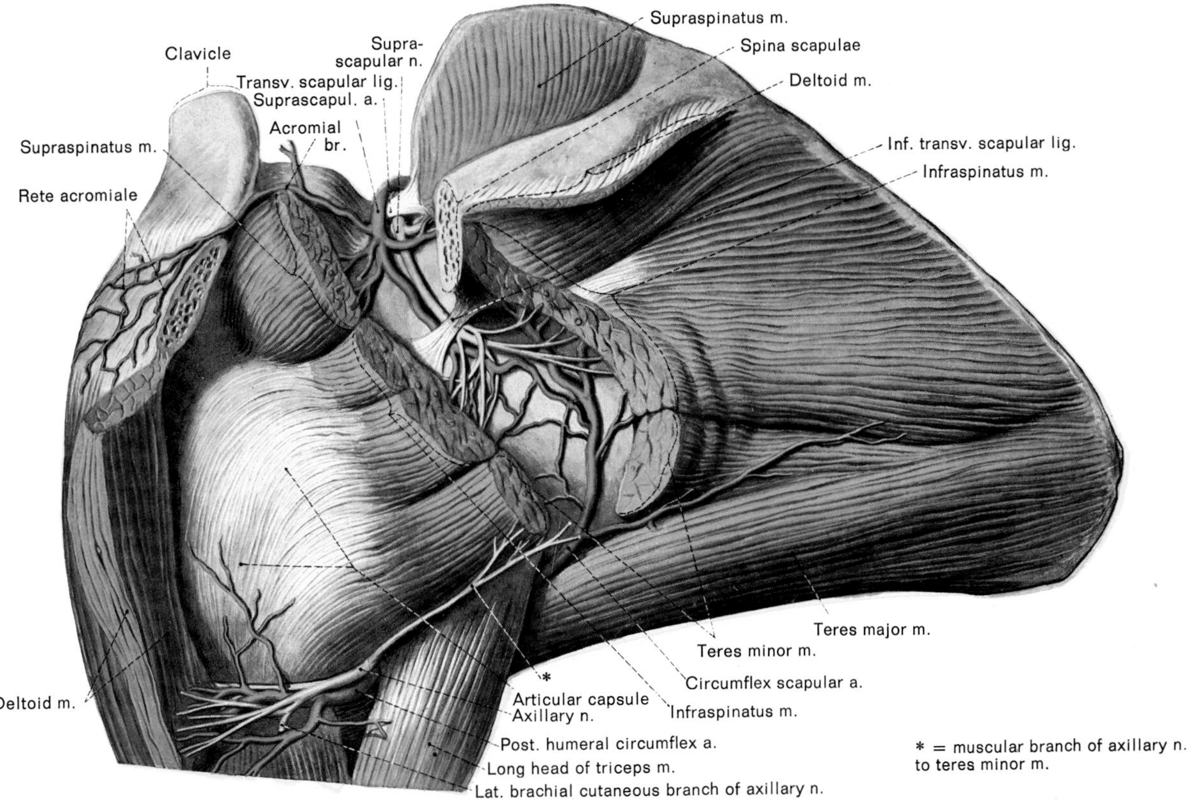
Supraspinatus m.
Spina scapulae
Deltoid m.
Clavicle
Supra-
scapular n.
Transv. scapular lig.
Suprascapul. a.
Acromial
br.
Supraspinatus m.
Rete acromiale
Inf. transv. scapular lig.
Infraspinatus m.
Teres major m.
Teres minor m.
Circumflex scapular a.
Infraspinatus m.
*
Articular capsule
Axillary n.
Deltoid m.
Post. humeral circumflex a.
Long head of triceps m.
Lat. brachial cutaneous branch of axillary n.
* = muscular branch of axillary n.
to teres minor m.

Fig. 381. Nerves and vessels of the left shoulder region, dorsal view. Deltoid muscle partially removed and reflected. Portion of the acromion removed; supraspinatus, infraspinatus and teres minor muscles sectioned and somewhat pulled apart.

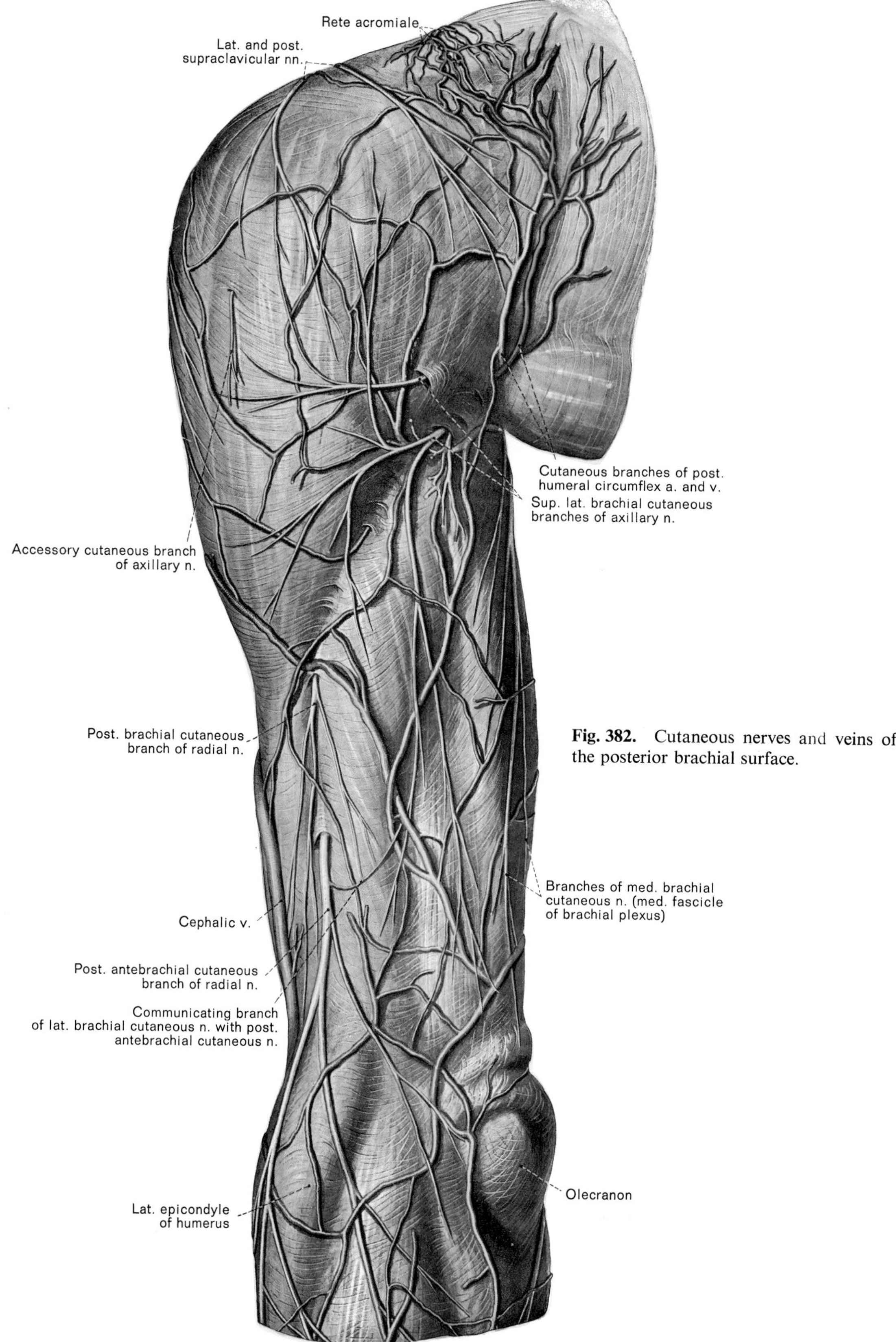
Rete acromiale
Lat. and post. supraclavicular nn.
Cutaneous branches of post. humeral circumflex a. and v.
Sup. lat. brachial cutaneous branches of axillary n.
Accessory cutaneous branch of axillary n.
Post. brachial cutaneous branch of radial n.
Branches of med. brachial cutaneous n. (med. fascicle of brachial plexus)
Cephalic v.
Post. antebrachial cutaneous branch of radial n.
Communicating branch of lat. brachial cutaneous n. with post. antebrachial cutaneous n.
Olecranon
Lat. epicondyle of humerus

Fig. 382. Cutaneous nerves and veins of the posterior brachial surface.

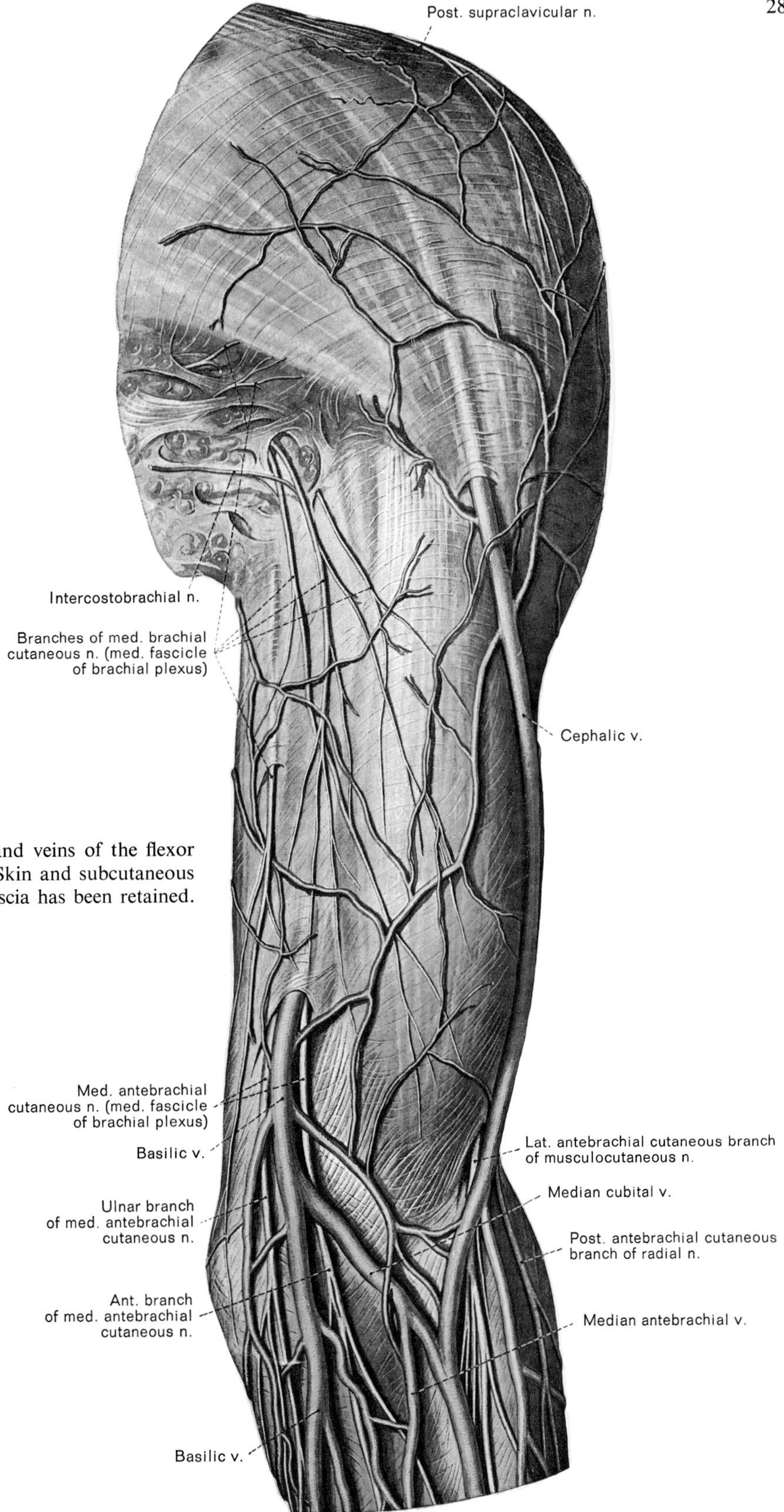
Post. supraclavicular n.
Intercostobrachial n.
Branches of med. brachial cutaneous n. (med. fascicle of brachial plexus)
Cephalic v.
Med. antebrachial cutaneous n. (med. fascicle of brachial plexus)
Basilic v.
Lat. antebrachial cutaneous branch of musculocutaneous n.
Median cubital v.
Ulnar branch of med. antebrachial cutaneous n.
Post. antebrachial cutaneous branch of radial n.
Ant. branch of med. antebrachial cutaneous n.
Median antebrachial v.
Basilic v.

Fig. 383. Cutaneous nerves and veins of the flexor surface of the left brachium. Skin and subcutaneous fat have been removed, the fascia has been retained.

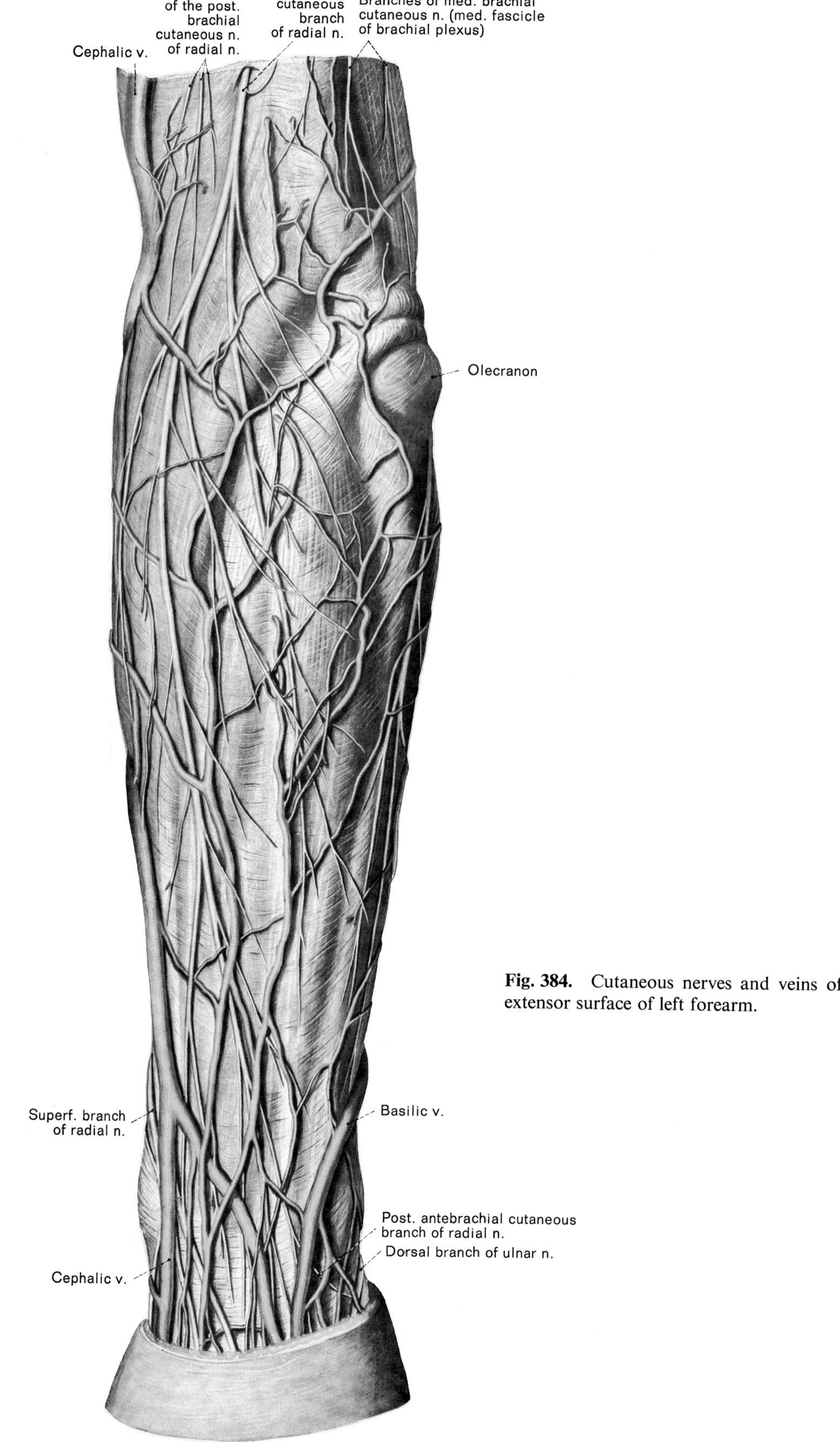
Branches of the post. brachial cutaneous n. of radial n.
Post. antebrachial cutaneous branch of radial n.
Branches of med. brachial cutaneous n. (med. fascicle of brachial plexus)
Cephalic v.
Olecranon
Superf. branch of radial n.
Basilic v.
Post. antebrachial cutaneous branch of radial n.
Dorsal branch of ulnar n.
Cephalic v.

Fig. 384. Cutaneous nerves and veins of extensor surface of left forearm.

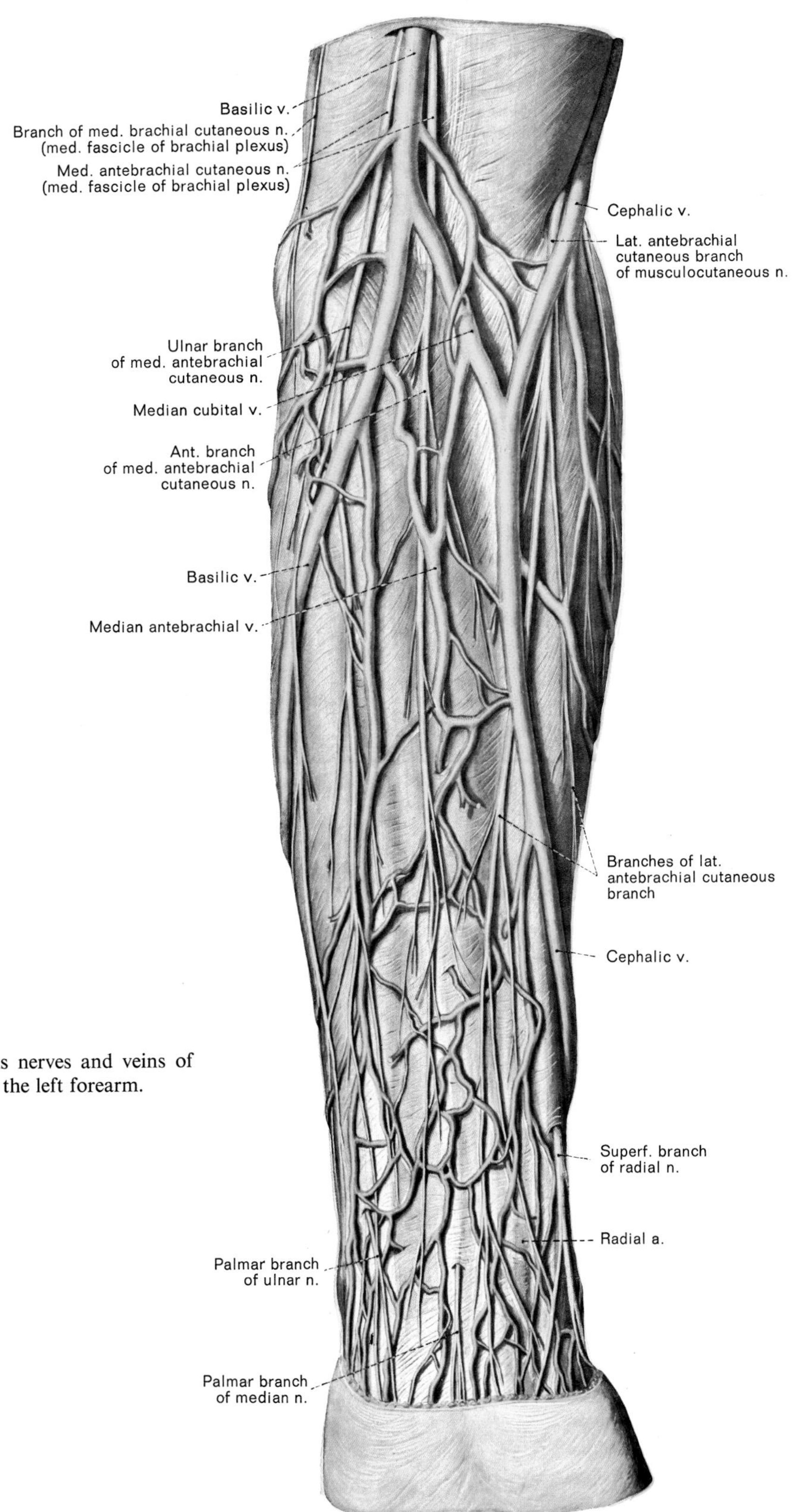
Basilic v.
Branch of med. brachial cutaneous n.
(med. fascicle of brachial plexus)
Med. antebrachial cutaneous n.
(med. fascicle of brachial plexus)
Cephalic v.
Lat. antebrachial
cutaneous branch
of musculocutaneous n.
Ulnar branch
of med. antebrachial
cutaneous n.
Median cubital v.
Ant. branch
of med. antebrachial
cutaneous n.
Basilic v.
Median antebrachial v.
Branches of lat.
antebrachial cutaneous
branch
Cephalic v.
Superf. branch
of radial n.
Radial a.
Palmar branch
of ulnar n.
Palmar branch
of median n.

Fig. 385. Cutaneous nerves and veins of the flexor surface of the left forearm.

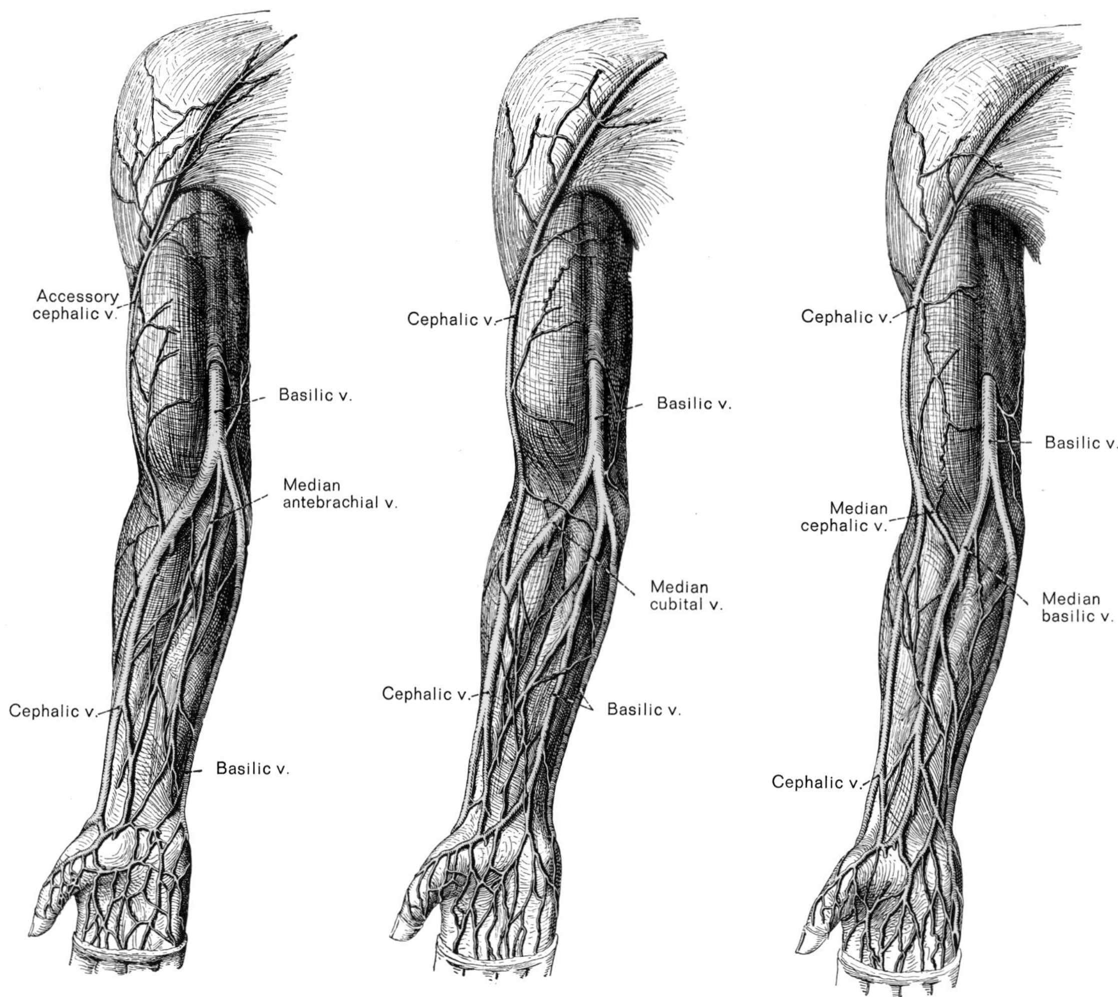
Accessory
cephalic v.
Basilic v.
Median
antebrachial v.
Cephalic v.
Basilic v.
Cephalic v.
Basilic v.
Median
cubital v.
Cephalic v.
Basilic v.
Cephalic v.
Basilic v.
Median
cephalic v.
Median
basilic v.
Cephalic v.

Fig. 386. Variations in venous pattern of upper extremity.

Cutaneous veins of the upper extremity

1. *Cephalic vein;* it begins at the radial half of the back of the hand from tributaries of the venous network; it receives blood from the palm of the hand via the intercapital veins (Fig. 387); ist courses proximally on the radial side of the antebrachium toward the cubital fossa where it anastomoses with the basilic vein. It continues through the lateral bicipital sulcus toward the deltoideopectoral triangle where it penetrates the fascia and empties into the axillary vein. Figs. 344–348, 379, 382, 383, 385–387.

2. *Basilic vein;* it originates from the ulnar side of the back of the hand and courses over the ulnar flexor side of the antebrachium toward the cubital fossa where it connects to the cephalic vein via the median cubital vein. In the brachial area it is, in most cases, larger than the cephalic vein. It runs in the medial bicipital sulcus to approximately the middle of the brachium where it penetrates the fascia and continues proximally as medial brachial vein. Figs. 383–388.

3. *Median cubital vein;* it is an oblique, highly variable, anastomosis between the basilic and cephalic veins and receives, in most instances, the median antebrachial vein which originates from veins of the palmar surface of hand and antebrachium. Figs. 383, 385, 386.

4. *Median basilic vein* and

5. *Median cephalic vein;* these are very variable and, if present, form connections between cephalic, basilic and median cubital veins. Fig. 386.

Clinical significance of the cutaneous veins in the cubital fossa: to draw blood or make intravenous injections.

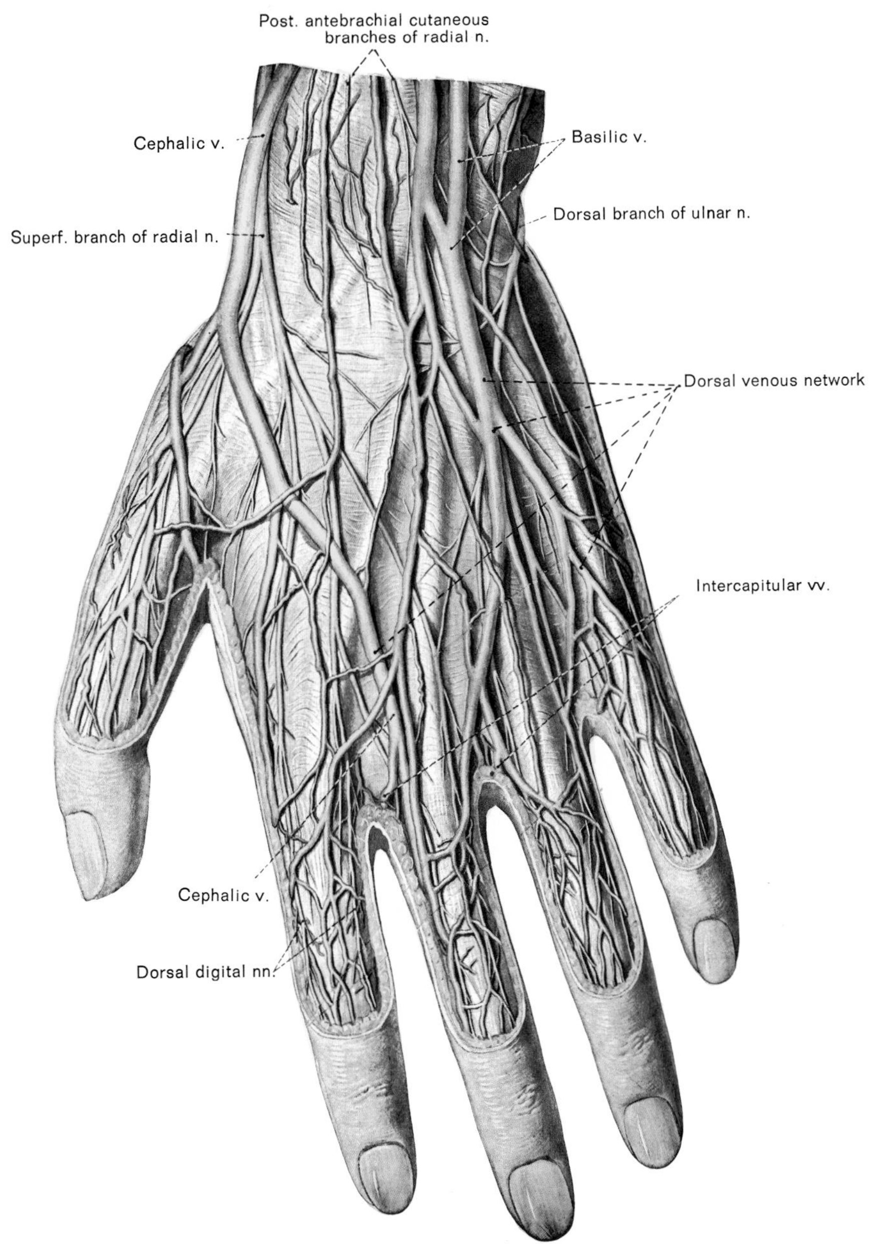
Post. antebrachial cutaneous
branches of radial n.
Cephalic v.
Basilic v.
Dorsal branch of ulnar n.
Superf. branch of radial n.
Dorsal venous network
Intercapitular vv.
Cephalic v.
Dorsal digital nn.

Fig. 387. Superficial nerves and veins of dorsum of hand.

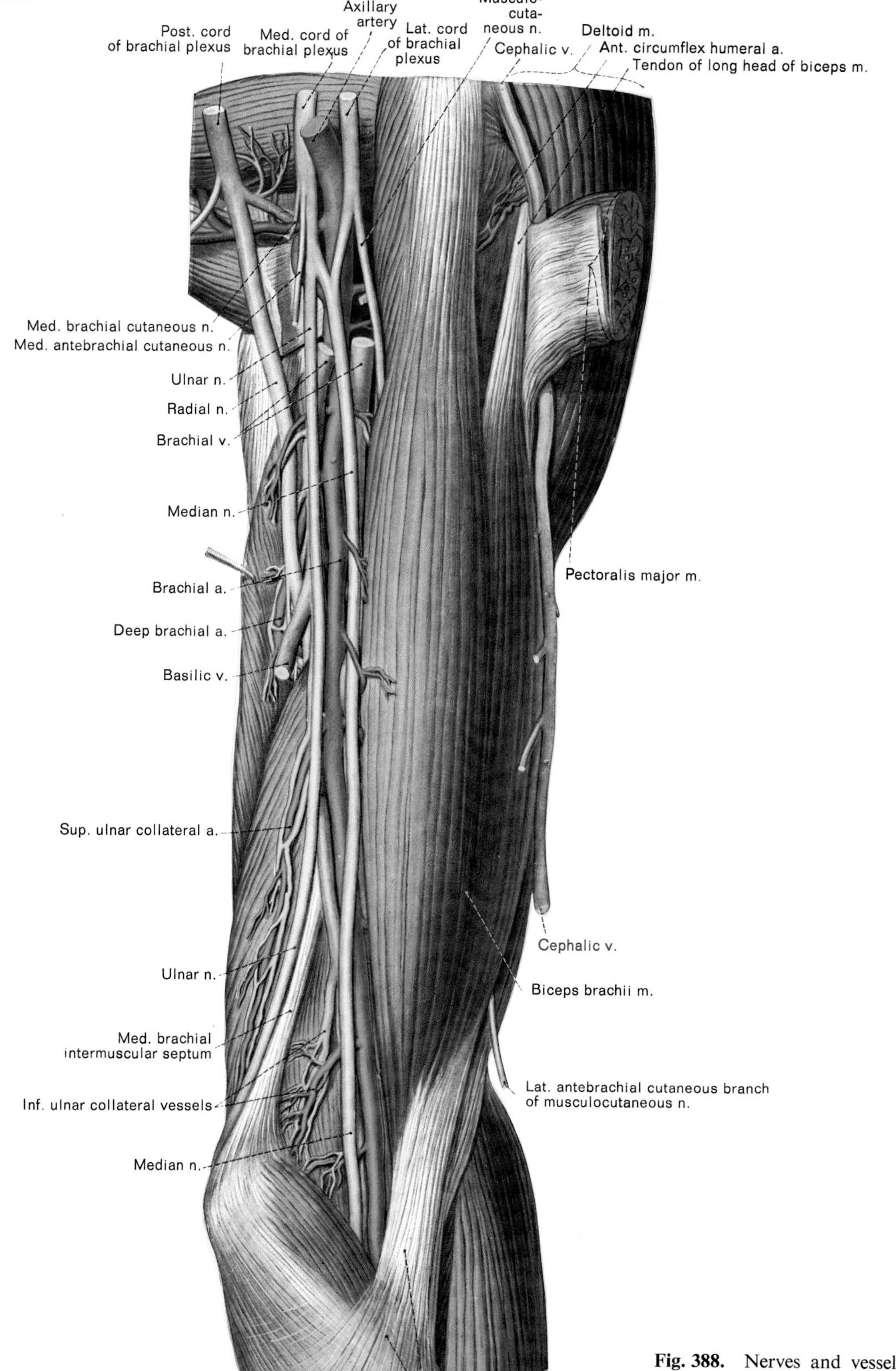
Post. cord of brachial plexus
Med. cord of brachial plexus
Axillary artery
Lat. cord of brachial plexus
Musculo-cuta-neous n.
Cephalic v.
Deltoid m.
Ant. circumflex humeral a.
Tendon of long head of biceps m.
Med. brachial cutaneous n.
Med. antebrachial cutaneous n.
Ulnar n.
Radial n.
Brachial v.
Median n.
Brachial a.
Deep brachial a.
Basilic v.
Pectoralis major m.
Sup. ulnar collateral a.
Cephalic v.
Ulnar n.
Biceps brachii m.
Med. brachial intermuscular septum
Lat. antebrachial cutaneous branch of musculocutaneous n.
Inf. ulnar collateral vessels
Median n.
Aponeurosis of biceps brachii m.

Fig. 388. Nerves and vessels of anterior surface of left arm.

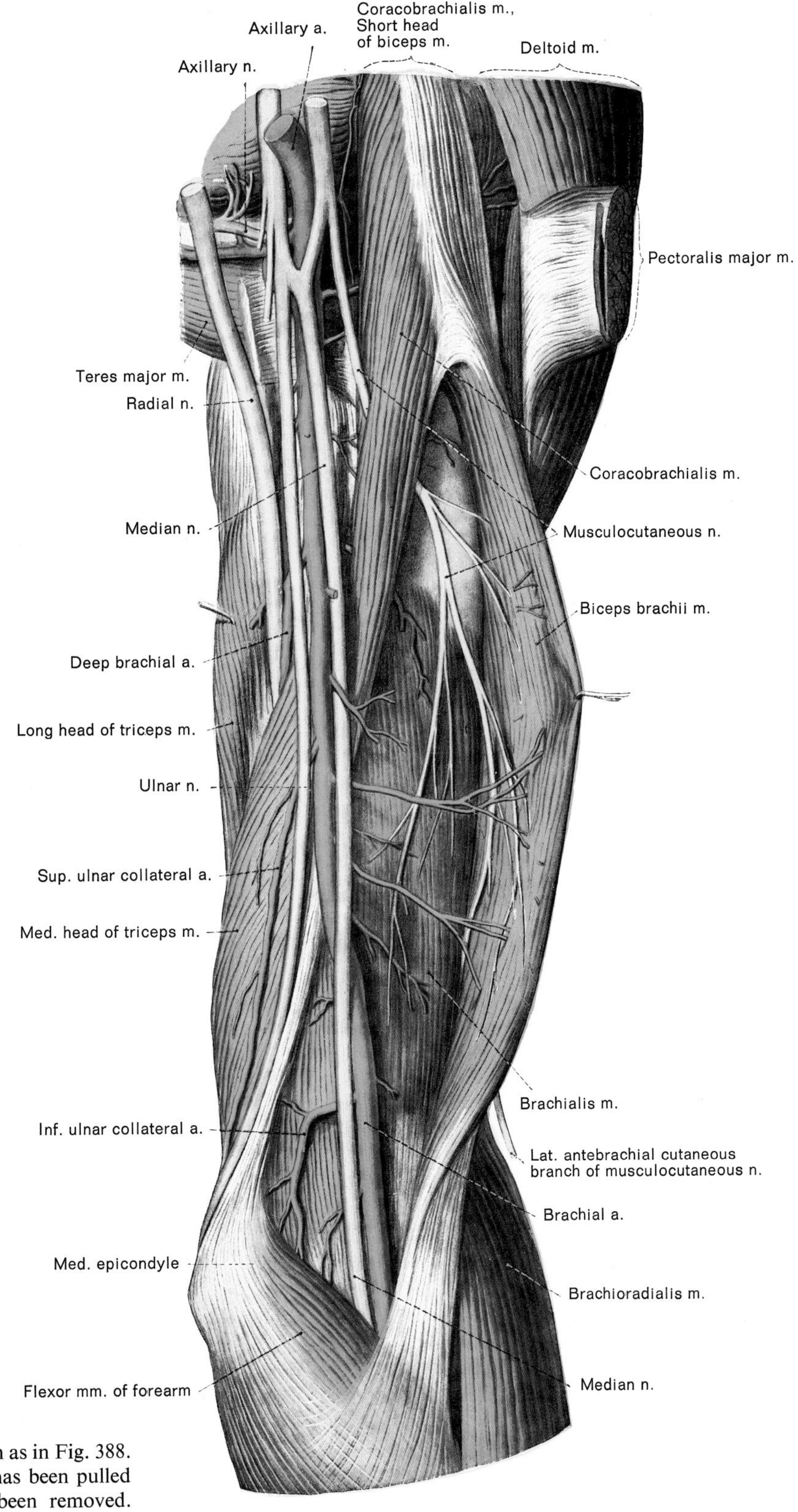
Axillary a.
Coracobrachialis m., Short head of biceps m.
Deltoid m.
Axillary n.
Pectoralis major m.
Teres major m.
Radial n.
Coracobrachialis m.
Median n.
Musculocutaneous n.
Biceps brachii m.
Deep brachial a.
Long head of triceps m.
Ulnar n.
Sup. ulnar collateral a.
Med. head of triceps m.
Brachialis m.
Inf. ulnar collateral a.
Lat. antebrachial cutaneous branch of musculocutaneous n.
Brachial a.
Med. epicondyle
Brachioradialis m.
Flexor mm. of forearm
Median n.

Fig. 389. Same preparation as in Fig. 388. The biceps brachii muscle has been pulled sideward, the veins have been removed.

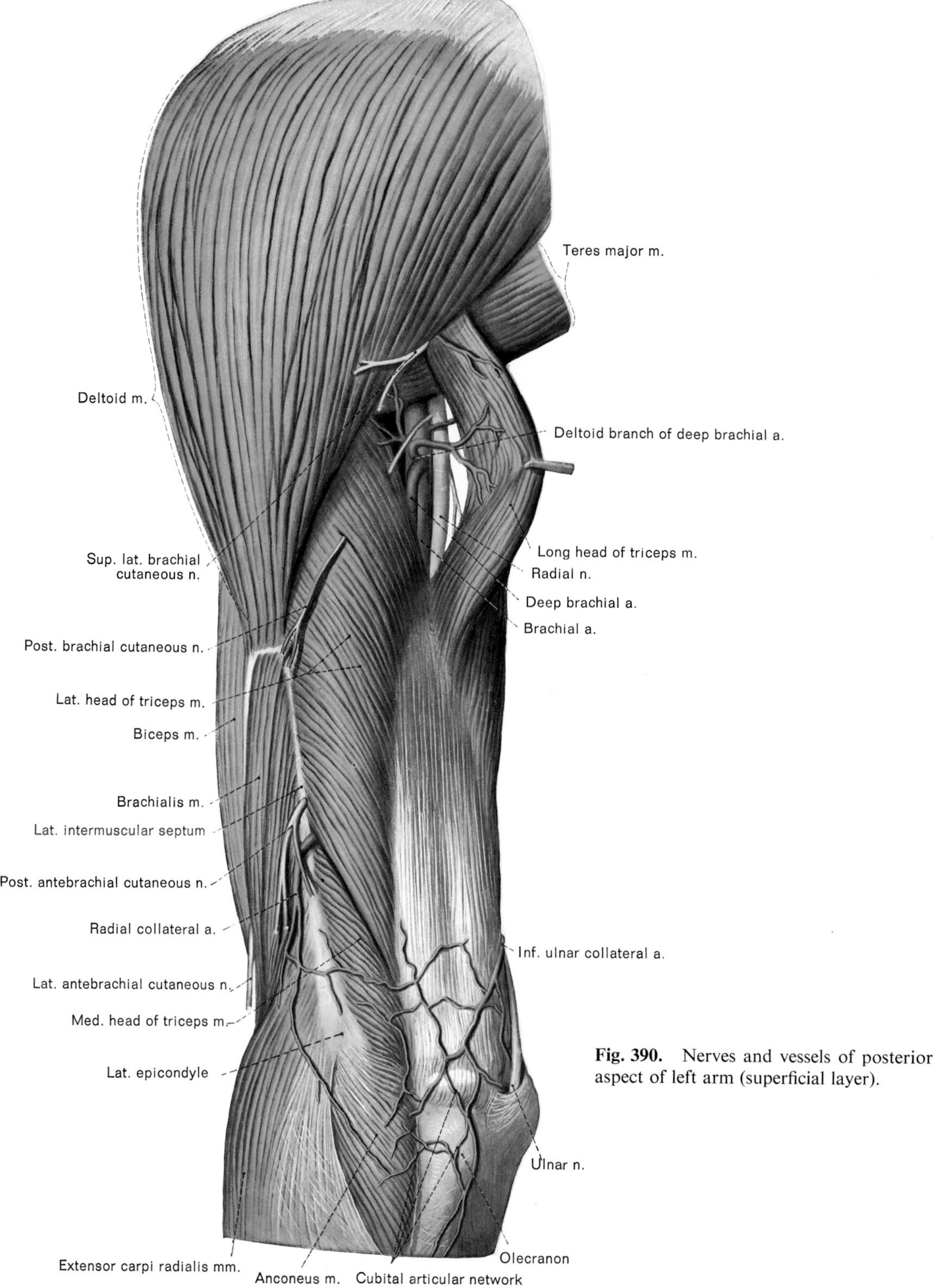
Teres major m.
Deltoid m.
Deltoid branch of deep brachial a.
Sup. lat. brachial cutaneous n.
Long head of triceps m.
Radial n.
Deep brachial a.
Brachial a.
Post. brachial cutaneous n.
Lat. head of triceps m.
Biceps m.
Brachialis m.
Lat. intermuscular septum
Post. antebrachial cutaneous n.
Radial collateral a.
Inf. ulnar collateral a.
Lat. antebrachial cutaneous n.
Med. head of triceps m.
Lat. epicondyle
Ulnar n.
Olecranon
Extensor carpi radialis mm.
Anconeus m.
Cubital articular network

Fig. 390. Nerves and vessels of posterior aspect of left arm (superficial layer).

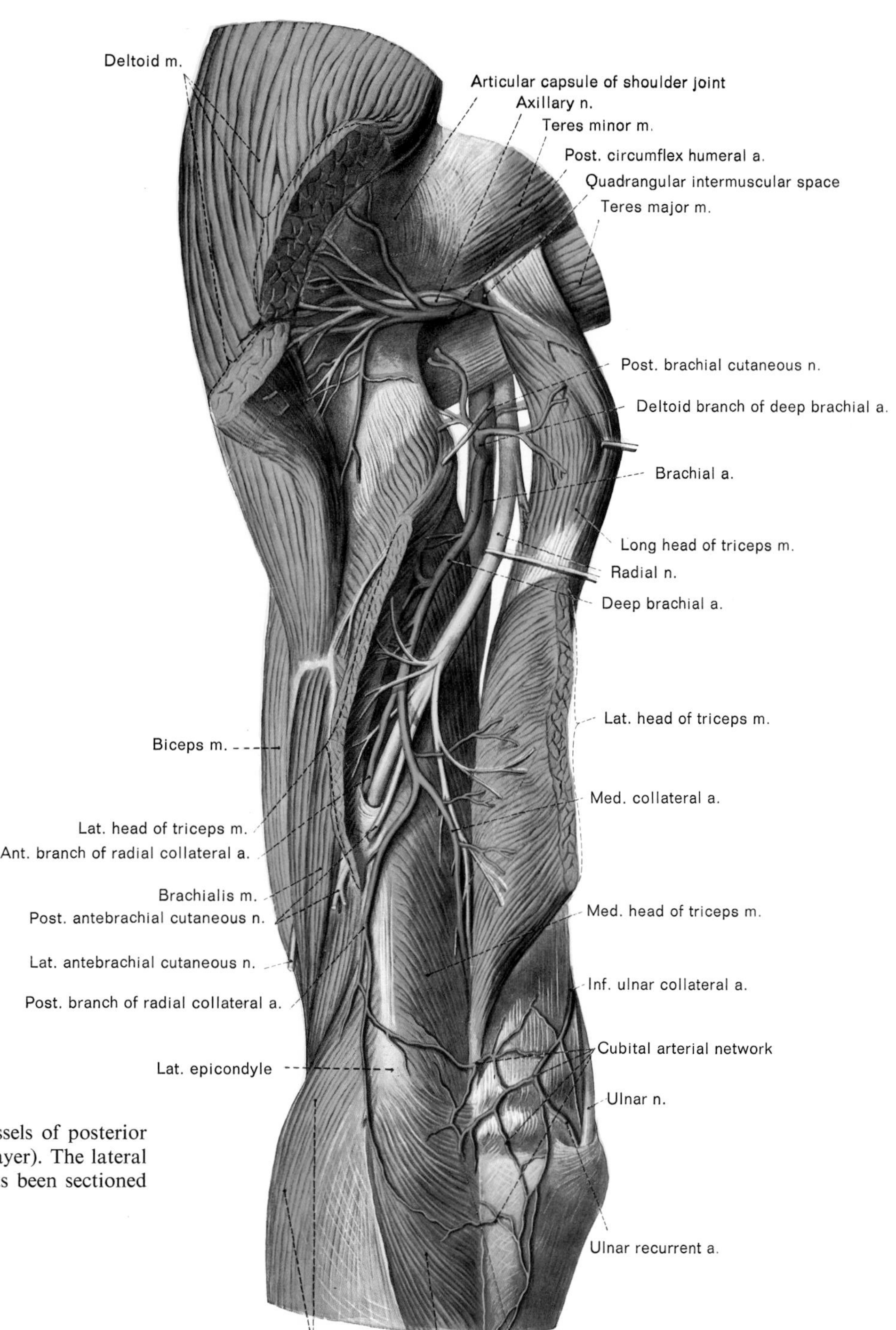
Deltoid m.
Articular capsule of shoulder joint
Axillary n.
Teres minor m.
Post. circumflex humeral a.
Quadrangular intermuscular space
Teres major m.
Post. brachial cutaneous n.
Deltoid branch of deep brachial a.
Brachial a.
Long head of triceps m.
Radial n.
Deep brachial a.
Lat. head of triceps m.
Biceps m.
Med. collateral a.
Lat. head of triceps m.
Ant. branch of radial collateral a.
Brachialis m.
Post. antebrachial cutaneous n.
Med. head of triceps m.
Lat. antebrachial cutaneous n.
Inf. ulnar collateral a.
Post. branch of radial collateral a.
Cubital arterial network
Lat. epicondyle
Ulnar n.
Ulnar recurrent a.
Extensor carpi radialis mm.
Anconeus m.

Fig. 391. Nerves and vessels of posterior aspect of left arm (deep layer). The lateral head of triceps muscle has been sectioned and reflected.

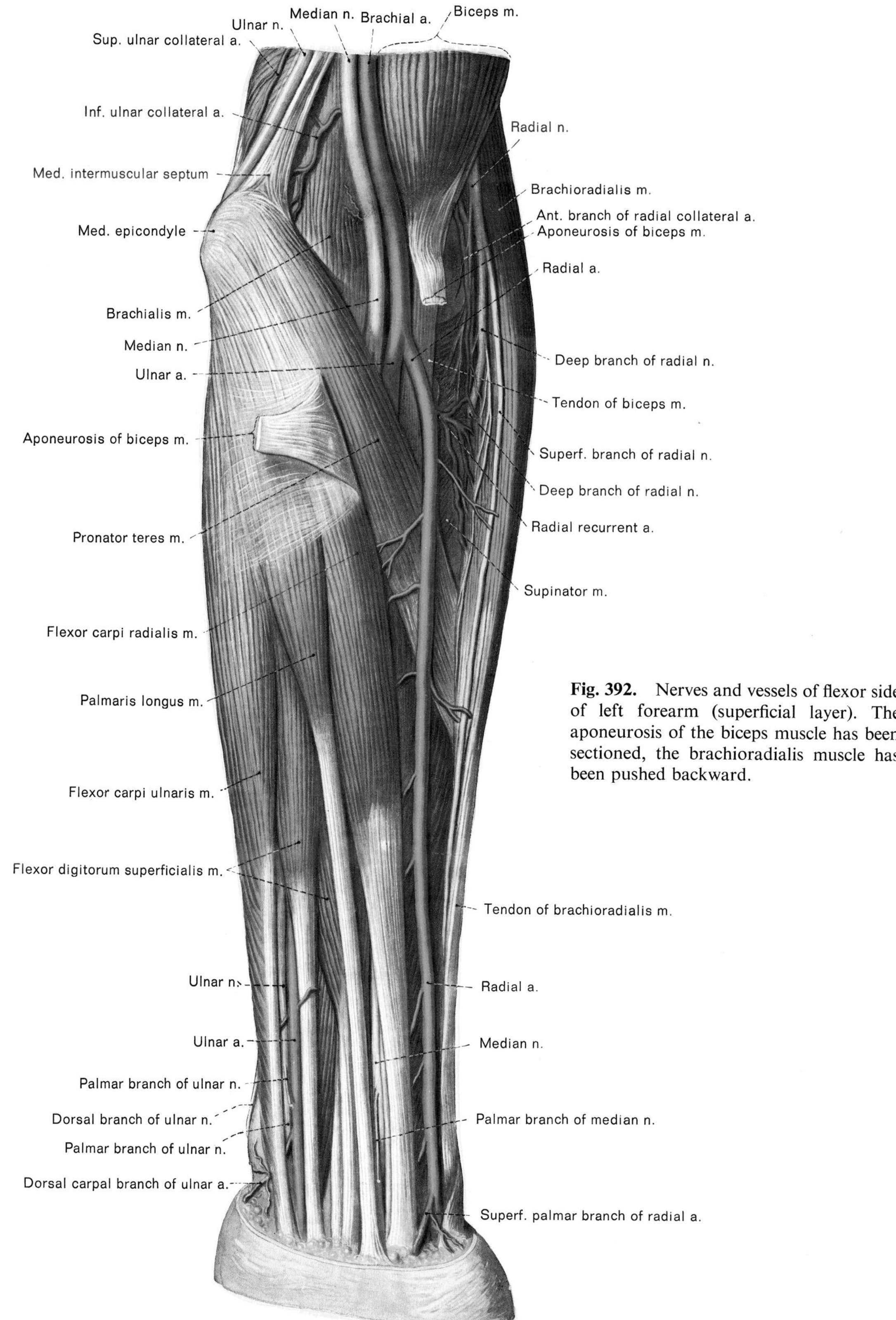
Ulnar n.
Median n.
Brachial a.
Biceps m.
Sup. ulnar collateral a.
Inf. ulnar collateral a.
Radial n.
Med. intermuscular septum
Brachioradialis m.
Ant. branch of radial collateral a.
Aponeurosis of biceps m.
Med. epicondyle
Radial a.
Brachialis m.
Median n.
Deep branch of radial n.
Ulnar a.
Tendon of biceps m.
Aponeurosis of biceps m.
Superf. branch of radial n.
Deep branch of radial n.
Radial recurrent a.
Pronator teres m.
Supinator m.
Flexor carpi radialis m.
Palmaris longus m.
Flexor carpi ulnaris m.
Flexor digitorum superficialis m.
Tendon of brachioradialis m.
Ulnar n.
Radial a.
Ulnar a.
Median n.
Palmar branch of ulnar n.
Dorsal branch of ulnar n.
Palmar branch of median n.
Palmar branch of ulnar n.
Dorsal carpal branch of ulnar a.
Superf. palmar branch of radial a.

Fig. 392. Nerves and vessels of flexor side of left forearm (superficial layer). The aponeurosis of the biceps muscle has been sectioned, the brachioradialis muscle has been pushed backward.

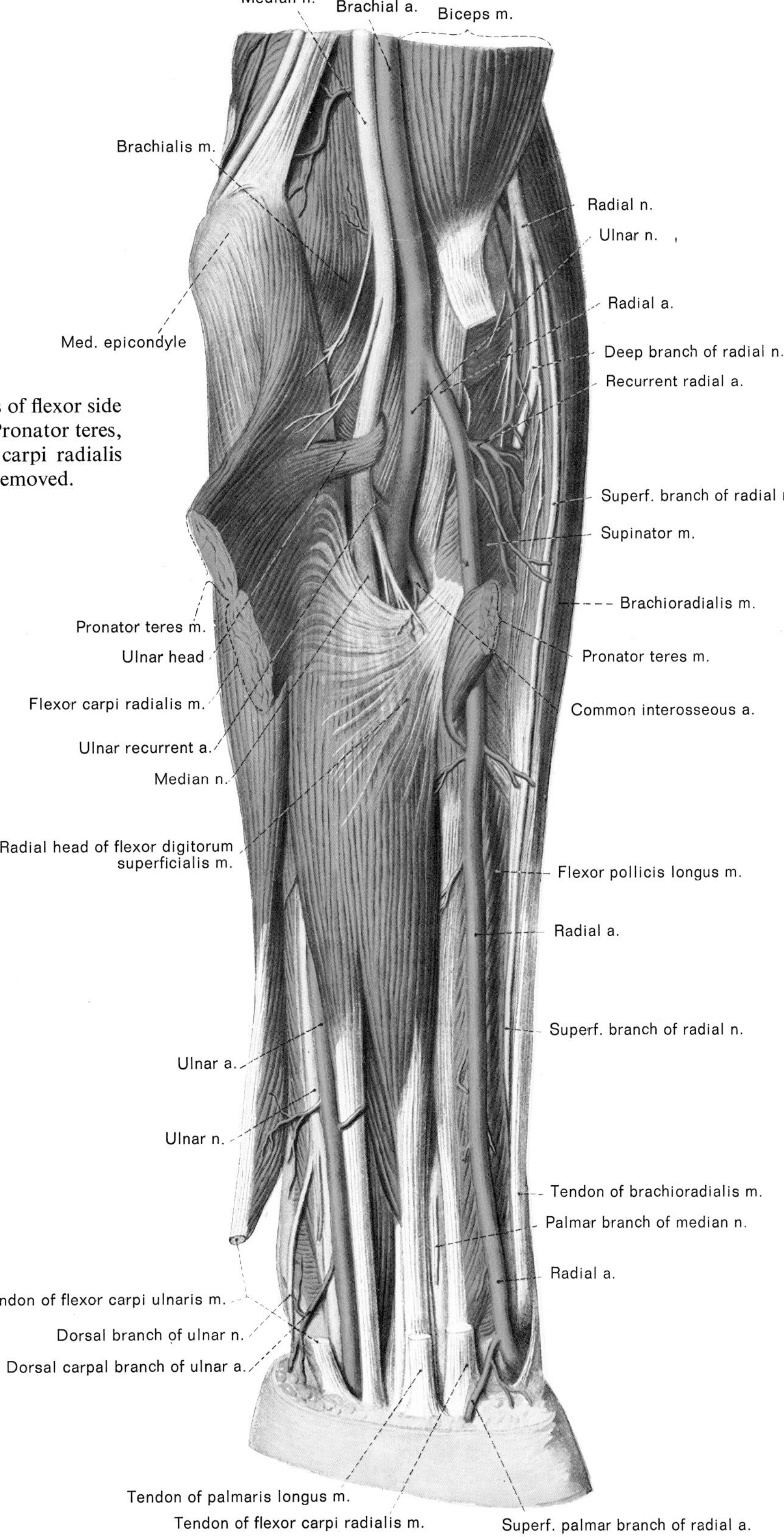
Median n.
Brachial a.
Biceps m.
Brachialis m.
Radial n.
Ulnar n.
Radial a.
Med. epicondyle
Deep branch of radial n.
Recurrent radial a.
Superf. branch of radial n.
Supinator m.
Brachioradialis m.
Pronator teres m.
Pronator teres m.
Ulnar head
Common interosseous a.
Flexor carpi radialis m.
Ulnar recurrent a.
Median n.
Radial head of flexor digitorum superficialis m.
Flexor pollicis longus m.
Radial a.
Superf. branch of radial n.
Ulnar a.
Ulnar n.
Tendon of brachioradialis m.
Palmar branch of median n.
Radial a.
Tendon of flexor carpi ulnaris m.
Dorsal branch of ulnar n.
Dorsal carpal branch of ulnar a.
Tendon of palmaris longus m.
Tendon of flexor carpi radialis m.
Superf. palmar branch of radial a.

Fig. 393. Nerves and vessels of flexor side of left forearm (deep layer). Pronator teres, palmaris longus, and flexor carpi radialis muscles have been partially removed.

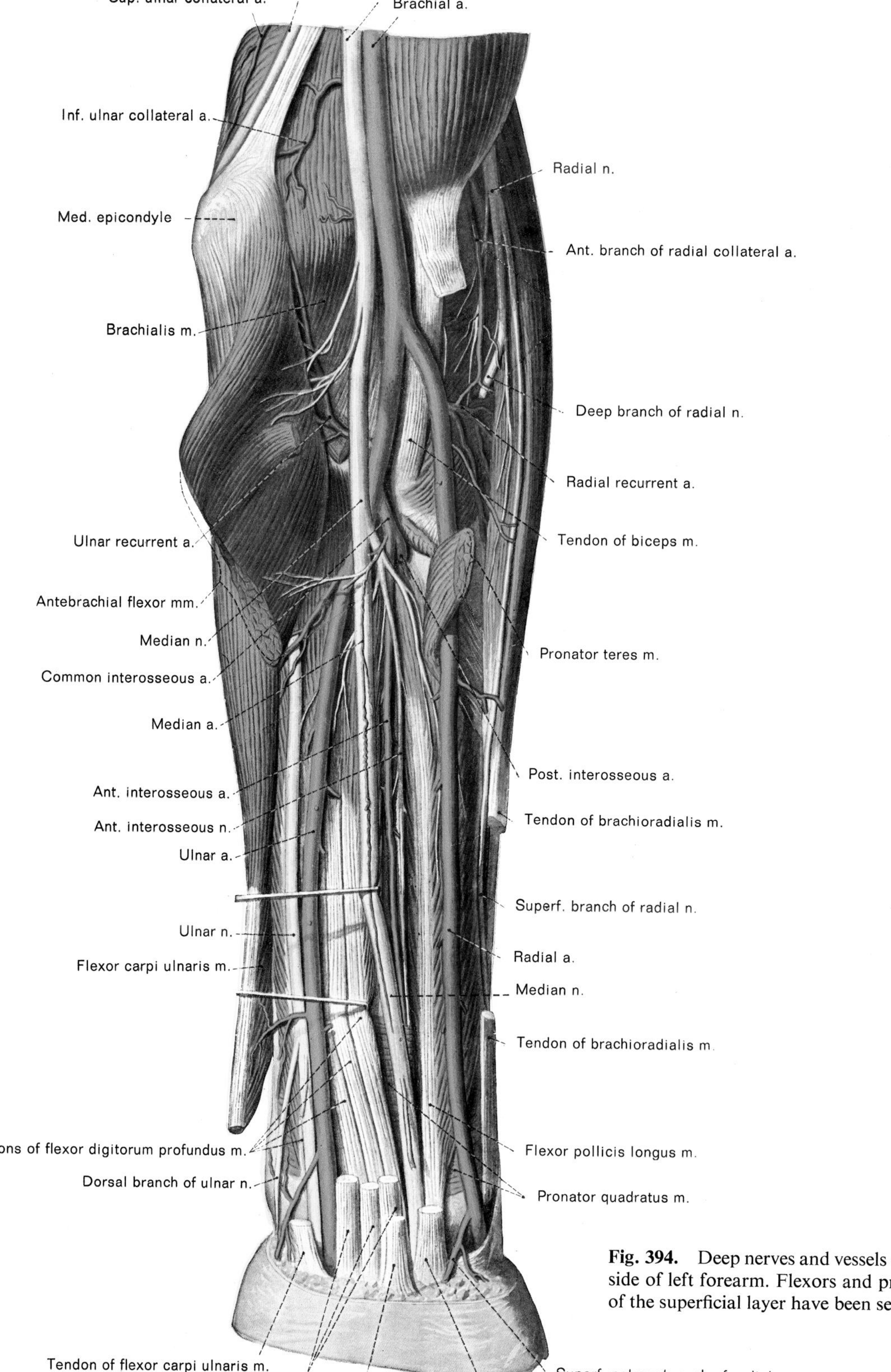
Sup. ulnar collateral a.
Ulnar n.
Median n.
Brachial a.
Inf. ulnar collateral a.
Radial n.
Med. epicondyle
Ant. branch of radial collateral a.
Brachialis m.
Deep branch of radial n.
Radial recurrent a.
Ulnar recurrent a.
Tendon of biceps m.
Antebrachial flexor mm.
Median n.
Pronator teres m.
Common interosseous a.
Median a.
Post. interosseous a.
Ant. interosseous a.
Tendon of brachioradialis m.
Ant. interosseous n.
Ulnar a.
Superf. branch of radial n.
Ulnar n.
Radial a.
Flexor carpi ulnaris m.
Median n.
Tendon of brachioradialis m.
Tendons of flexor digitorum profundus m.
Flexor pollicis longus m.
Dorsal branch of ulnar n.
Pronator quadratus m.
Tendon of flexor carpi ulnaris m.
Tendons of flexor digitorum superficialis m.
Tendon of palmaris longus m.
Superf. palmar branch of radial a.
Tendon of flexor carpi radialis m.

Fig. 394. Deep nerves and vessels of flexor side of left forearm. Flexors and pronators of the superficial layer have been sectioned.

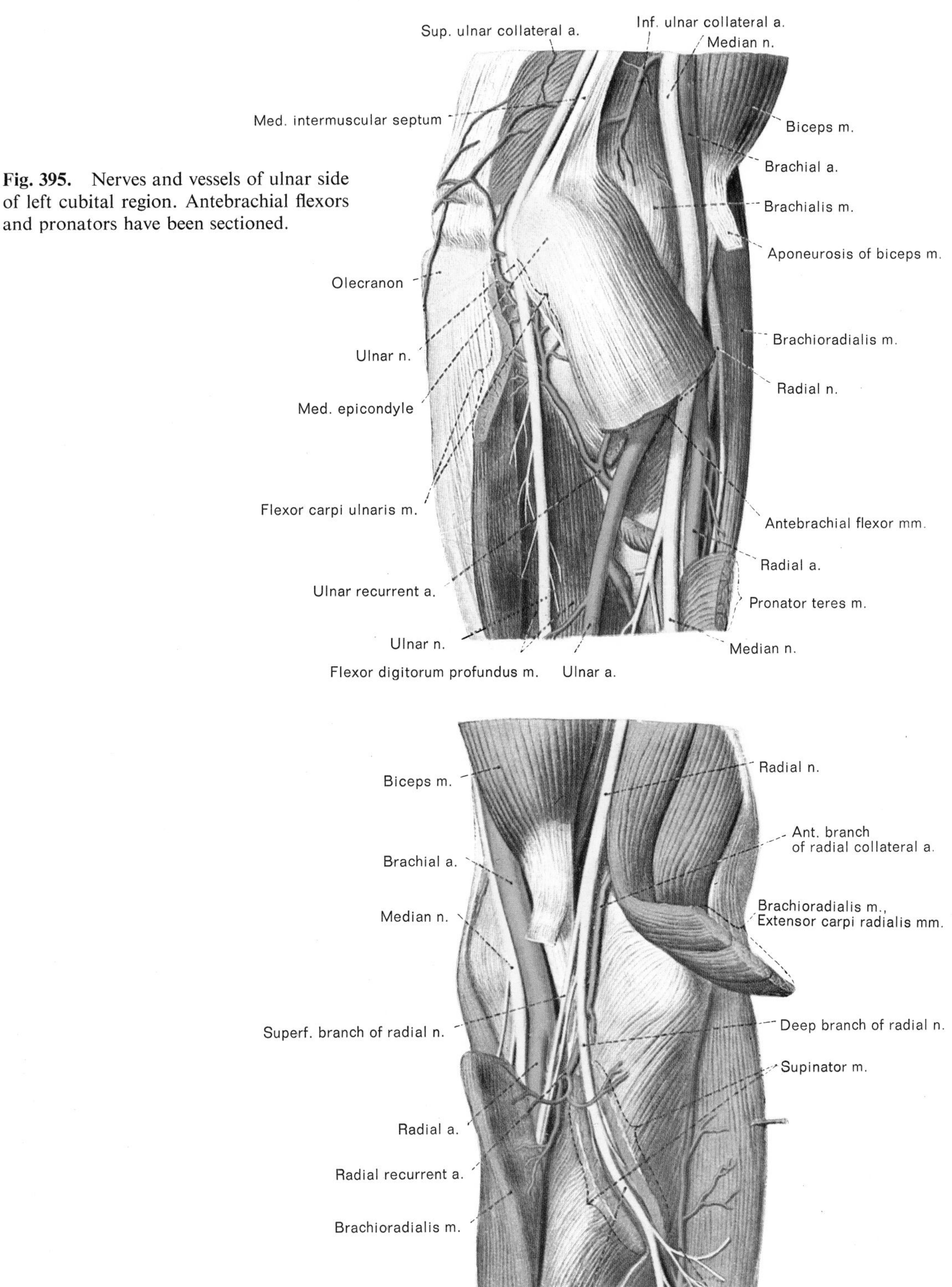

Sup. ulnar collateral a.
Inf. ulnar collateral a.
Median n.
Med. intermuscular septum
Biceps m.
Brachial a.
Brachialis m.
Aponeurosis of biceps m.
Olecranon
Brachioradialis m.
Ulnar n.
Radial n.
Med. epicondyle
Flexor carpi ulnaris m.
Antebrachial flexor mm.
Radial a.
Ulnar recurrent a.
Pronator teres m.
Ulnar n.
Median n.
Flexor digitorum profundus m.
Ulnar a.
Biceps m.
Radial n.
Ant. branch of radial collateral a.
Brachial a.
Median n.
Brachioradialis m., Extensor carpi radialis mm.
Superf. branch of radial n.
Deep branch of radial n.
Supinator m.
Radial a.
Radial recurrent a.
Brachioradialis m.
Deep branch of radial n.
Recurrent interosseous a.

Fig. 395. Nerves and vessels of ulnar side of left cubital region. Antebrachial flexors and pronators have been sectioned.

Fig. 396. Nerves and vessels of radial side of left cubital region. The radial group of antebrachial muscles has been sectioned, the supinator muscle has been split along the deep branch of radial nerve.

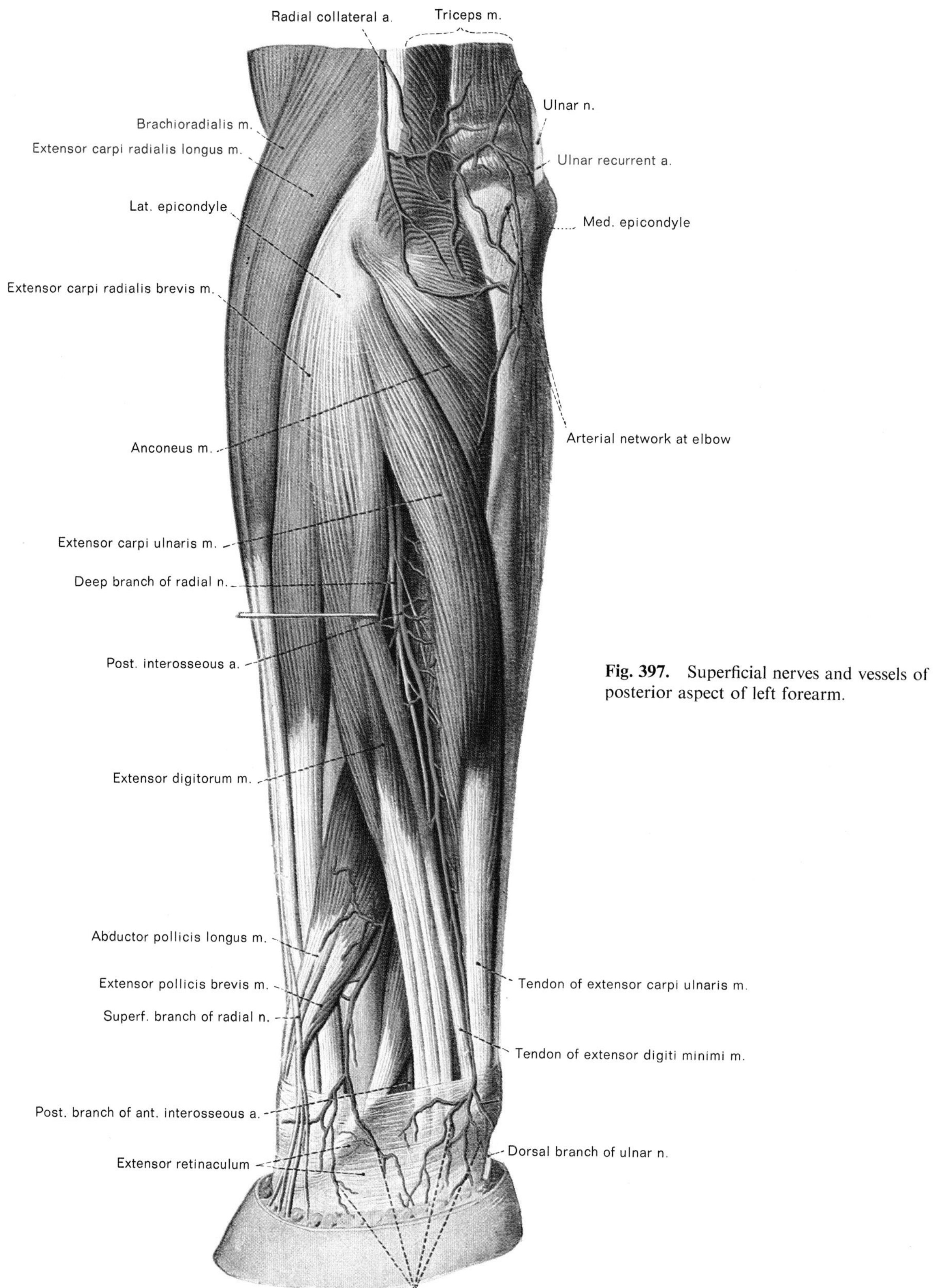
Radial collateral a.
Triceps m.
Ulnar n.
Brachioradialis m.
Extensor carpi radialis longus m.
Ulnar recurrent a.
Lat. epicondyle
Med. epicondyle
Extensor carpi radialis brevis m.
Arterial network at elbow
Anconeus m.
Extensor carpi ulnaris m.
Deep branch of radial n.
Post. interosseous a.
Extensor digitorum m.
Abductor pollicis longus m.
Extensor pollicis brevis m.
Tendon of extensor carpi ulnaris m.
Superf. branch of radial n.
Tendon of extensor digiti minimi m.
Post. branch of ant. interosseous a.
Dorsal branch of ulnar n.
Extensor retinaculum
Arterial network at wrist

Fig. 397. Superficial nerves and vessels of posterior aspect of left forearm.

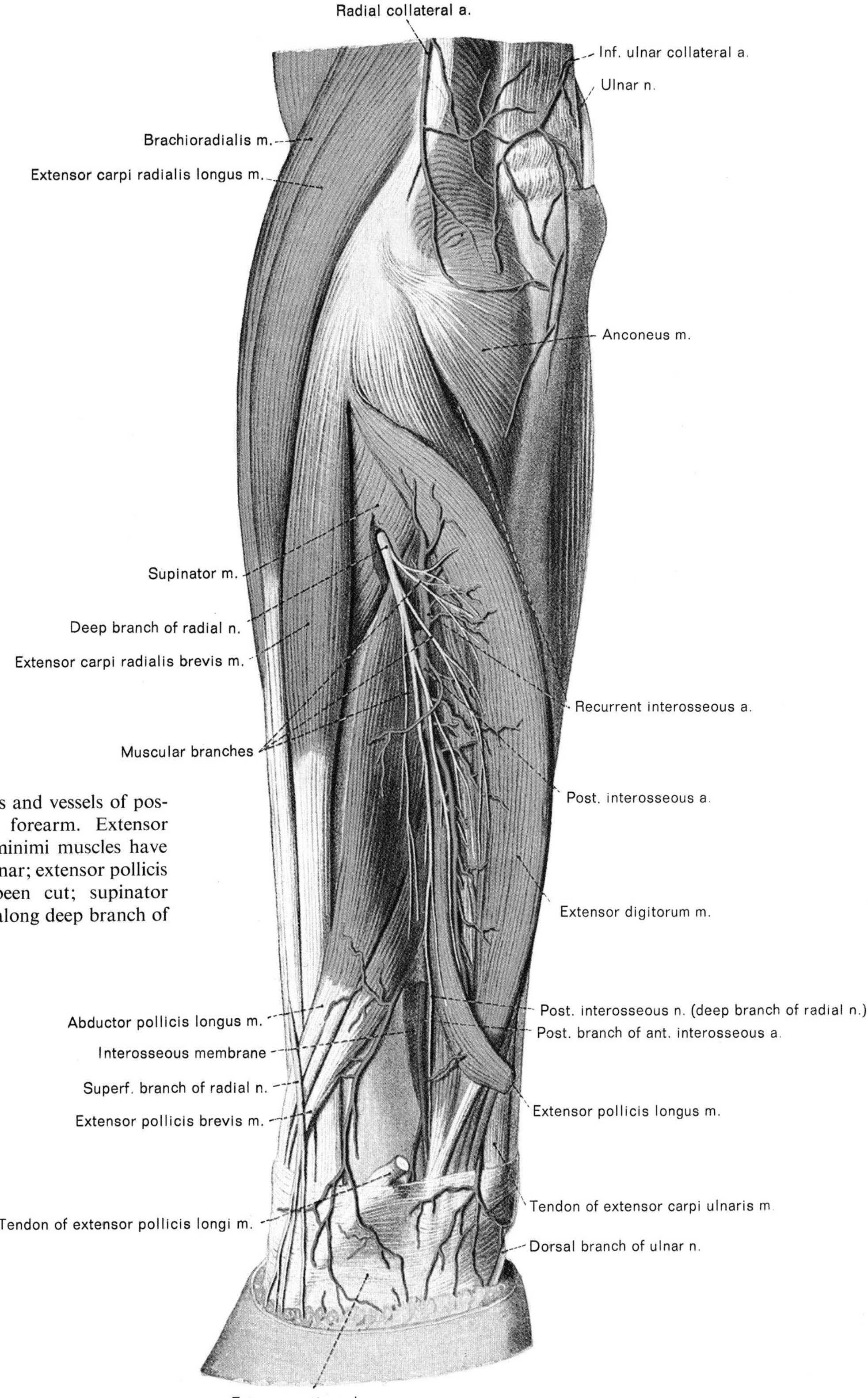
Radial collateral a.
Inf. ulnar collateral a.
Ulnar n.
Brachioradialis m.
Extensor carpi radialis longus m.
Anconeus m.
Supinator m.
Deep branch of radial n.
Extensor carpi radialis brevis m.
Recurrent interosseous a.
Muscular branches
Post. interosseous a.
Extensor digitorum m.
Abductor pollicis longus m.
Post. interosseous n. (deep branch of radial n.)
Post. branch of ant. interosseous a.
Interosseous membrane
Superf. branch of radial n.
Extensor pollicis brevis m.
Extensor pollicis longus m.
Tendon of extensor carpi ulnaris m.
Tendon of extensor pollicis longi m.
Dorsal branch of ulnar n.
Extensor retinaculum

Fig. 398. Deep nerves and vessels of posterior aspect of left forearm. Extensor digitorum and digiti minimi muscles have been pushed toward ulnar; extensor pollicis longus muscle has been cut; supinator muscle has been split along deep branch of radial nerve.

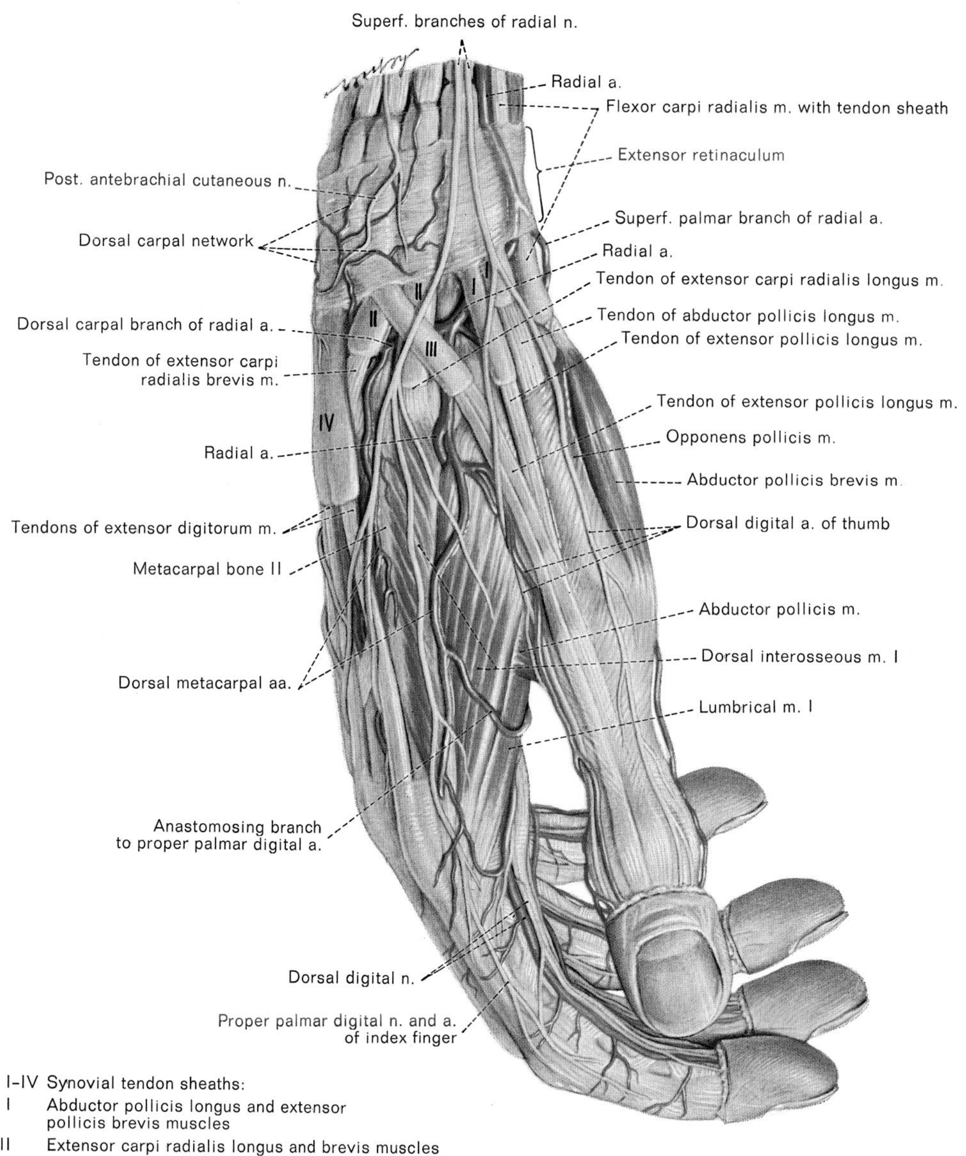
Superf. branches of radial n.
Radial a.
Flexor carpi radialis m. with tendon sheath
Extensor retinaculum
Post. antebrachial cutaneous n.
Superf. palmar branch of radial a.
Dorsal carpal network
Radial a.
Tendon of extensor carpi radialis longus m.
Dorsal carpal branch of radial a.
Tendon of abductor pollicis longus m.
Tendon of extensor pollicis longus m.
Tendon of extensor carpi radialis brevis m.
Tendon of extensor pollicis longus m.
Opponens pollicis m.
Radial a.
Abductor pollicis brevis m.
Tendons of extensor digitorum m.
Dorsal digital a. of thumb
Metacarpal bone II
Abductor pollicis m.
Dorsal interosseous m. I
Dorsal metacarpal aa.
Lumbrical m. I
Anastomosing branch to proper palmar digital a.
Dorsal digital n.
Proper palmar digital n. and a. of index finger
I
II
III
IV

I-IV Synovial tendon sheaths:
I Abductor pollicis longus and extensor pollicis brevis muscles
II Extensor carpi radialis longus and brevis muscles
III Extensor pollicis longus muscle
IV Extensor digitorum and extensor indicis muscles

Fig. 399. Superficial arteries and nerves of the right hand, radial view. Skin, subcutaneous tissue and fascia have been removed. Note the radial artery in the radial fovea which is bordered by the tendons of the extensor pollicis brevis and longus muscles.

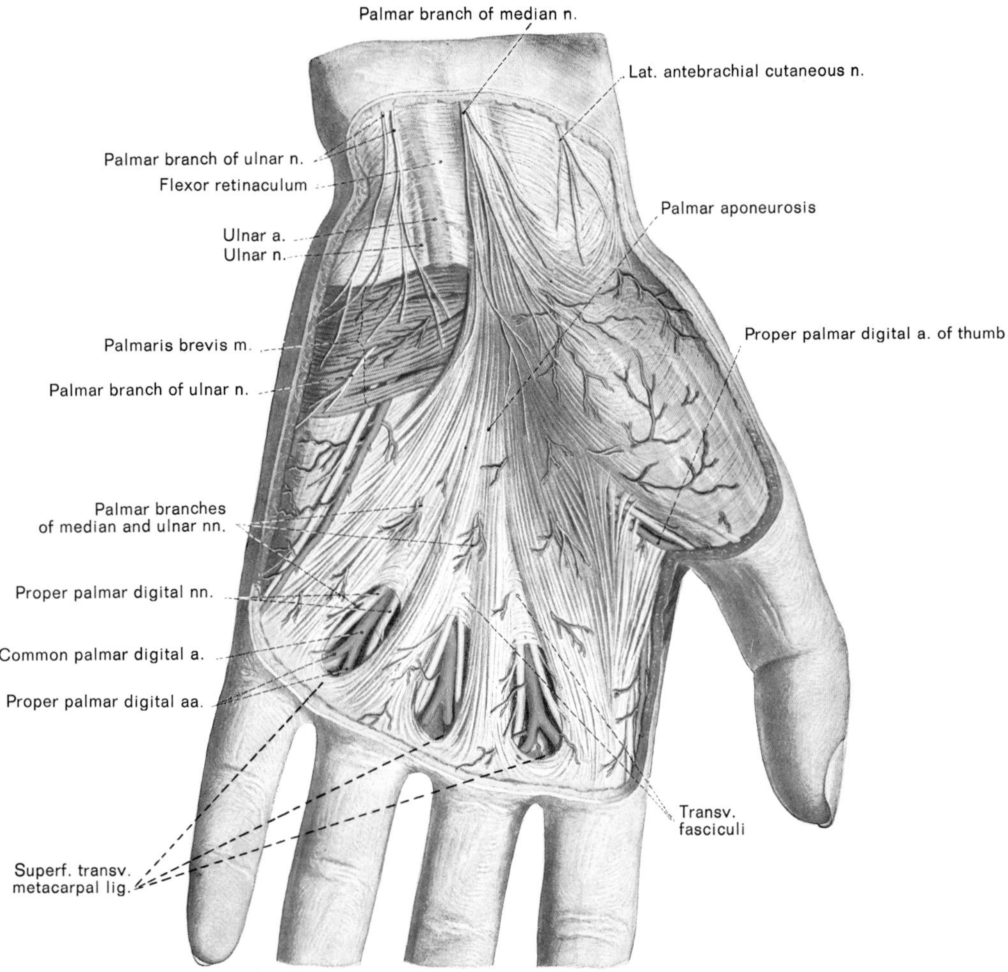
Palmar branch of median n.
Lat. antebrachial cutaneous n.
Palmar branch of ulnar n.
Flexor retinaculum
Palmar aponeurosis
Ulnar a.
Ulnar n.
Proper palmar digital a. of thumb
Palmaris brevis m.
Palmar branch of ulnar n.
Palmar branches
of median and ulnar nn.
Proper palmar digital nn.
Common palmar digital a.
Proper palmar digital aa.
Transv.
fasciculi
Superf. transv.
metacarpal lig.

Fig. 400. Superficial nerves and arteries of palm of left hand.

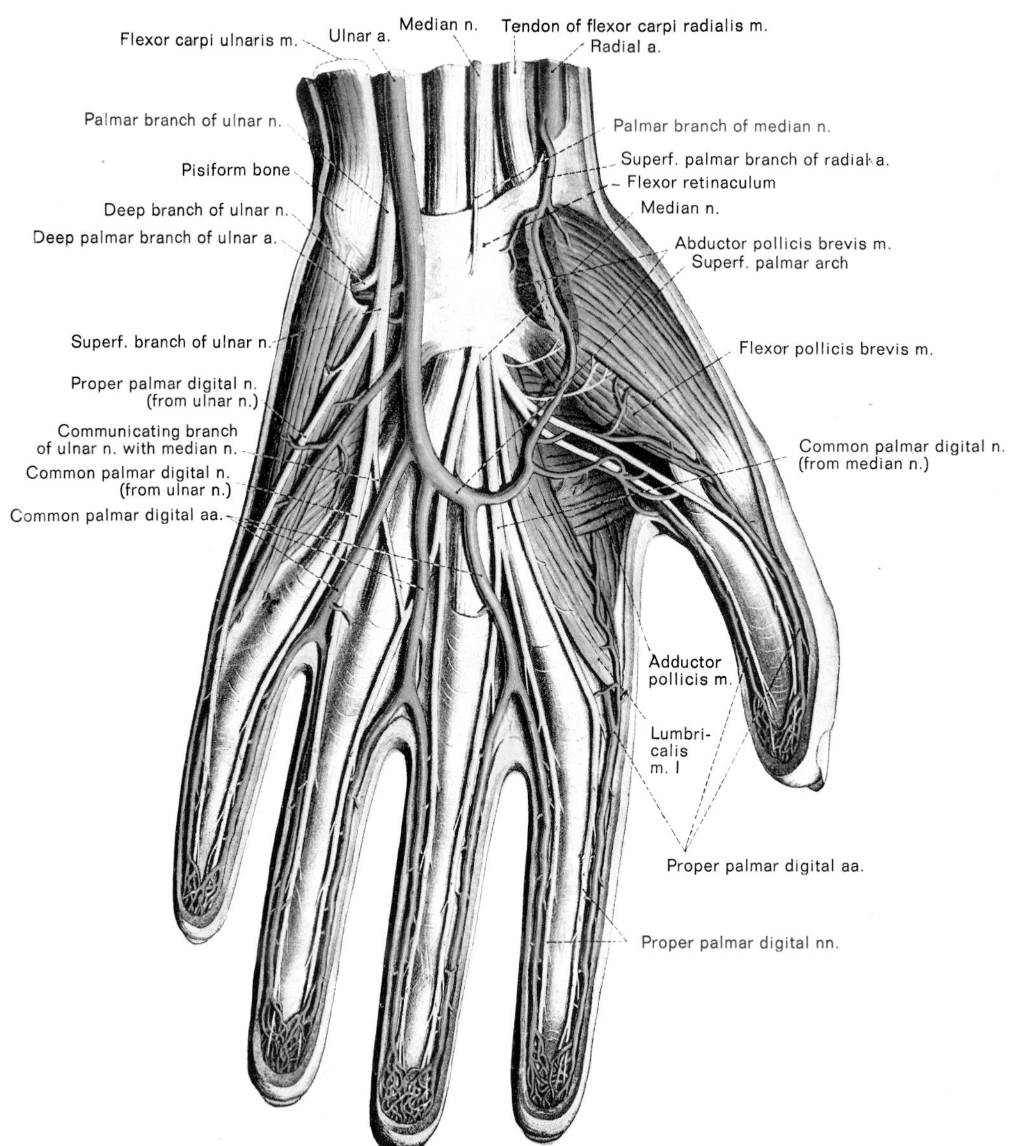
Flexor carpi ulnaris m.
Ulnar a.
Median n.
Tendon of flexor carpi radialis m.
Radial a.
Palmar branch of ulnar n.
Palmar branch of median n.
Pisiform bone
Superf. palmar branch of radial a.
Flexor retinaculum
Deep branch of ulnar n.
Median n.
Deep palmar branch of ulnar a.
Abductor pollicis brevis m.
Superf. palmar arch
Superf. branch of ulnar n.
Flexor pollicis brevis m.
Proper palmar digital n. (from ulnar n.)
Communicating branch of ulnar n. with median n.
Common palmar digital n. (from median n.)
Common palmar digital n. (from ulnar n.)
Common palmar digital aa.
Adductor pollicis m.
Lumbricalis m. I
Proper palmar digital aa.
Proper palmar digital nn.

Fig. 401. Nerves and arteries of palm of left hand. The palmar aponeurosis has been removed, the abductor pollicis brevis muscle has been split along the superficial palmar branch of the radial artery.

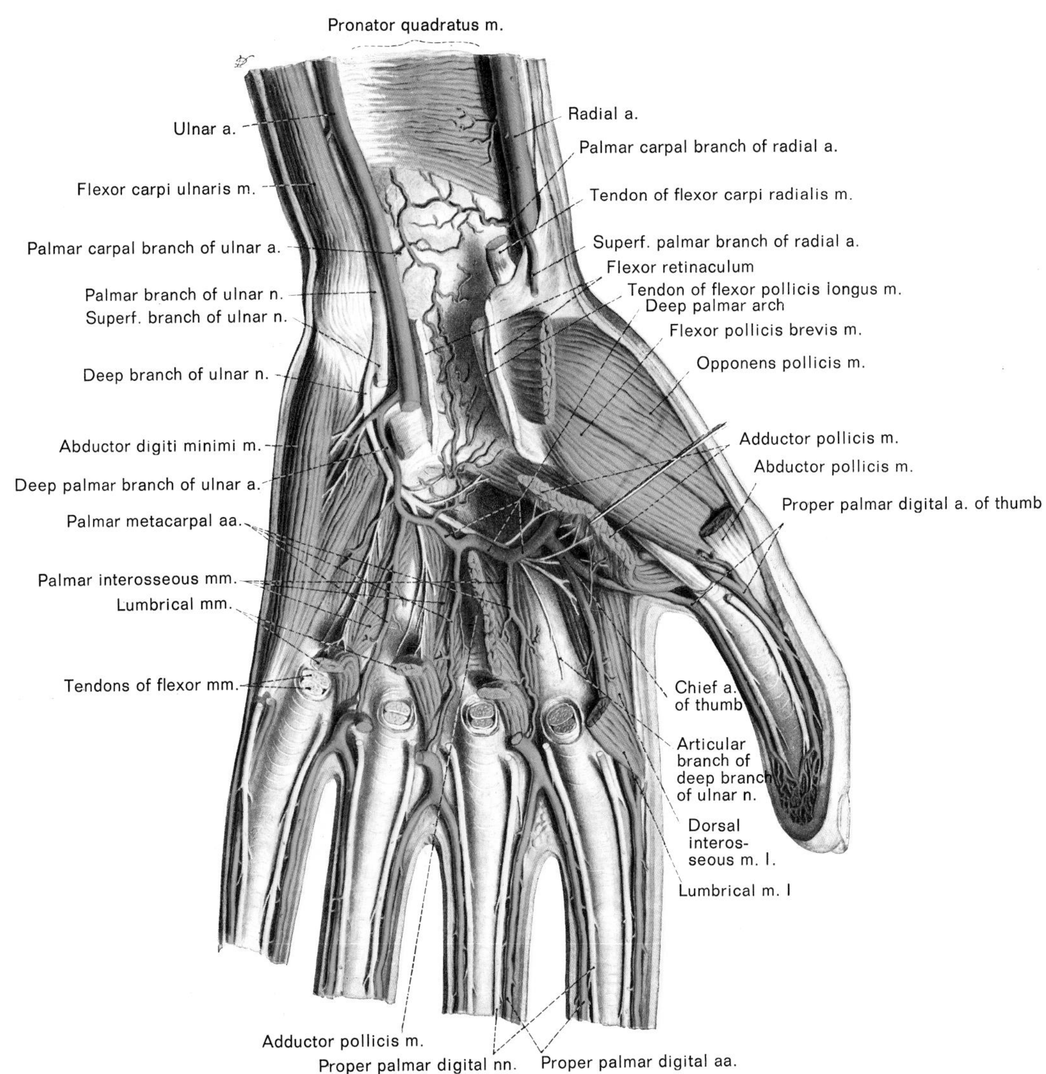
Pronator quadratus m.
Ulnar a.
Flexor carpi ulnaris m.
Palmar carpal branch of ulnar a.
Palmar branch of ulnar n.
Superf. branch of ulnar n.
Deep branch of ulnar n.
Abductor digiti minimi m.
Deep palmar branch of ulnar a.
Palmar metacarpal aa.
Palmar interosseous mm.
Lumbrical mm.
Tendons of flexor mm.
Radial a.
Palmar carpal branch of radial a.
Tendon of flexor carpi radialis m.
Superf. palmar branch of radial a.
Flexor retinaculum
Tendon of flexor pollicis longus m.
Deep palmar arch
Flexor pollicis brevis m.
Opponens pollicis m.
Adductor pollicis m.
Abductor pollicis m.
Proper palmar digital a. of thumb
Chief a. of thumb
Articular branch of deep branch of ulnar n.
Dorsal interos- seous m. I.
Lumbrical m. I
Adductor pollicis m.
Proper palmar digital nn.
Proper palmar digital aa.

Fig. 402. Nerves and arteries of palm of left hand, deep layer. Abductor pollicis brevis, adductor pollicis and flexor digiti minimi muscles have been sectioned; flexor tendons, median nerve, superficial branch of ulnar nerve and superficial palmar arch have been removed.

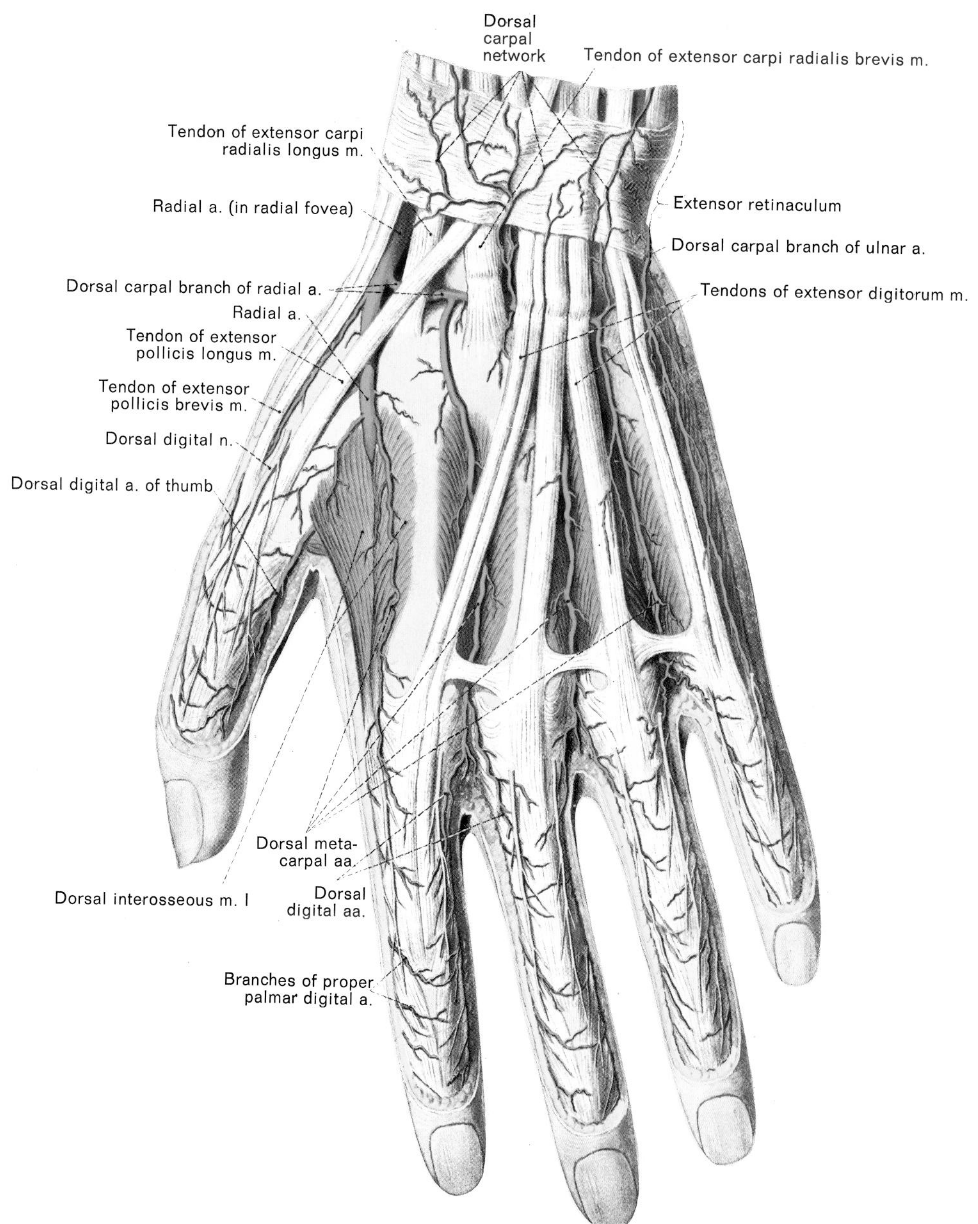
Dorsal
carpal
network
Tendon of extensor carpi radialis brevis m.
Tendon of extensor carpi
radialis longus m.
Radial a. (in radial fovea)
Extensor retinaculum
Dorsal carpal branch of ulnar a.
Dorsal carpal branch of radial a.
Tendons of extensor digitorum m.
Radial a.
Tendon of extensor
pollicis longus m.
Tendon of extensor
pollicis brevis m.
Dorsal digital n.
Dorsal digital a. of thumb
Dorsal meta-
carpal aa.
Dorsal interosseous m. I
Dorsal
digital aa.
Branches of proper
palmar digital a.

Fig. 403. Arteries of dorsum of left hand, superficial layer.

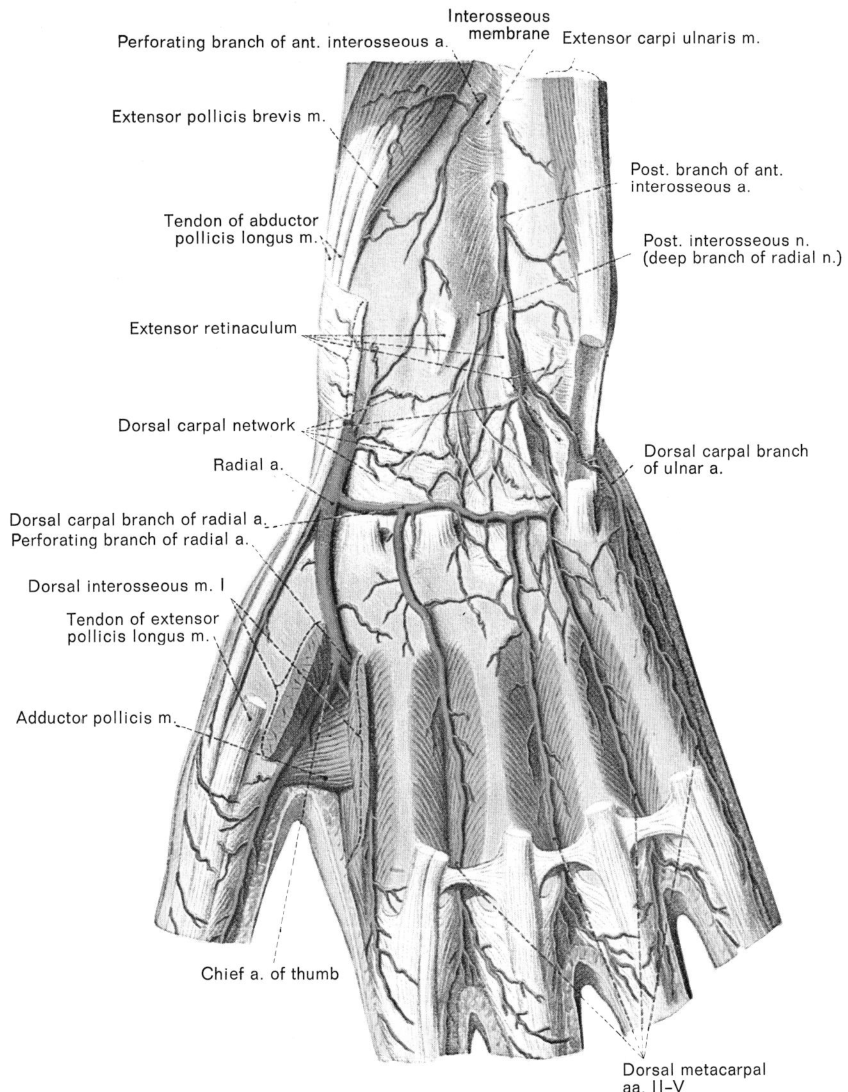
Interosseous membrane
Perforating branch of ant. interosseous a.
Extensor carpi ulnaris m.
Extensor pollicis brevis m.
Post. branch of ant. interosseous a.
Tendon of abductor pollicis longus m.
Post. interosseous n. (deep branch of radial n.)
Extensor retinaculum
Dorsal carpal network
Radial a.
Dorsal carpal branch of ulnar a.
Dorsal carpal branch of radial a.
Perforating branch of radial a.
Dorsal interosseous m. I
Tendon of extensor pollicis longus m.
Adductor pollicis m.
Chief a. of thumb
Dorsal metacarpal aa. II–V

Fig. 404. Arteries of dorsum of left hand and wrist. The extensor tendons with the exception of the abductor pollicis longus and extensor pollicis brevis muscles have been cut and partially removed; the extensor retinaculum has been opened and partially removed; the dorsal interosseous muscle I has been sectioned.

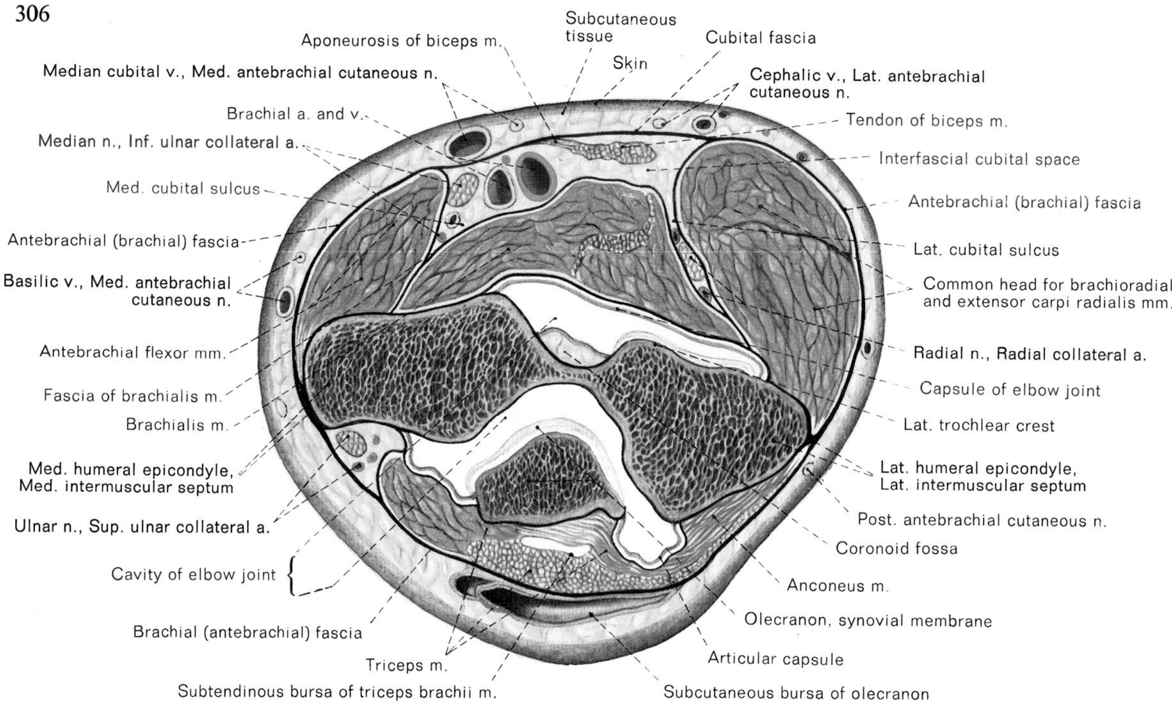

Subcutaneous tissue
Aponeurosis of biceps m.
Cubital fascia
Skin
Median cubital v., Med. antebrachial cutaneous n.
Cephalic v., Lat. antebrachial cutaneous n.
Brachial a. and v.
Tendon of biceps m.
Median n., Inf. ulnar collateral a.
Interfascial cubital space
Med. cubital sulcus
Antebrachial (brachial) fascia
Antebrachial (brachial) fascia
Lat. cubital sulcus
Basilic v., Med. antebrachial cutaneous n.
Common head for brachioradialis and extensor carpi radialis mm.
Antebrachial flexor mm.
Radial n., Radial collateral a.
Fascia of brachialis m.
Capsule of elbow joint
Brachialis m.
Lat. trochlear crest
Med. humeral epicondyle, Med. intermuscular septum
Lat. humeral epicondyle, Lat. intermuscular septum
Ulnar n., Sup. ulnar collateral a.
Post. antebrachial cutaneous n.
Coronoid fossa
Cavity of elbow joint
Anconeus m.
Olecranon, synovial membrane
Brachial (antebrachial) fascia
Articular capsule
Triceps m.
Subtendinous bursa of triceps brachii m.
Subcutaneous bursa of olecranon

Fig. 405. Cross section through the right arm at the level of the elbow joint. (Figs. 405–408 from *Pernkopf/Ferner:* Atlas der topographischen und angewandten Anatomie des Menschen, vol. 2. Urban & Schwarzenberg, München–Berlin 1963.)

Med. antebrachial cutaneous n.
Median n.
Pronator teres m.
Ulnar a.
Subcutaneous tissue
Cubital fascia
Interosseous a.
Skin
Median cubital v.
Ulnar a.
Antebrachial fascia
Radial a.
Flexor carpi radialis m., Palmaris longus m., Humeral head of flexor digitorum superficialis m.
Lat. antebrachial cutaneous n.
Tendon of biceps m., Bicipito-radial bursa
Superf. branch of radial n.
Ulnar n.
Cephalic v.
Med. antebrachial cutaneous n.
Brachioradial m.
Deep branch of radial n.
Basilic v.
Extensor carpi radialis longus m.
Post. antebrachial cutaneous n.
Flexor carpi ulnaris m.
Antebrachial fascia
Ulnar recurrent a.
Extensor carpi radialis brevis m.
Ulnar head of pronator teres m.
Radius
Tendon of brachialis m.
Intermuscular septum
Post. margin of ulna
Fascia of supinator m.
Supinator m.
Extensor carpi ulnaris m.
Antebrachial fascia
Post. antebrachial cutaneous n.
Extensor digitorum m., Extensor digiti minimi m.

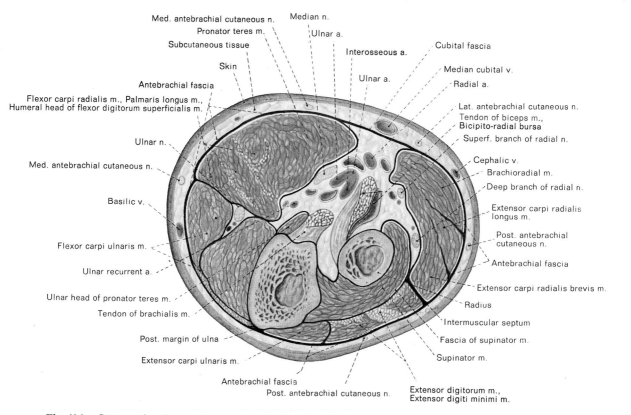

Fig. 406. Cross section through the proximal third of the right forearm.

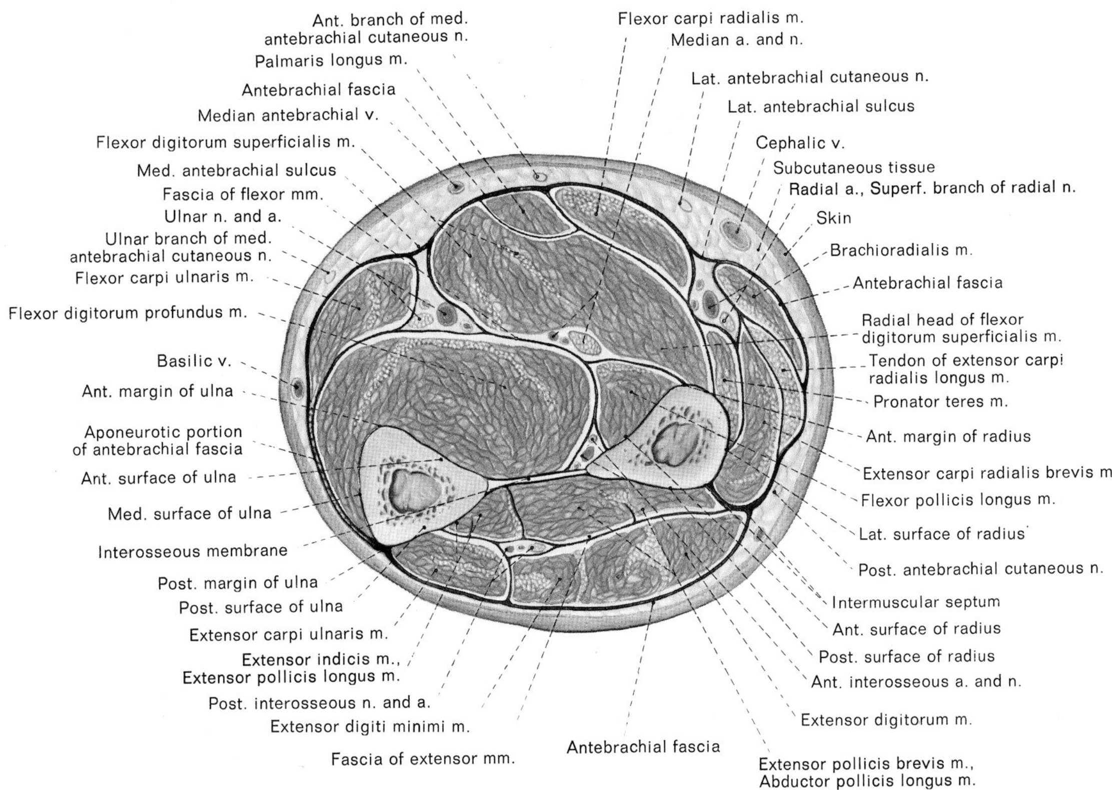
Ant. branch of med. antebrachial cutaneous n.
Palmaris longus m.
Antebrachial fascia
Median antebrachial v.
Flexor digitorum superficialis m.
Med. antebrachial sulcus
Fascia of flexor mm.
Ulnar n. and a.
Ulnar branch of med. antebrachial cutaneous n.
Flexor carpi ulnaris m.
Flexor digitorum profundus m.
Basilic v.
Ant. margin of ulna
Aponeurotic portion of antebrachial fascia
Ant. surface of ulna
Med. surface of ulna
Interosseous membrane
Post. margin of ulna
Post. surface of ulna
Extensor carpi ulnaris m.
Extensor indicis m., Extensor pollicis longus m.
Post. interosseous n. and a.
Extensor digiti minimi m.
Fascia of extensor mm.
Antebrachial fascia
Flexor carpi radialis m.
Median a. and n.
Lat. antebrachial cutaneous n.
Lat. antebrachial sulcus
Cephalic v.
Subcutaneous tissue
Radial a., Superf. branch of radial n.
Skin
Brachioradialis m.
Antebrachial fascia
Radial head of flexor digitorum superficialis m.
Tendon of extensor carpi radialis longus m.
Pronator teres m.
Ant. margin of radius
Extensor carpi radialis brevis m.
Flexor pollicis longus m.
Lat. surface of radius
Post. antebrachial cutaneous n.
Intermuscular septum
Ant. surface of radius
Post. surface of radius
Ant. interosseous a. and n.
Extensor digitorum m.
Extensor pollicis brevis m., Abductor pollicis longus m.

Fig. 407. Cross section through the middle third of the right forearm.

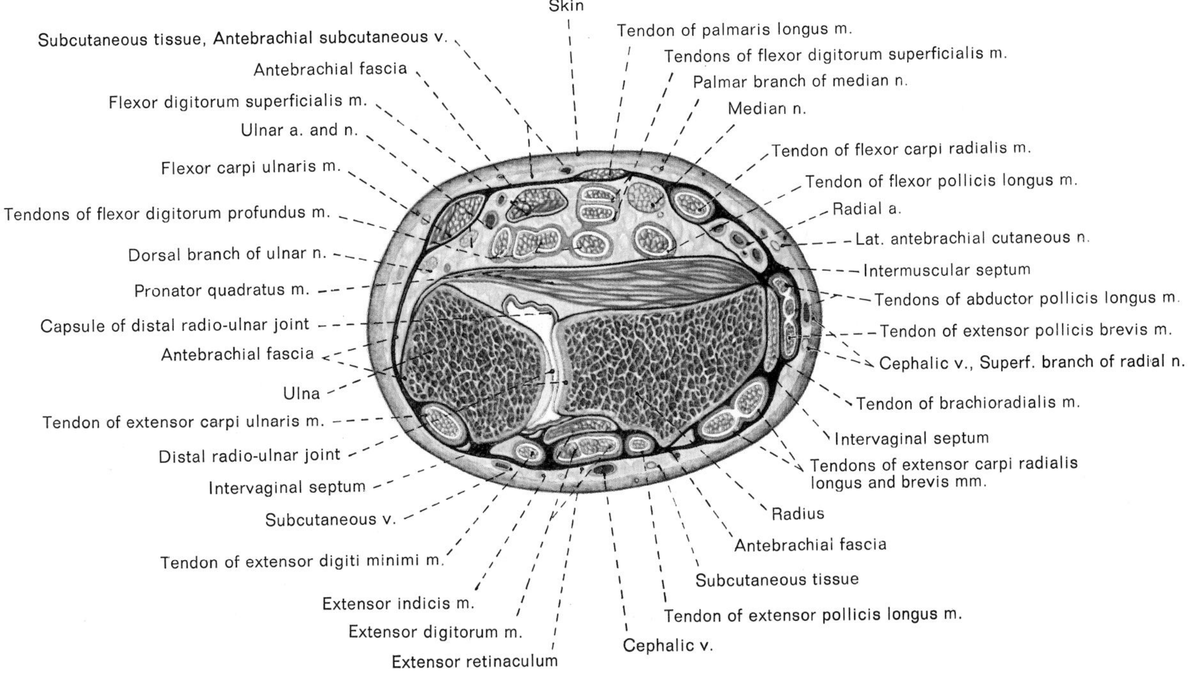
Skin
Subcutaneous tissue, Antebrachial subcutaneous v.
Antebrachial fascia
Flexor digitorum superficialis m.
Ulnar a. and n.
Flexor carpi ulnaris m.
Tendons of flexor digitorum profundus m.
Dorsal branch of ulnar n.
Pronator quadratus m.
Capsule of distal radio-ulnar joint
Antebrachial fascia
Ulna
Tendon of extensor carpi ulnaris m.
Distal radio-ulnar joint
Intervaginal septum
Subcutaneous v.
Tendon of extensor digiti minimi m.
Extensor indicis m.
Extensor digitorum m.
Extensor retinaculum
Tendon of palmaris longus m.
Tendons of flexor digitorum superficialis m.
Palmar branch of median n.
Median n.
Tendon of flexor carpi radialis m.
Tendon of flexor pollicis longus m.
Radial a.
Lat. antebrachial cutaneous n.
Intermuscular septum
Tendons of abductor pollicis longus m.
Tendon of extensor pollicis brevis m.
Cephalic v., Superf. branch of radial n.
Tendon of brachioradialis m.
Intervaginal septum
Tendons of extensor carpi radialis longus and brevis mm.
Radius
Antebrachial fascia
Subcutaneous tissue
Tendon of extensor pollicis longus m.
Cephalic v.

Fig. 408. Cross section through the distal third of the right forearm.

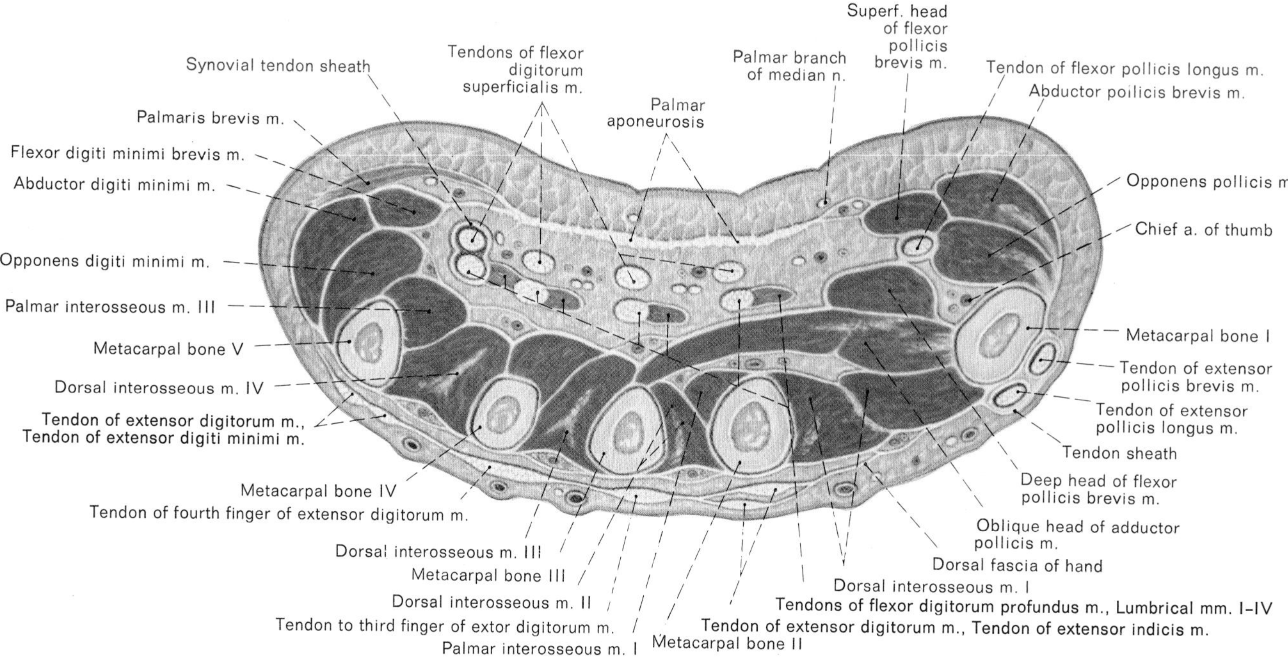
Synovial tendon sheath
Tendons of flexor digitorum superficialis m.
Palmar aponeurosis
Palmar branch of median n.
Superf. head of flexor pollicis brevis m.
Tendon of flexor pollicis longus m.
Abductor pollicis brevis m.
Palmaris brevis m.
Flexor digiti minimi brevis m.
Abductor digiti minimi m.
Opponens pollicis m.
Chief a. of thumb
Opponens digiti minimi m.
Palmar interosseous m. III
Metacarpal bone V
Dorsal interosseous m. IV
Tendon of extensor digitorum m., Tendon of extensor digiti minimi m.
Metacarpal bone I
Tendon of extensor pollicis brevis m.
Tendon of extensor pollicis longus m.
Tendon sheath
Deep head of flexor pollicis brevis m.
Metacarpal bone IV
Tendon of fourth finger of extensor digitorum m.
Oblique head of adductor pollicis m.
Dorsal interosseous m. III
Dorsal fascia of hand
Metacarpal bone III
Dorsal interosseous m. I
Dorsal interosseous m. II
Tendons of flexor digitorum profundus m., Lumbrical mm. I–IV
Tendon to third finger of extor digitorum m.
Tendon of extensor digitorum m., Tendon of extensor indicis m.
Palmar interosseous m. I
Metacarpal bone II

Fig. 409. Cross section through right metacarpus.

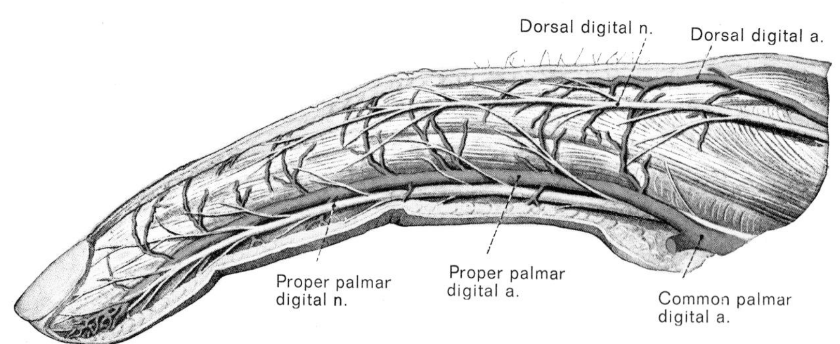
Dorsal digital n.
Dorsal digital a.
Proper palmar digital n.
Proper palmar digital a.
Common palmar digital a.

Fig. 410. Nerves and arteries of the index finger.

Figs. 411–413. Cross section through the middle finger: proximal phalanx (Fig. 411), middle phalanx (Fig. 412), distal phalanx (Fig. 413). Observe the location of the arteries and nerves lateral to the flexor tendons at the level of the proximal and middle phalanges (important for anesthesia and hemostasia).

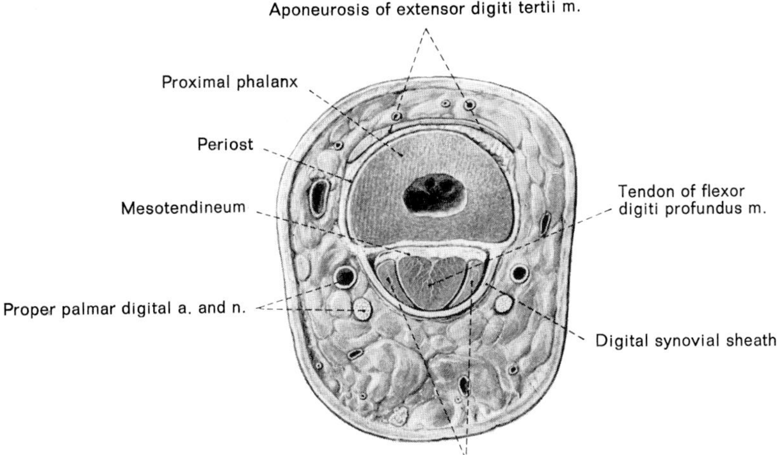
Aponeurosis of extensor digiti tertii m.
Proximal phalanx
Periost
Mesotendineum
Tendon of flexor digiti profundus m.
Proper palmar digital a. and n.
Digital synovial sheath
Tendon of flexor digiti superficialis m.

Fig. 411

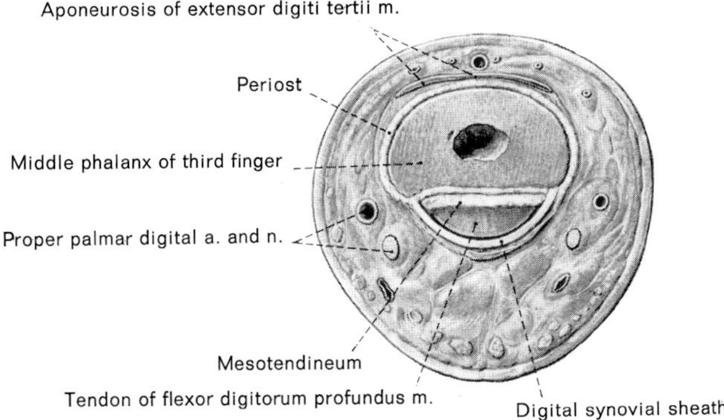
Aponeurosis of extensor digiti tertii m.
Periost
Middle phalanx of third finger
Proper palmar digital a. and n.
Mesotendineum
Tendon of flexor digitorum profundus m.
Digital synovial sheath

Fig. 412

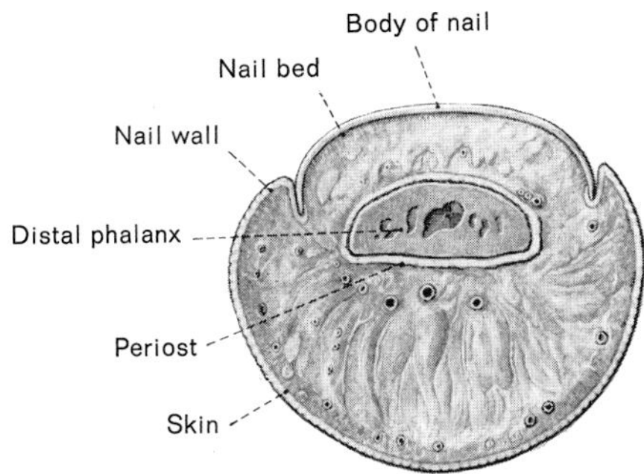
Body of nail
Nail bed
Nail wall
Distal phalanx
Periost
Skin

Fig. 413

Peripheral Nerves and Vessels

Nerves and Vessels of the Lower Extremity

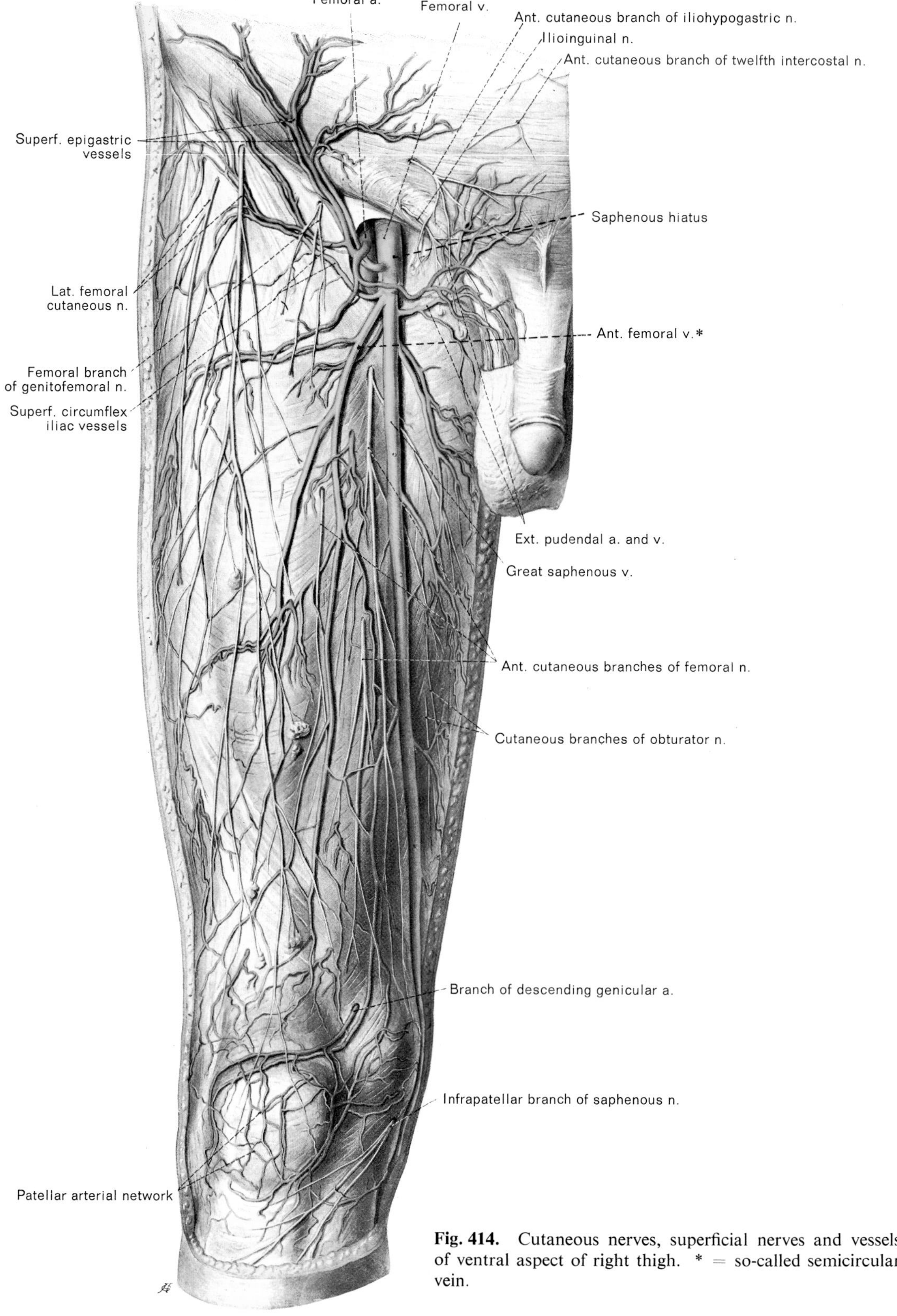
Femoral a.
Femoral v.
Ant. cutaneous branch of iliohypogastric n.
Ilioinguinal n.
Ant. cutaneous branch of twelfth intercostal n.
Superf. epigastric vessels
Saphenous hiatus
Lat. femoral cutaneous n.
Ant. femoral v.*
Femoral branch of genitofemoral n.
Superf. circumflex iliac vessels
Ext. pudendal a. and v.
Great saphenous v.
Ant. cutaneous branches of femoral n.
Cutaneous branches of obturator n.
Branch of descending genicular a.
Infrapatellar branch of saphenous n.
Patellar arterial network

Fig. 414. Cutaneous nerves, superficial nerves and vessels of ventral aspect of right thigh. * = so-called semicircular vein.

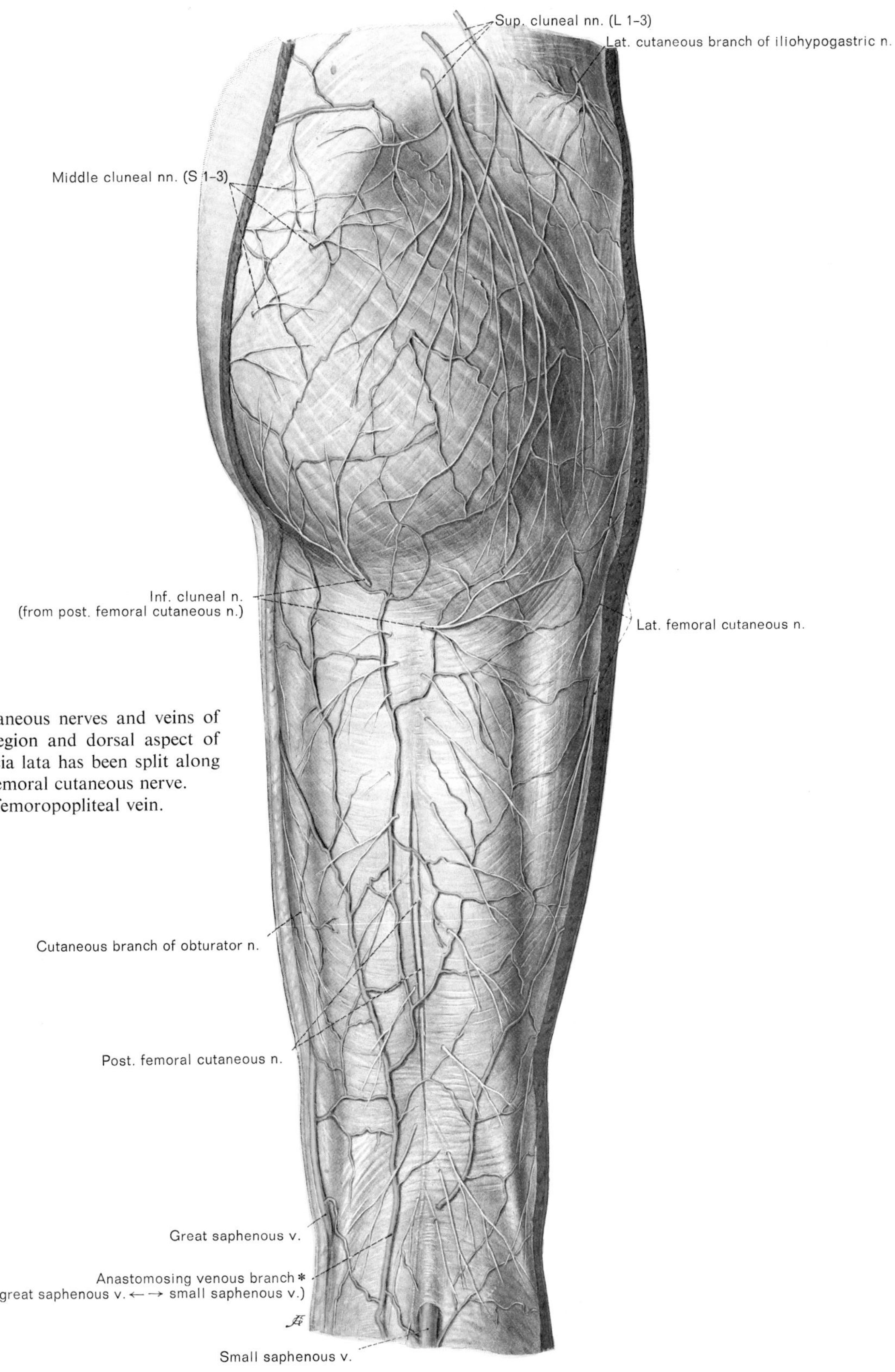
Sup. cluneal nn. (L 1-3)
Lat. cutaneous branch of iliohypogastric n.
Middle cluneal nn. (S 1-3)
Inf. cluneal n.
(from post. femoral cutaneous n.)
Lat. femoral cutaneous n.
Cutaneous branch of obturator n.
Post. femoral cutaneous n.
Great saphenous v.
Anastomosing venous branch *
(great saphenous v. ←→ small saphenous v.)
Small saphenous v.

Fig. 415. Cutaneous nerves and veins of right gluteal region and dorsal aspect of thigh. The fascia lata has been split along the posterior femoral cutaneous nerve.
* = so-called femoropopliteal vein.

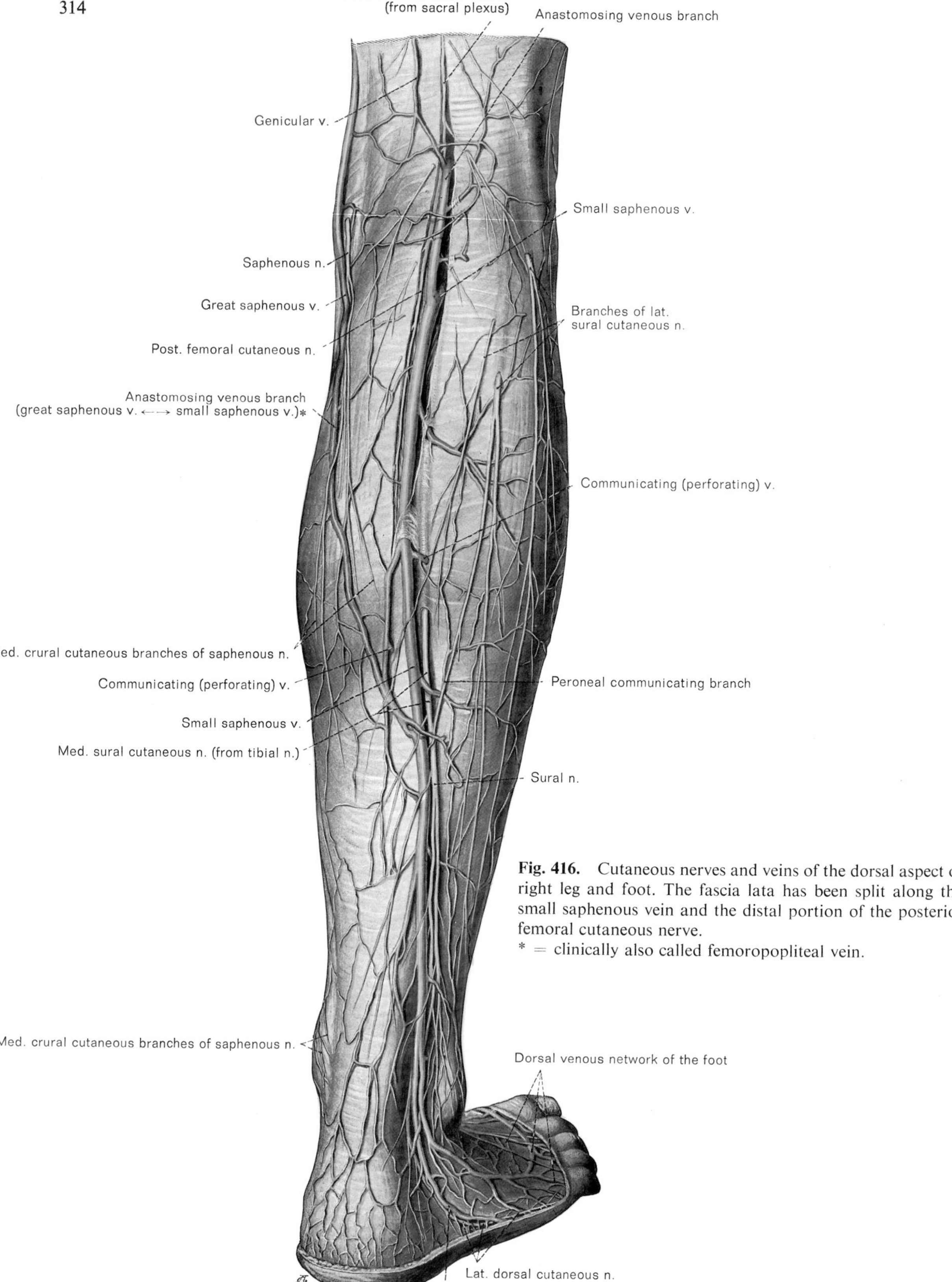
Post. femoral cutaneous n. (from sacral plexus)
Anastomosing venous branch
Genicular v.
Small saphenous v.
Saphenous n.
Great saphenous v.
Branches of lat. sural cutaneous n.
Post. femoral cutaneous n.
Anastomosing venous branch (great saphenous v. ←→ small saphenous v.)*
Communicating (perforating) v.
Med. crural cutaneous branches of saphenous n.
Communicating (perforating) v.
Peroneal communicating branch
Small saphenous v.
Med. sural cutaneous n. (from tibial n.)
Sural n.
Med. crural cutaneous branches of saphenous n.
Dorsal venous network of the foot
Lat. dorsal cutaneous n.
Small saphenous v.

Fig. 416. Cutaneous nerves and veins of the dorsal aspect of right leg and foot. The fascia lata has been split along the small saphenous vein and the distal portion of the posterior femoral cutaneous nerve.
* = clinically also called femoropopliteal vein.

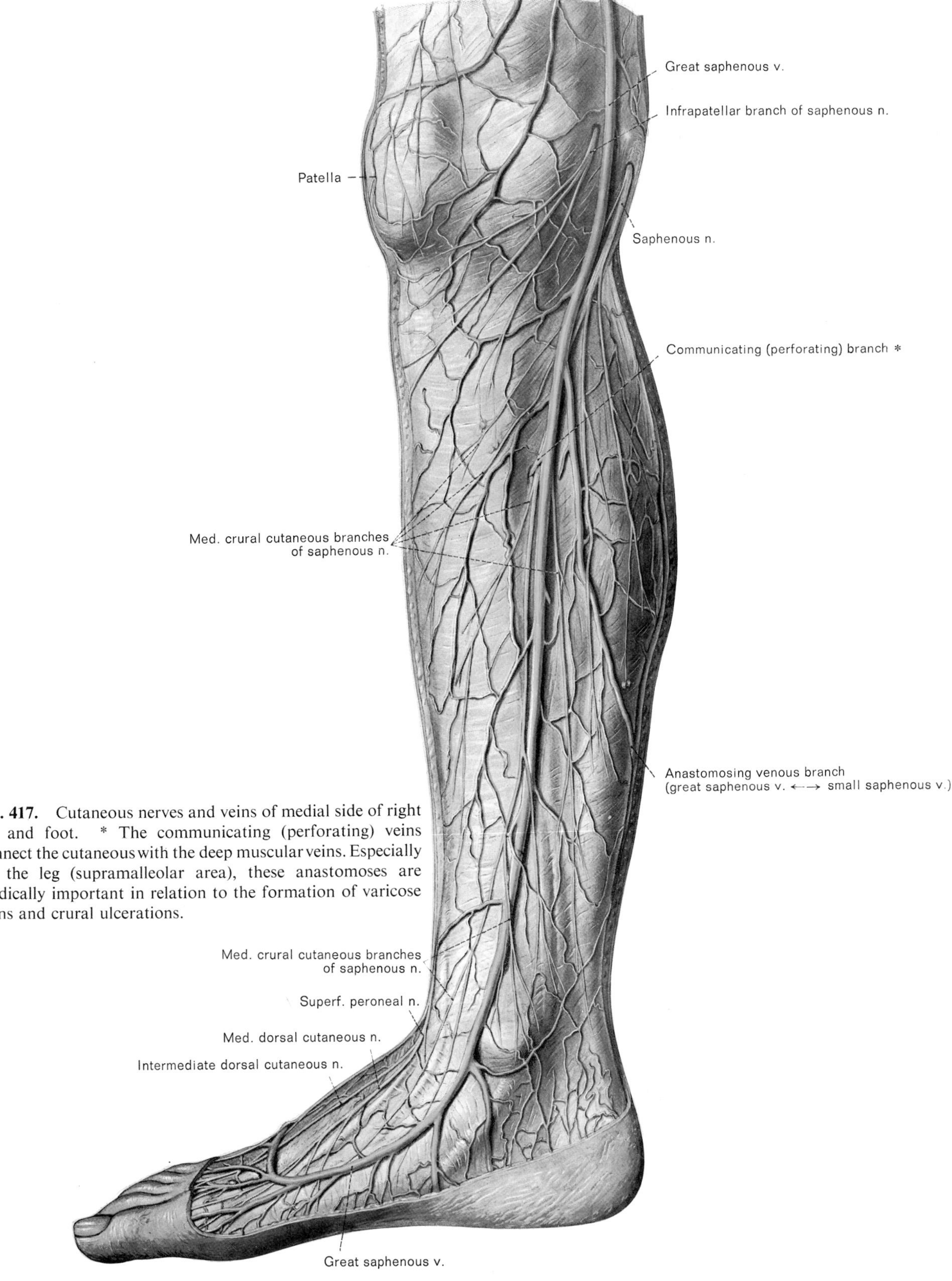
Great saphenous v.
Infrapatellar branch of saphenous n.
Patella
Saphenous n.
Communicating (perforating) branch *
Med. crural cutaneous branches of saphenous n.
Anastomosing venous branch (great saphenous v. ←→ small saphenous v.)
Med. crural cutaneous branches of saphenous n.
Superf. peroneal n.
Med. dorsal cutaneous n.
Intermediate dorsal cutaneous n.
Great saphenous v.

Fig. 417. Cutaneous nerves and veins of medial side of right leg and foot. * The communicating (perforating) veins connect the cutaneous with the deep muscular veins. Especially on the leg (supramalleolar area), these anastomoses are medically important in relation to the formation of varicose veins and crural ulcerations.

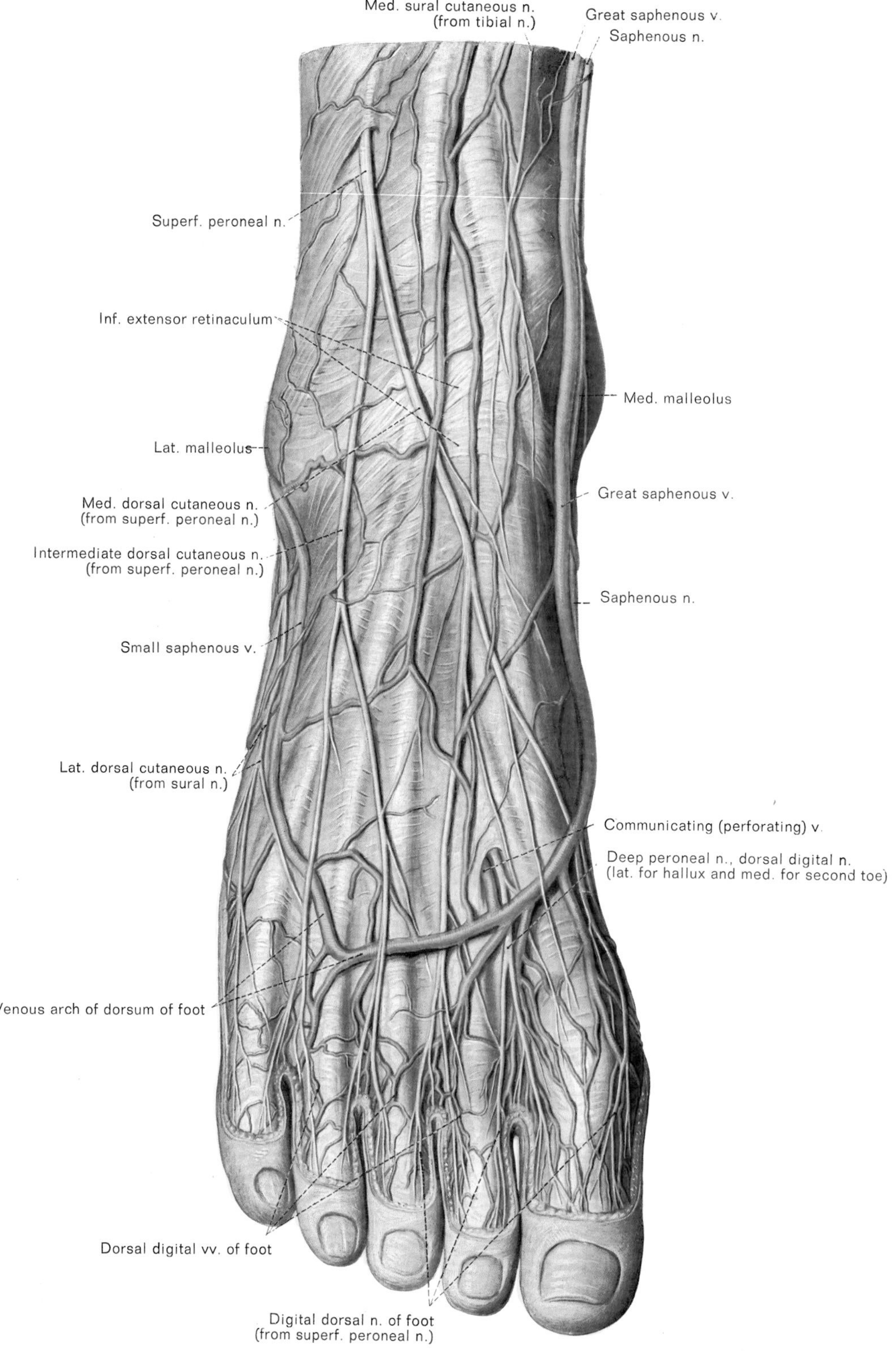

Med. sural cutaneous n.
(from tibial n.)
Great saphenous v.
Saphenous n.
Superf. peroneal n.
Inf. extensor retinaculum
Med. malleolus
Lat. malleolus
Med. dorsal cutaneous n.
(from superf. peroneal n.)
Great saphenous v.
Intermediate dorsal cutaneous n.
(from superf. peroneal n.)
Saphenous n.
Small saphenous v.
Lat. dorsal cutaneous n.
(from sural n.)
Communicating (perforating) v.
Deep peroneal n., dorsal digital n.
(lat. for hallux and med. for second toe)
Venous arch of dorsum of foot
Dorsal digital vv. of foot
Digital dorsal n. of foot
(from superf. peroneal n.)

Fig. 418. Cutaneous nerves and veins of dorsum of right foot.

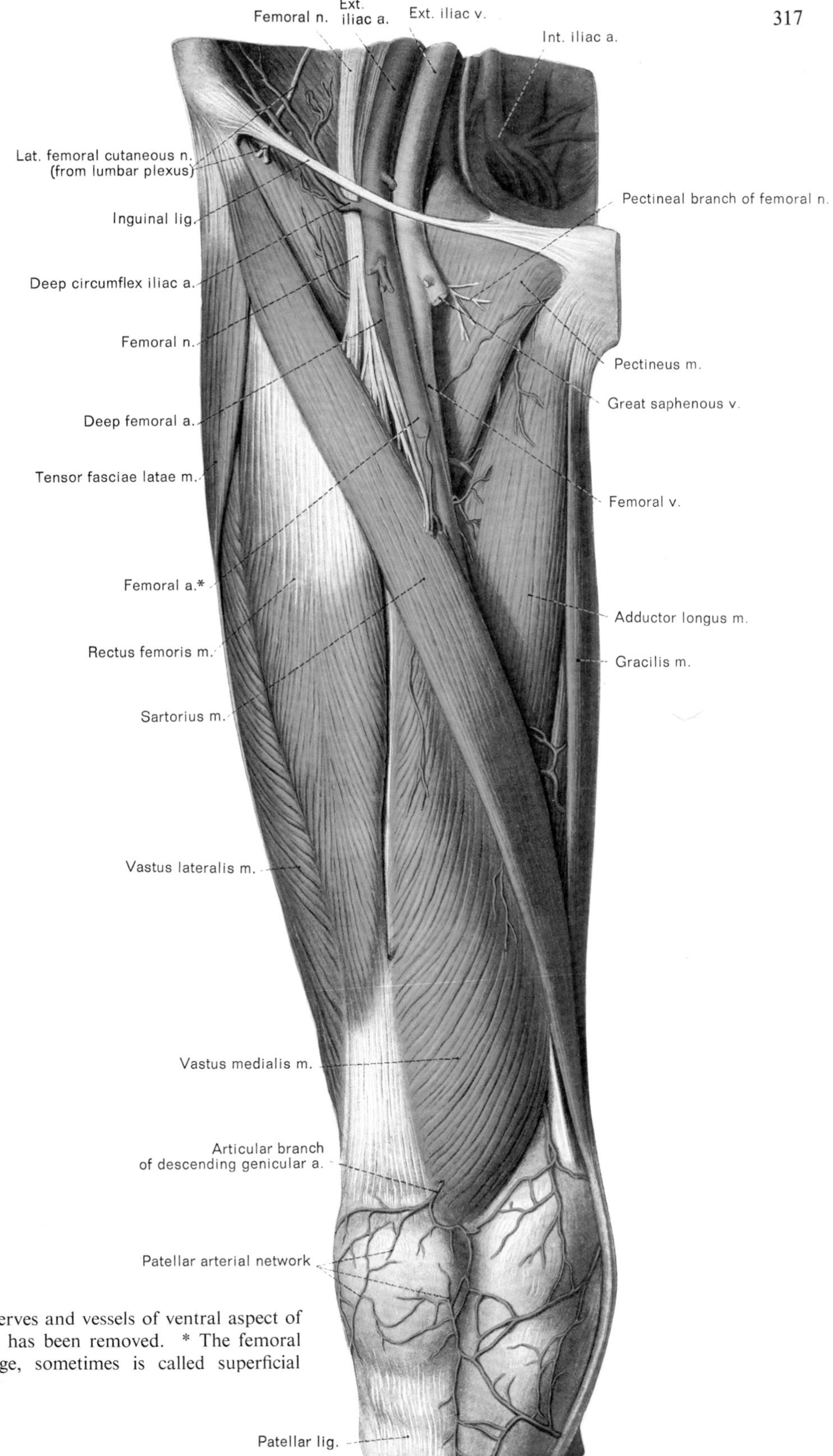
Femoral n.
Ext. iliac a.
Ext. iliac v.
Int. iliac a.
Lat. femoral cutaneous n. (from lumbar plexus)
Inguinal lig.
Deep circumflex iliac a.
Femoral n.
Deep femoral a.
Tensor fasciae latae m.
Femoral a.*
Rectus femoris m.
Sartorius m.
Vastus lateralis m.
Vastus medialis m.
Articular branch of descending genicular a.
Patellar arterial network
Patellar lig.
Pectineal branch of femoral n.
Pectineus m.
Great saphenous v.
Femoral v.
Adductor longus m.
Gracilis m.

Fig. 419. Superficial nerves and vessels of ventral aspect of right thigh. Fascia lata has been removed. * The femoral artery, in clinical usage, sometimes is called superficial femoral artery.

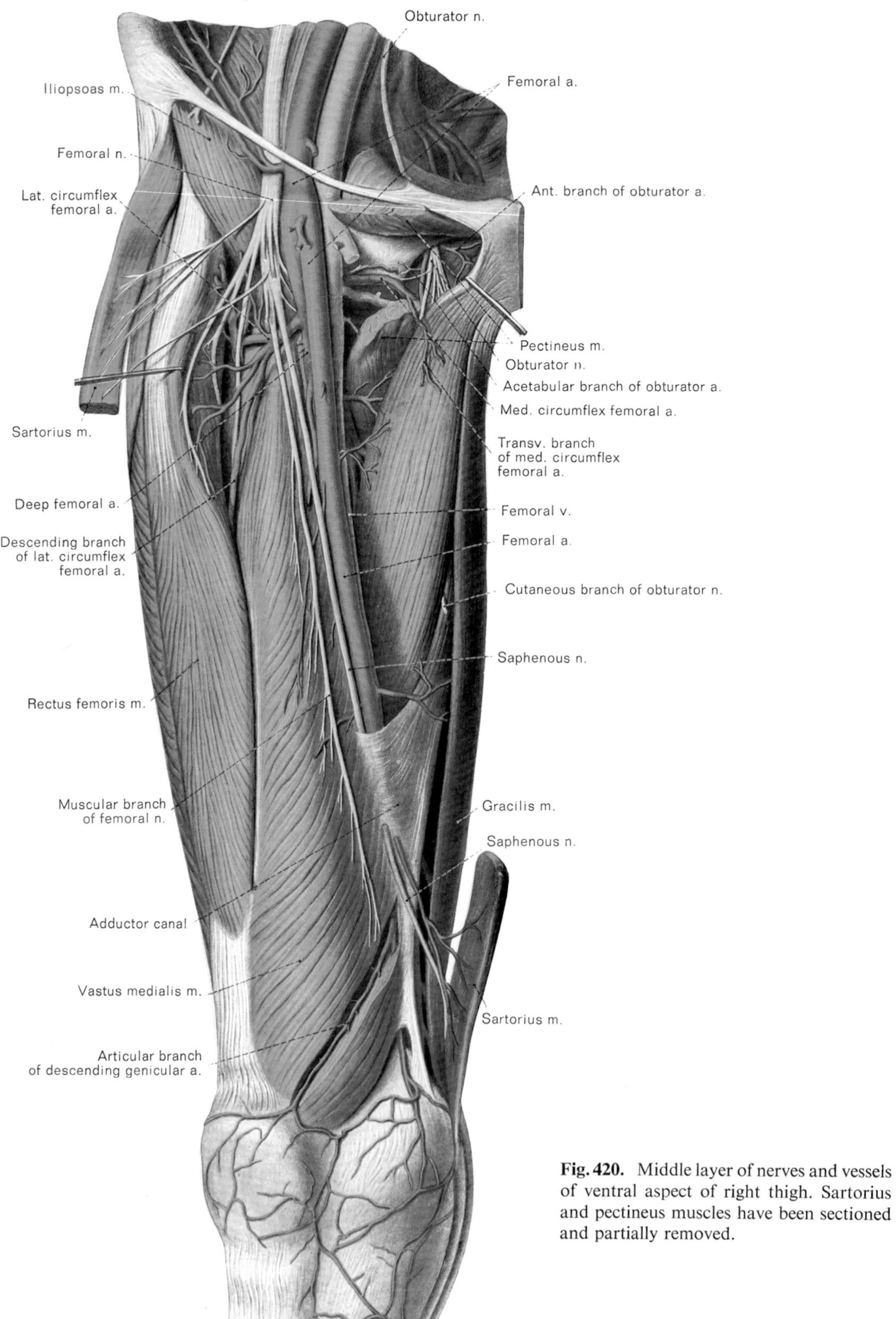
Obturator n.
Femoral a.
Iliopsoas m.
Femoral n.
Ant. branch of obturator a.
Lat. circumflex femoral a.
Pectineus m.
Obturator n.
Acetabular branch of obturator a.
Med. circumflex femoral a.
Sartorius m.
Transv. branch of med. circumflex femoral a.
Deep femoral a.
Femoral v.
Descending branch of lat. circumflex femoral a.
Femoral a.
Cutaneous branch of obturator n.
Saphenous n.
Rectus femoris m.
Gracilis m.
Muscular branch of femoral n.
Saphenous n.
Adductor canal
Vastus medialis m.
Sartorius m.
Articular branch of descending genicular a.

Fig. 420. Middle layer of nerves and vessels of ventral aspect of right thigh. Sartorius and pectineus muscles have been sectioned and partially removed.

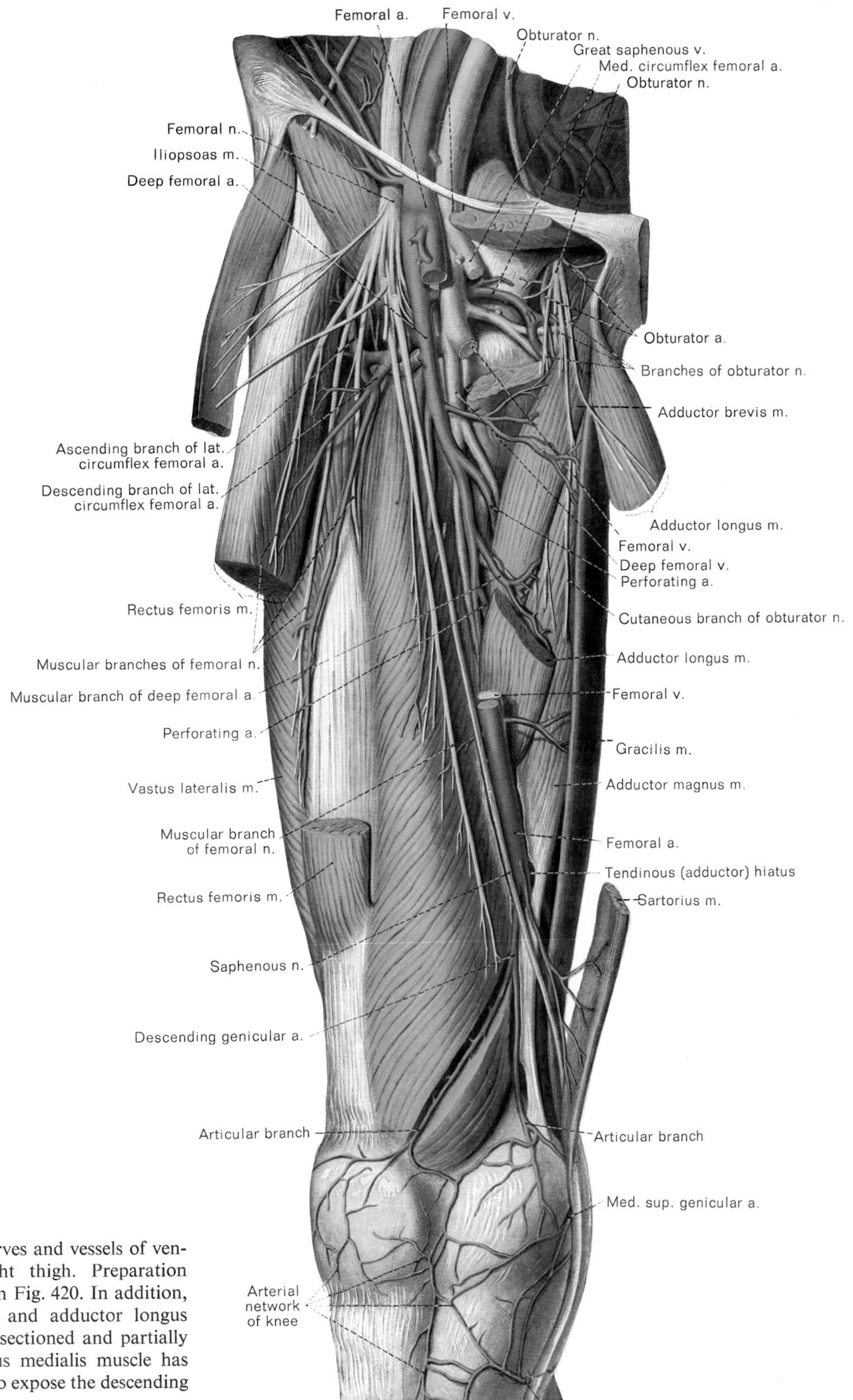
Femoral a.
Femoral v.
Obturator n.
Great saphenous v.
Med. circumflex femoral a.
Obturator n.
Femoral n.
Iliopsoas m.
Deep femoral a.
Obturator a.
Branches of obturator n.
Adductor brevis m.
Ascending branch of lat. circumflex femoral a.
Descending branch of lat. circumflex femoral a.
Adductor longus m.
Femoral v.
Deep femoral v.
Perforating a.
Rectus femoris m.
Cutaneous branch of obturator n.
Muscular branches of femoral n.
Adductor longus m.
Muscular branch of deep femoral a.
Femoral v.
Perforating a.
Gracilis m.
Vastus lateralis m.
Adductor magnus m.
Muscular branch of femoral n.
Femoral a.
Tendinous (adductor) hiatus
Rectus femoris m.
Sartorius m.
Saphenous n.
Descending genicular a.
Articular branch
Articular branch
Med. sup. genicular a.
Arterial network of knee
Med. inf. genicular a.

Fig. 421. Deep nerves and vessels of ventral aspect of right thigh. Preparation similar to the one in Fig. 420. In addition, the rectus femoris and adductor longus muscles have been sectioned and partially removed; the vastus medialis muscle has been split in order to expose the descending genicular artery.

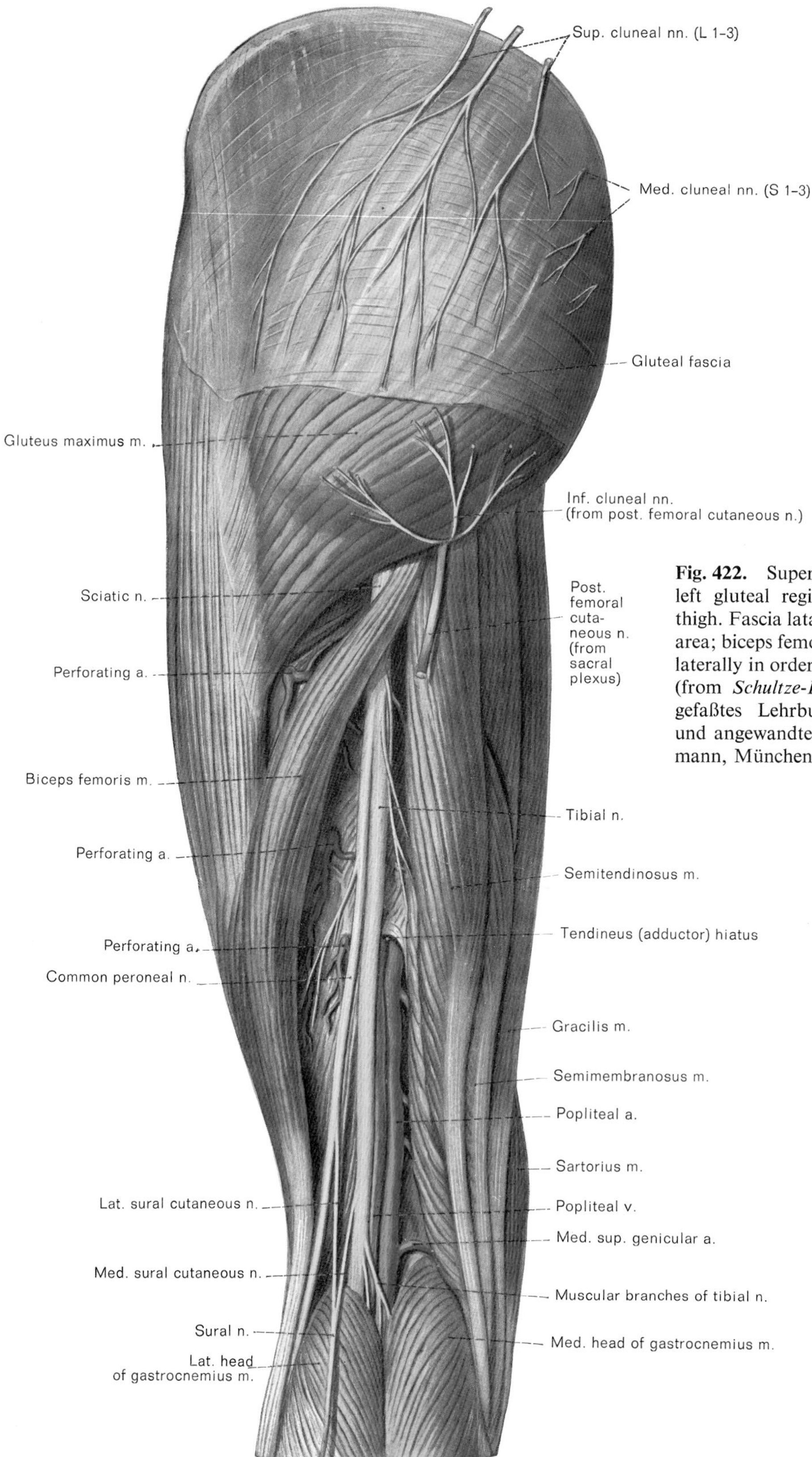
Sup. cluneal nn. (L 1-3)
Med. cluneal nn. (S 1-3)
Gluteal fascia
Gluteus maximus m.
Inf. cluneal nn.
(from post. femoral cutaneous n.)
Sciatic n.
Post. femoral cuta- neous n. (from sacral plexus)
Perforating a.
Biceps femoris m.
Tibial n.
Perforating a.
Semitendinosus m.
Tendineus (adductor) hiatus
Perforating a.
Common peroneal n.
Gracilis m.
Semimembranosus m.
Popliteal a.
Sartorius m.
Lat. sural cutaneous n.
Popliteal v.
Med. sup. genicular a.
Med. sural cutaneous n.
Muscular branches of tibial n.
Sural n.
Med. head of gastrocnemius m.
Lat. head of gastrocnemius m.

Fig. 422. Superficial nerves and vessels of left gluteal region and dorsal aspect of thigh. Fascia lata is retained only in gluteal area; biceps femoris muscle has been pulled laterally in order to expose the sciatic nerve (from *Schultze-Lubosch:* Atlas und kurzgefaßtes Lehrbuch der topographischen und angewandten Anatomie. 4th ed. Lehmann, München 1935).

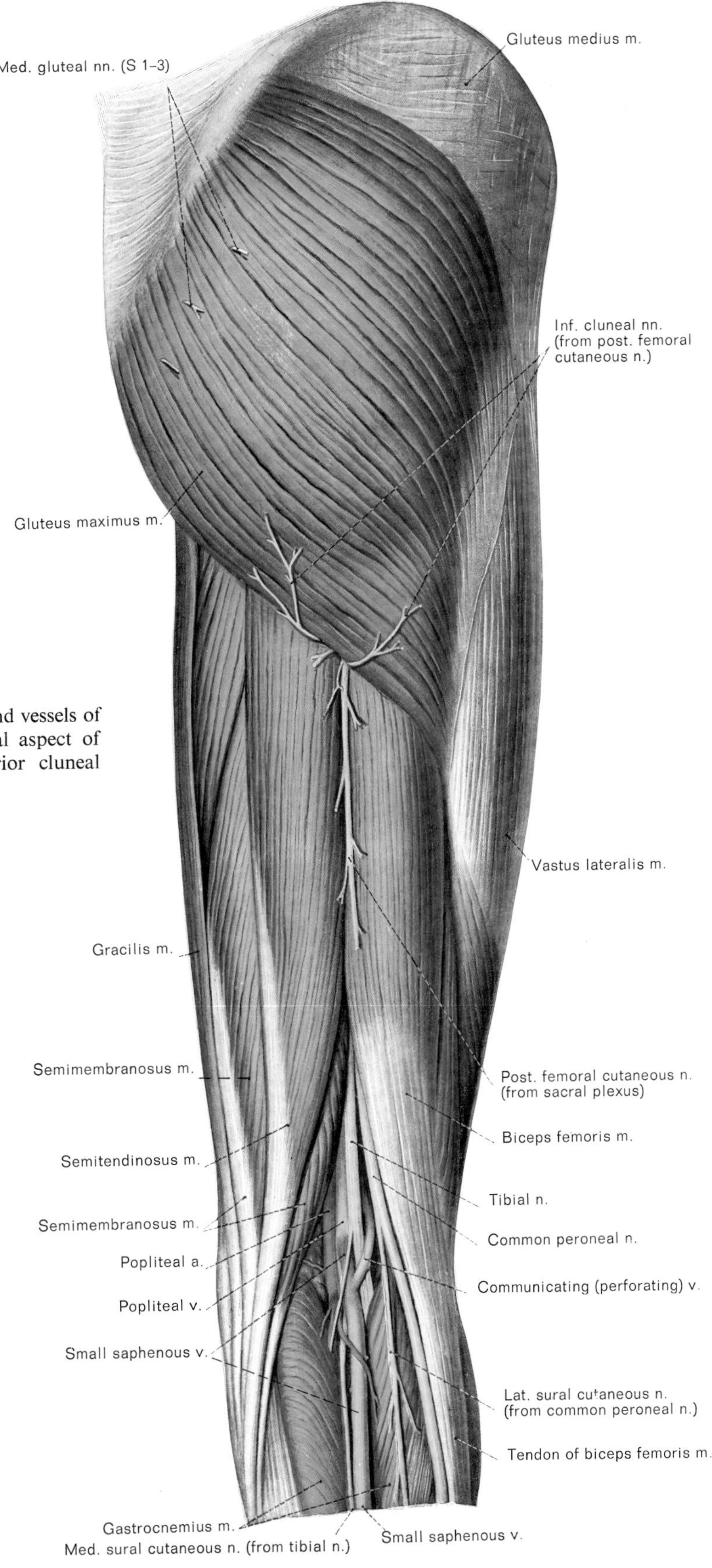
Med. gluteal nn. (S 1–3)
Gluteus medius m.
Inf. cluneal nn.
(from post. femoral
cutaneous n.)
Gluteus maximus m.
Vastus lateralis m.
Gracilis m.
Semimembranosus m.
Post. femoral cutaneous n.
(from sacral plexus)
Biceps femoris m.
Semitendinosus m.
Tibial n.
Semimembranosus m.
Common peroneal n.
Popliteal a.
Communicating (perforating) v.
Popliteal v.
Small saphenous v.
Lat. sural cutaneous n.
(from common peroneal n.)
Tendon of biceps femoris m.
Gastrocnemius m.
Med. sural cutaneous n. (from tibial n.)
Small saphenous v.

Fig. 423. Superficial nerves and vessels of right gluteal region and dorsal aspect of thigh. Fascia lata and superior cluneal nerves have been removed.

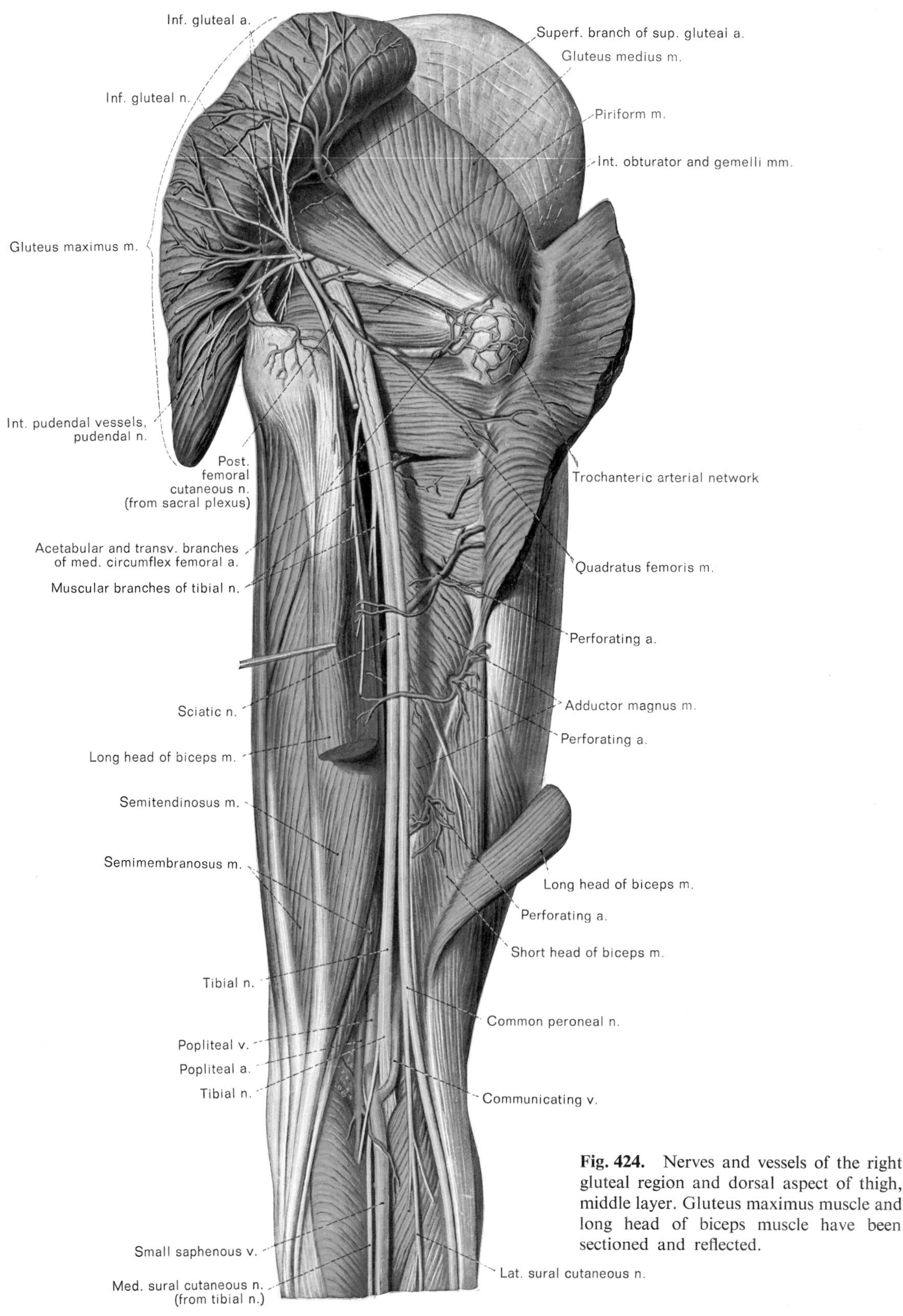

Inf. gluteal a.
Superf. branch of sup. gluteal a.
Gluteus medius m.
Inf. gluteal n.
Piriform m.
Int. obturator and gemelli mm.
Gluteus maximus m.
Int. pudendal vessels, pudendal n.
Post. femoral cutaneous n. (from sacral plexus)
Trochanteric arterial network
Acetabular and transv. branches of med. circumflex femoral a.
Quadratus femoris m.
Muscular branches of tibial n.
Perforating a.
Sciatic n.
Adductor magnus m.
Perforating a.
Long head of biceps m.
Semitendinosus m.
Semimembranosus m.
Long head of biceps m.
Perforating a.
Short head of biceps m.
Tibial n.
Common peroneal n.
Popliteal v.
Popliteal a.
Tibial n.
Communicating v.
Small saphenous v.
Med. sural cutaneous n. (from tibial n.)
Lat. sural cutaneous n.

Fig. 424. Nerves and vessels of the right gluteal region and dorsal aspect of thigh, middle layer. Gluteus maximus muscle and long head of biceps muscle have been sectioned and reflected.

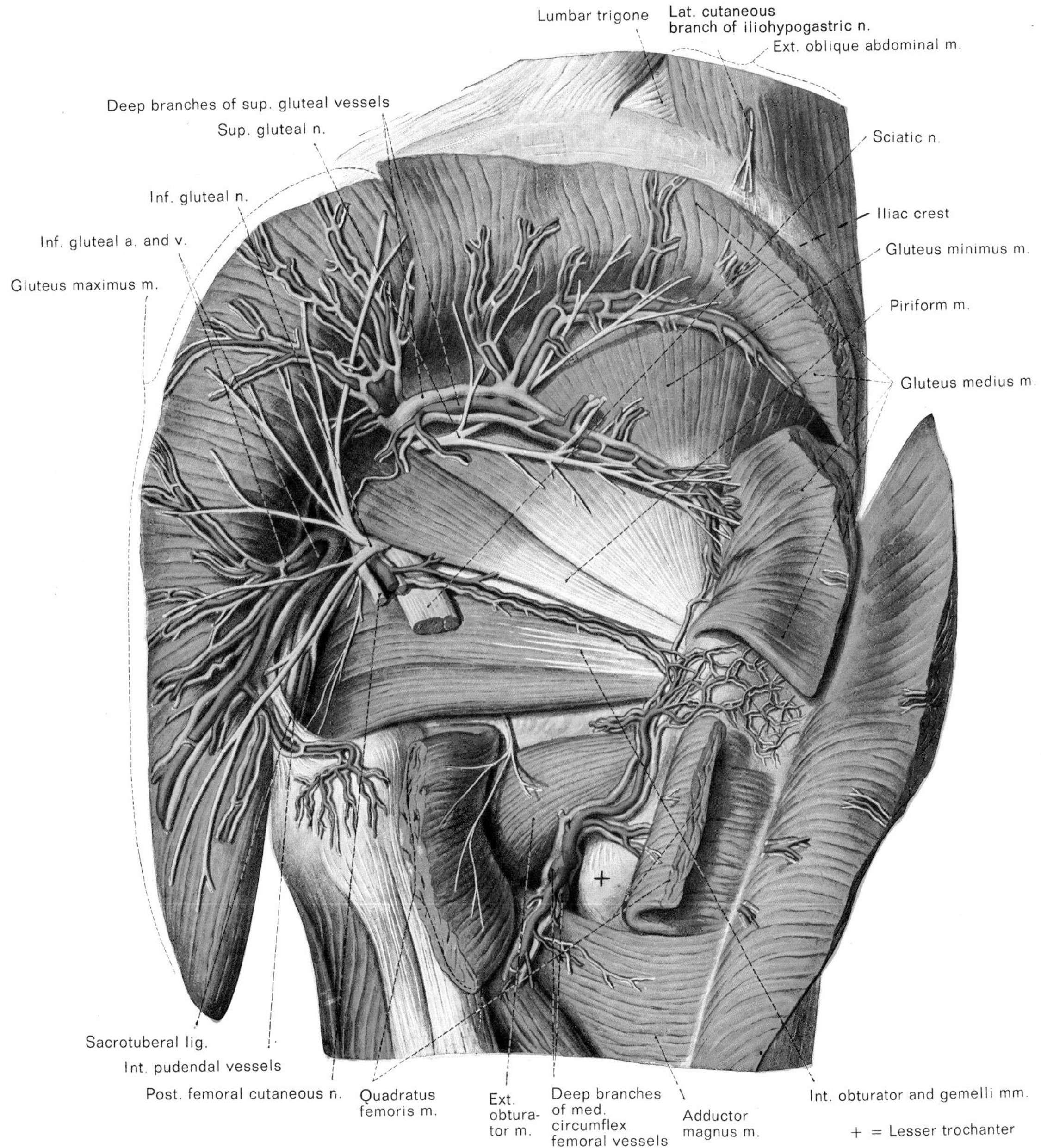
Lumbar trigone
Lat. cutaneous branch of iliohypogastric n.
Ext. oblique abdominal m.
Deep branches of sup. gluteal vessels
Sup. gluteal n.
Sciatic n.
Inf. gluteal n.
Iliac crest
Inf. gluteal a. and v.
Gluteus minimus m.
Gluteus maximus m.
Piriform m.
Gluteus medius m.
Sacrotuberal lig.
Int. pudendal vessels
Post. femoral cutaneous n.
Quadratus femoris m.
Ext. obtura- tor m.
Deep branches of med. circumflex femoral vessels
Adductor magnus m.
Int. obturator and gemelli mm.
+ = Lesser trochanter

Fig. 425. Deep nerves and vessels of gluteal region. Gluteus maximus, gluteus medius, quadratus femoris muscles and sciatic nerve have been sectioned and partially removed.

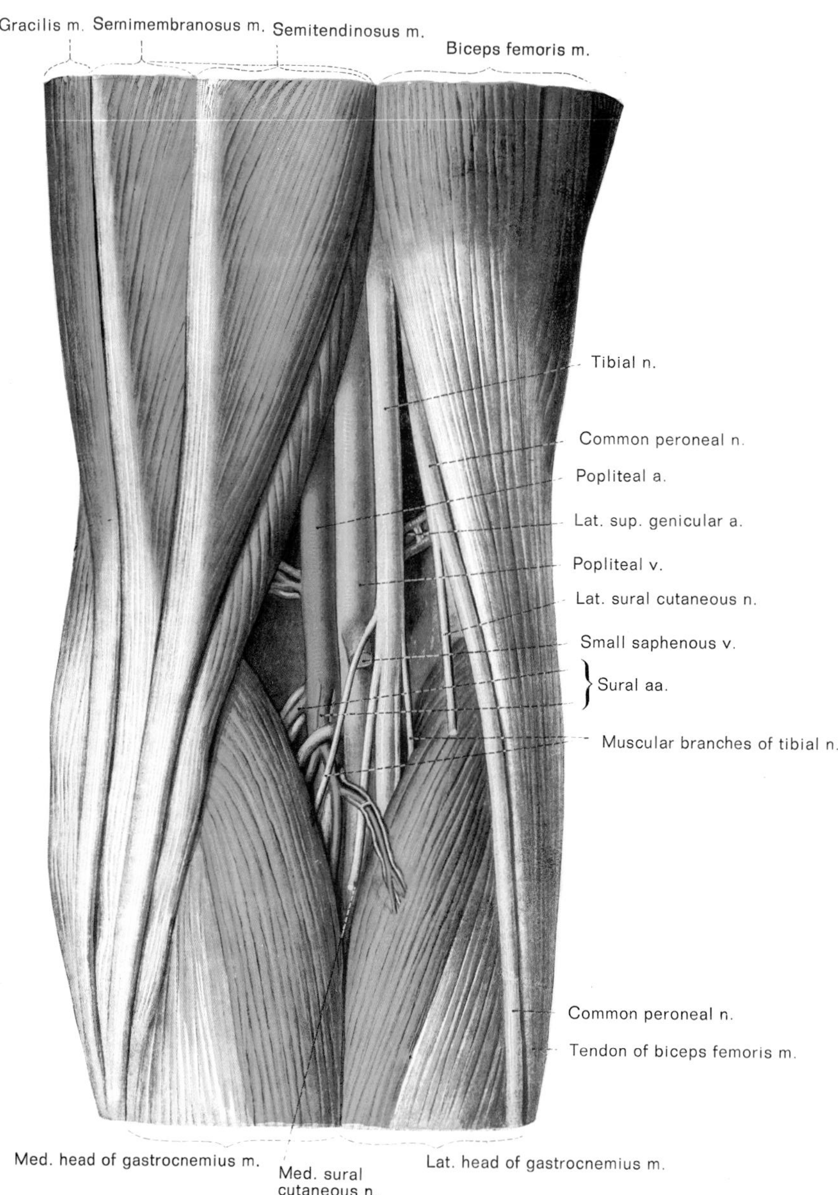
Gracilis m.
Semimembranosus m.
Semitendinosus m.
Biceps femoris m.
Tibial n.
Common peroneal n.
Popliteal a.
Lat. sup. genicular a.
Popliteal v.
Lat. sural cutaneous n.
Small saphenous v.
Sural aa.
Muscular branches of tibial n.
Common peroneal n.
Tendon of biceps femoris m.
Med. head of gastrocnemius m.
Med. sural cutaneous n.
Lat. head of gastrocnemius m.

Fig. 426. Superficial nerves and vessels of right popliteal fossa.

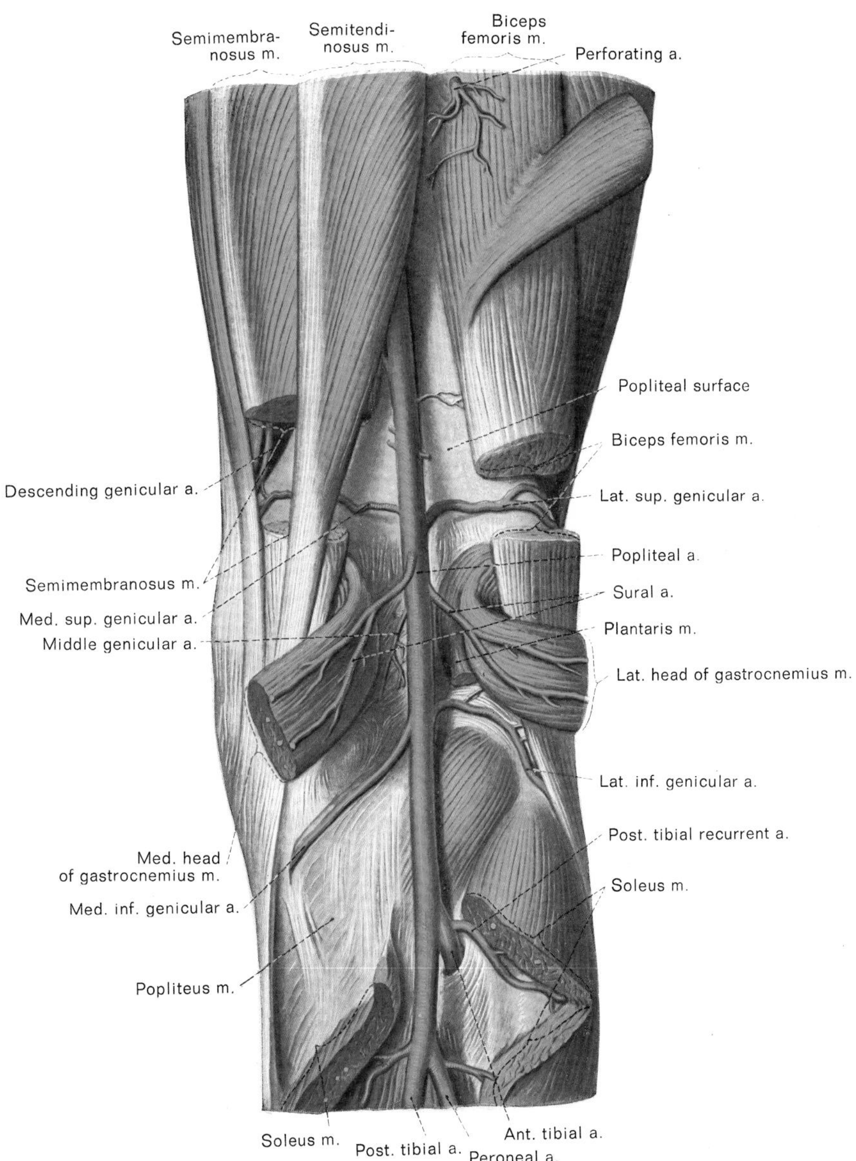
Semimembranosus m.
Semitendinosus m.
Biceps femoris m.
Perforating a.
Popliteal surface
Biceps femoris m.
Descending genicular a.
Lat. sup. genicular a.
Popliteal a.
Semimembranosus m.
Sural a.
Med. sup. genicular a.
Plantaris m.
Middle genicular a.
Lat. head of gastrocnemius m.
Lat. inf. genicular a.
Post. tibial recurrent a.
Med. head of gastrocnemius m.
Soleus m.
Med. inf. genicular a.
Popliteus m.
Soleus m.
Post. tibial a.
Ant. tibial a.
Peroneal a.

Fig. 427. Arteries of right popliteal fossa.

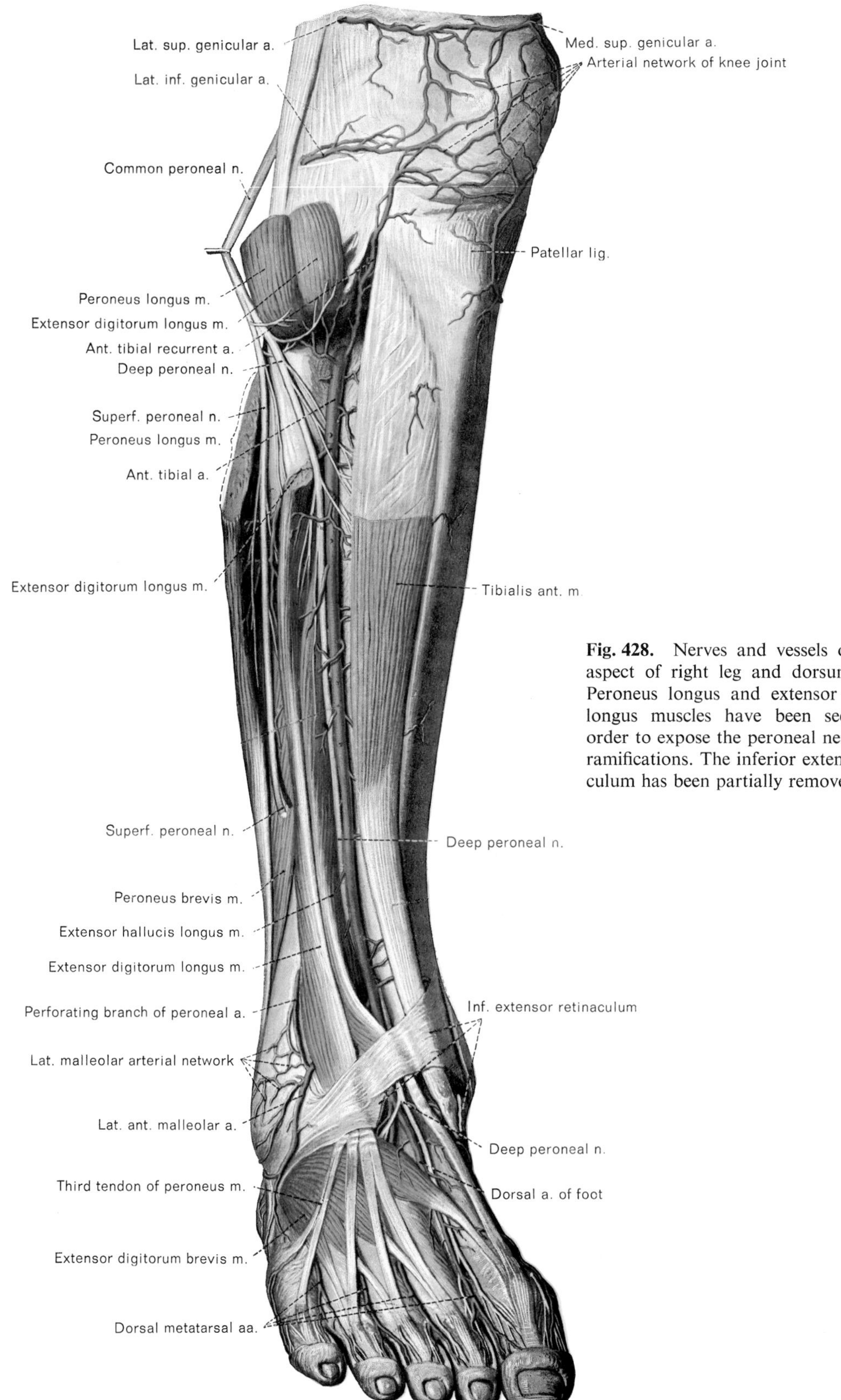
Lat. sup. genicular a.
Lat. inf. genicular a.
Med. sup. genicular a.
Arterial network of knee joint
Common peroneal n.
Patellar lig.
Peroneus longus m.
Extensor digitorum longus m.
Ant. tibial recurrent a.
Deep peroneal n.
Superf. peroneal n.
Peroneus longus m.
Ant. tibial a.
Extensor digitorum longus m.
Tibialis ant. m.
Superf. peroneal n.
Deep peroneal n.
Peroneus brevis m.
Extensor hallucis longus m.
Extensor digitorum longus m.
Perforating branch of peroneal a.
Inf. extensor retinaculum
Lat. malleolar arterial network
Lat. ant. malleolar a.
Deep peroneal n.
Third tendon of peroneus m.
Dorsal a. of foot
Extensor digitorum brevis m.
Dorsal metatarsal aa.

Fig. 428. Nerves and vessels of anterior aspect of right leg and dorsum of foot. Peroneus longus and extensor digitorum longus muscles have been sectioned in order to expose the peroneal nerve and its ramifications. The inferior extensor retinaculum has been partially removed.

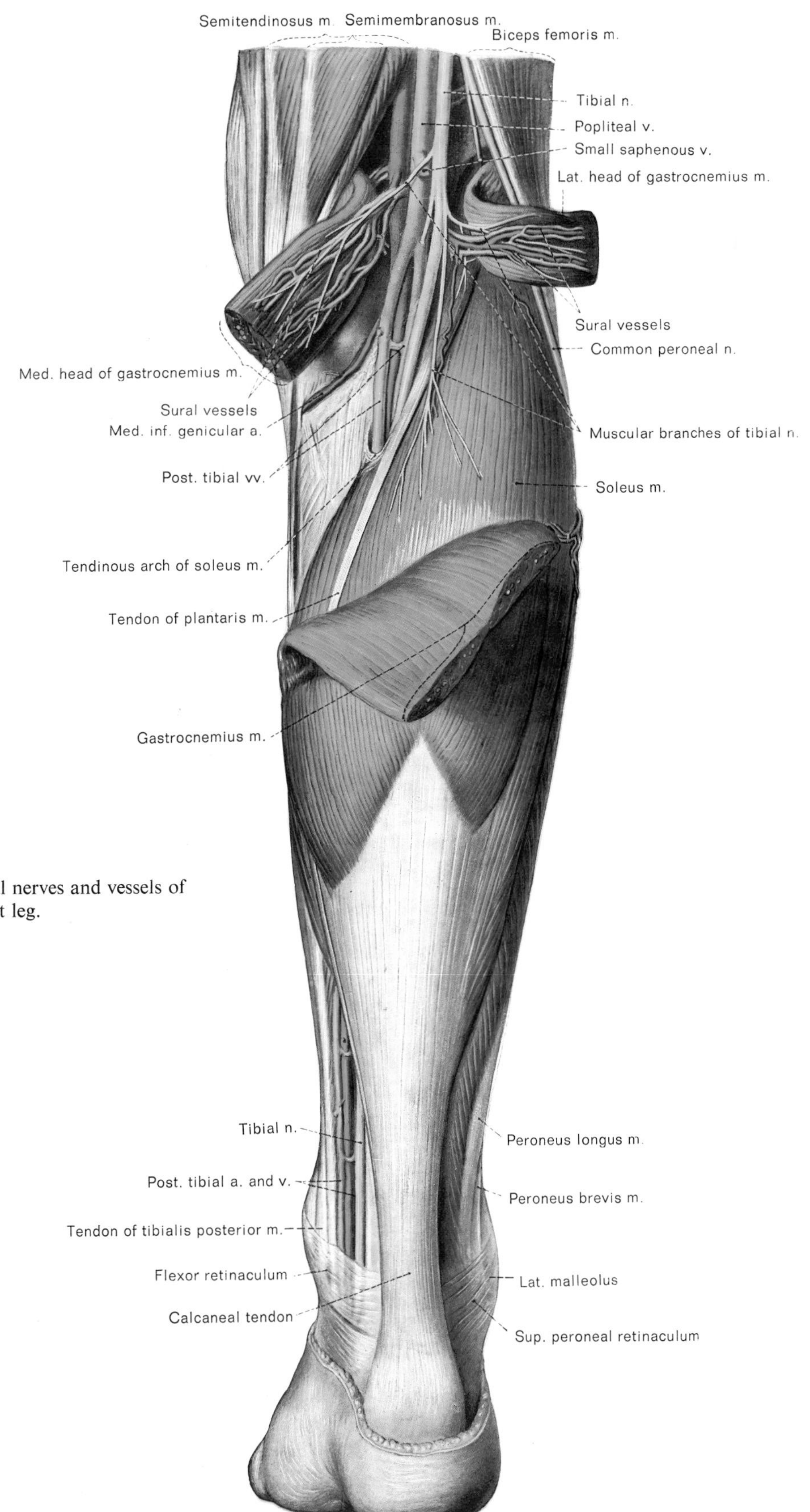
Semitendinosus m.
Semimembranosus m.
Biceps femoris m.
Tibial n.
Popliteal v.
Small saphenous v.
Lat. head of gastrocnemius m.
Sural vessels
Common peroneal n.
Med. head of gastrocnemius m.
Sural vessels
Med. inf. genicular a.
Muscular branches of tibial n.
Post. tibial vv.
Soleus m.
Tendinous arch of soleus m.
Tendon of plantaris m.
Gastrocnemius m.
Tibial n.
Peroneus longus m.
Post. tibial a. and v.
Peroneus brevis m.
Tendon of tibialis posterior m.
Flexor retinaculum
Lat. malleolus
Calcaneal tendon
Sup. peroneal retinaculum

Fig. 429. Superficial nerves and vessels of dorsal aspect of right leg.

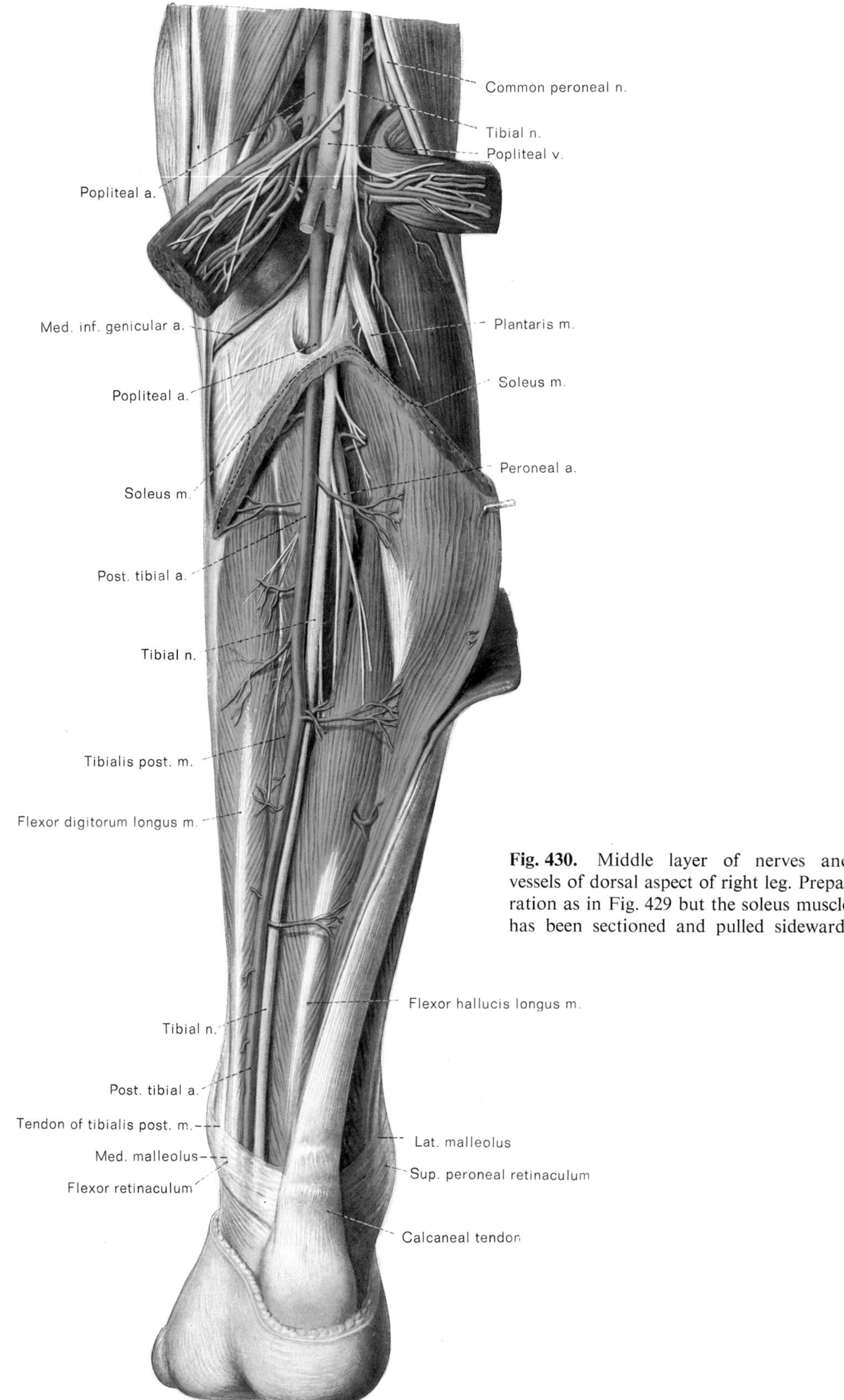
Common peroneal n.
Tibial n.
Popliteal v.
Popliteal a.
Med. inf. genicular a.
Plantaris m.
Popliteal a.
Soleus m.
Peroneal a.
Soleus m.
Post. tibial a.
Tibial n.
Tibialis post. m.
Flexor digitorum longus m.
Flexor hallucis longus m.
Tibial n.
Post. tibial a.
Tendon of tibialis post. m.
Lat. malleolus
Med. malleolus
Sup. peroneal retinaculum
Flexor retinaculum
Calcaneal tendon

Fig. 430. Middle layer of nerves and vessels of dorsal aspect of right leg. Preparation as in Fig. 429 but the soleus muscle has been sectioned and pulled sideward.

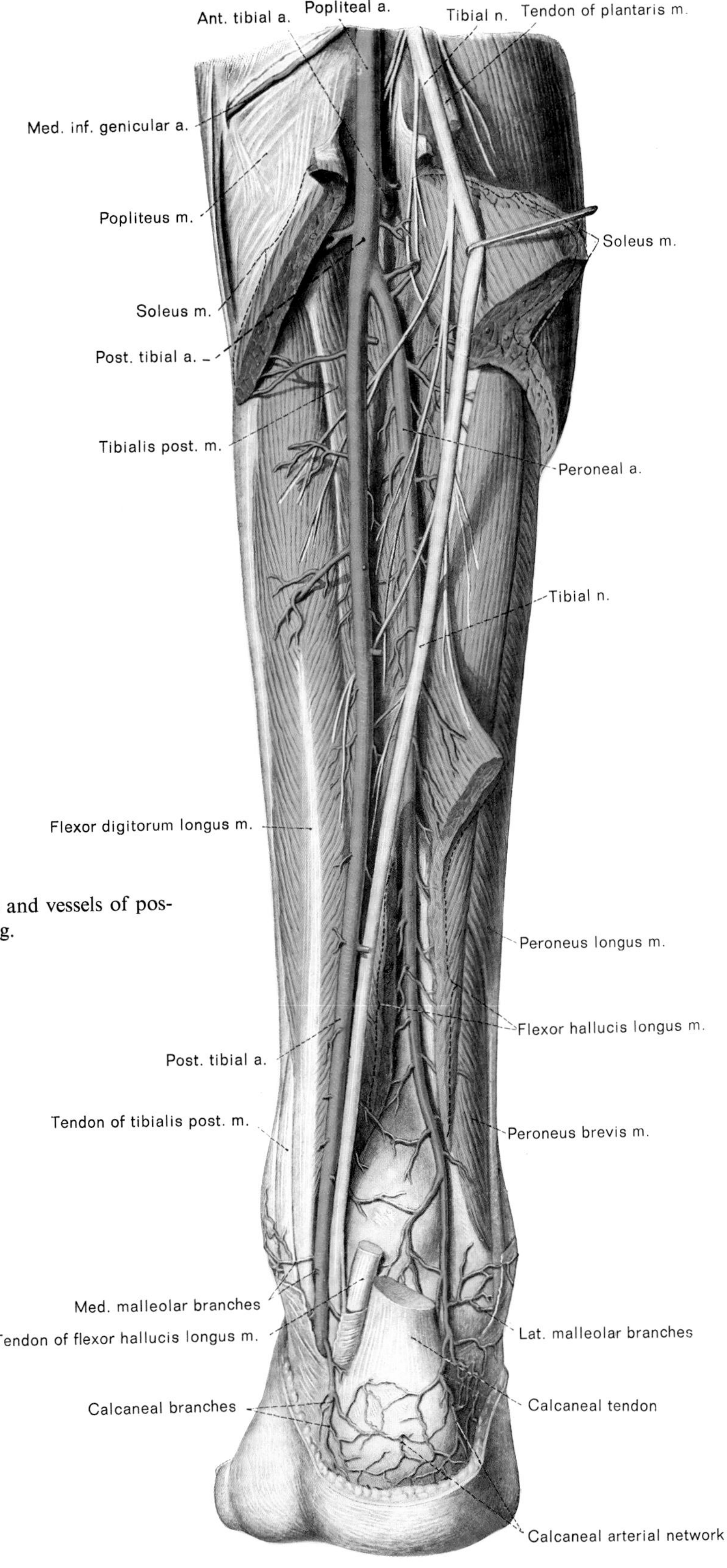
Ant. tibial a.
Popliteal a.
Tibial n.
Tendon of plantaris m.
Med. inf. genicular a.
Popliteus m.
Soleus m.
Soleus m.
Post. tibial a.
Tibialis post. m.
Peroneal a.
Tibial n.
Flexor digitorum longus m.
Peroneus longus m.
Flexor hallucis longus m.
Post. tibial a.
Tendon of tibialis post. m.
Peroneus brevis m.
Med. malleolar branches
Tendon of flexor hallucis longus m.
Lat. malleolar branches
Calcaneal branches
Calcaneal tendon
Calcaneal arterial network

Fig. 431. Deep nerves and vessels of posterior aspect of right leg.

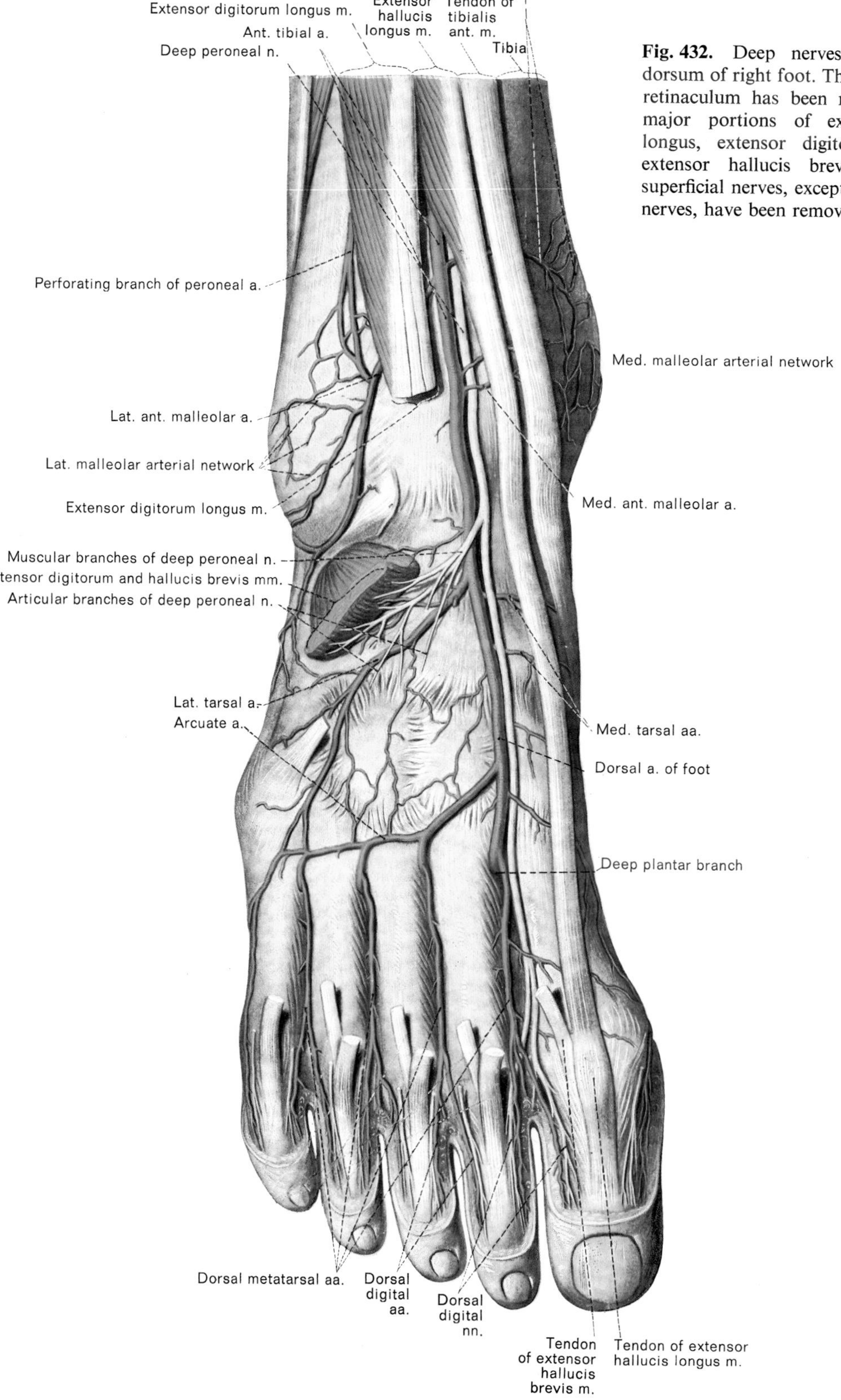
Med. ant. malleolar a.
Extensor digitorum longus m.
Extensor hallucis longus m.
Tendon of tibialis ant. m.
Ant. tibial a.
Deep peroneal n.
Tibia
Perforating branch of peroneal a.
Med. malleolar arterial network
Lat. ant. malleolar a.
Lat. malleolar arterial network
Extensor digitorum longus m.
Med. ant. malleolar a.
Muscular branches of deep peroneal n.
Extensor digitorum and hallucis brevis mm.
Articular branches of deep peroneal n.
Lat. tarsal a.
Arcuate a.
Med. tarsal aa.
Dorsal a. of foot
Deep plantar branch
Dorsal metatarsal aa.
Dorsal digital aa.
Dorsal digital nn.
Tendon of extensor hallucis brevis m.
Tendon of extensor hallucis longus m.

Fig. 432. Deep nerves and arteries of dorsum of right foot. The inferior extensor retinaculum has been removed, also the major portions of extensor digitorum longus, extensor digitorum brevis and extensor hallucis brevis muscles. The superficial nerves, except the dorsal digital nerves, have been removed.

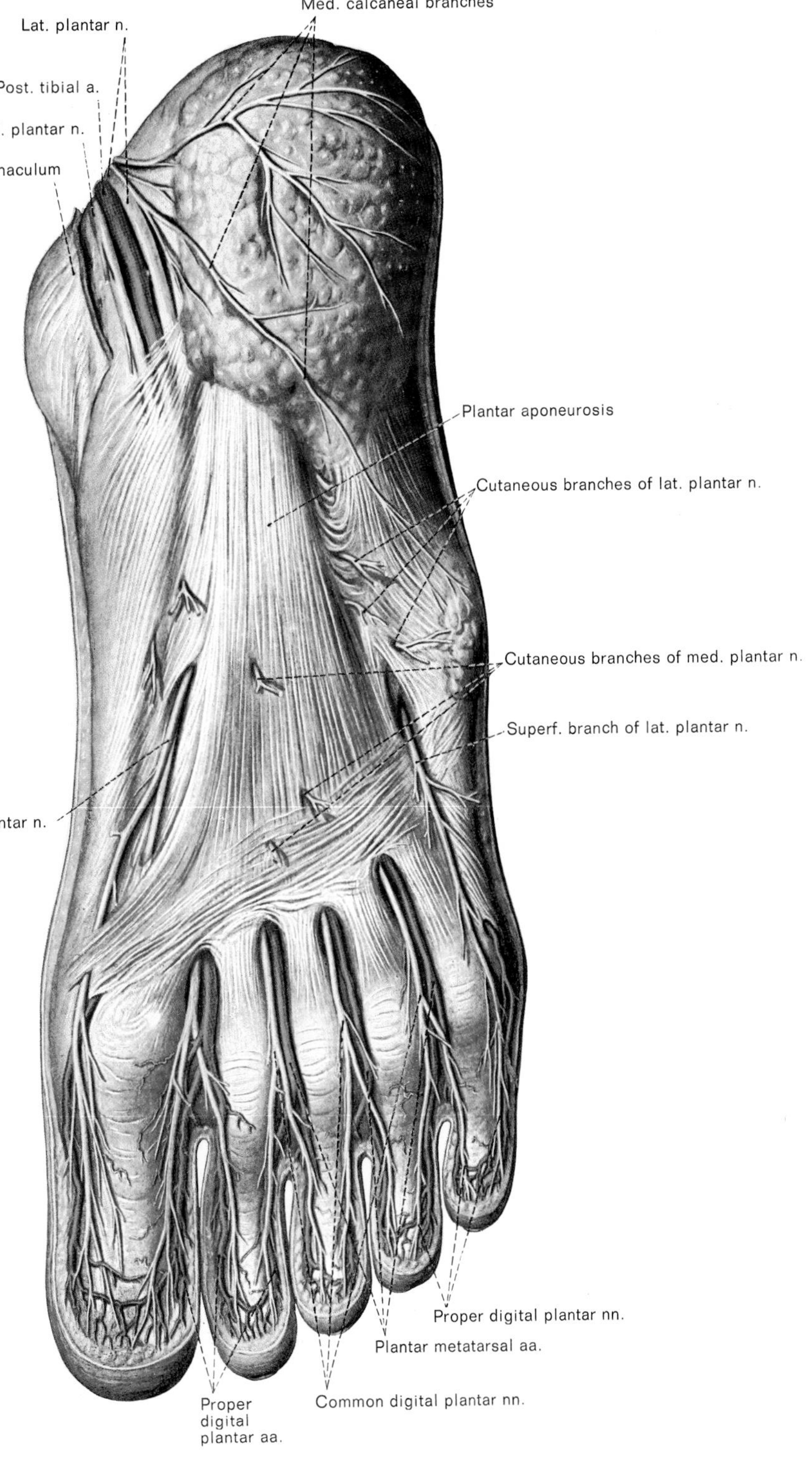
Med. calcaneal branches
Lat. plantar n.
Post. tibial a.
Med. plantar n.
Flexor retinaculum
Plantar aponeurosis
Cutaneous branches of lat. plantar n.
Cutaneous branches of med. plantar n.
Superf. branch of lat. plantar n.
Proper digital plantar n.
Proper digital plantar nn.
Plantar metatarsal aa.
Proper
digital
plantar aa.
Common digital plantar nn.

Fig. 433. Superficial nerves and arteries of sole of right foot. The flexor retinaculum has been split.

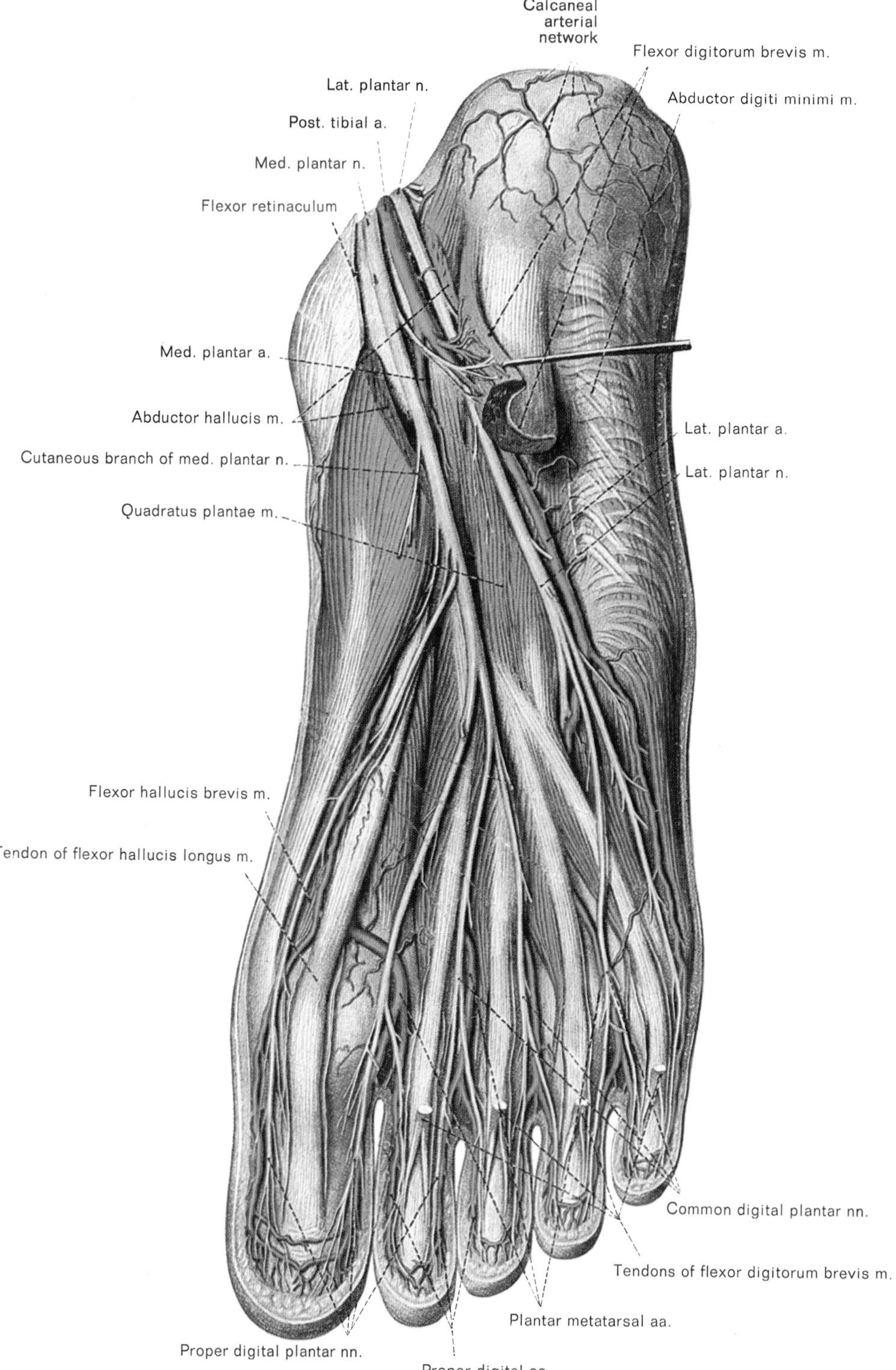

Calcaneal arterial network
Flexor digitorum brevis m.
Abductor digiti minimi m.
Lat. plantar n.
Post. tibial a.
Med. plantar n.
Flexor retinaculum
Med. plantar a.
Abductor hallucis m.
Cutaneous branch of med. plantar n.
Quadratus plantae m.
Lat. plantar a.
Lat. plantar n.
Flexor hallucis brevis m.
Tendon of flexor hallucis longus m.
Common digital plantar nn.
Tendons of flexor digitorum brevis m.
Plantar metatarsal aa.
Proper digital plantar nn.
Proper digital aa.

Fig. 434. Nerves and arteries of sole of right foot, intermediate layer. The abductor hallucis muscle has been sectioned, the flexor digitorum brevis muscle together with the plantar aponeurosis has been partially removed.

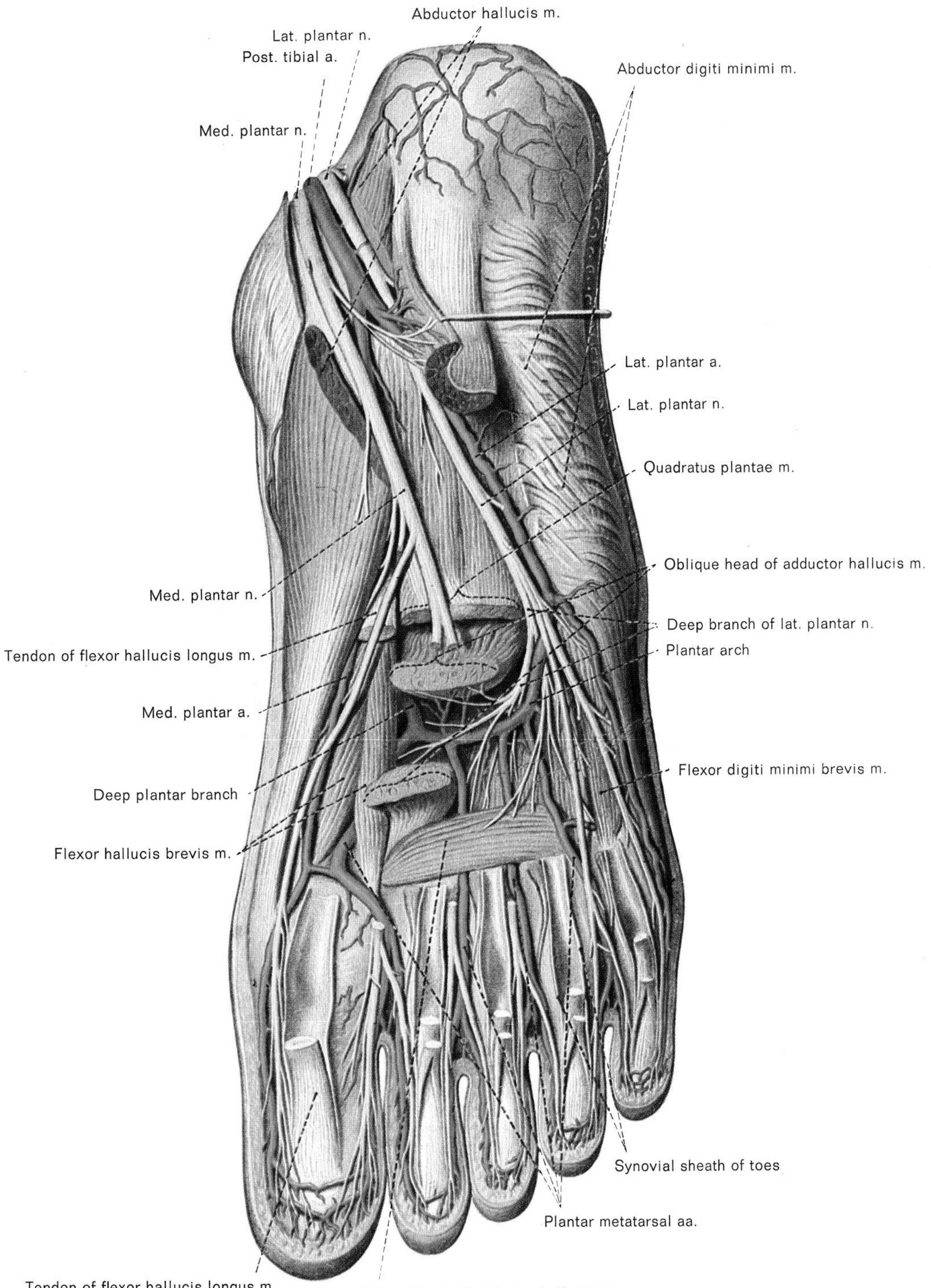
Abductor hallucis m.
Lat. plantar n.
Post. tibial a.
Abductor digiti minimi m.
Med. plantar n.
Lat. plantar a.
Lat. plantar n.
Quadratus plantae m.
Oblique head of adductor hallucis m.
Med. plantar n.
Deep branch of lat. plantar n.
Tendon of flexor hallucis longus m.
Plantar arch
Med. plantar a.
Flexor digiti minimi brevis m.
Deep plantar branch
Flexor hallucis brevis m.
Synovial sheath of toes
Plantar metatarsal aa.
Tendon of flexor hallucis longus m.
Transv. head of adductor hallucis m.

Fig. 435. Deep nerves and arteries of sole of right foot.

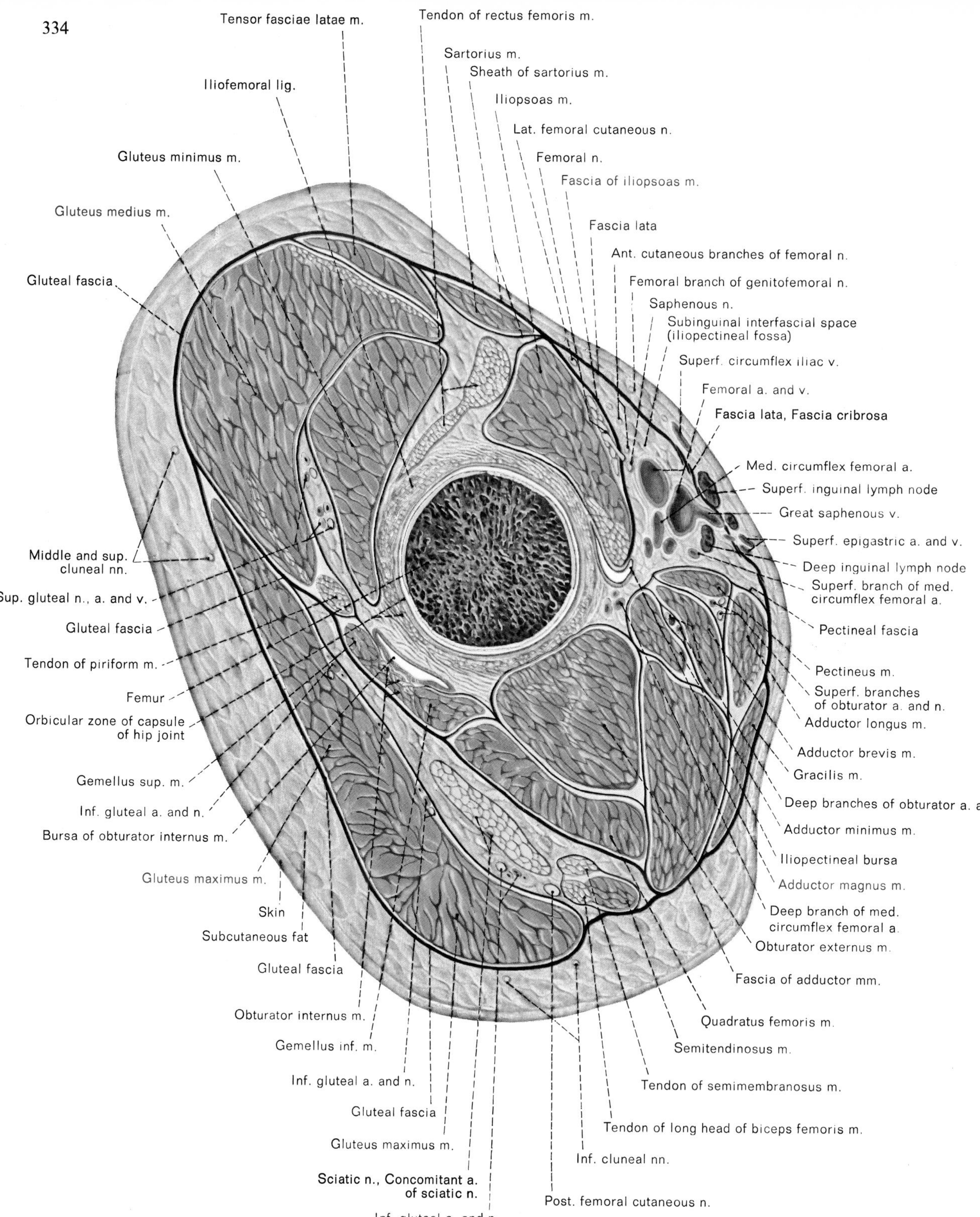
Tensor fasciae latae m.
Tendon of rectus femoris m.
Sartorius m.
Sheath of sartorius m.
Iliofemoral lig.
Iliopsoas m.
Lat. femoral cutaneous n.
Gluteus minimus m.
Femoral n.
Fascia of iliopsoas m.
Gluteus medius m.
Fascia lata
Ant. cutaneous branches of femoral n.
Gluteal fascia
Femoral branch of genitofemoral n.
Saphenous n.
Subinguinal interfascial space (iliopectineal fossa)
Superf. circumflex iliac v.
Femoral a. and v.
Fascia lata, Fascia cribrosa
Med. circumflex femoral a.
Superf. inguinal lymph node
Great saphenous v.
Superf. epigastric a. and v.
Middle and sup. cluneal nn.
Deep inguinal lymph node
Superf. branch of med. circumflex femoral a.
Sup. gluteal n., a. and v.
Pectineal fascia
Gluteal fascia
Tendon of piriform m.
Pectineus m.
Superf. branches of obturator a. and n.
Femur
Adductor longus m.
Orbicular zone of capsule of hip joint
Adductor brevis m.
Gracilis m.
Gemellus sup. m.
Deep branches of obturator a. ar
Inf. gluteal a. and n.
Adductor minimus m.
Bursa of obturator internus m.
Iliopectineal bursa
Gluteus maximus m.
Adductor magnus m.
Skin
Deep branch of med. circumflex femoral a.
Subcutaneous fat
Obturator externus m.
Gluteal fascia
Fascia of adductor mm.
Obturator internus m.
Quadratus femoris m.
Gemellus inf. m.
Semitendinosus m.
Inf. gluteal a. and n.
Tendon of semimembranosus m.
Gluteal fascia
Tendon of long head of biceps femoris m.
Gluteus maximus m.
Inf. cluneal nn.
Sciatic n., Concomitant a. of sciatic n.
Post. femoral cutaneous n.
Inf. gluteal a. and n.

Fig. 436. Section through the distal region of the right hip joint perpendicular to the axis of the femoral neck. Cut surface seen from distal. In Figs. 436–443 the fasciae are shown in black, tendons and ligaments in violet (from *Pernkopf/Ferner:* Atlas der topographischen und angewandten Anatomie des Menschen. vol. 2. Urban und Schwarzenberg, München–Berlin 1964).

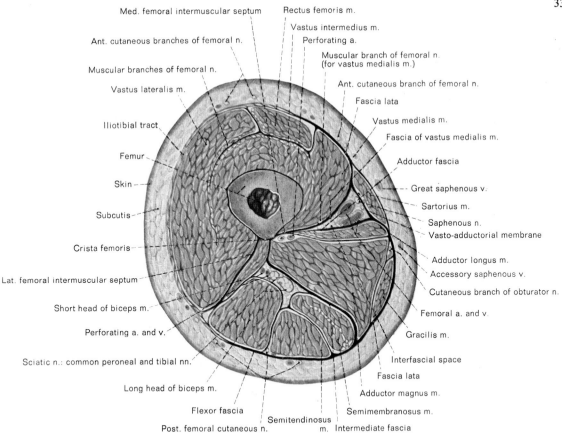

Med. femoral intermuscular septum
Rectus femoris m.
Vastus intermedius m.
Ant. cutaneous branches of femoral n.
Perforating a.
Muscular branch of femoral n. (for vastus medialis m.)
Muscular branches of femoral n.
Ant. cutaneous branch of femoral n.
Vastus lateralis m.
Fascia lata
Iliotibial tract
Vastus medialis m.
Fascia of vastus medialis m.
Femur
Adductor fascia
Skin
Great saphenous v.
Sartorius m.
Subcutis
Saphenous n.
Vasto-adductorial membrane
Crista femoris
Adductor longus m.
Accessory saphenous v.
Lat. femoral intermuscular septum
Cutaneous branch of obturator n.
Short head of biceps m.
Femoral a. and v.
Perforating a. and v.
Gracilis m.
Interfascial space
Sciatic n.: common peroneal and tibial nn.
Fascia lata
Long head of biceps m.
Adductor magnus m.
Flexor fascia
Semimembranosus m.
Semitendinosus m.
Post. femoral cutaneous n.
Intermediate fascia

Fig. 437. Cross section through middle third of right thigh. Sectioned surface seen from distal.

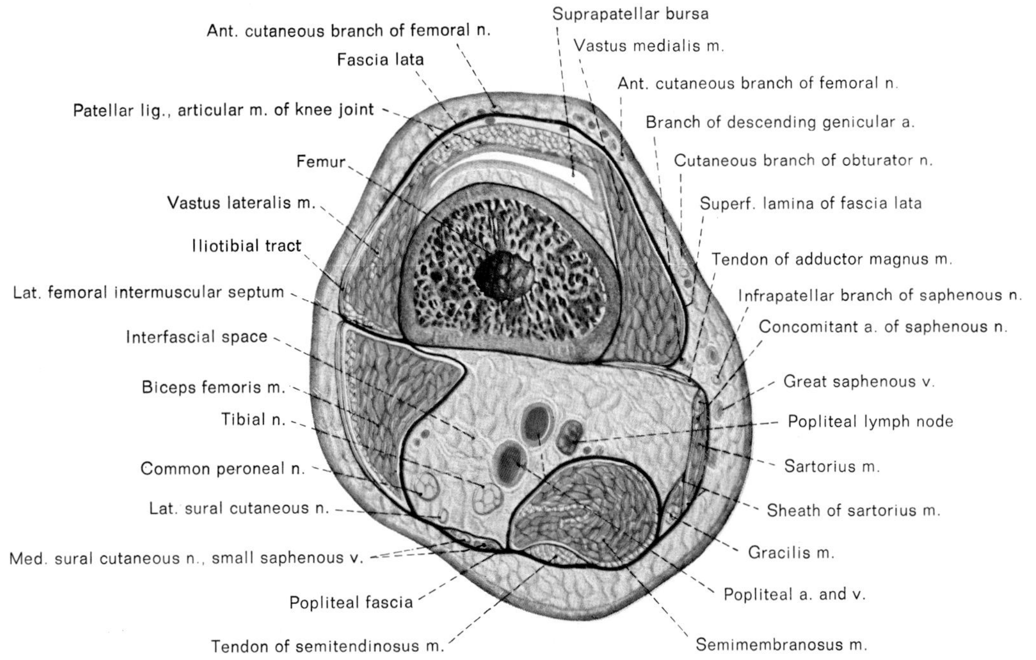
Suprapatellar bursa
Ant. cutaneous branch of femoral n.
Vastus medialis m.
Fascia lata
Ant. cutaneous branch of femoral n.
Patellar lig., articular m. of knee joint
Branch of descending genicular a.
Femur
Cutaneous branch of obturator n.
Vastus lateralis m.
Superf. lamina of fascia lata
Iliotibial tract
Tendon of adductor magnus m.
Lat. femoral intermuscular septum
Infrapatellar branch of saphenous n.
Concomitant a. of saphenous n.
Interfascial space
Great saphenous v.
Biceps femoris m.
Popliteal lymph node
Tibial n.
Sartorius m.
Common peroneal n.
Lat. sural cutaneous n.
Sheath of sartorius m.
Med. sural cutaneous n., small saphenous v.
Gracilis m.
Popliteal a. and v.
Popliteal fascia
Tendon of semitendinosus m.
Semimembranosus m.

Fig. 438. Cross section through the distal third of the right thigh. Sectioned surface seen from distal.

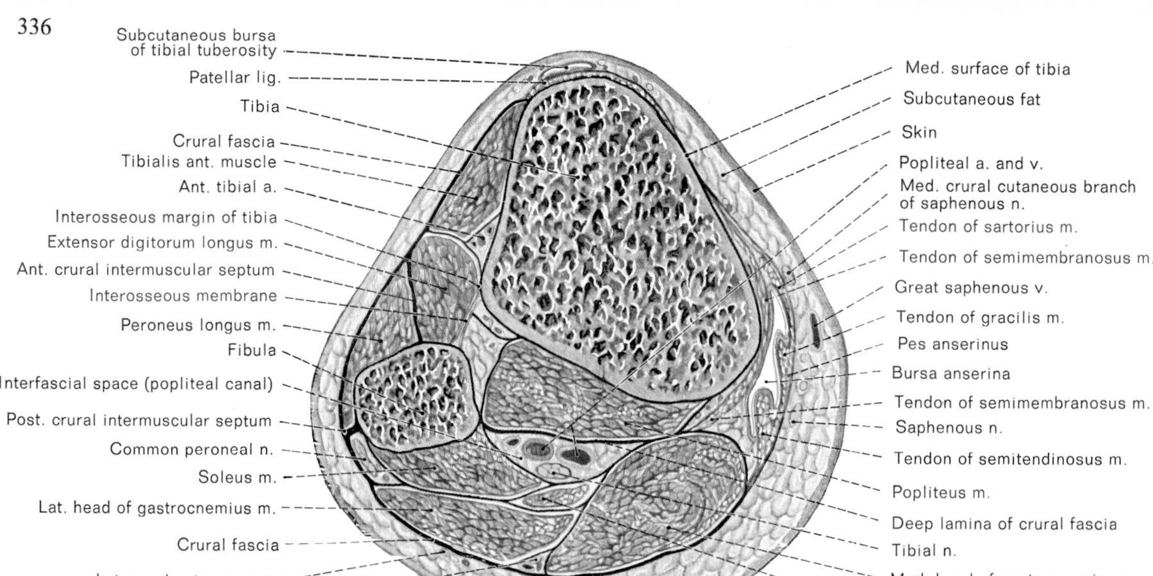
Subcutaneous bursa of tibial tuberosity
Patellar lig.
Tibia
Crural fascia
Tibialis ant. muscle
Ant. tibial a.
Interosseous margin of tibia
Extensor digitorum longus m.
Ant. crural intermuscular septum
Interosseous membrane
Peroneus longus m.
Fibula
Interfascial space (popliteal canal)
Post. crural intermuscular septum
Common peroneal n.
Soleus m.
Lat. head of gastrocnemius m.
Crural fascia
Lat. sural cutaneous n.
Med. sural cutaneous n., Small saphenous v.
Med. surface of tibia
Subcutaneous fat
Skin
Popliteal a. and v.
Med. crural cutaneous branch of saphenous n.
Tendon of sartorius m.
Tendon of semimembranosus m.
Great saphenous v.
Tendon of gracilis m.
Pes anserinus
Bursa anserina
Tendon of semimembranosus m.
Saphenous n.
Tendon of semitendinosus m.
Popliteus m.
Deep lamina of crural fascia
Tibial n.
Med. head of gastrocnemius m.
Plantaris m.

Fig. 439. Cross section through proximal third of right leg. Sectioned surface seen from distal.

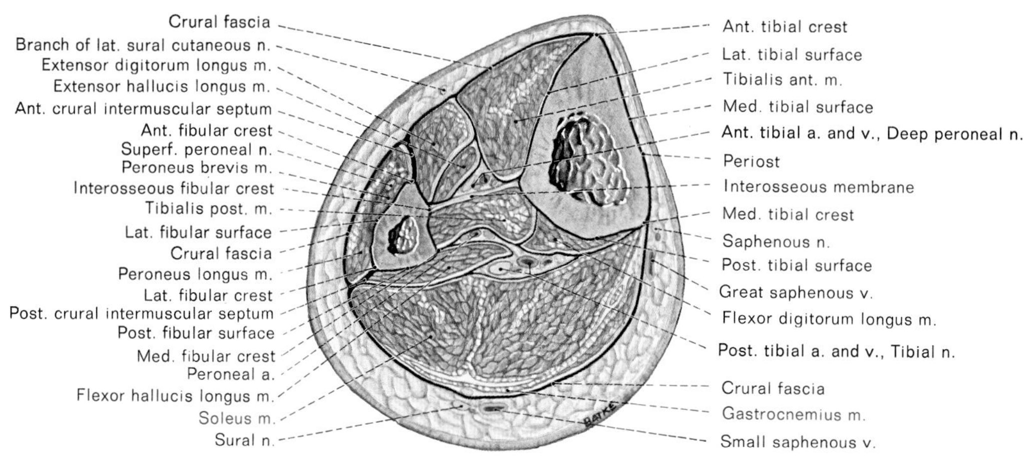
Crural fascia
Branch of lat. sural cutaneous n.
Extensor digitorum longus m.
Extensor hallucis longus m.
Ant. crural intermuscular septum
Ant. fibular crest
Superf. peroneal n.
Peroneus brevis m.
Interosseous fibular crest
Tibialis post. m.
Lat. fibular surface
Crural fascia
Peroneus longus m.
Lat. fibular crest
Post. crural intermuscular septum
Post. fibular surface
Med. fibular crest
Peroneal a.
Flexor hallucis longus m.
Soleus m.
Sural n.
Ant. tibial crest
Lat. tibial surface
Tibialis ant. m.
Med. tibial surface
Ant. tibial a. and v., Deep peroneal n.
Periost
Interosseous membrane
Med. tibial crest
Saphenous n.
Post. tibial surface
Great saphenous v.
Flexor digitorum longus m.
Post. tibial a. and v., Tibial n.
Crural fascia
Gastrocnemius m.
Small saphenous v.
BATKE

Fig. 440. Cross section through middle third of right leg. Sectioned surface seen from distal.

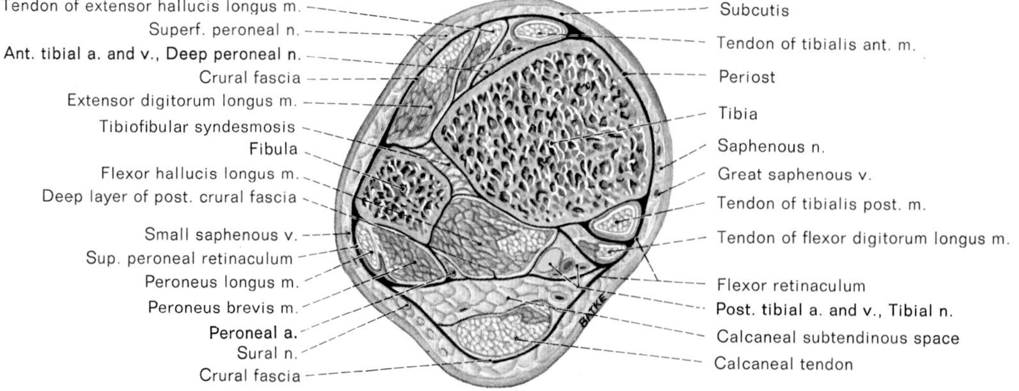
Tendon of extensor hallucis longus m.
Superf. peroneal n.
Ant. tibial a. and v., Deep peroneal n.
Crural fascia
Extensor digitorum longus m.
Tibiofibular syndesmosis
Fibula
Flexor hallucis longus m.
Deep layer of post. crural fascia
Small saphenous v.
Sup. peroneal retinaculum
Peroneus longus m.
Peroneus brevis m.
Peroneal a.
Sural n.
Crural fascia
Subcutis
Tendon of tibialis ant. m.
Periost
Tibia
Saphenous n.
Great saphenous v.
Tendon of tibialis post. m.
Tendon of flexor digitorum longus m.
Flexor retinaculum
Post. tibial a. and v., Tibial n.
Calcaneal subtendinous space
Calcaneal tendon
BATKE

Fig. 441. Cross section through the right leg above the malleoli. Sectioned surface seen from distal.

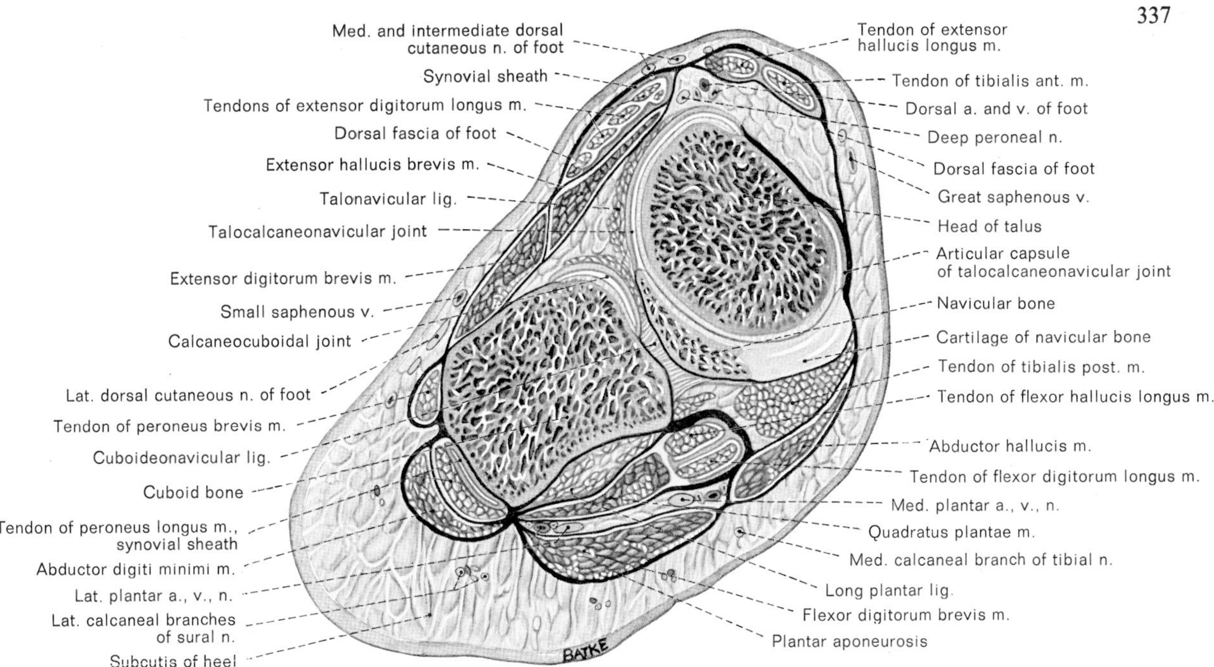
Med. and intermediate dorsal cutaneous n. of foot
Synovial sheath
Tendons of extensor digitorum longus m.
Dorsal fascia of foot
Extensor hallucis brevis m.
Talonavicular lig.
Talocalcaneonavicular joint
Extensor digitorum brevis m.
Small saphenous v.
Calcaneocuboidal joint
Lat. dorsal cutaneous n. of foot
Tendon of peroneus brevis m.
Cuboideonavicular lig.
Cuboid bone
Tendon of peroneus longus m., synovial sheath
Abductor digiti minimi m.
Lat. plantar a., v., n.
Lat. calcaneal branches of sural n.
Subcutis of heel
Tendon of extensor hallucis longus m.
Tendon of tibialis ant. m.
Dorsal a. and v. of foot
Deep peroneal n.
Dorsal fascia of foot
Great saphenous v.
Head of talus
Articular capsule of talocalcaneonavicular joint
Navicular bone
Cartilage of navicular bone
Tendon of tibialis post. m.
Tendon of flexor hallucis longus m.
Abductor hallucis m.
Tendon of flexor digitorum longus m.
Med. plantar a., v., n.
Quadratus plantae m.
Med. calcaneal branch of tibial n.
Long plantar lig.
Flexor digitorum brevis m.
Plantar aponeurosis
BATKE

Fig. 442. Cross section through the right tarsus in the area of the talus head. Sectioned surface seen from distal. Tendon sheaths and synovial membrane of joint capsules are shown in light blue.

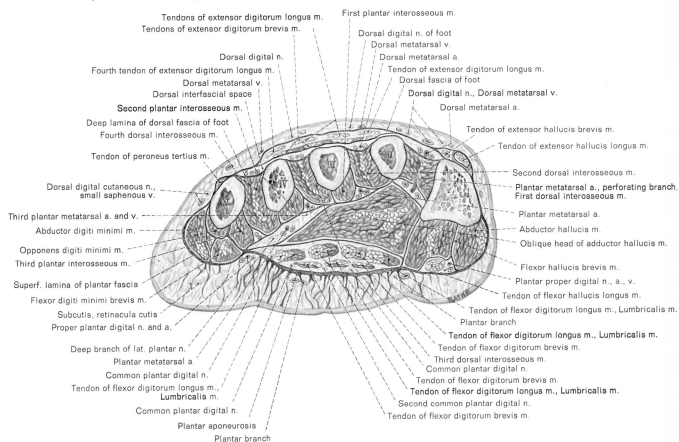

Tendons of extensor digitorum longus m.
Tendons of extensor digitorum brevis m.
Dorsal digital n.
Fourth tendon of extensor digitorum longus m.
Dorsal metatarsal v.
Dorsal interfascial space
Second plantar interosseous m.
Deep lamina of dorsal fascia of foot
Fourth dorsal interosseous m.
Tendon of peroneus tertius m.
Dorsal digital cutaneous n., small saphenous v.
Third plantar metatarsal a. and v.
Abductor digiti minimi m.
Opponens digiti minimi m.
Third plantar interosseous m.
Superf. lamina of plantar fascia
Flexor digiti minimi brevis m.
Subcutis, retinacula cutis
Proper plantar digital n. and a.
Deep branch of lat. plantar n.
Plantar metatarsal a.
Common plantar digital n.
Tendon of flexor digitorum longus m., Lumbricalis m.
Common plantar digital n.
Plantar aponeurosis
Plantar branch
First plantar interosseous m.
Dorsal digital n. of foot
Dorsal metatarsal v.
Dorsal metatarsal a.
Tendon of extensor digitorum longus m.
Dorsal fascia of foot
Dorsal digital n., Dorsal metatarsal v.
Dorsal metatarsal a.
Tendon of extensor hallucis brevis m.
Tendon of extensor hallucis longus m.
Second dorsal interosseous m.
Plantar metatarsal a., perforating branch, First dorsal interosseous m.
Plantar metatarsal a.
Abductor hallucis m.
Oblique head of adductor hallucis m.
Flexor hallucis brevis m.
Plantar proper digital n., a., v.
Tendon of flexor hallucis longus m.
Tendon of flexor digitorum longus m., Lumbricalis m.
Plantar branch
Tendon of flexor digitorum longus m., Lumbricalis m.
Tendon of flexor digitorum brevis m.
Third dorsal interosseous m.
Common plantar digital n.
Tendon of flexor digitorum brevis m.
Tendon of flexor digitorum longus m., Lumbricalis m.
Second common plantar digital n.
Tendon of flexor digitorum brevis m.
I II III IV V
BATKE

Fig. 443. Cross section through the right metatarsus. Sectioned surface seen from distal. I–V = first to fifth metacarpal bones.

Subject Index

(All numbers refer to the numbers of pages)

B

C

D

G

H

M

O

P

Q

R

S

T

U

V

W

Z

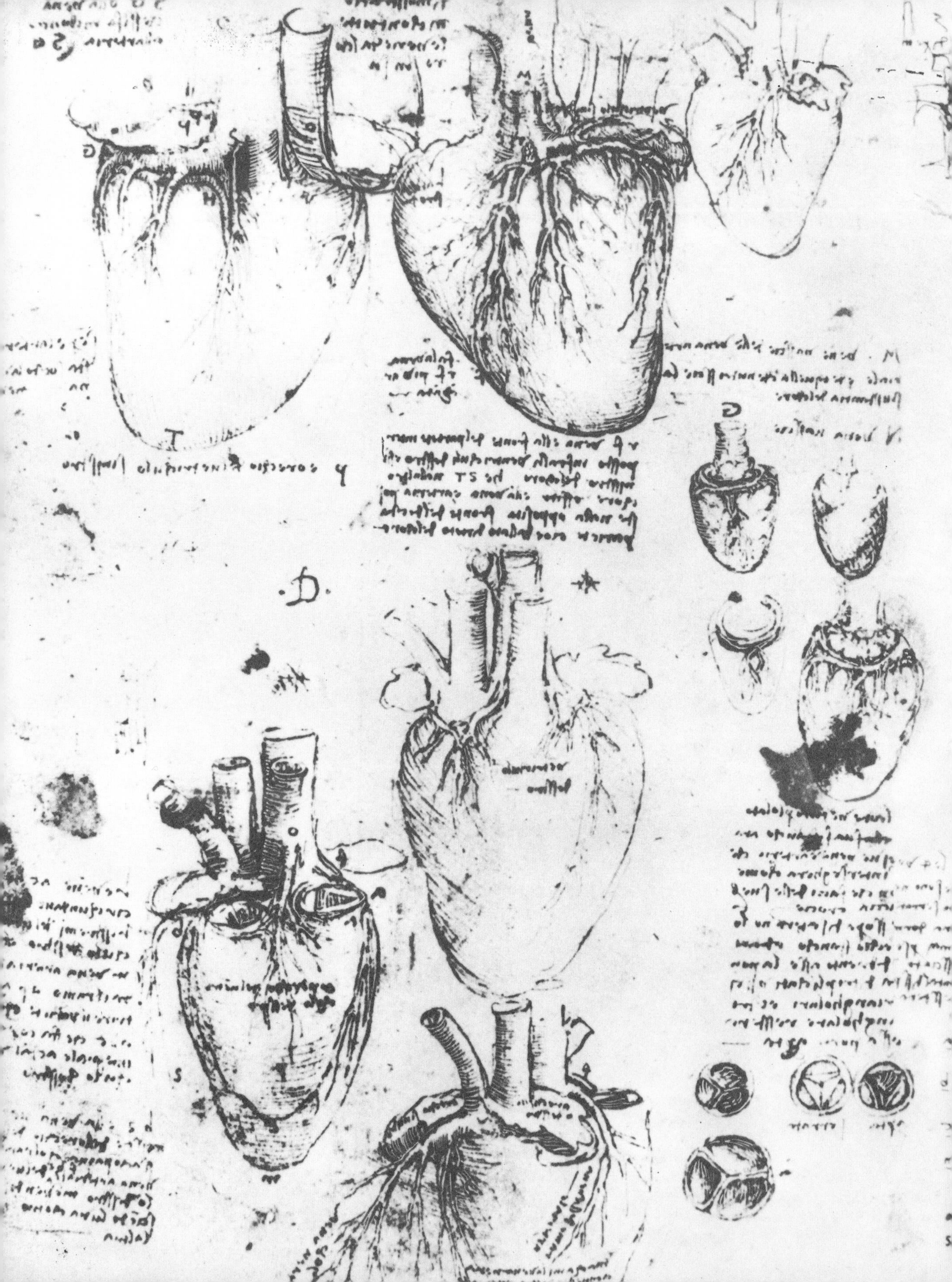